Modeling Techniques and Tools for Computer Performance Evaluation

Modeling Techniques and Tools for Computer Performance Evaluation

Edited by

Ramon Puigjaner

University of the Balearic Islands
Palma, Spain

and

Dominique Potier

Thomson CSF
Orsay, France

PLENUM PRESS • NEW YORK AND LONDON

Library of Congress Cataloging in Publication Data

International Conference on Modeling Techniques and Tools for Computer Performance
  Evaluation (4th: 1988: Palma, Spain)
  Modeling techniques and tools for computer performance evaluation / edited by Ramon
Puigjaner and Dominique Potier.
     p.   cm.
  "Proceedings of the Fourth International Conference on Modeling Techniques and Tools
for Computer Performance Evaluation, held September 14–16, 1988, in Palma, Balearic
Islands, Spain"—T.p. verso.
  Includes bibliographical references.
  ISBN-13: 978-1-4612-7853-5   e-ISBN-13: 978-1-4613-0533-0
  DOI: 10.1007/ 978-1-4613-0533-0
  1. Digital computer simulation—Congresses. 2. Electronic digital computers—Evaluation
—Congresses. I. Puigjaner, Ramon. II. Potier, D. III. Title.
QA76.9.C65I54   1988   89-22866
003.3—dc20   CIP

Proceedings of the Fourth International Conference on Modeling
Techniques and Tools for Computer Performance Evaluation,
held September 14–16, 1988, in Palma, Balearic Islands, Spain

© 1989 Plenum Press, New York
Softcover reprint of the hardcover 1st edition 1989
A Division of Plenum Publishing Corporation
233 Spring Street, New York, N.Y. 10013

Organized by:

- Associació de Tècnics d'Informàtica
- Universitat de les Illes Balears

in cooperation with:

- Association for Computing Machinery (ACM)
- Association Française pour la Cybernetique Economique et Technique (AFCET)
- Federación Española de Sociedades de Informática (FESI)
- Institute of Electrical and Electronic Engineers, Computer Society (IEEE-CS)
- Institut National de Recherche en Informatique et Automatique (INRIA)
- International Federation for Information Processing, Working Group 7.3 (IFIP-WG 7.3)
- SEDISI

with the sponsorship of:

- CIRIT, Generalitat de Catalunya
- Consell Insular de Mallorca

with the financial support of:

- Caixa d'Estalvis de Balears, "Sa Nostra"
- Caixa d'Estalvis de Catalunya
- Caixa de Pensions per a la Vellesa i d'Estalvis de Catalunya i Balears, "La Caixa"
- Digital Equipment Corporation
- IBM, S.A.E.
- Unisys, S.A.

and with the assistance in equipments of:

- Equipos Informáticos SUN, S.A.
- Matra España, S.A.

PROGRAM COMMITTEE

D. Potier (F), Chairman
R. J. Walstra (USA), America representative
Y. Takahashi (J), Asia representative
S. Agrawal (USA)
B. Aladjem (E)
G. Balbo (I)
H. Beilner (D)
P. J. Courtois (B)
D. Ferrari (USA)
G. S. Graham (CDN)
U. Herzog (D)
P. Hughes (GB)
P. Kritzinger (SA)
J. Labetoulle (F)
R. Marie (F)
H. Perros (USA)
R. Puigjaner (E)
G. Pujolle (F)
M. Reiser (CH)
G. Serazzi (I)
O. Spaniol (D)

ORGANIZING COMMITTEE

A. Bennàssar
B. Bennasar
G. Fontanet
R. Puigjaner
B. Serra

PREFACE

There is a growing perception that the succesful design and exploitation of complex information systems is critically dependant on the level of methods and support for performance modelling. Fast technological evolution creates a strong demand for analysis techniques which can handle new hardware and software organisations. Performance modelling users are expecting improved tools in terms of their user friendliness and their integration in the system design and operation process.

Providing an image as clear as possible of the recent advances in these areas is the objective of the serie of **International Conference on Modelling Techniques and Tools for Computer Performance Evaluation**. We believe thst the 4th edition does respond to the objective. It illustrates the most recent trends in our domain and gives insight into what we may expect in terms of new modelling techniques, tools and practices in the future years.

The proceedings include the twenty seven papers accepted by the Program Committee (out of sixty six submitted) and three invited papers presented at the Conference. They cover the following topics:

* Modelling Tools

* Networking

* Architecture and Workload

* Protocols

* Architecture Configuration

* Parallelism

* Performability

* Algorithms

We would like to express our sincere appreciation and gratitude to the members of the *Program Committee* and to the reviewers for their time and effort. Without their kind cooperation, the Conference would not have been possible.

Also, we wish to thank all the cooperating and sponsoring organizations for their help and support in setting up the Conference.

Dominique Potier
Program Committee Chairman

Ramon Puigjaner
Conference Chairman

CONTENTS

REGULAR AND INVITED PAPERS

Modelling Tools

Networking

Architecture and Workload

Protocols

Architecture Configuration

Parallelism

Performability

Algorithms

THE CHALLENGE OF COMBINING TEXT AND GRAPHICS

IN MODELING SUPPORT ENVIRONMENTS

Benjamin Melamed

Robbe J. Walstra

AT&T Bell Laboratories
Holmdel, New Jersey 07733

Hewlett-Packard Laboratories
Palo Alto, California 94304

ABSTRACT

Considerable effort is being expended worldwide towards the design and implementation of modeling support environments (MSEs). Efforts range from simulation to analytical support environments, and combinations of the two. Originally text-only, MSEs are increasingly designed to incorporate extensive graphics to facilitate user interactions with the software.

The pursuit of MSEs is economically motivated and aims at increasing the productivity of modelers by enabling them to concentrate on modeling, without the distraction of undue programming detail. An MSE provides facilities and services that help create models, test and debug them, run computations and interpret the results. Increased modeler satisfaction is an important benefit of an MSE. We argue that market pressures resulting in shortened life cycles of computer-related products are putting a premium on good and efficient modeling during the design, development and operation of systems.

The purpose of this paper is to present and discuss issues germane to the design of MSEs and their facilities. We present a framework for an integrated-services MSE as a software platform for applications (tools) which share a high level of commonality. The theme binding the discussion is the synergetic integration of text and graphics to deliver better MSEs.

INTRODUCTION

A modeling support environment (MSE) is a software system designed to facilitate modeling activities on a digital computer. This includes model specification and alteration, model execution, and output display and analysis. The better MSE provides services and facilities which allow the user to concentrate on modeling activities without being distracted by undue programming detail. To attain this laudable goal, the better MSE must have:

- integrated services which speed up modeling and modification cycles;

- a user interface that is easy to use, flexible and protective;

- a useful modeling paradigm which minimizes the gap between computational models and their computer representation(s).

1

A computational model is a formal representation of the system under study which is used to estimate its performance measures. In the sequel, any allusion to a model without qualification will mean a computational model including its computer representation. Finally, a visual model refers to the visual representation of entities which form part of the user interface; the full interface consists of both text and graphics.

Based on their model solution method, MSEs can be classified in two broad categories: simulation systems and analytical methods. In this paper we limit the discussion to process-oriented discrete event Monte Carlo simulation languages, even though most of the issues to be raised also apply to continuous simulation languages or hybrid languages.

A simulation approach to modeling is empirical in nature, and has a strong statistical flavor [BRAT83]. In this approach, the modeler creates a program that computes sample paths (histories) of the system under study. Statistics collected within and across sample paths are used to estimate various performance measures such as mean queue lengths, server utilization factors, and customer time-in-queue distributions. Random phenomena are simulated through pseudo-random number generators. Some well-known simulation languages include GPSS, SIMSCRIPT, SIMULA, SIMAN and SLAM. Simulation models are driven by time-ordered events whose execution causes the model to change state; in between events the model is considered quiescent. A simulation language provides an MSE with a world view which usually includes resources and consumers, and supports facilities for generating pseudo-randomness, for ordering events, and for controlling their execution.

An analytical method is a mathematical algorithm that generates a performance measure or an approximation thereof based on a mathematical theory which postulates a certain model structure (e.g. Markovian processes). The computation is mostly numerical rather than logical and often involves the solution of systems of equations. In this paper we confine ourselves to queueing network models. We mention as examples BEST/1^{TM} [BGS82], PANACEA [RAMA82], QNA [WHIT85] and QNAP2^{TM} [VERA85].

Generally, simulation has a broad modeling scope, but tends to require extensive computational resources (memory and time). In contrast, analytical methods have a far smaller modeling scope, but when applicable, can require only a fraction of the resources used by a simulation model. This duality drives the choice of a particular modeling paradigm for a given system. Because a simulation can incorporate fine model details, there is often a temptation to create an "over-modeled" simulation, giving the impression of false fidelity. Conversely, analytical methods can bring about over-simplification, and consequently poor fidelity. Good modeling is still an art, and a difficult art to master.

We emphasize that an MSE is just what the name implies: an environment to aid a modeler in translating a computational model into a computer representation, then executing it and and interpreting its output. We think that intelligent MSEs which guide the modeling process using reasoning mechanisms from the domain of Artificial Intelligence are still largely visionary. Rather, we will confine ourselves to MSEs that increase a modeler's productivity by speeding up the model creation, verification, and validation cycles. The contention is that by shortening those cycle turnaround times, the feedback provided by the computer will speed up the modeling process.

ADVENT OF GRAPHICS

The proliferation of affordable and powerful desktop computers with graphics capabilities has brought about important changes in the way users interact with computers. Many people are now familiar with the use of a mouse and menu-driven interfaces to communicate with a computer and instruct it to do useful work [BENZ85]. From the office to CAD, CAM, and CAE systems, combined text and graphics environments are now becoming commonplace. This state of affairs is receiving increasing attention not only from industry but also from government. A case in point is VISC (Visual Initiative in

2

Scientific Computing) - an NSF iniative announced in 1987 and designed to support computer-based visualization tools. The VISC panel recommended [MCCO87]

"... to get visualization tools into the hearts and minds of scientists.
Scientists and engineers would team up with visualization researchers to
solve graphics, image processing, human/computer interface, or representational
problems grounded in the needs and methods of an explicit discipline."

Certainly, the areas of system modeling and performance analysis are instances of an "explicit discipline" within the scope of VISC .

It is not surprising that both industry and academia have also responded in kind. Recently, workers have begun to incorporate graphics into MSEs. Among the earliest ones are SEE-WHY^{TM} [FIDD81] (by BLSL), PAW [MELA85] (by AT&T) and RESQ [KURO86] (by IBM); a more recent effort is PME [WALS87] (by HP). In addition, a number of simulation languages have also added a graphics component for specification, animation, and statistical display. Examples include CINEMA^{TM} [HEAL86] (added to SIMAN), SIMANIMATION^{TM} [MULL87] (added to SIMSCRIPT II.5®) and TESS^{TM} [STAN85] (added to SLAM II^{TM}). Further examples are IMSE [HUGH87] - the European ongoing effort to build an MSE as part of the Esprit Project; and TANGRAM [MUNT88] - an AI-flavored MSE currently under construction at UCLA. This list is merely a sample; the interested reader is referred to [BELL85] for a more comprehensive survey.

To understand the prominence of graphics in MSEs one need only note that the vast majority of systems requiring performance analysis contain a marked visual component. Computer systems, communication networks, and manufacturing lines can often be described as networks of interconnected components which provide service to dynamic entities (transactions). Queueing in these systems is a prevalent phenomenon. Note also the common practice in system design of representing components and relations among them by nodes and arcs, while actions appear as text inserts. Not only are graphics natural for specifying system topology, they are useful in animating traffic flows and the dynamics of congestion [JOHN88], and for pictorially packaging statistics (histograms, time series, pie charts and plots) which are invaluable for grasping the computed statistics. A visual model constitutes a "transparent box" which allows users to observe model internals as well as model dynamics, in contrast to the traditional "black box" approach. The visual approach is extremely effective in enhancing user confidence in models, in communicating their details, and in encouraging tinkering and experimentation.

We hasten to add that graphics should supplement, not supplant text. In the better MSE, these two modes of communication between Man and Machine should blend together with smooth transitions from text to graphics and vice versa. There is a fundamental tradeoff between text and graphics. If one wishes to specify a procedure or a list of declarations, then text has a higher information density than an equivalent flowchart. That is, flow-charting minute instructions takes more room, is tedious to carry out, and beyond a certain complexity level, is hard to understand. Experience with entirely graphical procedural routines suggests that most of their value lies in instructing novices about programming [GLIN84]. On the other hand, graphic icons are highly efficient in encapsulating objects, ideas, and concepts. This is mostly due to their mnemonic quality, and the ease of locating them on screen and referring to them by pointing and clicking. In short, graphics are good for representing chunks of information, while the use of text prevails in spelling out the gory details. In line with this fact, one can expect novices to prefer extensive iconic interfaces, while experienced users tend to gravitate to the more concentrated expressive power of text. The point we make is that a designer of an MSE should not be a purist, but should exploit text or graphics as necessary to build a better MSE.

The theme, then, of this paper is the synergetic blending of text and graphics. We present our views on how to combine effectively text and graphics in a better MSE.

OBSERVATIONS, PREMISES AND GOALS

By way of motivation, we first make a number of observations and state our premises and goals.

a. We observe that the increasing complexity of systems requires the predictive power of models to make cost-effective decisions. Such decisions must be made at every stage of the system life cycle: from design and prototyping through manufacturing and enhancement to operation and maintenance. We also note that the primary cost in modeling is the modeler's time. This includes investigating and understanding the system (a human thinking activity little aided by an MSE), and the manipulation of a model on the computer (where the bulk of MSE interaction takes place). The goal of an MSE is ultimately underpinned by economic considerations. More specifically, an MSE aims at increasing the productivity of modelers by enabling them to concentrate on modeling, without the distraction of undue programming detail.

b. We discern two distinct phases of modeling activities: model development and production runs. Model development activities consist of model creation and specification followed by cycles of verification and validation punctuated by specification changes (refinement, debugging etc.). This phase is characterized by extensive interaction with the MSE. Production run activity takes place when the model is stable. It consists in the main of number crunching resulting in massive amounts of data. Production runs are carried out to compute analytical models or to run simulation replications; they are launched to compute statistics, to explore an area in parameter space for optimality of a given performance measure, or to conduct a sensitivity analysis of model parameters and performance indices. Beyond generating production run scripts, launching them, and examining output statistics, this modeling phase requires little interaction with the MSE. In fact, most of these activities could be carried out outside the MSE, or even in the background, without the modeler's presence.

c. We expect that an MSE will run on a powerful personal computer or workstation with a high resolution color display, and to operate in a networked configuration. We further assume that the cost of hardware/software is secondary. This assumption appears justified based on the current trend of declining hardware cost.

d. In view of the preceding discussion, the model development phase is particularly suitable to be carried out on a desktop computer - essentially a single user resource. Extensive production runs, however, will execute locally, often in the background, or will be uploaded and run remotely on a mainframe or supercomputer.

With these observations and premises in mind, we proceed with a description of the goals and requirements of a better MSE.

a. Increased modeling productivity is the fundamental goal of an MSE. In our view, the bulk of productivity gain is achieved by shortening interaction cycles with the MSE, particularly during the development phase. Of special importance is the modeler's ability to harness the power of the MSE to respond quickly to "what-if" questions. The MSE will facilitate the timely generation and presentation of options to the decision maker. Where possible, decision making algorithms or expert reasoning can be incorporated, but we do not view these as crucial.

b. A better MSE affords the modeler a good quality of (modeling) life. By this we mean an MSE with a truly easy-to-use user interface and extensive services, to be discussed later. The MSE's role is, like a good cop, to "serve and protect". The better MSE should make modeling a fun activity, not drudgery, and should facilitate rapid learning by novices. Here, good human factors and reasonable modeling paradigms are crucial. Furthermore, the MSE should have the look and feel of an integrated system rather than a loose collection of tools. Smooth transitions among modeling activities and short response times are the keys to user satisfaction.

MSE ISSUES

Guided by the points raised above, we proceed with a review of the salient issues in devising better MSEs.

MSE Architecture

Ideally, an MSE allows the modeler to describe a model in a language that employs both text and graphics; then, under modeler guidance, the MSE would bring to bear a battery of tools (simulation, analysis etc.) on the model. Unfortunately, the principle of one-specification-many-tools can merely be approximated. The trouble is, of course, that different tools can have drastically different world views and domains of applicability. For example, a simulation model requires computer code to drive model components, while an analytic model requires equations and/or sets of parameters. A partial solution is to translate from one domain to another; but unless the modeling domain is suitably restricted, this can rarely be done automatically. Generally, it is easier to translate an analytical specification to a simulation specification than vice versa. In addition, an attempt to translate in the other direction may well result in assumptions outside the solvable domain.

More often, a many-specifications-many-tools approach will have to be adopted. Nevertheless, an MSE can still maintain a common look and feel across tools. At least as far as entering, deleting and modification operations are concerned, all tools can share common graphics and text editors. Furthermore, there is a simple way to organize composite models as a tree in a natural way: submodels at the same level constitute sibling nodes while constituent submodels form children nodes. In fact, a directory and file structure (such as in the UNIX® operating system†) is a universal way of organizing information, including model information. Whether a component contains code (possibly entered by a syntax-directed or other text editor), parameters (possibly entered by a form editor) or merely children nodes and other icons (possibly entered by a graphics editor) is immaterial as far as this high-level paradigm for organizing information is concerned.

Consistent with this view is the requirement that an MSE should erect a software platform - a kernel of text, graphics and database services - common to all applications. All tools are instances of applications and are built on top of the kernel. Though users will have to master the semantics of each individual tool, routine operations on code, data, and images can be common to all. Again, we advocate an integrated environment with strong "operational" commonalities rather than a toolkit with loosely connected tools.

Object Management

An object-oriented approach [COX86] meshes nicely with a visual environment, especially in system modeling. Psychologically, objects can be better comprehended when their visualization (an icon or other pictorial representation) is displayed on the screen within their visual context. Both the iconic representation itself and its visual context are helpful in organizing information, creating and filing it and, later on, retrieving and modifying it. We allude to charting methods as an effective way to represent gross structure and relations; fine structural and interaction details are better left to text. We return to this point in the next section.

An object in a visual environment can be referred to in three ways: by its logical name, its address, or its icon. The first two references belong to the domain of traditional programming and are accomplished by entering a text string; the iconic reference mode is achieved by using a pointing device and is in the exclusive province of a visual environment. Reference by pointing and clicking is convenient and fast; it is particularly helpful for browsing through complex data structures and for debugging code.

---

† UNIX is a Registered Trademark of AT&T

The object-oriented approach is also useful to the implementer of an MSE. The notions of class and instance facilitate the implementation of such pervasive actions as printing an object, drawing its icon, storing submodels and retrieving them. We advocate the object-oriented approach both for user [COX86] and implementer [STRO86].

Model Construction

Model building is inherently object-oriented, the objects being models, submodels, attributes, parameters and fragments of code, to mention a few of the most fundamental ones. A natural way to build a top-down visual model is to visually create "boxes" on the screen. Each box represents a submodel and outlines its boundary. Here, the term "box" is used to connote a minimal or stripped-down icon; more elaborate icons can be used, but one should beware of overly ornate pictorial displays which distract rather than inform [TUFT83]. Initially empty, a "box" will be fleshed out with attributes and actions (in a simulation model) or with equations and parameters (in an analytical model). Hybrid models are naturally accomodated in this paradigm. We mention that a bottom-up visual model construction is also feasible. The bottom-up approach is employed by assembly operations of "cutting and pasting", possibly using model libraries. A typical scenario of visual model building is likely to be a mixture of top-down and bottom-up styles with the first style predominating.

Other icons can be used to represent submodel attributes: queues, variables or parameters. A standard graphic interface provides facilities for icon creation, reuse of extant icons, display layout, and general graphics editing. Zooming is an important standard operation. For example, zooming on a submodel will make it the current submodel and thereby display its constituent submodels. This and similar standard operations are menu-driven in a windowing environment.

A good metaphor for a modeler's activities is an electrical engineer tinkering with electronic parts on a board, trying to create a new system from off-the-shelf or custom-tailored components. Once functional, the new board itself can become an off-the-shelf piece. We point out that this approach is conducive to creating libraries. These libraries will consist of useful submodels that can be reused both as entire models or as constituent submodels of larger composite ones. The economy underlying model libraries is obvious.

An interesting application is automatic model building where real-life data determine the particular structure and/or parameters of a model selected from a sufficiently restricted class. An example is PET (Performance Engineering/Management Tool), developed in AT&T [FARR86]. PET analyzes UNIX statistics files and pipes the data to a workload builder which parametrizes a PAW model of a UNIX system; the model is used to estimate in real time performance measures not collected by UNIX, such as response times.

Text Entry

Text entry is needed to enter code and data. Code is required for simulation models; data is required for both analytical and simulation models.

A comprehensive MSE will have a programming language that can be either interpreted or translated into an established language, preferably with an optimizing compiler. During model development, user-generated code will run via the interpreter. At this stage, the flexibility gained outweighs the relative slowness of the interpreter. The number-crunching phase is better served by compiled and optimized binaries. The MSE language need not be brand new; an implementation of a good procedural language, preferably object-oriented, will do nicely. Whatever the choice, a syntax-directed editor, with rudimentary knowledge of the MSE world view, will be a welcome facility. The "look over the shoulder" mode will be especially helpful to beginners, though probably annoying to experienced users. The latter will be allowed to use a text editor of their choice. Of course, in this case they assume the burden of producing syntactically correct code.

The MSE should similarly provide facilities for setting program variables or parameters of pre-programmed submodels. A pre-programmed submodel is one whose code (rules of operations) are predefined, so no explicit procedural programming is called for. The only leeway accorded the modeler is entry of agreed on parameters (possibly with default values). For example, if the modeling domain is restricted to queueing networks, the modeler can specify for a given queue its discipline, capacity, number of servers etc. Form editors (preferably syntax-directed) are again useful and should be provided by the MSE.

Database Services

Database services such as a query language are of considerable value to modelers. How to organize an MSE as a database manager is a major issue which is outside the scope of this paper. We merely use this opportunity to raise the issue in passing.

Testing and Debugging

Good testing and debugging facilities are essential for increased modeler productivity. The usefulness of code debugging facilities such as tracing statements, setting breakpoints and inspecting variables is clear; these facilities must be provided by the MSE.

The availability of graphics enhances debugging and testing in a number of ways. First, objects can be refered to through their icons as discussed before. Second, program models can be coded to display system states, traffic flows, and output statistics. In the case of queueing networks, system states can be shown by displaying the queues at network nodes, while traffic flows can be visualized by animating the movement of transactions among nodes. Network congestion in a visual model can then be grasped at a glance. In addition, output statistics can also be animated, as discussed in the next subsection. These facilities go far beyond syntactic debugging as they embed modeling semantics invaluable in model verification - the activity of checking that a computational model was correctly translated to its computer representation.

Pursuing the engineering metaphor, an MSE should support testbed environments. Just as faulty components can be removed by the engineer from their board and tested in isolation to pinpoint failures, any submodel should be testable in isolation. This may not detect bugs due to interactions beyond the submodel boundary, but it would simplify the identification of bugs resulting from internal interactions and dependencies. As with electrical components, after isolated debugging, the tested submodel will be inserted to its original place for further testing in a broader context.

Output Analysis

The correct analysis and interpretation of model predictions is the payoff of modeling. While this activity is as much an art as model construction, an MSE should provide services to extract information from data.

First, a report generator will assist in organizing output statistics displays. The most common ways of visualizing statistics include histograms, time-series, and bar and pie charts. Performance mesures can be effectively compared by plotting them on a common chart.

Second, in simulation models we can easily implement animation of dynamic statistics. A dynamic statistic is a display of intermediate results while an animated statisic refers expressly to the successive display of intermediate pictorial displays in real time. The value of animated statistics lies in the time sequencing of statistical information. For example, instability can manifest itself in a histogram when the probability mass is seen to move to the right.

Third, the MSE can provide statistical tests and models similar to the S language [BECK84]. At the minimum, one should be able to pipe output data to established statistical facilities.

Finally, the MSE can support exploration of parameter spaces. A more intelligent MSE will also help in guiding searches for optimal or near optimal performance measures.

<u>Applications and Programming Styles</u>

We have already described a visual style for organizing submodels as "boxes within boxes", and argued that it is general enough to encompass all important model categories. We now turn to styles of text programming - the contents of the constituent submodels ("boxes").

Both procedural and non-procedural style programming are useful in modeling. (Again, we exclude logic programming from the discussion). General purpose simulation modeling will primarily employ procedural code fragments to drive submodel components (usually representing site-oriented static entities such as network nodes, resources etc.) as well as transactions (usually representing dynamic entities such as customers, packets etc.). For certain modeling domains (queueing networks, protocols, Petri nets, Markov processes) with substantially fixed semantics, the MSE could provide predefined submodels which are merely parametrizable. From the modeler's point of view, combining predefined submodels and parametrizing them is non-procedural programming. Predefined submodels may or may not be modifiable. Thus, simulation programming could span the spectrum of styles: from purely procedural to purely non-procedural as well as hybrids in between.

The situation in analytical models is reversed. One can usually expect an MSE application to come with a full-fledged world view and a set of pre-programmed (but parametrizable) components. But user-supplied algorithms can typically expected to be procedural.

CONCLUSION

We have argued that current modeling needs amply justify the construction of powerful and versatile MSEs. Furthermore, the right blend of text and graphics will greatly enhance the Man-Machine interaction and enable the modeler to concentrate on the creative side of modeling.

Technologies already exist to build the components of MSEs along the lines described in this paper. These technologies include graphics and text editors, browsers, compilers, debuggers, and statistical-analysis programs. The challenge is to put all pieces together and deliver an integrated-services MSE which "serves and protects", is easy-to-use, yet possesses the power and versatility to model efficiently a wide variety of systems in the best possible modeling paradigm.

ACKNOWLEDGEMENTS

We gratefully acknowledge the comments of Bryn C. Ekroot and Robert T. J. Morris.

REFERENCES

[BECK84]   Becker R. A. and Chambers J. M., *S : An Interactive Environment for Data Analysis and Graphics*, Wadsworth, 1984.

[BELL85]   Bell P. C. and O'Keefe R. M., "Visual Interactive Simulation - History, Recent Developments, and Major Issues", *Simulation*, Vol. 49, No. 3, 1987, 109-116.

[BENZ85]   Benzon B., "The Visual Mind and the Macintosh", *Byte*, Jan. 1985, 113-130.

[BGS82]   BGS Systems Inc., *The BEST/1 User Guide*, 1982.

[BRAT83]   Bratley P., Fox B. L. and Schrage L. E., *A Guide to Simulation*, Springer Verlag, 1983.

[COX86]   Cox B. J., *Object Oriented Programming*, Addison-Wesley, 1986.

[FARR86]   Farrel B. L. and Ramamurthy G., "A Prototype Performance Engineering/Management Tool for UNIX Based Systems", *Proceedings of the International Conference on Management and Performance Evaluation of Computer Systems*, Las Vegas, Nevada, 1986, 345-352.

[FIDD81]   Fiddy E., Bright J. G. and Hurrion R. D., "SEE-WHY: Interactive Simulation on the Screen", *Proceedings of the Institute of Mechanical Engineers*, C293/81, 1981, 167-172.

[GLIN84]   Glinert E. P. and Tanimoto S. L., "Pict: An Interactive Graphical Programming Environment", *IEEE Computer*, Vol. 17, No. 11, 1984, 7-25.

[HEAL86]   Healy K. J., "Cinema Tutorial", *Proceedings of the Winter Simulation Conference*, SCS, 1986, 207-211.

[HUGH87]   Hughes P. and Potier D., "Integrated Modeling Support Environment", *Esprit II Proposal, Project Overview (third version)*, May 1987.

[JOHN88]   Johnson E. M. and Poorte J. P., "A Hierarchical Approach to Computer Animation in Simulation Modeling", *Simulation*, Vol. 50, No. 1, 1988, 30-36.

[KURO86]   Kurose J. F., Kurtiss G. J., Gordon R. F., MacNair E. A. and Welch P. D., "A Graphics-Oriented Modeler's Workstation Environment for the RESearch Queueing Package (RESQ)", *Proceedings of the Fall Joint Computer Conference*, Dallas, Texas, 1986, 719-728.

[MCCO87]   McCormick B. H., DeFanti T.A. and Brown M. D. (editors), "Visualization in Scientific Computing - A Synopsis", *IEEE Computer Graphics and Applications*, Vol. 7, No. 6, 1987, 61-70.

[MELA85]   Melamed B. and Morris R. J. T., "Visual Simulation: The Performance Analysis Workstation", *IEEE Computer*, Vol. 18, No. 8, 1985, 87-94.

[MULL87]   Mullarney A., *SIMANIMATION User's Guide and Casebook*, CACI Products Co., 1987.

[MUNT88]   Muntz R. R. and Parker D. S., "Tangram: Project Overview", *Technical Report CSD-880032*, UCLA, Computer Science Department, 1988.

[RAMA82]   Ramakrishnan K.G. and Mitra D., "An Overview of PANACEA: A Software Package for Analyzing Markovian Queueing Networks", *Bell System Technical Journal*, Vol. 61, No. 10, 1982, 2849-2872.

[STAN85]   Standridge C. R., "Performing Simulation Projects with the Extended Simulation System (TESS)", *Simulation*, Vol. 45, No. 6, 1985, 283-291.

[STRO86]   Stroustrup B., *The C++ Programming Language*, Addison-Weseley, 1986.

[TUFT83]   Tufte E. R., *Visual Display of Quantitative Information*, Graphics Press, 1983.

[VERA85]   Veran M. and Potier D., "QNAP2 : A Portable Environment for Queueing Systems Modelling", *Proceedings of the International Workshop on Modelling Techniques and Performance Evaluation*, Paris, France, 1985,

[WALS87]   Walstra, R. J., "Composite Models of System Performance", *Proceedings of the International Workshop on Modelling Techniques and Performance Evaluation*, Paris, France, 1987, 195-203.

[WHIT85]   Whitt W., "The Queueing Network Analyzer", *Bell System Technical Journal*, Vol. 62, No. 9, 2779-2815.

COMPILING TECHNIQUES FOR THE ANALYSIS

OF STOCHASTIC PETRI NETS

Giovanni Chiola

Dipartimento di Informatica
Universita` di Torino
Torino, Italy

ABSTRACT

The performance of Stochastic Petri Net models can be estimated either by Monte-Carlo simulation or by construction and evaluation of Markov chains isomorphic to their reachability graphs. In both cases, the efficiency of the algorithms used to compute the marking sequences reachable by a model is crucial for the applicability of this methodology in practical cases. It is claimed that an organic approach based on ad-hoc techniques is needed to improve the efficiency of the software used for the analysis and to allow the solution of problems of realistic size. A set of compiling techniques is presented to produce Petri net analysis or simulation programs tailored on the specific characteristics of individual models. The proposed approach allows to improve on the performance of currently used packages of up to one order of magnitude in both space and time efficiency of reachability algorithms and in time efficiency of event-driven simulation of Petri nets.

1. INTRODUCTION

One of the limiting factors in the practical usability of Stochastic Petri Nets (SPN) [1, 2, 3, 4] is the lack of efficient exact analysis techniques that overcome the construction and numerical solution of their isomorphic Markov chain (MC). No break-through result comparable with efficient algorithms developed for product-form queueing networks is likely to be proposed in the near future, so that either exact numerical solutions based on a "brute-force" attack or Monte-Carlo simulation have to be considered. Decomposition/aggregation techniques can certainly be exploited to partition large models in smaller submodels, but even individual submodels can very easily turn out to be too complex to be analyzed with the available tools at acceptable costs.

The size of the state space of an SPN model can hardly be related to the "size" of the model description. It is possible to prove that in the worst case the number of markings of an SPN increases exponentially with the number of places. On the other hand, it is possible to find many favorable cases in which the size of the state space increases polynomially with the number of places and transitions of the net. Experience suggests that a reasonable number of interesting models (usually coming from a preliminary decomposition and/or simplification of complex actual models) yield reachability graphs of size ranging from a few hundred to a few hundred thousand of markings. Therefore, an algorithm for the computation of the reachability graph of an SPN should be able to handle at least 100,000 states on a workstation or a minicomputer, subject to both space and time constraints.

It is not difficult to understand that the most limiting factor is the amount of memory used by the program, rather than the actual CPU time needed to run it. This is true even in the case of machines using virtual memory: if the size of the program working set exceeds the size of the machine physical memory, the elapsed time of the program is increased of a factor that may easily approach the ratio between the secondary memory access time and the main memory access time, thus causing the execution time to become unacceptably long even if the algorithm is not theoretically compute-bound.

Selecting an appropriate data structure to achieve both space and time efficiency becomes thus a challenging task. Existing implementations of reachability analysis for Petri nets try to achieve the best compromise between these two conflicting constraints [5, 6, 7, 8]. For instance, the reachability graph analyzer included in the *GreatSPN* package [6] allows the generation of some ten thousand markings using data structures not exceeding 2 Mbytes in size. Most of the memory is used in this case to store the encoded markings and a balanced binary tree used to speed-up their searching. Using a balanced tree allows a theoretical time complexity of $N\log_2 N$, if N is the number of markings of the model. This complexity computation assumes that all the data structures can be kept in main memory. Whenever these memory requirements exceed the main memory size, since the working set of the algorithm tend to coincide with the whole data structure used to implement the searching of markings, the time complexity count mentioned previously no longer holds. Therefore, the $N\log_2 N$ time complexity cannot be achieved if the data structures are scaled up of one order of magnitude, unless a machine with a substantially larger main memory is used to run the computation, because of the effect of the size of the program working set on the performance of the virtual memory of the system.

Another issue that is usually neglected in the evaluation of the performance of a program, but that can considerably affect both the program elapsed time and the global level of system software overhead, is the amount of input/output (I/O) performed. Computing the reachability graph of a Petri net is of little use if the graph generated is not stored on a file to be analyzed by other programs. The amount of space required to encode the reachability graph can thus indirectly affect the time efficiency of a program implementing the analysis algorithm also on machine having substantial main memory space. Decreasing the marking encoding of, for example, one order of magnitude would result also in decreasing of one order of magnitude the I/O operations required to store the results, and thus the total execution time.

In the case of event-driven simulation, memory space is usually not a problem. The execution time of a simulation experiment depends mainly on the overhead induced by event-list management operations. Considerable optimizations can be performed on specific simulation programs, when knowledge exist of the behavior of the particular system being simulated. In a general purpose simulation program instead, little can be done to improve the efficiency of such event management.

The normal approach followed in the implementation of computer packages for performance evaluation, no matter whether based on numerical or simulation techniques, is to implement an analysis or simulation program capable of dealing with an entire class of models such as, for example, product-form queueing networks. The description of the model is reflected in some internal data structure, whose dimension is either predefined at compile time or, in some more sophisticated cases, allocated at run time after reading the dimension of the model to be analyzed. Event-driven simulation is in this case obtained through what in the Computer Science jargon is called an ''interpretation'' of the model description. In the case of numerical solution, the solver must be prepared to deal with the most general model that can be contained in the class of models to be solved; data-dependent optimizations are cumbersome to implement, so that general algorithms are usually applied also to cases that could be attacked using simpler, special case techniques.

In this paper a quite different approach is proposed, in which techniques inspired by well established compiler construction methods are used to produce either a reachability graph construction program or an event-driven simulation program, whose code and data structure are optimized for the specific net to be analyzed/simulated. In particular, both marking encodings and transition operation implementations are chosen from a set of predefined patterns in order to adapt the analysis or simulation program to the peculiar characteristics of a given net. At the cost of some preprocessing which involves a preliminary structural analysis of the net, the generation of a portion of analysis/simulation code dependent on the structural properties of the net, the compilation of the model-dependent code, and its linking with a model-independent analysis/simulation core, the solution of the net is subject to a ''not so brute-force'' attack, which can exploit some implicit information embedded in the PN structure to reduce its computational effort.

It should be observed that this strategy is reasonable in the case of large models, in which the preprocessing needed to set up the analysis/simulation program (which may take a few minutes of CPU time) is negligible compared to the total solution cost; in case of very simple models the overhead introduced by the use of a system compiler may exceed the CPU time of the solution itself, but the aim of this work is to address the problem of the analysis of large models that would be otherwise unsolvable. Experiments conducted on a significant sample of "real" cases have shown the possibility of gaining up to one order of magnitude in both time and space requirements over the previous approach.

2. CODING THE MARKING OF A PN

The first problem to be tackled in devising a data structure for the reachability analysis of a Petri net is the choice of a good coding schema for markings. An efficient marking coding can sometimes be required also in the case of simulation in at least two occasions: when a trace of a simulation run has to be recorded to perform, e.g., an animation of the model; when an automatic search for regeneration states is performed in a "pilot" simulation run. Theoretically, the problem may be solved using a prime number encoding; in practice this cannot be easily (and efficiently) implemented because of arithmetic overflow problems. Alternatively, one can choose to limit the analysis to PN in which all places are k-bounded, and use an array of numbers coded in $\lceil \log_2(k+1) \rceil$ bits dimensioned after the number of places. In the reachability graph constructor included in the *GreatSPN* package, the latter alternative was chosen, with $k=127$, thus coding a marking with as many bytes as the number of places of the net, and allowing at most 127 tokens to accumulate in each place.

2.1. Actual Bounds for Places

A first improvement on this method can be achieved by considering the actual limit k_i on the number of tokens that may accumulate in each place p_i of a particular net, assigning exactly $\lceil \log_2(k_i+1) \rceil$ bits to its coding in markings. The problem is then reduced to the determination of the actual k-bounding for each place of the PN, *before* the enumeration of the reachability set.

No algorithm is known to solve this problem in general; however it is possible to obtain an upper bound for the place k-bounding from the analysis of minimal-support linear place-invariants [9]. When an upper bound can be obtained from linear invariant analysis (i.e. when a place is contained in at least one minimal-support place-invariant), the experience shows that most of the times such bound is tight. This kind of analysis is implemented by a very fast algorithm [10], whose elapsed time is usually several orders of magnitude lower than that of the reachability graph construction. Pathological cases exist in which the number of minimal-support place-invariants becomes comparable with the number of markings of the net; on the other hand, such unfortunate patterns can be easily recognized on the net structure, and are hardly found in PN models that are not deliberately constructed with the goal of making the invariant computation algorithm fail. A linear invariant analysis can provide useful results even in the case of extended Petri nets with inhibitor arcs and different transition priorities [11].

Minimal-support place-invariants are defined as the (finite) set PI of non-negative integer vectors $\mathbf{p}$ whose components are minimal, and that are solution of the matrix equation

$$\mathbf{C}^T \; \mathbf{p} \; = \; 0 \quad ,$$

where $\mathbf{C}$ is the incidence matrix of the net. The key characteristics of place-invariants is that their scalar product times any reachable marking of the net yields a constant, whose value can be determined from the initial marking of the net. Therefore, the set of minimal-support place-invariants together with the initial marking of the net yields a finite set of linear equations in the non-negative integer domain, from which an upper bound of the k_i-bounding of a place p_i of the net can be determined as:

$$k_i \; \leq \; \min_{\mathbf{p} \in PI \, : \, \mathbf{p}_i > 0} \; \frac{\mathbf{p} \bullet M_0}{\mathbf{p}_i}$$

(provided that p_i is included in at least one place-invariant). This technique was already exploited in the RDPS package [5].

2.2. Linear Place-Invariants

A second improvement in the coding of place markings can be obtained in many cases by observing that place-invariants may be considered as closed paths followed by the tokens when flowing through the net, much in the same way as chains [12] in closed queueing networks. This is not the case for arbitrary subsets of places in a generic Petri net, in which one can only say that tokens are added in a given place by the firing of its input transitions and destroyed by the firing of its output transitions. The computation of place-invariants highlights the conservative components of a Petri net, and can then be compared to the identification of closed chains of customers visiting the service stations in a queueing network.

Having identified a subset of places among which tokens are moved, an alternative way of representing the contribution that these tokens give to the state of the net is that of encoding their position within their subsets of places, rather than the number of tokens in each of these places.

For instance, let's consider the case of the net depicted in Figure 1. The four places p_1, p_2, p_3, and p_5 form a minimal-support place-invariant, among which only one token is present. The first alternative would require 4 bits to encode the number of tokens in the four places. The second alternative requires that a single 2-bit number is associated with the set of places, encoding the position of the single token in one of the four places. The fifth place p_4 is contained into another 1-bounded place-invariant (together with p_1, and p_5), so that its marking can be encoded in one bit. Therefore it is possible to use only three bits to encode the whole marking of the net of Figure 1.

Note that this strategy can actually eliminate some redundant places from the coding: a place in which the number of tokens is constant in all reachable markings constitutes a place-invariant by itself, therefore the position of its tokens can be coded in $\log_2(1) = 0$ bits.

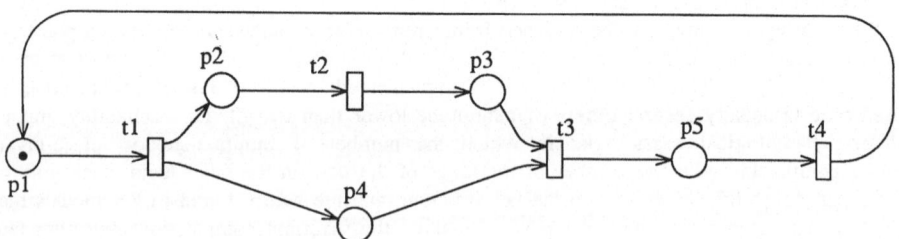

Figure 1. *An example of a Petri net.*

2.3. Redundant Places

Another kind of redundancy can be eliminated by testing for the presence of *implicit* places [13]. A place is said to be implicit when its marking can be obtained as a linear combination (with non-negative integer coefficients) of the marking of a set of other places, that are called implicant. Implicit places, together with their implicant sets, can be recognized automatically by a slight modification of the algorithm used to compute place-invariants [13]. It is therefore easy to eliminate implicit places from the marking to be encoded, and substitute the decoding of their marking with the computation of the linear combination of the marking of their implicants.

For example, in the net of Figure 1 place p_4 can be easily recognized to be implicit, since its marking can always be obtained as the sum of the markings in places p_2 and p_3. Eliminating place p_4 from the marking coding of the net in Figure 1 happens to yield *the optimal coding,* since only two bits are used and the reachability set of the net contains four markings.

2.4. Non-Linear Place-Invariants and Redundancy

Consider the Petri net depicted in Figure 2, which represents a trivial modification of the one shown in Figure 1. In particular, place p_4 in Figure 1 is substituted by places p_4 and p_6, and by transition t_5 in Figure 2. In this case neither p_4 nor p_6 are implicit places, so that a coding based on linear place invariants requires, for instance, two bits to encode the position of the token in the place-invariant p_1, p_2, p_3, p_5, and two bits to encode the marking in places p_4, and p_6, which are also 1-bounded due to the place-invariant p_1, p_4, p_6, p_5.

Clearly the two above mentioned minimal-support place-invariants p_1, p_2, p_3, p_5, and p_1, p_4, p_6, p_5 are not independent of each other, since they share the two places p_1 and p_5. The dependence between different minimal-support place-invariants cannot be expressed in terms of linear equations in non-negative integer arithmetics. One possible non-linear representation of this interdependency is:

$$\text{if } p_1+p_5 > 0 \quad \text{then} \quad p_1+p_5 = 1 \ \wedge \ p_2+p_3+p_4+p_6 = 0$$
$$\text{else} \quad p_2+p_3 = 1 \ \wedge \ p_4+p_6 = 1$$

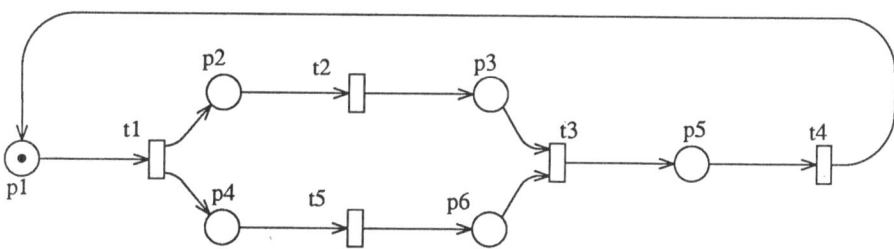

Figure 2. *An example of a Petri net without implicit places.*

This non-linear invariant expression can be obtained easily by combination of linear invariant expressions that have common elements. A compact coding can be constructed based on this non-linear invariant expression, by encoding separately the position of tokens inside conditional invariants. If we denote with cc the coding of the common part (places p_1 and p_5), and with $cs1$ and $cs2$ the codings of the two disjoint subparts (places p_2 and p_3, and places p_4 and p_6, respectively), in terms of token position within a portion of linear invariants, a compound coding may be defined as the union of subcoding cc with the Cartesian product of the two subcodings $cs1 \times cs2$. The number of configurations required by this compound coding is the sum of the number of configurations for encoding cc (i.e. 2), plus the product of the number of configurations required by subcoding $cs1$ and $cs2$ (i.e. 2×2 in this case). In the particular case depicted in Figure 2, only six coding configurations (that can be represented using three bits) are thus required if the mutual relation among overlapping minimal-support place-invariants is considered, instead of the sixteen coding configurations (that can be represented using four bits) that would result by considering the individual linear invariants separately.

It is interesting to note that, in this particular case, the proposed compound marking encoding is optimal, since six coding configurations can be used while the net happens to have a reachability set comprising exactly six different markings. Indeed, the example in Figure 2 happens to be a net of type "safe marked graph" [14], and the optimality of this encoding scheme can be proved in the case of Petri nets that fit into this restricted class.

Another interesting property of this compound marking encoding scheme is that it can automatically avoid the encoding of redundant places. In the case of the net depicted in Figure 1 the subcoding corresponding to the implicit place p_4 has a single configuration, so that its Cartesian product times the subcoding corresponding to places p_2 and p_3 does not increase the total number of configurations in the compound encoding.

2.5. A Linear Place-Invariant Based Heuristics for Marking Encoding

Given a particular set *PI* of place-invariants, it is possible to organize a heuristics to minimize the marking encoding of the net as follows.

(1)   Delete places that are contained in place-invariants containing only one place.

(2)   Delete all implicit places that are found in the net, and substitute them with the linear combination of their implicants.

(3)   Compute the minimal-support place-invariants on the resulting net.

(4)   Sort the place-invariants for increasing token count in the initial marking first, and then (in case of place-invariants with the same token count) for decreasing support (i.e., number of places covered by the invariant).

(5)   While there are places not yet encoded and place-invariants not yet considered
   • consider the places contained in the first place-invariant that are not yet encoded;
      if the invariant encoding is convenient (i.e. if the token count of the place-invariant is less than the number of places to be encoded due to the invariant itself)
      then encode the considered places by token position in the invariant
      else encode each considered place singularly with the bounding determined by the first invariant.
   • delete the first place-invariant and re-sort the remaining place-invariants by increasing token count and then by decreasing number of not yet encoded places in the support.

(6)   Encode all not yet coded places (the ones not included in any place-invariant) by considering them K-bounded, with some arbitrarily chosen reasonable value of K (possibly 255).

Since most machine architectures implement efficient instructions to access main memory at an 8-bit byte level, in the actual implementation of the proposed algorithms a grouping of different codings in sets so that the representation of each set of encodings fits an 8-bit byte boundary is introduced. Different encodings are then grouped in *coding chunks* (or byte) (implemented as "unsigned char" in the C programming language [15]) for programming convenience. Individual codings can be retrieved very efficiently by using mask and shift machine instructions.

3. ORGANIZING A TIME AND SPACE EFFICIENT MARKING SEARCH TREE

The main loop of a reachability graph algorithm is usually organized as depicted in Figure 3, to implement an exhaustive breadth-first search into the state space. As one can realize, the data structure used to encode the reachability set is crucial for the performance of the algorithm: it must allow a very efficient test for inclusion (to be performed as many times as the product of the number of reachable markings times the average number of transitions enabled in a marking), an efficient insertion of a new element (to be performed as many times as the number of markings in the reachability set), and, last but not least, it must fit in a few Mbytes of core memory in order not to incur in the virtual memory penalty that would result from a working set larger than the physical memory available on a minicomputer or a workstation.

The solution adopted in a previous reachability graph constructor [16], and that was found to work satisfactorily on a 4 Mbyte UNIX machine in case of reachability sets comprising up to 10 thousands markings, was organized as follows. The actual marking coding (the number of tokens in the places of the net for each marking) was stored in a large array of bytes. A second data structure organized as a balanced binary tree was used to maintain a lexicographic order between

```
        <let NM be an ordered list of markings>;
        <let RS be the reachability set of the net>;
        NM := [M₀] (* the initial marking *);
        RS := [M₀];
        while <NM is not empty> do begin
                <let CM be the first element of NM>;
                <remove CM from NM>;
                foreach <transition t enabled in CM> do begin
                        <let MM be the marking obtained by firing t in CM>;
                        if <MM is not in RS> then begin
                                <insert MM at the end of NM>;
                                <add MM to RS>
                        end
                end
        end;
```

Figure 3. *A sketch of the reachability graph algorithm.*

markings, with the nodes of the tree pointing to the first bytes of the actual marking encodings into the array. The complexity of a search was thus logarithmic in the number of markings already stored in the reachability set, and linear in the number of bytes of the marking encoding. The ordered insertion into the balanced tree was implemented by a standard rebalance algorithm [17]. The total memory requirement was of the order of $n \times (k+p)$, where n is the number of markings, p is the number of places, and k is a constant accounting for the dimension of the nodes of the tree (something like 20 bytes in the actual implementation), resulting in a memory requirement of about 1 Mbyte for a typical net with some 10 thousand markings and some fifty places.

We are now proposing a different coding structure based on a multiple tree, that allows reducing substantially both the search and insert time as well as the total memory requirement. The idea is similar to that exploited by Vaishnavi [18] to generalize a rebalance algorithm for multiple dimensional binary trees. The proposed data structure is best explained by an example. Assume that the marking of the net can be coded with three bytes according to the compact coding heuristics described in the previous section, and suppose to encode the following five markings:

	markings		
#	b0	b1	b2
M1	0	0	1
M2	0	0	2
M3	0	1	1
M4	1	0	2
M5	0	0	4

The coding can be organized into a three-level tree (associating one byte of coding with each depth level of the tree) as:

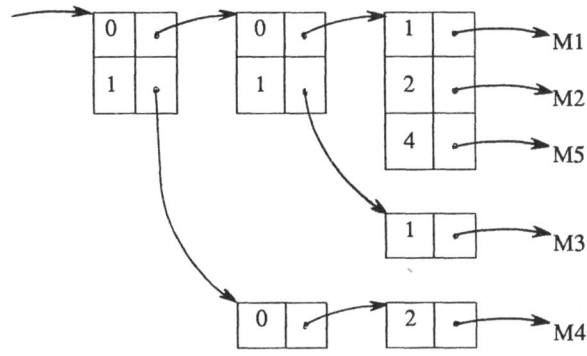

Note that, with this tree organization the first two byte representation of the codings of markings M1, M2, and M5 are merged together; similarly, the first byte representation of marking M3 is shared with the three above listed markings.

It is apparent that such a data structure has the potential of saving a substantial amount of memory space with respect to the binary tree coding previously used. It is not too difficult to prove that the maximum benefit is obtained when the chunks of marking encodings are sorted in increasing order of number of possible different values. Such an optimal sorting can be approximated by the knowledge of the k-bounding of the places whose marking is encoded in the bytes.

Another advantage of the above sketched data structure is that the search complexity becomes a function of the number of coding bytes, rather than of the logarithm of the number of markings. In the case considered in the example, a maximum of three tests is required in the worst case to determine whether a given marking is already in the reachability graph, independently of the number of markings itself (which is limited by the number of different codings that can be contained in three bytes, i.e. 2^{24}). Moreover, the search procedure may be interrupted at the level corresponding to the first chunk that doesn't match. For instance, the presence of marking M=(2,0,5) can be excluded after the test on the first byte, and the presence of marking (1,1,0) can be excluded after the test of the second byte. This is not the case in a balanced binary tree, were the presence of a given marking may not be excluded until reaching a leaf of the tree (after at least $d-1$ tests if d is the current depth of the tree).

A practical problem remains in the implementation of the nodes of the search tree. There is no reason to use the same node structure at different depth levels in the tree. Using a preprocessing phase it is possible to automatically generate the code that is most appropriate for the encoding of the reachability set of a particular net, and then compile a "tailored" version of the reachability constructor. Selecting the C programming language [15] for implementation, it is possible to produce very efficient ad-hoc code, that can easily access the most efficient machine instructions needed to encode/decode and handle pointers of different ranges.

Depending on the number of possible values that the chunk associated with a given tree depth may assume, different data structures may be used to implement the tree nodes. In the above example, at the third level of the tree a single node is used to encode the three markings M1, M2, and M5. The node must contain three pointers, each one corresponding to a different value of the coding byte. Either an array of pointers to the next chunk with as many elements as the range of possible values (four in this case), or a binary balanced subtree with as many subnodes as the actual number of possible values (three in the example) may be most appropriate, in order to trade-off memory space requirements and insertion/search time.

The array solution has the advantage of requiring a single subscript evaluation to implement both search and insertion, and eliminates the need for two pointers (the left and right "children" pointers) and of the byte value encoding for each value of the byte itself. On the other hand, it requires the preallocation of the complete array, even if only a small part of the range of possible values of the chunk is actually needed to encode the reachability set.

In case a binary tree structure is chosen, the worst case search and insert time is bounded by $\log_2(v)$ tests, where $v \leq 256$ is the maximum number of different values that the byte may assume. Only the chunk values actually present in the reachability set need to be allocated as subtree nodes, but each node is much more complex than an array item, since it must hold the information needed to traverse and maintain balance in the tree.

After having tuned the trade-off on some representative sample of the class of nets to be analyzed, the above sketched data structure has experimentally proved an improvement of up to one order of magnitude in both time and space requirements with respect to the previous general purpose algorithm.

4. EXPLOITING STRUCTURAL PROPERTIES TO OPTIMIZE TRANSITION FIRING

From the reachability graph algorithm outlined in Figure 3 in the previous section, one can realize that another key factor in the efficiency of the implementation is the firing of a transition and the computation of the next marking, that are contained in the inner "foreach" loop.

The same problem appears in the implementation of a Monte-Carlo simulator for an SPN model, in which many hundred thousands transition firings may be necessary in order to reach the desired confidence interval for the estimated results. In this case, the classical event list structure can be augmented in order to relate each event notice to a net transition, thus obtaining a two-dimensional structure linked both by simulation time and by transition identity. Scheduling of events is implemented using simulation time links, while de-scheduling of events can be performed following transition links corresponding to transitions that are disabled by conflict situations.

The first technique used to speed up the transition firing is the automatic creation of enabling and firing procedures starting from the marking encoding and the actual arc connections. The procedures implement both the enabling test and the next marking computation directly on the compact encoding for the sake of efficiency. As many C functions are produced as the number of transitions in the net, each one specialized in the firing of a particular transition in the compact encoding.

The second technique is the reduction of the number of transitions to be tested for enabling, by considering only a subset of transitions that are likely to be enabled in the current marking. This screening can be implemented based on the knowledge of some precomputed transition structural properties.

A list of the enabled transitions in the current marking (which normally is substantially smaller than the whole set of transitions, and that in case of event-driven simulation corresponds to the event-list) is maintained. After the firing of transition t, the list of transitions enabled in the new marking may be computed from the previous list by deleting all transitions that have been disabled by the firing of t, and adding all transitions that have been enabled by the firing of t. Since the number of transitions affected by the firing of t is usually much smaller than the number of transitions enabled in a marking, not to mention the total number of transitions in the net, this method has the potential of greatly reducing the time needed to compute the set of enabled transitions with respect to the trivial approach of testing all transitions of the net for enabling in each marking, that was used in previous implementations of the reachability construction [16].

Some of the transition structural properties proposed in [11] can be used for this purpose. In particular, a necessary condition for a transition t_k to be enabled by the firing of t is that t be causally connected to t_k (denoted as $t \ CC \ t_k$). On the other hand, a necessary condition for a transition t_k to be disabled by the firing of t is that the two transitions are not mutually exclusive (not $t \ ME \ t_k$), and that t_k is in structural conflict with t ($t_k \ SC \ t$). Formal definitions of the three above relations are given in [11] as functions of the place-invariants and the structure of the net, and their computation is easily coded into a computer program. An enabled list manipulation function can be generated in C language, according to the structural relations of the transition currently firing.

5. PRODUCING A BAND-DIAGONAL STATE-TRANSITION MATRIX

It is well known that the efficiency of algorithms implementing a numerical solution of sparse matrix linear equations can be improved by some matrix patterns. In particular, the inversion of large sparse matrices becomes efficient in case of band-diagonal patterns [19]. Some routine packages use sophisticated heuristics to rearrange the matrix shape before tackling its solution, trying to approach a band-diagonal form. In the case of the state-transition matrix of the Markov chain generated by the reachability graph of an SPN, we can try to exploit the information implicit in the structure of the underlying PN to generate a matrix whose shape is as close as possible to a band-diagonal permutation.

Due to the choice of a breadth-first search algorithm, reachable markings are generated in such an order that the state-transition matrix is guaranteed to be band-lower-triangular. The claim can be proved by the following reasoning. Markings are numbered in the order in which they are generated, starting from the initial marking. A marking M_i which is not reachable by the first k markings is certainly generated after any marking M_j reached by one of the first k markings, so that $i>j$. This is true for every possible choice of $i>k$, so that the state-transition matrix is band-lower-triangular by definition. As an example, Figure 4 depicts the non-zero entry shape of a typical 1350-state MC state-transition matrix generated by a breadth-first firing algorithm from an SPN specification.

In order to transform a band-lower-triangular matrix into a band-diagonal shape, we have to "control" in some way the returns to previously generated states. In particular, we have to minimize the distance between the indices of any two markings M_i and M_j such that $i>j$ and M_i returns in M_j.

In a Petri net, a necessary condition to return in a previous marking is that a *transition-invariant* exist. Minimal-support transition-invariants are the dual of place-invariants, being defined as the minimal non-negative integer vectors which are solutions of the matrix equation

$$C \ t \ = \ 0$$

A necessary condition for a bounded SPN to have a recurrent initial marking (and thus to be ergodic) is that all transitions in the net are contained in some minimal-support transition-invariant. All well-behaved SPN are thus covered by transition-invariants, and we may establish a connection between the transition-invariants of the underlying PN and the shape of the state-transition matrix of

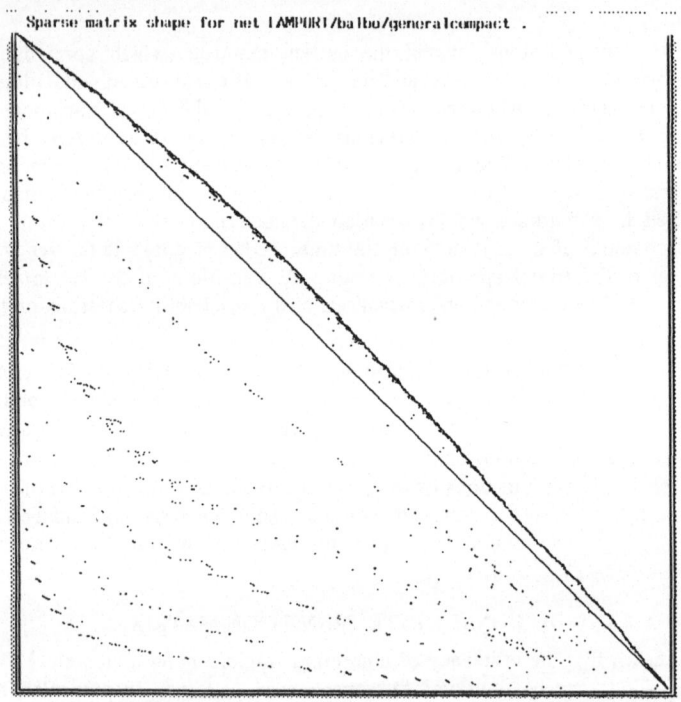

Figure 4. *The shape of non-zero items of a typical MC generated by breadth-first search.*

the MC generated by the SPN. The problem is that the presence of a transition-invariant in the underlying PN is a necessary, but not a sufficient condition for the MC to have a return in a state with lower ordinal number. It may be the case that a transition sequence corresponding to a given transition-invariant is not enabled in the PN. Therefore a shaping method based on the knowledge of transition-invariants is only a heuristics, that may fail in some unfortunate cases. It must be observed, however, that the vast majority of transition-invariants correspond to enabled transition sequences in real cases, so that the heuristics is expected to work reasonably well.

In order to reduce the distance between the markings that return in the current marking, a counter is associated with each transition in each transition-invariant, recording the number of firings from the initial marking to reach the current marking. A counter is reset as soon as the firing of a transition-invariant is completed. When more than one transition is enabled in the current marking, the transitions are ordered by decreasing number of firings still required to complete the .longest transition-invariant involving the transition. In this way, exploiting the marking order that results from the breadth-first transition firing strategy, the markings that are likely to have the longest return path to a previously generated marking are generated first, reducing the maximum distance from the diagonal of the non-null return items in the matrix.

Sorting the list of enabled transitions in the current markings contributes marginally to the complexity of the reachability program, due to the usually small number of transitions that are enabled in each marking. Moreover, it should be noted that only transitions that are added to the enabled list of the previous marking (following the enabled list management suggested in the previous section) actually need to be inserted in a sorted form; transitions that were already enabled in the previous marking were already sorted correctly, so that only the ordered insertion of a few transitions is actually needed at each step, rather than a complete sort of the list.

6. IMPLEMENTATION AND RESULTS

Most of the optimization techniques proposed in this paper have been already implemented in a new version of the *GreatSPN* package. In particular, the marking coding heuristics of section 2.5, the marking search tree described in section 3, and the optimization of the transition operations of section 4, have been implemented both for simulation and reachability graph construction. The simulation or solution phase is preceded by a structural analysis and the generation of some net specific portion of code that is then compiled and linked with the core of the solution package. Some other optimizations have been implemented to reduce the size of intermediate result files by means of compact coding techniques. The new version of the numerical solver based on the construction and solution of the underlying Markov chain has been successfully run on a workstation with models yielding up to 100,000 tangible markings. Comparisons with the old implementation of the *GreatSPN* package have been carried out on a SUN 3/50 diskless workstation with 4 Mbytes of main memory and without floating-point co-processor.

Figure 5 depicts a GSPN model that was presented in [20] Figure 11 to model a 3-processor multiprocessor architecture at the level of inter-process communication. A configuration with two tasks allocated on two processors, and one task allocated on the third one (see the initial marking of places "runtask1", "runtask2", and "runtask3") yields 10,710 tangible and 8,139 vanishing markings, and represents the largest system of this class that can be analyzed by the previous version of the *GreatSPN* reachability graph generator. Its solution takes 630 seconds of CPU time for the reachability graph construction with the previous version, while the new version requires 30 seconds of code generation and compile time and 57 seconds of execution time. The previous version requires 1,822,771 bytes of file storage to hold intermediate results, while the new one only 502,748 bytes. Moreover, the new implementation allows the analysis of a larger configuration with 2 tasks per processor (two tokens in the initial marking of place "runtask3" instead of one), which yields 48,399 tangible markings, almost five times the limit of the previous version using approximately the same amount of virtual memory. The construction of the reachability graph of this larger system requires 40 seconds of code generation and compile time, and 320 seconds of execution time. The file storage needed in this case amounts to 2,934,375 bytes. A four-processor configuration with one task per processor, which yields 15,933 tangible and 13,020 vanishing markings [20], shows a speed-up of about 25 times in the CPU time of the new version of the reachability graph constructor (including code generation and compiling) with respect to the old version.

As an example of the improvements that can be obtained in simulation with the proposed techniques, we present a comparison on the model of Figure 6, which was presented in [21, 22] Figure 1 to model a 6-station CSMA/CD local area network at the level of the bus access contention. This model is not particularly well suited to the new marking coding heuristics, since about half of the places that represent the signal propagation through the LAN bus, although 6-bounded, are not covered by place-invariants. Nevertheless the simulation of 20 regeneration cycles (corresponding to roughly 20,000 transition firings) takes 300 seconds of CPU time for the code generation and compilation and 420 seconds of CPU time for the execution with the new version, while the old one require 4250 seconds of CPU time to run a simulation of the same length.

21

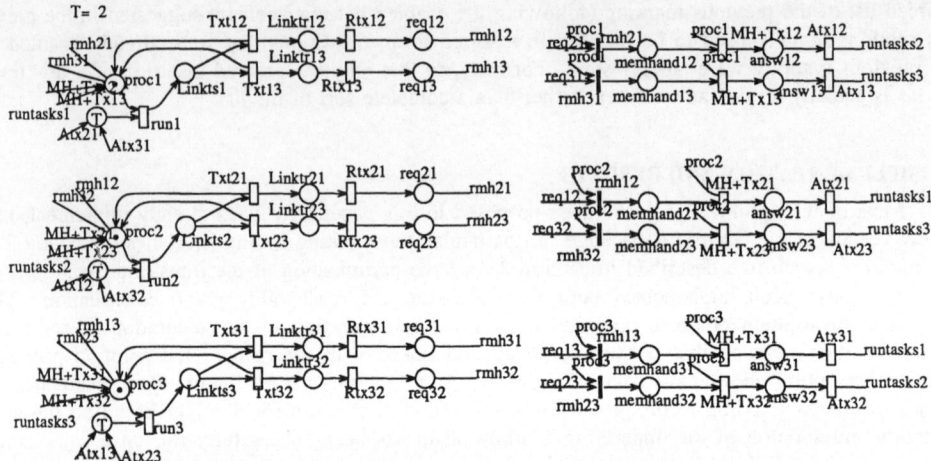

Figure 5. *GSPN model of a 3-processor PADMAVATI architecture.*

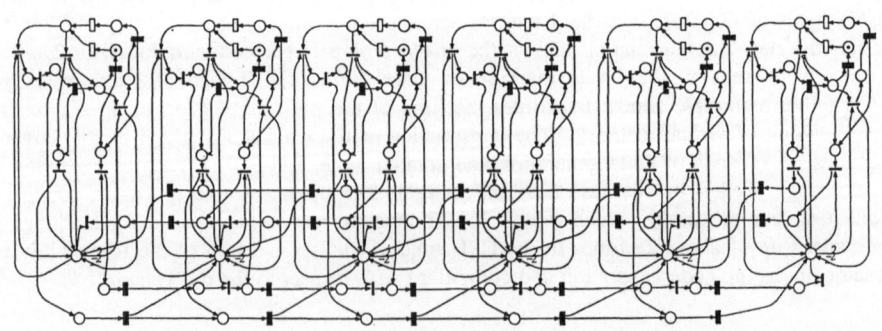

Figure 6. *GSPN model of a 6-station Ethernet-like LAN.*

7. CONCLUSIONS

The earlier analysis and simulation programs for stochastic Petri nets tackled the problem of efficiency in the implementation by using standard programming techniques. Different subproblems appearing at different stages of the algorithms were solved using the approach that was thought to be best suited for the solution of the particular subproblem, thus failing to recognize that the analysis of Petri nets is a complex problem in itself that, like many other Computer Science issues, deserves the development of an organic approach. Such an "unconscious" approach led to software that performed reasonably well on small to medium size cases, but that can hardly be scaled up any further, without improvements in the computer hardware technology.

The main purpose of this study is to point out that, as in the case of compiler technology, some ad-hoc optimization techniques may help substantially in improving the quality of the analysis software. The underlying model of SPN is a graph, with a proper structure. Moreover, a number of structural analysis techniques have already been developed for Petri nets, that can help in recognizing the embedded structure of the problem. Structural properties of the underlying Petri nets can provide enough information to guide optimizations and heuristics.

A new approach is proposed here, in which the analysis or simulation program for a given SPN model is produced automatically, taking into account the optimization and heuristics that can be based on a preliminary structural analysis of the model. This approach is contrasted to the standard approach, in which a single, general purpose, analysis/simulation program is written, that is intended to apply to an entire class of models. Using the standard approach, the efficiency of the implementation must be traded for the generality of the approach. With the proposed approach, the generality is provided by the ability of the program generator to deal with different models, while the individual instances of the analysis/simulation programs need not be general at all; algorithms and data structures can be tailored to the specific characteristics of the particular model for which the program is generated, so that substantial optimization can be achieved by using ad-hoc techniques.

Measures taken on an experimental implementation of the proposed techniques encourage to think that the approach is worthy to follow, and that a scale-up of one order of magnitude in the size of solvable problems is possible with respect to the software previously available, without changing the machine hardware configuration.

Having implemented an automatic reduction of the redundancy of the model description also improves the usability of the tool. Redundancy in the net description can in some cases help the definition of the model and of the performance indices to be measured. If this redundancy at the level of the user interface is not reflected in the efficiency of the simulation/solution of the model, the user is not discouraged to use model descriptions that are easier for him/her to handle.

Of course, the same philosophy could be applied to different models besides Petri nets, provided that appropriate structural properties are defined that can guide the application of heuristics or optimization techniques. It might be interesting to investigate the possibility of developing techniques similar to those proposed in this paper for the optimization of numerical algorithms or simulation programs for queueing networks as well, trying to exploit the intrinsically simpler structure of queueing models as compared to Petri net models.

REFERENCES

[1] G. Florin and S. Natkin, "Les Reseaux de Petri Stochastiques," *Technique et Science Informatiques* 4(1)(February 1985).

[2] M.K. Molloy, "Performance Analysis using Stochastic Petri Nets," *IEEE Transaction on Computers* C-31(9) pp. 913-917 (September 1982).

[3] M. Ajmone Marsan, G. Balbo, and G. Conte, "A Class of Generalized Stochastic Petri Nets for the Performance Analysis of Multiprocessor Systems," *ACM Transactions on Computer Systems* 2(1)(May 1984).

[4] M. Ajmone Marsan, G. Balbo, G. Chiola, and G. Conte, "Generalized Stochastic Petri Nets Revisited: Random Switches and Priorities," pp. 44-53 in *Proc. Int. Workshop on Petri Nets and Performance Models*, IEEE-CS Press, Madison, WI, USA (August 1987).

[5]   G. Florin and S. Natkin, "RDPS: a Software Package for the Evaluation and the Validation of Dependable Computer Systems," in *proc. SAFECOMP86*, , Sarlat, France (1986).

[6]   G. Chiola, "A Graphical Petri Net Tool for Performance Analysis," in *proc. 3rd Int. Workshop on Modeling Techniques and Performance Evaluation*, AFCET, Paris, France (March 1987).

[7]   M.A. Holliday and M.K. Vernon, "The GTPN Analyzer: Numerical Methods and User Interface," Tech. Rep. #639, Dept. Computer Science, University of Wisconsin, Madison, WI (April 1986).

[8]   R.R. Razouk, "A Guided Tour of P-NUT," Tech. Rep. #86-25, Dept. Information & Computer Science, University of California, Irvine, CA (January 1987).

[9]   K. Lautenbach, "Linear Algebraic Technique for Place/Transition Nets," in *Proc. Advanced Course on Petri Nets*, Springer Verlag, Bad Honnef, West Germany (September 1986).

[10] J. Martinez and M. Silva, "A Simple and Fast Algorithm to Obtain All Invariants of a Generalized Petri Net," in *Proc. 2nd European Workshop on Application and Theory of Petri Nets*, Springer Verlag, Bad Honnef, West Germany (September 1981).

[11] G. Chiola, "Structural Analysis for Generalized Stochastic Petri Nets: Some Results and Prospects," pp. 317-332 in *proc. 8th European Workshop on Application and Theory of Petri Nets*, , Zaragoza, Spain (June 1987).

[12] M. Reiser and H. Kobayashi, "Queueing Networks with Multiple Closed Chains: Theory and Computational Algorithms," *IBM Journal of R. & D.* **19**(3) pp. 283-294 (May 1975).

[13] M. Silva, *Las Redes de Petri en la Automatica y la Informatica,* Editorial AC, Madrid, Spain (1985). (in Spanish)

[14] F. Commoner, A. Holt, S. Even, and A. Pnueli, "Marked Directed Graphs," *Journal of Computer and System Sciences* **5**(5) pp. 511-523 (October 1971).

[15] B.W. Kernighan and D.M. Ritchie, *The C Programming Language,* Prentice-Hall, Englewood Cliffs, NJ (1978).

[16] G. Chiola, "A Software Package for the Analysis of Generalized Stochastic Petri Net Models," in *proc. Int. Workshop on Timed Petri Nets*, IEEE-CS Press, Torino, Italy (July 1985).

[17] D.E. Knuth, *The Art of Computer Programming,* Addison-Wesley, Reading, MA (1973).

[18] V.K. Vaishnavi, "Multidimensional Height-Balanced Trees," *IEEE Transactions on Computers* **C-33**(4) pp. 334-343 (April 1984).

[19] R.P. Tewarson, *Sparse Matrices,* Academic Press, New York (1973).

[20] M. Ajmone Marsan, G. Balbo, G. Chiola, and G. Conte, "Modeling the Software Architecture of a Prototype Parallel Machine," in *Proc. 1987 SIGMETRICS Conference*, ACM, Banf, Alberta, Canada (May 1987).

[21] M. Ajmone Marsan, G. Chiola, and A. Fumagalli, "An Accurate Performance Model of CSMA/CD bus LAN," pp. 146-161 in *Advances on Petri Nets '87*, ed. G. Rozenberg,Springer Verlag (1987).

[22] M. Ajmone Marsan, G. Chiola, and A. Fumagalli, "Timed Petri Net Model for Accurate Performance Analysis of CSMA/CD Bus LAN," *Computer Communications* **10**(6) pp. 304-312 (December 1987).

PANACEA: AN INTEGRATED SET OF TOOLS FOR PERFORMANCE ANALYSIS

K. G. Ramakrishnan and D. Mitra

AT&T Bell Laboratories
Murray Hill, New Jersey 07974

ABSTRACT

PANACEA is a collection of UNIX^{TM} tools for analyzing the performance of computer systems, communication networks, manufacturing lines, etc. This paper gives a brief overview of PANACEA, its various versions, and its language. PANACEA incorporates a new theory of asymptotic expansions, for analyzing large systems. There are three versions of PANACEA:

- PANACEA/Analytic solves a class of analytically tractable queueing models arising in on-line computer systems, communication networks with window flow control, and manufacturing systems involving pallets or kanbans. This version incorporates the asymptotic expansions technique for solving large networks. Fast response times are assured for all models.

- PANACEA/Analytic_Approximations incorporates analytic approximations to solve queueing networks that are otherwise intractable. Queueing models with general service and arrival processes fall into this category. This version also gives fast response times, since analytical formulas are used to solve the model.

- PANACEA/Simulation is a discrete event simulator for simulating complex systems with finite waiting rooms, blocking, product priorities, etc. Using a built-in tool called "user escapes", PANACEA/Simulation can be customized to model many unique features of real-world systems, such as machine breakdowns, product-aging, and multiple-access nodes.

A special purpose language, PML (PANACEA Model Language) is a common user interface to all three versions of PANACEA. This symbolic language has features such as macros, include files, and regular expressions commonly found in higher level languages. All PANACEA tools have built-in sensitivity analysis and graphical output. Recently, parallel algorithms for PANACEA/Analytic and PANACEA/Simulation have been developed for the BALANCE 21000 multiprocessor.

1. INTRODUCTION

PANACEA is an integrated set of software tools for performance analysis. Currently there are three versions of PANACEA:

- PANACEA/Analytic is a fast analytic solution package for exact analysis of models arising in computer and communication systems.

- PANACEA/Analytic_Approximations is also a fast solution package incorporating methods for approximate analysis of models with general service and arrival processes. These models commonly arise in the analysis of manufacturing systems.

- PANACEA/Simulation is a simulation package for simulating complex systems that are analytically intractable.

All versions of PANACEA run on any UNIX^{TM} operating system (SYSTEM V, BSD, Ultrix, UTS, etc.). PANACEA has been ported to many machines ranging from PCs to mainframes. Examples of machines that PANACEA runs on are

- VAX family of computers.

- 3B family of computers.

- Amdahl and IBM family mainframes.

- SUN 2 and SUN 3 workstations.

- CRAY/XMP computer.

PANACEA/Analytic solves *product-form* queueing networks. The qualifier *Analytic* implies that the performance measures are analytically obtained. The most *unique* feature of PANACEA/Analytic is its ability to solve *large* closed queueing networks. Using the new theory of asymptotic expansions, and integral representations [MCK81, MCK82, MCK84], PANACEA/Analytic solves *large* closed queueing networks. As described in Section 2.1, the convolutional and mean value analysis [REI75, REI80] algorithms are of limited utility in this case, because of their memory requirements and computational complexity.

To illustrate the power of PANACEA/Analytic, consider a real-world model (described in [RAM82]) with eight nodes, nine closed classes and a total population of 700. The convolutional and mean value analysis algorithms require 10^{17} arithmetic operations to analyze this queueing network, whereas the asymptotic expansions method incorporated in PANACEA/Analytic requires 10^7 arithmetic operations(This is with four terms in the expansions and errors which are insignificant as indicated by the computed lower and upper bounds. The concepts of asymptotic expansions and error bounds for them are explained later). At a gigaflop processing rate, these numbers translate to three cpu-years and Thus the convolutional and mean value analysis algorithms, and the software packages based on them, are impractical to solve this model. PANACEA/Analytic was able to sovle this model in two minutes on a VAX 11/780. In fact, PANACEA/Analytic was born through the challenge of being able to solve such large models which are quite commonly encountered in current computer and communication networks and systems.

Thus, an advantage of PANACEA/Analytic in comparison to other systems like RESQ [SAU82], and BEST/1 [BES83], is its ability to analyze large closed queueing networks efficiently. Another advantage of PANACEA system as a whole is its versatility; i.e., being able to move from analysis to simulation and vice versa, without substantial changes to the model description.

PANACEA/Analytic also incorporates convolutional algorithms for the following reasons:

i)   Convolutional algorithms are computationally efficient in producing exact performance measures (up to numerical round-off errors), for small networks.

ii) The asymptotic expansions, though much faster than convolutions even for small networks, may require too many terms in the expansion for these small networks. Another potential difficulty is the premature divergence of the asymptotic series. In general, we have found the asymptotic expansions to work well for medium to large networks, and the convolutions to work well for small networks.

Automatic decisions are made inside PANACEA/Analytic as to the choice of the solution technique, based on the size of the network. These decisions, of course, can be overridden by user-specified options on the command line.

PANACEA/Analytic_Approximations (abbreviated sometimes to PANACEA/AA), is a package for *approximately* solving multi-class, open, queueing networks with general interarrival time and service time distributions. The package incorporates the approximations developed by Whitt [WHI83], to derive expressions for first and second moments of arrival time processes, when general arrival processes are superposed. After this, PANACEA/AA approximates the point arrival process by a renewal process with the estimated parameters above, and uses formulas developed by Nozaki and Ross [NOZ78] to estimate the congestion measures of GI/G/s systems.

There is a fundamental difference between PANACEA/Analytic and PANACEA/AA. While PANACEA/Analytic gives *exact* bounds for the performance measures (in case the asymptotic expansions are used to solve the network), PANACEA/AA gives *no guarantees* as to the goodness of approximations; i.e., no bounds are given. It may be pointed out that this is an inherent difficulty with the approximations used in PANACEA/AA. One possible remedy, to gain confidence in the approximate answers, is to conduct simulations, using PANACEA/Simulation, and validate the approximate answers. We have experimented widely on many classes of networks and found the agreement between PANACEA/AA, and PANACEA/Simulation to be almost always good.

PANACEA/Simulation is a discrete-event simulator for an extended class of queueing networks with features which make them analytically intractable. Features such as priorities, blocking, general service time distributions, etc., which are commonly encountered in real world systems, are simulated by PANACEA/Simulation. Since this version has the same user interface as the other two versions (as explained later), validation of models is easily accomplished by simulating the same models on PANACEA/Simulation. This nice feature of interchangeability between versions has potential benefits, beyond the obvious. One could envision decomposing a complex queueing network into parts simulated by PANACEA/Simulation and parts analyzed by PANACEA/Analytic (or by PANACEA/AA) and iterated over, until convergence is achieved. Such fixed-point models have been used by us in modeling complex multiprocessor systems [MIT83].

PANACEA/Simulation gives, besides the mean performance measures, some distribution statistics on queue lengths, response times, and sojourn times. The user has the ability to conduct independent replications, restart the simulation from a previously terminated point, and remove transient bias from the statistics. All these options are specifiable on the command line.

At the present time, PANACEA/Simulation does not give any confidence intervals. One can use post-processing routines to accomplish the same.

The user interface to PANACEA is common to all three versions. A new special purpose language, PML (Panacea Model Language) is used to compactly describe the queueing networks. PML has language constructs for describing queueing networks in a natural manner. Many constructs that are standard in programming languages, like

- Macros
- Include files
- Regular expressions

are integral to PML. It also has other language constructs specific to describing queueing networks. The output produced by PANACEA are the congestion measures of the queueing network. These measures include, on a per class per node basis

- Utilizations
- Mean sojourn times

- Mean and standard deviation of queue lengths

- Mean throughputs

- Mean response times

PANACEA/Simulation, besides these measures, also produces histograms of queue lengths, sojourn times, and response times.

Figure 1 shows the common input/output interface of PANACEA versions. The user describes the queueing network in PML; based on the shell variable *VERSION*, one of the three versions of PANACEA is invoked to analyze the queueing network. The version invoked produces the output in a standard manner. Another way to describe the queueing network is through PAW, the Performance Analysis Workstation [MEL85]. This is a graphical animation tool in which the user graphically inputs the queueing network on a DMD 5620 [WES84]. As shown in Fig. 1, PAW optionally produces a PML program description of the network which can then be interfaced with PANACEA.

PANACEA has a built-in tool, PANACEA/Graphics, for graphically displaying the output produced by PANACEA. A high resolution graphical output is produced on a DMD 5620, and a character resolution graphical output is produced in a non-graphics terminal.

PANACEA also has a built-in sensitivity analysis tool. The user describes the variations of a particular input parameter, using the *for* language statement available in PANACEA. For example, the statement

> *for (cputime = 50.0; cputime <= 100; cputime*
>
> *= cputime + 10.0) do*
>
> *service time cpu cputime;*

varies the cpu service time from 50.0 to 100.0, in increments of 10.0. For each assignment of *cputime*, one queueing network model is solved. Thus one invocation of PANACEA solves, in this case, 6 models. The *for* statements can be nested to any degree, giving the user capabilities to vary many input parameters simultaneously. For example, the doubly nested *for* statements

> for ($i = 1$; $i <= 5$; $i = i + 1$) do
>
> begin
>
> > degree i;
> >
> > for (rate = 15.0; rate <= 25.0;
> > rate = rate + .5) do
> >
> > begin
> >
> > > service rate dbp rate;
> >
> > end;
>
> end;

vary both *degrees of multiprogramming* (in the outer loop) as well as the service rate of a node (dbp). Thus, a total of 100 PANACEA models would be solved in one invocation of PANACEA.

2. VARIOUS VERSIONS OF PANACEA

This section describes the three versions of PANACEA; the class of queueing networks

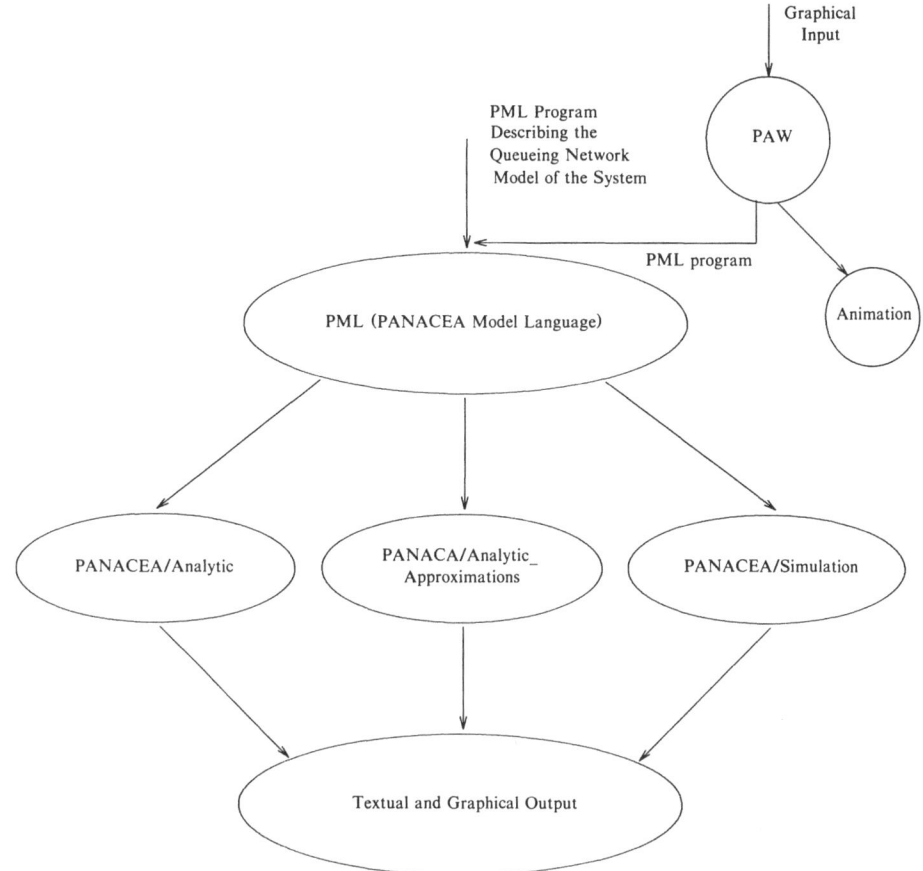

Fig. 1 . PANACEA Input/Output Interface

they solve, the underlying theory they use, and the algorithms for their implementation.

2.1 PANACEA/Analytic

PANACEA/Analytic solves a class of open, closed, or mixed product-form queueing networks, which form a major subset of the BCMP class of queueing networks [BAS75]. A unique feature of PANACEA/Analytic is its ability to analyze large closed queueing networks. By *large*, we mean

— large populations in each closed class; there is no restriction on the population size.

— moderately large number of job classes, in the 40-50 range.

— moderately large number of nodes, also in the 40-50 range.

The analysis of these large networks is made feasible by the asymptotic expansion method [MCK81, MCK82, MCK84].

Many computer and communication networks in real life can be modeled as closed queueing networks [BAS75, KEL79, KLE76, SCH77]. Despite this utility of closed queueing networks, only a small collection of these are computationally tractable using established algorithms. There are two such algorithms: convolutional method [REI75, BUZ71, BRU80], and Mean Value Analysis [REI80]. Both of these methods require arithmetic operations and virtual memory, proportional to

$$p\,(1+2q)\ \prod_{j=1}^{p}\ (K_j+1) \qquad\qquad (1)$$

where

p is the number of closed classes in the queueing network

q is the number of processing nodes, and .

K_j is the population of closed class j, $1 \leqslant j \leqslant p$

(1) clearly shows the exponential (in p) behavior of convolution and mean value analysis algorithms. Thus, the models solvable by these algorithms have small numbers of classes and a small population in each customer class.

The asymptotic expansion method, incorporated in PANACEA/Analytic, extends the class of computationally tractable closed queueing networks by several orders of magnitude. This method obtains solutions to closed queueing networks with p closed classes and q processing nodes in $O(qp^t)$ arithmetic operations. The virtual memory requirements are about 20q kilobytes. Here t denotes the number of terms in the asymptotic expansions of the first and second moments of performance measures (utilizations, queue lengths, sojourn times, etc.). Many computational experiments demonstrate that four terms ($t = 4$) are usually more than adequate to produce accurate results. But more importantly, the number of operations and the amount of virtual memory are both **independent of the population sizes** of closed classes. This is in sharp contrast to the convolutional methods and mean value analysis.

Despite the efficient computational complexity of the asymptotic expansions method, there are two drawbacks of the method as it is currently incorporated in PANACEA/Analytic:

i)   There should be at least one infinite server (IS) node present in the network, and

ii)   The normal usage constraint: this constraint states that all processing centers of the queueing network operate at a *normal usage* range. Generally, this implies utilizations of processing centers below 90%. The constraint occurs because of the assumption of non-negativity of a certain parameter α used in the asymptotic expansions, as discussed later.

Item i) above poses no serious difficulty in modeling real systems. Usually, in real systems, the closed classes arise in modeling on-line, terminal generated traffic. Thus the terminals can be modeled as one or more IS nodes. In our work we have rarely encountered closed models with no IS nodes. For these exceptional circumstances PANACEA/Analytic provides an alternative, the convolutional method.

Item ii) poses a more serious challenge. When any processing node of the queueing network goes beyond normal usage, the asymptotic expansions break down, and PANACEA/Analytic issues a diagnostic message and terminates. The user now has two options:

a)   If the queueing network is small enough, invoke PANACEA/Analytic again and force it to use convolutional algorithms.

b)   Increase the service rates of those processing nodes that are operating beyond normal usage.

Recently, many approximate algorithms have been proposed for analyzing large closed queueing networks [CHA82, EAG86, CHI87]. Most of these methods are approximate MVA algorithms. It will be an interesting research project to compare these methods with the asymptotic expansion method, both for accuracy of solution and the computational efficiency.

2.1.1 Asymptotic Expansions of Performance Measures for Closed Queueing Networks.
We will now describe the main results on the asymptotic expansions of performance measures of the closed queueing networks [MCK81, MCK82, MCK84, RAM82]. For brevity, we omit the detailed description of the implementation for evaluating the asymptotic expansions.

Our discussion of the asymptotic expansions is necessarily brief; for a more complete treatment of the asymptotic expansions, the reader may refer to [MCK81, MCK82, MCK84]. In addition, we restrict our descriptions to the first and second moments of individual queue lengths in the processors; various other performance measures, such as processor utilizations, throughput, are also evaluated in PANACEA/Analytic, but omitted in our discussion as they are either simply derived from, or closely related to, the measures discussed. The theoretical underpinning, for the asymptotic expansions method is the integral representation of the normalization constant G, occurring in the stationary probability expression

$$\pi(\mathbf{n}) = \frac{1}{G} \Pi \, \pi_i(\mathbf{n}_i) . \tag{2}$$

In [MCK82] G was shown to have the integral representation

$$G(\mathbf{K}) = \frac{1}{\Pi K_\sigma !} \int_{Q^+} e^{-1'\mathbf{u}} \Pi (\sum \rho_{\sigma\tau} u_\tau + \rho_{\sigma 0})^{K_\sigma} d\mathbf{u} \tag{3}$$

where

p = number of classes of jobs

q = number of number of processing nodes

K_σ = population of jobs of class σ

$\rho_{\sigma\tau}$ = $\dfrac{\text{relative number of visits of class } \sigma \text{ jobs to node } \tau}{\text{mean service rate of class } \sigma \text{ jobs at node } \tau}$

$\rho_{\sigma 0}$ = $\displaystyle\sum_{\tau \in \{\text{IS nodes}\}} \left[\dfrac{\text{relative number of visits of class } \sigma \text{ jobs to node } \tau}{\text{mean service rate of class } \sigma \text{ jobs at node } \tau} \right]$

and $1 \leqslant \sigma \leqslant p$, $1 \leqslant \tau \leqslant q$. The moments of queue lengths are computed as ratios of moment partition functions, $G^{(m)}(\mathbf{K})$ [MCK84], which can also be represented as integrals similar to (3). These integrals are expanded in inverse powers of a large parameter, to obtain the performance measures.

Denoting $n_{\sigma\tau}$ as the random variable defining the number of jobs of class σ in node τ, we simply give below the expressions for the leading moments of the stationary distributions of individual queue lengths.

$$\langle n_{\sigma\tau} \rangle (\mathbf{K}) = \left\{ \frac{r_{\sigma\tau} K_\sigma}{\alpha_\tau} \right\} \frac{I_{\sigma,\tau}^{(1)}(N)}{I(N)} \qquad 1 \leqslant \sigma \leqslant p$$

$$\langle n_{\sigma\tau}(n_{\sigma\tau} - 1) \rangle (\mathbf{K}) = \left\{ \frac{r_{\sigma\tau}^2 K_\sigma (K_\sigma - 1)}{\alpha_\tau^2} \right\} \frac{I_{\sigma,\tau}^{(2)}(N)}{I(N)} \qquad 1 \leqslant \tau \leqslant q$$

where

$$r_{\sigma\tau} = \rho_{\sigma\tau} / \rho_{\sigma 0}$$

$$\alpha_\tau = 1 - \sum_\sigma K_\sigma r_{\sigma\tau} \quad (> 0 \text{ for } normal \text{ usage})$$

$$I_{\sigma,\tau}^{(m)}(N) = \begin{array}{l} \text{integrals parameterized by} \\ N, \quad m = 0, 1, 2; \quad 1 \leqslant \sigma \leqslant p; \quad 1 \leqslant \tau \leqslant q \end{array}$$

$$I(N) = I_{\sigma,\tau}^{(0)}(N) \quad \text{(for } m = 0, \text{ there is no dependence on } \sigma \text{ or } \tau\text{)}.$$

In the above expressions N is a large parameter. PANACEA/Analytic chooses $N = 1/\min_{\sigma,\tau} r_{\sigma\tau}$. While this choice of N is not at all critical, theoretical reasons corroborated by computational experience indicate that this choice serves very well to keep all terms in the expansions within machine precision. It is shown in [MCK84] that $I_{\sigma,\tau}^{(m)}$ can be asymptotically expanded as

$$I_{\sigma,\tau}^{(m)} \sim \sum_{k=0}^{t-1} A_{\sigma,\tau,k}^{(m)} / N^k \tag{4}$$

where

$$A_{\sigma,\tau,k}^{(m)} = \int e^{-1'v} \, v_{\tau}^m \, h_k^m(v) dv \tag{5}$$

Equation (5) defines $A_{\sigma,\tau,k}^{(n)}$ as an integral. We identify this integral as a partition function of another network, the *pseudonetwork*. This identification results in an efficient divide-and-conquer computational procedure.

Let us now consider t in (4), the number of terms in the asymptotic expansion. The error in the calculation of the integrals, and therefore of the queue length moments in (3) from using only t terms, is $0(1/N^t)$. In PANACEA/Analytic, generally,

$$t \leqslant 4. \tag{6}$$

However, PANACEA/Analytic has the facility to automatically select t to be less than the maximum. There are two reasons for this. First, if the user desires a guaranteed response time, the detailed computational complexity analysis allows PANACEA/Analytic to fulfill the guarantee by calculating the appropriate value of t. As all output quantities are typically accompanied by lower and upper bounds, this facility leading to small t is both useful and often exercised. The user typically starts with a small t and increases it until the bounds are *tight*. This approach of starting with a small t and increasing it appropriately is especially crucial in analyzing large networks. The user usually automates the procedure of varying t, by a simple shell script such as

for t in 1 2 3 4; do

panacea   *−n t* $\cdots$

post process the output

done

The *panacea*   *−n t* line above invokes panacea with the number of terms set to t.

The second reason for selecting t to be less than the maximum is that PANACEA/Analytic automatically looks for departure from monotonicity of the series in (4), and in the event of its occurrence, PANACEA/Analytic truncates the series at the turning point.

2.2 PANACEA/Simulation

PANACEA/Simulation is a continuous-time, discrete-event simulator of queueing networks. The class of queueing networks that PANACEA/Simulation can simulate is an

32

extended class of queueing networks, which includes, of course, all the product-form queueing networks. This extended class of queueing networks is almost identical to the class defined by Sauer and McNair [SAU80]. This extended class not only includes all the product-form queueing networks, but also networks that have features that are analytically intractable (like blocking, general service times, etc.). A potentially useful feature of PANACEA/Simulation is the *User Escapes*. This feature enables the user to write event routines in C language [KER78], and interface them with the PANACEA/Simulation package, every time the state of the queueing network changes. Almost **any queueing network** can be simulated using this feature. We have successfully simulated multiprocessor models with constrained arrivals [MIT83] (every time a *read* request arrives, a *write* request arrives as well, at a different node), and slotted aloha models, some of whose nodes have "collision disciplines" [SEE87] (when more than one job arrives at a node at the same time, all jobs are lost).

PANACEA/Simulation is implemented in *C* language [KER78].

2.3 *PANACEA/Analytic_Approximations*

PANACEA/Analytic_Approximations (abbreviated PANACEA/AA) is the third member of the PANACEA family of software tools. It was motivated mainly by the need to analyze manufacturing systems. These systems are generally modelled as open queueing networks with multiple server nodes and general interarrival time and service time distributions. At the heart of PANACEA/AA is a set of approximations to convert G/G/s nodes to GI/G/s nodes and solving the GI/G/s system using modified M/G/s formulas. These approximations are used to analyze the queueing network, producing mean performance measures of utilization, queue lengths, throughputs, and sojourn times.

PANACEA/AA solves a class of queueing networks, with the following features:

- Multiple open classes.
- FCFS queueing discipline.
- Probabilistic routing with or without class hopping.
- General service time distributions for each class and each node.
- General inter-arrival distributions for all classes.
- Multiple servers for each node.
- Job spawning

The general service and interarrival time distributions in PANACEA/AA are characterized by the first two moments of the distributions. This is because the formulas in the analytic approximations require only the first two moments of these distributions. PANACEA/AA *does not* give any error bounds for the performance measures.

Since PANACEA/AA involves only evaluation of closed form expressions, it is very fast. The most time consuming operation in PANACEA/AA is solving two linear systems for each class, one for each moment of the approximating renewal point process submitted to each queueing node in the network. Thus the computational complexity is in LU factorization of a stochastic matrix and the backward solution of the resulting upper triangular system. The following may be a guide to the execution time of PANACEA/AA: a queueing network with 50 classes and 50 nodes takes about 5 cpu minutes to execute on a VAX 11/780. This fast execution permits sensitivity analysis of the output measures. PANACEA/Graphics can then be used to display the results graphically.

2.3.1 Decomposition of the Original Queueing Network into a Set of GI/G/S Nodes. As mentioned before, the analytic approximations used in PANACEA/AA consist of two major steps:

i)   Decomposition of the original queueing network into a set of isolated GI/G/s nodes.

ii) Modifying M/G/s measures to approximately evaluate the GI/G/s system.

The approximations used in step i) are mainly due to Whitt [WHI82, WHI83]. Approximations in step ii) are due to Nozaki and Ross [NOZ78], and modified by us [RAM85]. PANACEA/AA owes most of its theoretical underpinnings to the work of Whitt [WHI83]. Some minor modifications to Whitt's formulas used in step i) have been made by us. These modifications have to do mainly with class disaggregation in the evaluation of internal flow parameters.

Decomposition of the queueing network into a collection of independent GI/G/s nodes is accomplished by solving for internal traffic rates, and their variability. The variability parameters for internal flows are obtained by using the general framework of Whitt [WHI83] for approximating point processes, as well as incorporating refinements suggested by Albin [ALB81] for merging. As stated by Whitt [WHI83], the decomposition procedure is best described as a parametric decomposition method. Once decomposed, the nodes are treated as stochastically independent. The dependence between the nodes is approximated through the internal flow parameters.

3. SOFTWARE STRUCTURE OF PANACEA

PANACEA is a UNIX-based software tool. It has been developed to be portable to all versions of UNIX. Recently, parallel algorithms have been developed for PANACEA, and implemented on the Balance 21000 [BAL85].

All the PANACEA software has been written in C-language [KER78]. The parser and the lexical analyzer for the PML have been machine generated, using the UNIX tools YACC [YAC75] and LEX [LES75]. The source code of PANACEA for various versions are controlled by the Source Code Control system [SCC75]. The compilation procedure for various versions of PANACEA is controlled by a shell script, and the *make* file mechanism [MAK78].

Thus, as can be seen from the above description, PANACEA utilizes the existing UNIX tools effectively in writing the software, controlling its evolution, and compiling it into process images.

During the design phase of PANACEA, careful thought was given to the process architecture, so that PANACEA could be ported to a wide range of hardware ranging from personal computers (PCs) to super computers. Thus the design had to account for small non-virtual memory UNIX systems running on PCs to the full 32-bit virtual memory UNIX systems running on mainframes. To accomplish this wide portability, PANACEA was partitioned functionally into four primary UNIX processes: These processes are i) the parser and controller process (PCP), ii) the computational process (CP), iii) the graphics process (GP), and iv) the throughput-solver process (TP). Each of these processes can be configured to meet any memory requirements. These processes communicate with each other using standard UNIX interprocess communication.

The software structure of Parallel-PANACEA is similar, except for the multiple copies of the CP. Coordination between these CPs, if necessary, is accomplished by the use of shared-memory data structures.

Parallel-PANACEA/Simulation employs a simple form of marco-parallelism: each replication of the simulation is executed concurrently. If the user requests r replications of the simulation, r CPs are created. Since the Balance 21000 processor has 30 PEs (Processing Elements), 30 replications can proceed in parallel (assuming stand-alone environment). No coordination or synchronization is needed between the independent replications. Each CP generates an independent random stream of interarrival times and service times, conducts the simulation, and outputs the results. The speed up of Parallel-PANACEA/Simulation is about $\dfrac{r}{\left\lceil \dfrac{r}{30} \right\rceil}$ over PANACEA/Simulation.

The algorithm used in the asymptotic expansions (in PANACEA/Analytic) also lends itself to natural parallelization. The cpu-intensive part of this algorithm is the computation of the normalization constant G, for $\binom{p}{4}$ small queueing networks. These queueing networks are called pseudonetworks [MCK81, MCK82, RAM82]. These pseudonetworks have the same number of processing nodes as the original network, but have at most four classes, and at most a total of eight jobs. Each pseudonetwork has a unique 4-tuple of class indices (i, j, k, l), $1 \leq i < j < k < l \leq p$ (this accounts for $\binom{p}{4}$ pseudonetworks).

Parallel-PANACEA/Analytic parallelizes the solution of these pseudonetworks. Initially, n CPs are created (n depends on the number of PEs on the multiprocessor; usually it is 30 for the BALANCE 21000). There are two ways of allocating the $\binom{p}{4}$ pseudonetworks to the n CPs: dynamic, and static. In the dynamic allocation scheme a global task queue consisting of $\binom{p}{4}$ tasks is created in shared memory. Each CP, when ready to execute the next task, examines the task queue and removes a task, and performs the computation for that pseudonetwork. The CP then accumulates the result in a shared memory data structure. Each CP concurrently goes through this cycle of

- removing a task from task queue,
- performing convolutions on the pseudonetwork, and
- accumulating the results in shared memory,

until the task queue becomes empty.

Semaphores and locks ensure exclusive updates to shared memory.

This parallel algorithm was observed to have excessive synchronization delays, in waiting for exclusive access to shared memory. To ameliorate this overhead in synchronization, a static allocation scheme was proposed. In this scheme, the $\binom{p}{4}$ tasks are allocated apriori, to the n CPs. Each CP proceeds completely in parallel to solve these $\left\lceil \binom{p}{r} / n \right\rceil$ pseudonetworks, accumulating the results in its "local memory". After all n CPs complete execution, the local memories are transferred to "shared memory". We found the static allocation algorithm to be superior, in speed up, to the dynamic allocation algorithm (at the expense of replicating the shared memory data structure).

Both versions of Parallel-PANACEA/Analytic have a speed up over PANACEA/Analytic that depends on the number of classes and number of nodes. Typically, we have observed a speed up of about 20 (on a 30 PE machine; thus an efficiency of 66%) for a 25 class, 40 node problem.

4. PANACEA MODEL LANGUAGE (PML)

As mentioned in the introduction, PML is a high level language for describing queueing networks. The language has been designed to efficiently and compactly encode queueing network parameters, such as routing probabilities, service times, etc. Considerable thought has been given to designing PML to be easy to use, compact, self-documenting, and extensible.

PML can be thought of as a core-oriented language, like C [KER78] and Pascal [WIR76]. A small well-defined set of statements has been designed as the core of the language. Other statements, if and when needed, are added to the core, thus extending the language.

PML is a descriptive language. There is no thread of program control that flows through a PML program executing statements in it. Instead, the statements merely describe various entities of the queueing network. Consequently, there is no ordering of statements in PML. The statements can appear in any order, natural to the description of the queueing network.

PML is a symbolic language. User-defined symbols of arbitrary length identify various entities of the queueing network, such as servers, customer classes, etc. Higher level language constructs are available in PML to collectively identify these symbols for instance, in the statement

$$service \ time \quad \hat{} cpu.*` \quad 15.0;$$

the regular expression $\hat{} cpu.*`$ collectively identifies all nodes in the network whose names start with a prefix *cpu*. Other constructs, like macros and include files also help in compact description of queueing networks.

We will now discuss some properties of PML.

4.1 Properties of PML

PML strives to achieve the elegance and sophistication of many high level languages. We shall follow the guidelines set by G. M. Weinberg [WEI71] in describing PML.

4.1.1 Compactness. A distinct advantage of the computational algorithms in PANACEA is their ability to solve **large** networks. This advantage would be nullified if the user had to describe the queueing network in a cumbersome and verbose manner. Hence, it is crucial for PML to provide the user with tools that aid in compact description of networks, whenever possible. These language tools are discussed below.

4.1.1.1 Generalized Macros with Parameters. PML has facilities for defining and using macros. The syntax and usage of the macros in PML are derived primarily from the UNIX macro facility M4 [UNI85]. Macros in PML provide the ability to replace a large body of repeating text by just the name of a macro. Optionally, the user can give macro parameters to accommodate small variations in the body of the text. For example,

$$#define \quad abc \ (x, y, z) \quad cpu, disk : terminal \ \{x, y, z\}$$

defines a macro *abc* with three parameters *x, y, and z*. The text of the macro is

$$cpu, disk : terminal \ \{x, y, z\} \ .$$

If the macro is invoked somewhere in the PML program as *abc (1.0, .5, .3);*, then the PML parser will substitute the string *cpu, disk : terminal {1.0, .5, .3};* in its place.

Macros can be nested.

4.1.1.2 Include Files. The include file mechanism allows the user to partition the model description into several files and include them in one run by merging-them together. Alternatively, it allows the description of the model by several independent model developers, each familiar with the detailed workings of a part of the network. For example, consider a nationwide network that has three large subnetworks. Suppose node1.pml, node2.pml and node3.pml are pml programs describing the detailed inner workings of the three subnetworks.

Then, one can write a pml program describing the whole network by simply including the three pml programs together, as shown below:

> # include   node1.pml
>
> # include   node2.pml
>
> # include   node3.pml
>
> *additional statements describing*
> *the interconnection between the subnetworks*

4.1.1.3 Regular Expressions. Regular expressions aid in collectively identifying entities in the network. For example, the regular expression ʻʻdisk.*ʻ collectively identifies all the nodes in the network that are labelled with the symbols starting with *disk*. The regular expression ʻ.*ʻ that matches every node symbol can be used to identify all the nodes in the queueing network (PML provides a more readable synonym, *all_nodes*, for this regular expression). For example, the statement

> *external arrival time all_nodes 25.3;*

defines an interarrival time of 25.3 (exponentially distributed, by default) to **all** open classes, in **every** node of the queueing network.

4.1.1.4 Multiple Node and Edge Descriptions. As a universal rule in PML, a **list** of entities can be specified, whenever the syntax requires a single entity to be specified. The parameters will propagate to all members in the list. As an example

> *cpu1, disk, link, data_base FCFS;*

will assign the node discipline of *FCFS* to all the nodes in the list. As another example,

> *bus, memory : cpu, disk .5;*

will assign a transition probability of .5 to the transitions bus $\rightarrow$ cpu, memory $\rightarrow$ cpu, bus $\rightarrow$ disk, and memory $\rightarrow$ disk.

4.1.2 Uniformity. PML is characterized by the uniformity property. By uniformity, we mean that a feature of the language available in the statement, should be available everywhere else. Thus the language has no restrictions. The following list gives some uniformity properties of PML:

a)   Integer and real data types can be freely used anywhere. Mixed expressions in PML are permitted as well.

b)   Arithmetic expressions of arbitrary complexity can be specified whenever a number is required to be given in the syntax.

c)   A list of entity symbols separated by commas, can be specified whenever a single entity symbol is to be given.

4.1.3 Extensibility. The PML parser and lexical analyzer have been machine generated. Once the grammar rules and lexical tokens are specified, the parser and lexical analyzer can be generated by existing automated tools (YACC [YAC75] and Lex [LES75]). Thus it is easy to extend the language by adding additional grammar rules and lexical tokens. The feature of extensibility of PML was exploited in expanding the language to describe the queueing networks simulated by PANACEA/Simulation, and the queueing networks approximated by PANACEA/Analytic-Approximations.

5. CONCLUSION

PANACEA is evolving. A promising direction it is taking is the development of Parallel PANACEA. Some interesting new algorithmic innovations are possible here. Another direction of development is PANACEA/Analytic-glds, the generalized load-dependent server.

Currently there are many AT&T projects using PANACEA. It is also being used by several universities in U.S.A., for research and teaching.

6. ACKNOWLEDGEMENTS

The large body of PANACEA software and theory are due to many contributions. J. McKenna (along with Debasis Mitra) developed the theory of asymptotic expansions and integral representations. B. D. McClusky wrote many routines in PANACEA/Simulation. J. B. Seery contributed in the development of the sensitivity analysis tool. She also continues to maintain, distribute and consult on all of the PANACEA software. Finally, D. G. Gordon was responsible for writing some software for PANACEA/Graphics.

REFERENCES

[ALB81] Albin, S. L., *Approximating Queues with Superposition Arrival Processes*, Ph.D Dissertation, Dept. of Industrial Eng. and Operations Research, Columbia University, 1981.

[BAL85] *Balance 8000 System Technical Summary*, Sequent Computer Systems, Inc., 14360 N. W. Science Park Drive, Portland, Oregon.

[BAS75] Baskett, F., Chandy, K. M., Muntz R. R., and Palacios, F. G., "Open, Closed, and Mixed Networks of Queues with Different Classes of Customers", J. of the ACM, 22, No. 2 (April 1975), pp. 248-260.

[BES83] BEST/1-MVS User's Guide, BGS Systems, Inc., Waltham, MA, 1983.

[BRU80] Bruell, S. C., and Balbo, G., *COMPUTATIONAL ALGORITHMS FOR CLOSED QUEUEING NETWORKS*, Elsevier North Holland, 1980.

[BUZ71] Buzen, J., *Queueing Network Models of Multiprogramming*, Ph.D Thesis, Div. of Engineering and Applied Science, Harvard University, Cambridge, Mass., 1971.

[CHA82] Chandy, K. M., and Neuse, D., "Linearizer: A heuristic Algorithm for Queueing Network Models of Computer Systems", Comm. ACM, Vol. 25, No. 2, Feb. 1982, pp. 126-134.

[CHI87] Ching-Tarng Hsieh, and Lam, S. S., "PAM – A Noniterative Approximate Solution Method for Closed Multichain Queueing Networks", Tech. Report TR-87-28, Dept. of Computer Sciences, The University of Texas at Austin, Austin, TX 78712-1188.

[EAG86] Eager D. L., and Sevcik, K. C., "Bound Hierarchies for Multiple-Class Queueing Networks", J. of ACM, Vol. 33, No. 1, Jan. 1986, pp. 179-206.

[KEL79] Kelly, F. P., *Reversibility and Stochastic Networks*, John Wiley, New York, 1979.

[KER78] Kernighan, B. W., and Ritchie, D. M., *The C Programming Language*, Prentice-Hall, New Jersey, 1978.

[KLE76] Kleinrock, L., *Queueing Systems, Volume 2: Computer Applications*, John Wiley, New York, 1976.

[LES75]   Lesk, M. E., and Schmidt, E., Unpublished work.

[MAK78]   Make Command, *UNIX System V Release 2.0,* User Reference Manual, Section 1, AT&T Bell Laboratories, 1985.

[MCK81]   McKenna, J., and Mitra D., and Ramakrishnan, K. G., "A Class of Closed Markovian Queueing Networks: Integral Representations, Asymptotic Expansions, Generalizations, Bell Syst. Tech. J., 60, 5 (May-June 1981), 599-641.

[MCK82]   McKenna, J., and Mitra D., "Integral Representations and Asymptotic Expansions for Closed Markovian Queueing Networks: Normal Usage", Bell Syst. Tech. J., 61, 5 (May-June 1982), 661-683.

[MCK84]   McKenna, J., and Mitra D., "Asymptotic Expansions and Integral Representations of Moments of Queue Lengths in Closed Markovian Networks", J. ACM, 31, 2 (April 1984), 346-360.

[MEL85]   Melamed, B., and Morris, R. J. T., "Visual Simulation: The Performance Analysis Workstation", IEEE Computer, 1985.

[MIT83]   Mitra, D., Ramakrishnan, K. G., and Zee B., "Performance Analysis of Intercept 25", Unpublished work, Oct. 7, 1983.

[MIT86]   Mitra, D., and McKenna, J., "Asymptotic Expansions for Closed Markovian Networks with State-Dependent Service Rates", J. ACM, 33, 3 (July 1986), 568-592.

[NOZ78]   Nozaki, S. A., and Ross, S. M., "Approximations in Finite Capacity Multi-Server Queues with Poisson Arrivals", J. Appl. Prob., 15, (1978), pp. 826-834.

[QNA80]   Queueing Network Analysis Package, Copyright CII-Honeywell Bull and INRIA, 1980.

[RAM82]   Ramakrishnan, K. G., and Mitra, D., "An Overview of PANACEA, A Software Package for Analyzing Markovian Queueing Networks", Bell Syst. Tech. J., 61, 10 (Dec. 1982), 2849-2872.

[RAM85]   Ramakrishnan, K. G., and Mitra, D., "A Short User's Manual for PANACEA 4.1 (Analytic Approximations), Unpublished Work, Jan. 3, 1985.

[REI75]   Reiser, M., and Kobayashi, H., "Queueing Networks with Multiple Closed Chains: Theory and Computational Algorithms", IBM J. of Res. and Dev., 19, No. 3 (May 1975), 283-294.

[REI80]   Reiser, M., and Lavenberg, S. S., "Mean Value Analysis of Closed Multichain Queueing Networks", J. of ACM, 27, No. 2 (April 1980), pp. 313-322.

[SAU80]   Sauer, C. H., MacNair, A. E., and Salza, S., "A Language for Extended Queueing Network Models", IBM Journal of Research and Development, 24, No. 6 (Nov. 1980), pp. 747-755.

[SAU82]   Sauer, C. H., MacNair, A. E., and Kurose, J. F., "The Research Queueing Package: Past, Present, and Future", AFIPS, Proceedings of the National Computer Conference, 1982.

[SCC75]   *Source Code Control System User Guide,* UNIX System User Guide.

[SCH77]   Schwartz, M., *Computer-Communications Network Design and Analysis,* Prentice-Hall, Englewood Cliffs, 1977.

[SEE87]   Seery, J. B., Private Communication, 1987.

[UNI85]   *UNIX System V Release 2.0,* User Reference Manual, AT&T Bell Laboratories, 1985.

[WEI71]   Weinberg, G. M., *Psychology of Computer Programming,* Van Nostrand, New York, 1971.

[WES84]   5620 Dot-Mapped Display, User Guide, Western Electric, 306-120 issue 1, March, 1984.

[WHI82]   Whitt, W., *"Approximating a point process by a renewal process, I: Two basic Methods,"* Opers. Research, 30, No. 1 (Jan.-Feb. 1982), pp. 709-745.

[WHI83]   Whitt, W., "The Queueing Network Analyzer", BSTJ, 62, No. 9, Nov. 1983, pp. 2779-2815.

[WIR76]   Wirth, N., *Algorithms + Data Structures = Programs,* Prentice-Hall, New Jersey, 1976.

[YAC75]   YACC - Yet Another Compiler Compiler, *UNIX System Support Tools Guide.*

DISTRIBUTED SYSTEMS DESIGN:

AN INTEGRATED SOFTWARE TOOL FOR PERFORMANCE ANALYSIS

Michel Feuga and Yves Raynaud

Matra Espace
Z1 du Palays, 31077 Toulouse, France

Laboratoire Cerfia, équipe SIERA
Université Paul Sabatier 31 Toulouse, France

INTRODUCTION

In an operational context, designing sophisticated data processing systems involves a lot of difficulties such as choosing the good hardware components, dispatching the tasks on the various computers... But, above all, one of the most critical problem is to predict system's performances; that means to evaluate, before construction, the architecture behavior under processes loading.

An integrated software providing capabilities to easily define (or modify) an hardware architecture, describe all the running processes and give performance evaluations might be very useful during the earliest design steps to reduce development risks. It should be designed to be used directly by system engineers without any help, neither from a performance evaluation specialist nor a programmer; that means that it should include a means to automatically predict any system's performances only from its "physical" description.

This paper first examines the users' requirements for such a tool, describes the choice of an adapted solution for the performance evaluation functions. In a second part, this paper proposes briefly some solutions to hide these techniques to the final user and to insert them in an integrated software. Finally, after a description of the chosen solution for model generation, a work–station based software tool, developed at Matra Espace, is presented; some examples of its utilization are given too.

OBJECTIVES

As it has been rapidly presented in the introduction, the matter is to give to a system engineer a simple and quick means to help him designing a distributed architecture. This should be done in several steps:
    . develop a man/machine interface for hardware and software components description, recording and representation; including:

- graphic representation of the hardware architecture,
- menu and mouse choices for the management functions (create, modify...),
- hardware components library with dynamic creation of new units,
- aid during processes description,

. choose and implement performance evaluation facilities,
. develop a software module to expound performance results,
. integrate these functions in a single interactive software package.

During the first system design stages, we do not need very accurate estimates; what is more interesting is to reject the worst designs (but not selecting the best). In this context, queuing network modeling should be used and will give good results, even if the used models are built at a macroscopic level (4). Furthermore, during the early stages of the conception, a system engineer is not able to obtain very detailed designs, therefore a detailed model is not necessary.

Some modeling experiences, with queuing networks, on several existing distributed systems showed us that very abstract and simplistic models can provide good estimates of system performance. One of them is presented in the following example concerning a case study on a distributed data multiplexing system.

This experience, intended to verify the accuracy of a macroscopic model, consisted in finding the maximum input data rate without overflow; as it has been done on an existing system, modeling results could have been compared with measurement.
. the entire system is composed of five processors connected on a single data bus (multiplexed bus); four of them receive input data to be multiplexed (slaves), the fifth sends the multiplexed data (master),
. there are four kinds of processes:

- data receipt (slaves),
- data packets preparing (slaves),
- packets collecting (master),
- packets transmission (master),

. each computer has been modeled with a single queue and its server to which we associated estimates of the operating system and bus access overheads,
. the data bus has also been modeled with a single server.

The entire hardware architecture and the associated model are given in figure 1.

The results obtained with such a simple model are quite interesting:
. maximum input rate measured: 32 Kbps,
. maximum input rate obtained with modeling: 35 Kbps.

Furthermore, this evaluation permitted bottleneck identification which allowed improvements in the concerned software modules (resulting in performance improvements).

Several other similar studies have been carried out to evaluate the required modeling level; this permitted to define some typical models of elementary hardware components, such as computers or disk units, with a granularity adapted to our requirements. During these steps, simulation was always used due to the various modeled mechanism (5) (inter-process communication or synchronization, scheduling algorithms, ...) and because it has not any theoretical limitation (6).

As developing a specific software for the simulation capabilities would have been too long and costly, an existing software has been chosen: QNAP2 (Queuing Network Analysis Package; INRIA, Bull, Simulog). This package includes a high level language for model description and various methods for its resolution:

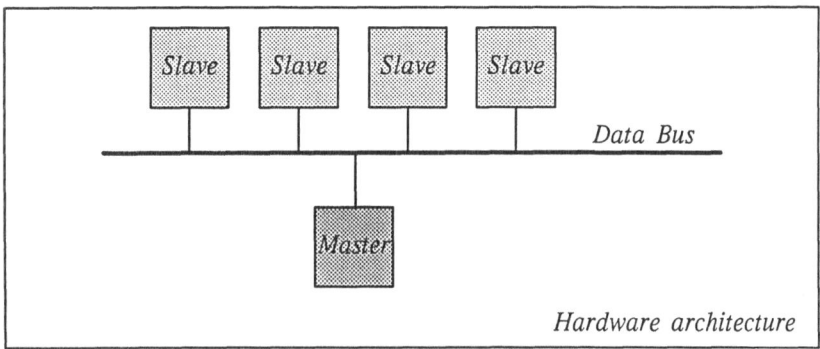

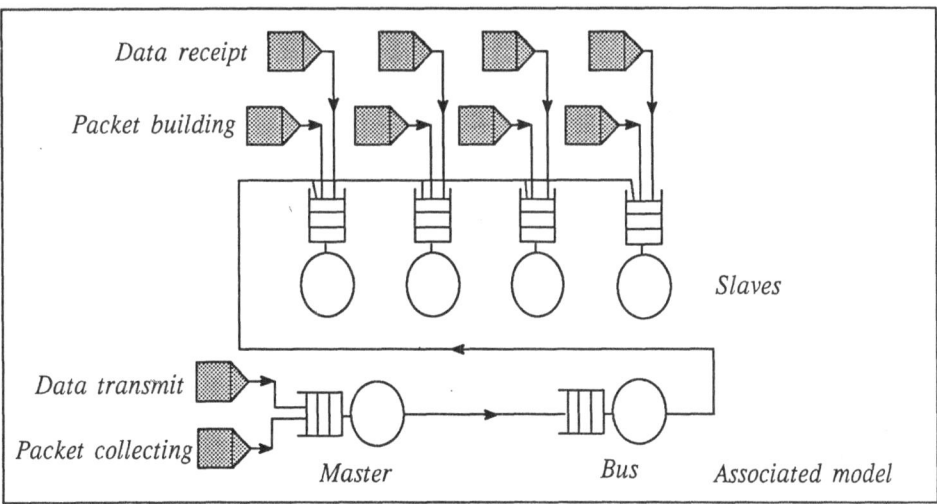

Figure   1

analytical solvers, simulation kernel, ... This permitted to quickly obtain validated modeling facilities and furthermore to have a well suited model representation formalism (8).

Once the required modeling level has been defined and when the model resolution software has been chosen, the remaining thing to do to reach our objectives is to develop around Qnap2 a "software shell" for architecture describing, automatic model generating and simulation results interpretation.

Although developing modules to describe architecture and interpret simulation results can be a relatively long job, it does not involve any particular difficulty; but it is not the same for automatic model generation for which a suitable method should be chosen. The following paragraph explains our choice after examining briefly four possible approaches.

MODEL GENERATION

At a macroscopic level, every data processing system can be considered as a set of two kind of components: resources (hardware units, software drivers, ...) and processes; resources give "work units" to the processes whereas processes consume resources. So, to generate a model, we will distinguish two steps:
. resources modeling (model topology),
. processes modeling (model population).

A process is always modeled by a queuing network customer to which we associate a set of attributes in order to reflect the characteristics of the modeled process. These attributes are used to perform transitions between the queues and to manage the work demands all over the different stations; they may be directly obtained from a simple description of the processes, given through a pre-established "process skeleton". Details concerning model population are given within the description of a specific software tool (last part).

On the other side, the model topology has to be obtained from a physical description of the various hardware units composing an architecture; several solutions may be used to do this "model generation"; the following part presents briefly four of them and mainly, explains our choice for the development of a specific tool.

Artificial Intelligence Techniques

An inventory of the multiple model constitution rules, collected from experts in modeling techniques, might constitute the knowledge base of an expert system for help in model designing. This method, already experimented on specific types of problems such as architecture configuration or model simulation (7), seems to be maladjusted to our requirements which specify a "user friendly" tool including configuration, modeling, simulation and results interpreting; furthermore, such an approach appears too ambitious in our operational context.

General Model

An other solution may consist in building a general model, including all the possible hardware components and able to unify with all the possible situations. For a particular system, the specific model is obtained by parameter setting on the general one; this allows to cut off all the useless branches of the global model with the object of reducing it to the studied system. For this method, the global model should include as many queues as necessary to cover all the components; also, every transition should be possible between queues. This approach is reasonable only if we can identify all the possible architectures and consider that each of them is a sub-set of a single one; however, it might be interesting for a generator intended to be used on a known set of data processing systems (based on a similar architecture) or on a specific architecture to generate automatically new models after each architecture evolution (disks adding, computing power increasing...). However, this method is too rigid for our application and might result in important difficulties during general model development.

<u>Sub-models Data Base</u>

A hierarchical approach may also allow automatic model constitution by aggregation of elementary sub-models. An inventory of the possible hardware components is done and a sub-model is constituted for each of them. These elementary models are built by modeling specialists, according to several rules defining for example the interfaces between sub-models, the modeling granularity... A data base, associated to the entire software tool might be used to organize the various models created; then they may be used by referencing directly the associated hardware component; this means that the final user (i.e. system engineer) only manipulates hardware components and knows nothing about the sub-models.
Sub-models aggregation enables global model construction and the produced model is only a set of independent sub-models; i.e. none pre-defined transition is present between sub-models after global model construction. Customers, which model processes, perform transitions according to a path given during processes description (the same method is used for the fourth solution and is described more precisely in the next part).

<u>Components Families</u>

For the last solution, let us consider that any hardware unit can be classified as a member of a components family which can be:
  - processors (processing units) for each unit able to give compute time to any customer (computers, I/O controlers, gateways...),
  - storage devices for all the disks and magnetic tapes,
  - arbitrary devices such as printers, user terminals...,
  - communication devices (buses, serial links).

A general sub-model is associated to each family; various parameters enable its unification with any member of the considered family; so, modeling a particular component model is done in two steps:
  - choice among the families,
  - parameter setting.

Each time a new component is taken into account, it may automatically enrich a component library including hardware characteristics and descriptions of the associated sub-models.
Once more, the entire model is built by aggregation of elementary ones.

For our application, the third and the fourth solutions might be used but, because of the large variety of possible components and as we want capabilities to create dynamically any component model (without any help from a modeling specialist), the last one has been chosen. Furthermore, we do not need such a level of detail than we can obtain with the third solution.
The following paragraph examines the main characteristics of the chosen solution and explains how hardware architecture and processes description are interpreted to perform model generation.

<u>Chosen Solution</u> (components families)

As it has been explained in the previous parts, the model of a specific data processing system is built in two steps:

– hardware components inventory to generate model topology (stations and queues declaration),
– processes description interpreting to generate model population (customers).

Model topology. One or several sub–models are associated to each components family, depending on the complexity of the corresponding components. These sub models might be very simplistic (i.e. a single queue for I/O devices such as printers or terminals) or might be a sophisticated "sub–network" of queues including different kind of servers (to model an ethernet local area network for example).

Anyway, in all cases, each sub–model has one input point and one output point with which it may cooperate with the others; this simplifies aggregation phase.

So, the model topology generation consists in declaring sub–models, according to the physical description of the hardware architecture. For each hardware component, an instance of the associated sub–model is created by means of a Qnap2 "macro call"; macros have been defined at once during tool development, they must be able to unify with any possible component of the associated family.

During this phase, there is not any path description between the declared sub–models, so, customers transitions between them will be done according to model population description (see next part); on the contrary inside a sub–model, paths between queues are pre–defined and depend on the type of the sub–model.

Model population. To perform system modeling, processes are represented by queuing network customers, so, this phase consists in declaring the source stations which generate customers, according to processes description given by a system engineer.

For each process, a "source type" station is created and the pre–defined customer attributes are set to memorize process characteristics such as the priority level, the number of instructions, the I/O requests... Inside sub–models, algorithmic language manipulates these attributes to represent resources occupation, delays, or synchronization primitives and to perform transition between aggregated sub–models. To be very simple, we may say that every customer "carries" all over the queues the characteristics of the process which it models.

This method has been implemented for the development of a dedicated software tool for help in designing distributed systems. The following chapter presents this development and the general software architecture of the tool.

DEDICATED TOOL DESCRIPTION

To satisfy the requirements described in the "objectives" part, three steps have been identified:
– operator interface for hardware and processes definition,
– sub–models definition and module for automatic model generation,
– simulation monitoring and results interpreting.

Remark: As in the models we use algorithmic language facilities of Qnap2, customers attributes and various synchronization mechanisms; simulation was the only way to solve our models even if it is sometimes long (and costly)...

The purpose of this chapter is to examine the various modules implemented for automatic model generation, simulation monitoring and architecture description. Examples of execution steps are given as a description of the user interface.

Figure 2 provides an overview of the entire software tool architecture hosted on a UNIX based Workstation. Interactive graphic capabilities of the SUN worksta-

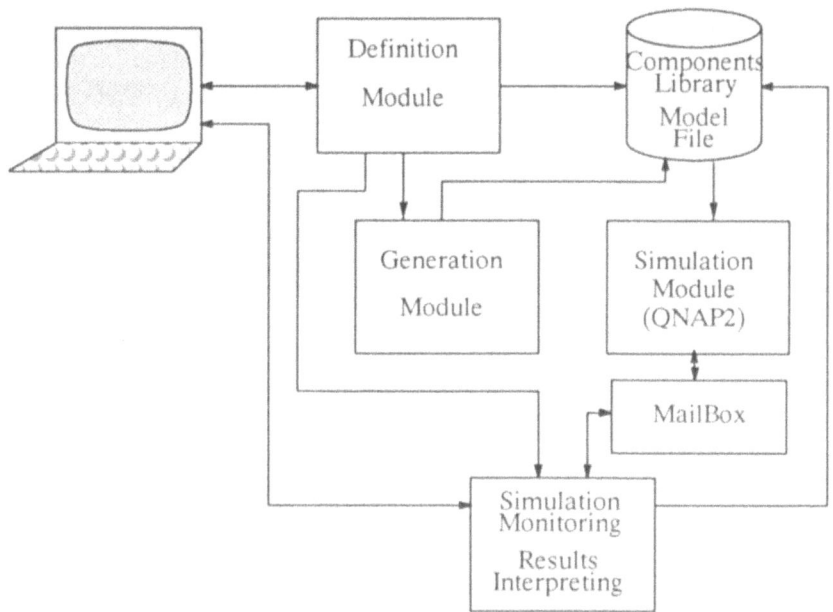

Figure   2   MAITE software architecture

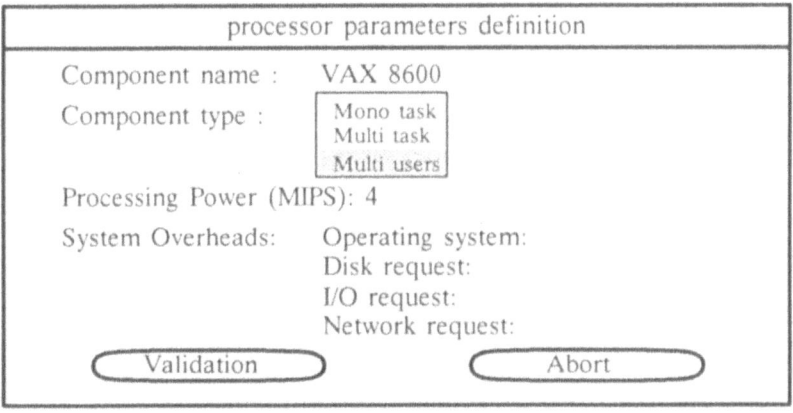

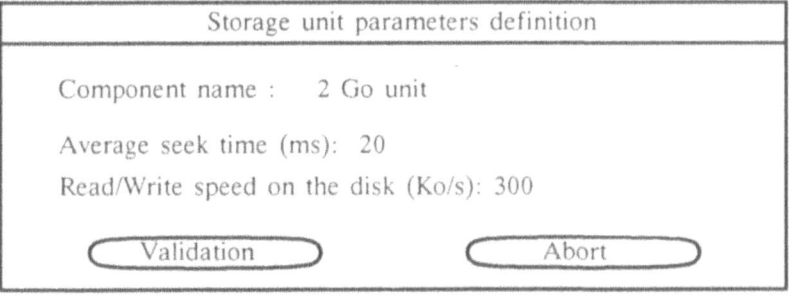

Figure   3   Templates to create hardware components

tion have been employed to define hardware and software components (processes); the principal development language for this tool is the C language, graphics and multi-windowing facilities are provided by Suncore and Sunview software packages.

The definition module manages the user interface by giving graphical means to build and maintain a file which comprise the components library; it also provides help for architecture and processes description. The generator module, builds a model according to the architecture defined before. This model is then resolved with Qnap2 simulation facilities, hosted on the same computer. The simulation monitoring module is intended to control simulation length, display intermediate results and expound final results.

Definition Module

A "user friendly" interface allows hardware architecture and processes description; it is a menu driven interface using the full graphic capabilities of the SUN workstation; an intensive use of the mouse reduces data input from the keyboard which is only used to specify numeric values or components names. The operator interface is divided in two modules, one to graphically describe the hardware architecture, the other for processes description.

Hardware definition module. This module provides the tools to define and maintain static performance characterization data (power, size, ...) for each hardware component included in the studied architecture.
Description of system topology is graphically done by selecting icons with the mouse; examples of a description in progress are given on figure 4. Figure 3 shows examples of data templates used to capture components parameters; these templates are brought up by using the mouse, each of them is associated to a particular component family.
A set of general functions allows drawing management (move or remove components, create a link between components...) and offers capabilities to manage the components library associated with the tool (according to the fourth method). When describing the hardware topology, a consistency check is automaticaly performed to prevent the user from creating impossible links (e.g. from Disk to Disk, Network to Disk...) or describe non valid units.

Processes definition module. This module is intended to provide help during processes definition. New processes are implanted on the architecture by using the mouse; then, a "process skeleton", closely linked to the customers attributes of the associated model (see previous chapter), is used to help the designer. Processes are always described as consumers of resources. The description is done in several steps: first the processing characterization (number of instructions, priority, ...), then, the requests to others devices such as disks, network, ... and finally the inter-process communication mechanisms. Figures 5 gives examples of the data templates used for processes description (distant processing template is intended to describe requests coming from the network).

Model Generation Module

Once the entire architecture has been described (hardware and processes), an associated model is generated according to the method presented in the previous chapter. The generator proceeds in two steps to write down a file containing the associated Qnap2 model; this generation is fully automatic, so the user does not see neither any Qnap2 language nor any queuing network.

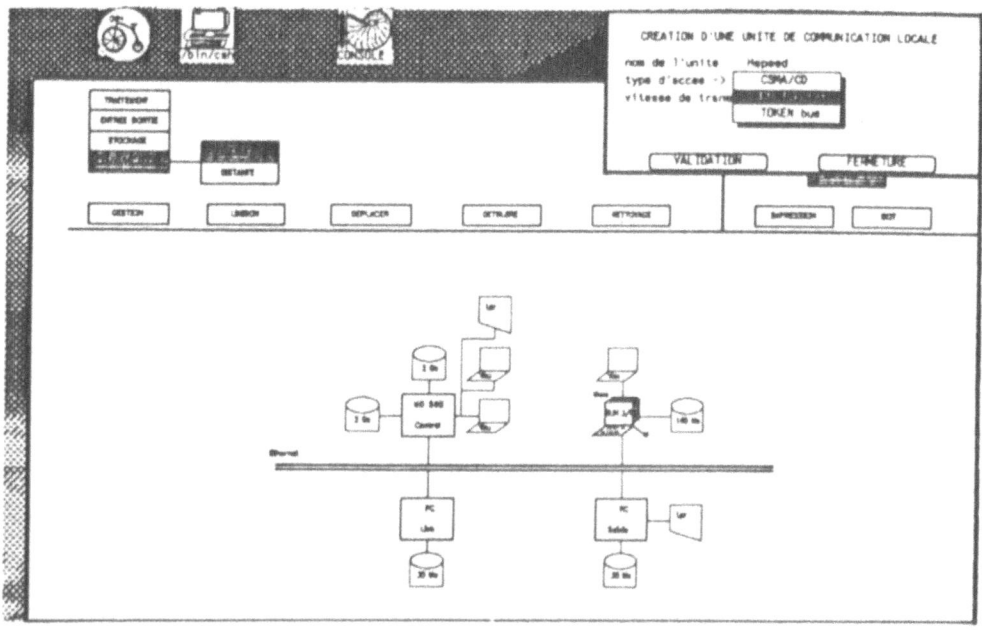

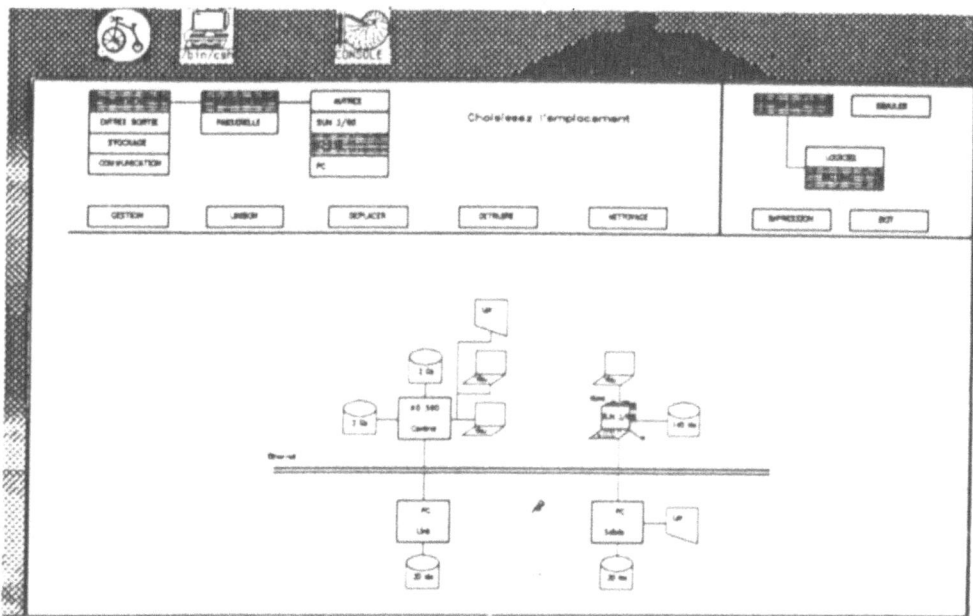

Figure   4   Hardware architecture description (examples)

```
┌─────────────────────────────────────────────────────────────┐
│                   processing description                      │
├─────────────────────────────────────────────────────────────┤
│ Associated processor name: VAX 8600                           │
│ Execution priority (up to 20): 3                              │
│ Activation type:        ┌──────────┐                          │
│                         │  cyclic  │                          │
│                         ├──────────┤                          │
│                         │  Random  │                          │
│                         ├──────────┤                          │
│                         │  Event   │                          │
│                         └──────────┘                          │
│ Instruction amount: 12000        ┌──────────────────────────┐ │
│ Execution priority (up to 20): 3 │          DISK            │ │
│                                  ├──────────────────────────┤ │
│ External requests............... │          I/O             │ │
│                                  ├──────────────────────────┤ │
│                                  │        Network           │ │
│                                  ├──────────────────────────┤ │
│                                  │   Communication event    │ │
│   ( Validation )                 └──────────────────────────┘ │
│                                          Abort                │
└─────────────────────────────────────────────────────────────┘

┌─────────────────────────────────────────────────────────────┐
│               Distant processing specification                │
├─────────────────────────────────────────────────────────────┤
│ Maximum access amount: 2                                      │
│ Minimum acces amount: 1                                       │
│ Kilo bytes on the network:  request: 0.5                      │
│                             return: 20                        │
│ Instruction amount: 12000        ┌──────────────────────────┐ │
│ Execution priority (up to 20): 1 │          DISK            │ │
│                                  ├──────────────────────────┤ │
│                                  │          I/O             │ │
│ External requests............... ├──────────────────────────┤ │
│                                  │   Communication event    │ │
│                                  └──────────────────────────┘ │
│       ( Validation )                   ( Abort )              │
└─────────────────────────────────────────────────────────────┘
```

Figure   5   Data templates for processes description

Model topology. Each hardware component is identified as a member of a family (see previous chapter), the parameters values given by the designer are used to set the associated sub-model parameters; this sub-model instance is written on the model file (see figure 2).

Model population. Qnap2 language is automatically generated to affect customers attributes according to the processes description; this step consists in associating each process skeleton with the pre-defined customer attributes which models it; these description are appended to the model file.

Figure 6 shows the general mechanism used during automatic model generation, in case of an inconsistency detected during interpretation step, an error is reported and the generation process is aborted.

Simulation Monitoring

Once the model is generated, the operator may activate a resolution phase in batch or in interactive mode. In batch mode, the control is given to the Qnap2 software after defining the length of the simulation run (this is done with a specific template, see figure 7); at the end of the simulation the standard results given by Qnap2 may be interpreted to produce curves or histograms as shown on figure 9. In batch mode no interaction is possible between the operator and the simulation run.

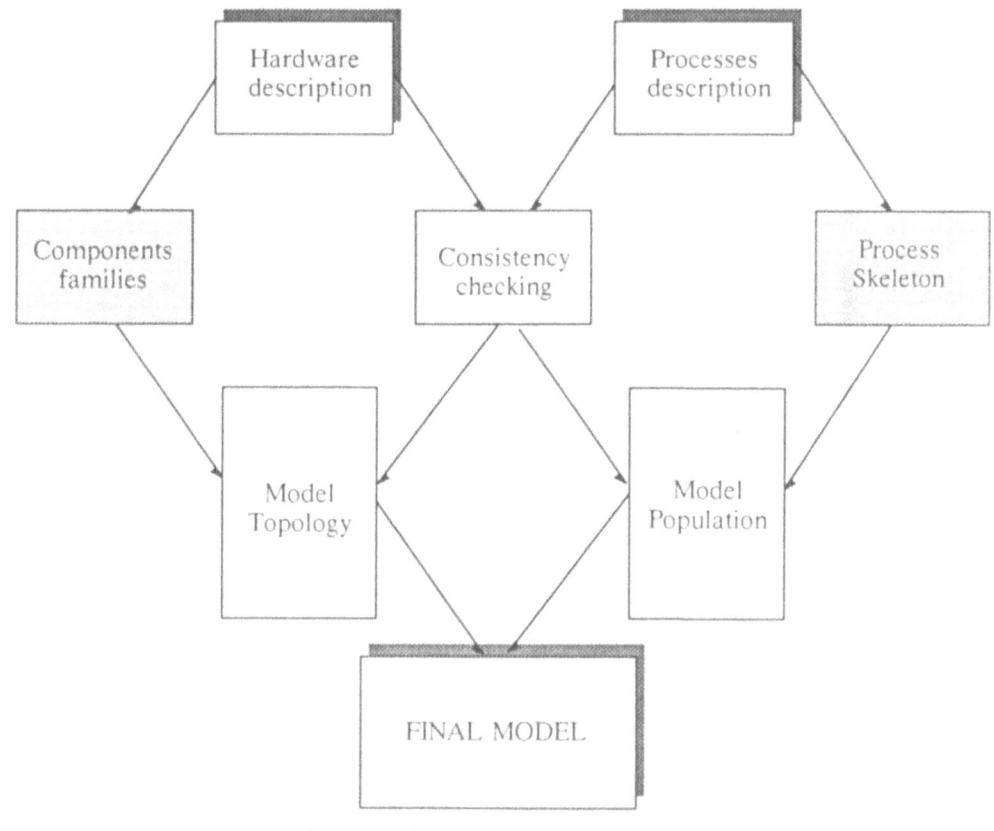

Figure   6   Model generation

In interactive mode, three operations are accessible to the designer: he may observe the system behavior by means of a real time loading rate display for each hardware unit (architecture animation), he may also activate a new process or simply stop the simulation run. To provide this interaction, Inter Process Communication (IPC) facilities of UNIX system V have been used (10).

Activating a simulation in interactive mode will result in the execution of three processes which are closely linked:
. The qnap2 simulation kernel which is directly activated to solve the model,
. A simulation monitoring process which displays loading rates for up to five selected units and allows inputs from the mouse to control the simulation flow. (a copy of an interactive display is given on figure 8)
. A management process used to acquire user's commands.

A programming hook called "utilit" included in the qnap2 software package has been used to produce intermediate simulation results according to a period defined by the user. The "utilit" procedure is part of Qnap2 software and is fully customizable; it has been used to directly access a 'Unix defined" mailbox. So, during the simulation run, this procedure is called and performs two functions:
. periodic storage of intermediate simulation results in the mailbox (in order to display them),
. periodic reading of an other mailbox to get user's commands (activate process or abort simulation).
On the other hand, the monitoring process reads the intermediate results in the mailbox and posts user commands which are generated by mouse selection. The

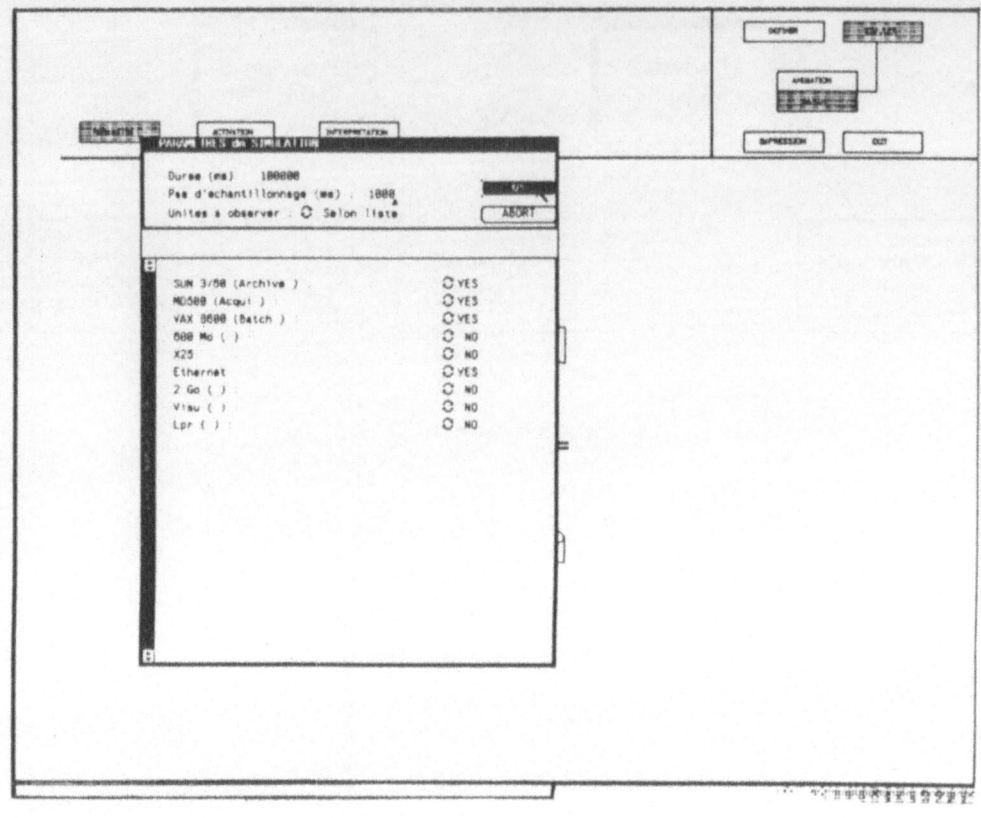

Figure   7   Data template to set simulation parameters

mailbox is constituted by a shared memory structure which is managed by sema-phores, this allows inter process communication at the rate of the simulation run.

CONCLUSION

An incomplete initial version of the tool (without simulation monitoring and results interpreting) became operational in October 1987 and is currently used at Matra Espace to evaluate newly designed distributed systems. A final version, including all the modules described above, will be operational in june 88.

With the current version, systems engineers are able to describe and model quickly a sophisticated data processing network and obtain accurate estimates of system's performances. Furthermore, the performance evaluation is obtained without any help neither from a modeling specialist nor a programmer.

Our short experience of its use has shown that application of such a tool may, on one hand, reduce development risks and cost owing to the capability to study various solutions for the same system; and, on the other hand, help system engineers understanding the system behavior under processes loading (that may allow design improvements).

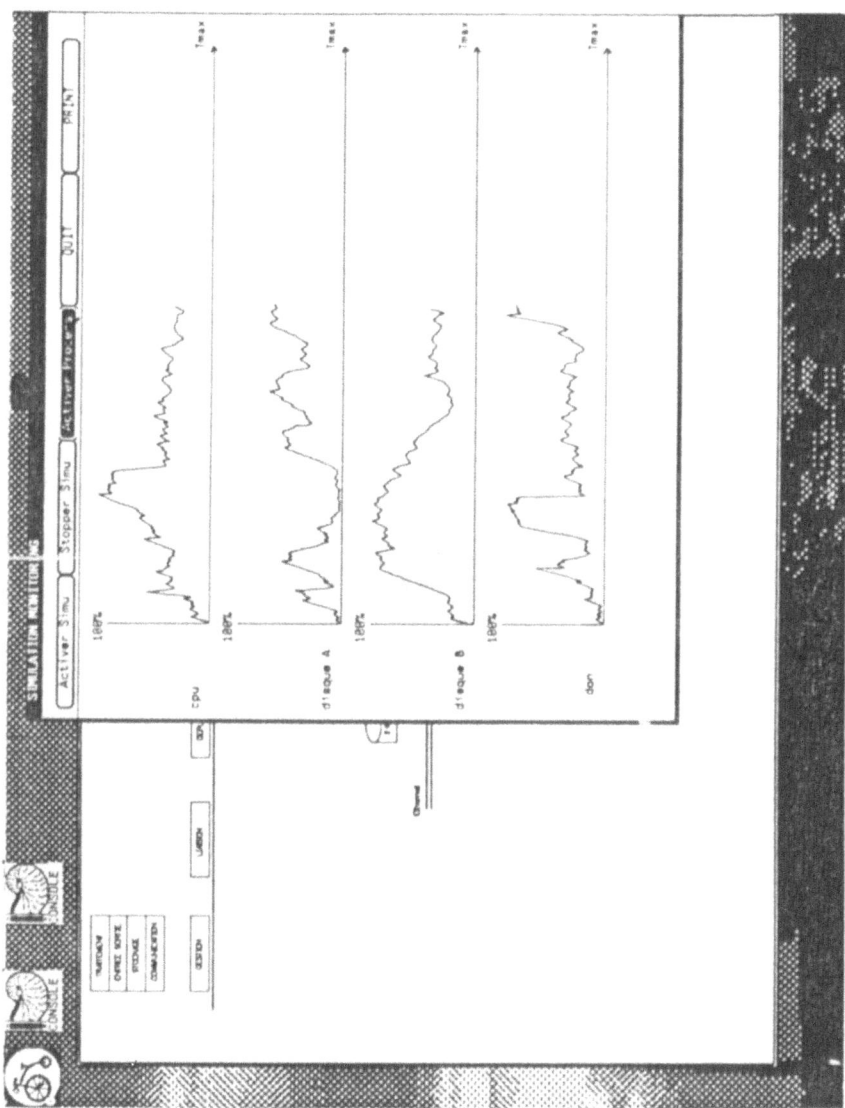

figure   8   Interactive simulation mode

53

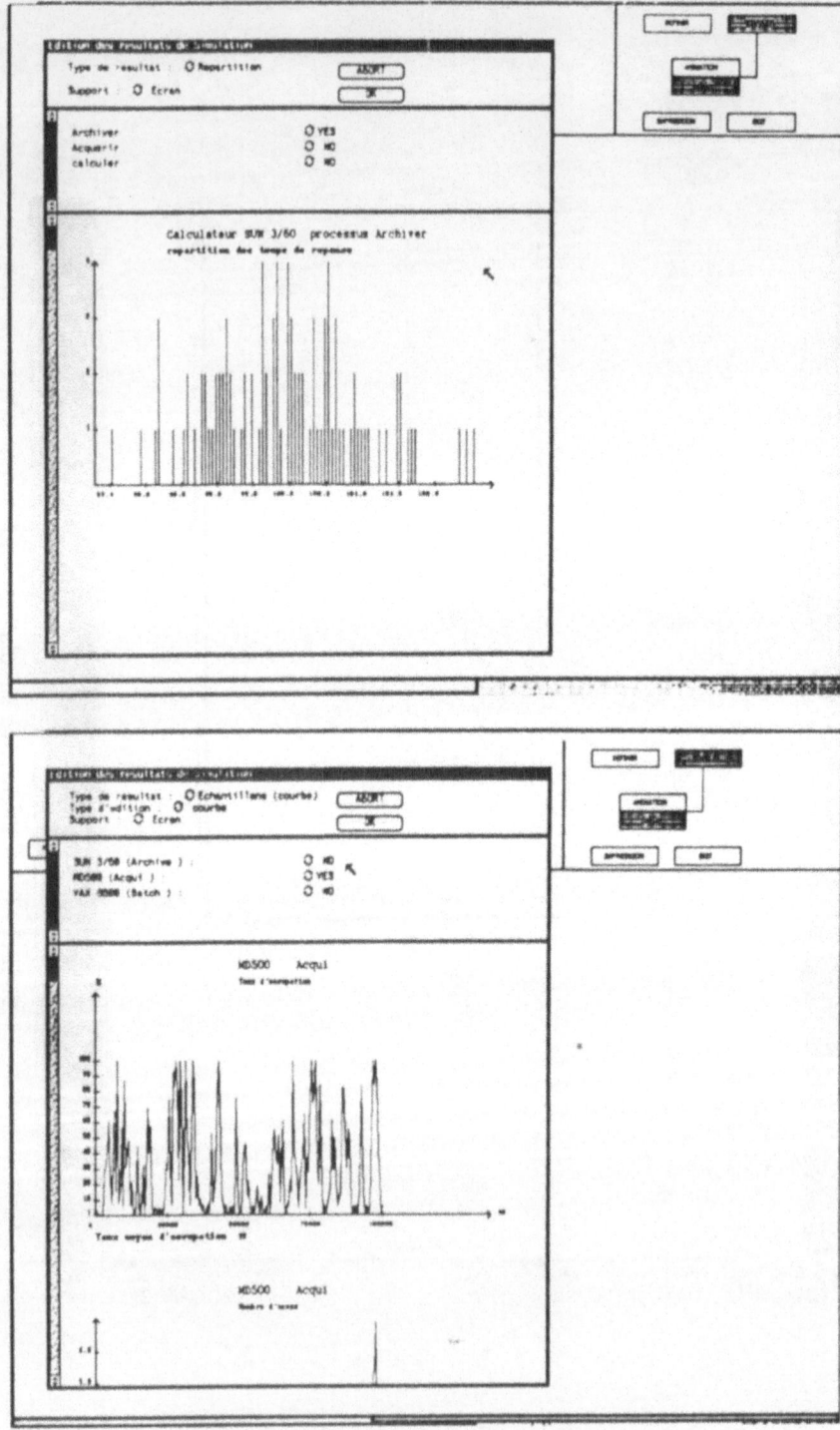

Figure 9   Simulation results interpreting

REFERENCES

(1)   Jhon F Soch and Jon A Hupp: "Measured performance of an Ethernet local network" (Communication of the ACM 12–80).

(2)   Ahmed Patel and Michael Purser: "Systems progamming for data communications on minicomputers" (Software practice and Experience).

(3)   "International Workshop on modeling techniques and performance evaluation" (AFCET 87).

(4)   CH Sauer and KM Chandy: "Computer systems performance modeling".

(5)   H Kobayashi: "Modeling and analysis: an introduction to performance evaluation methodology".

(6)   Proceedings, Symposium international: "La simulation dans les sciences pour l'ingénieur" (1983).

(7)   D Potier: "Computer performance evaluation and expert systems: a survey"

(8)   "Qnap2 reference manual V4.0" (1984)

(9)   Proceedings: "IEEE Compcon'84 Fall conference on the small computer (r)evolution" (September 16–20, 1984 Arlington, VA).

(10)   Unix system V programmer's manual (system calls) SUN Microsystems April 1986.

(11)   R. Nelson, D. Towsley and A. N. Tantawi: "Performance analysis of parallel processing systems" (IEEE Software April 88)

(12)   D. A. Reed, A. D. Malony and B. D. McCredie: "Parallel discrete event simulation using shared memory" (IEEE Software April 88)

(13)   T. J. McCabe, F. C. Joh Jr., K A. Adams and A. M. Sturgill: "Structured real time analysis and design" (IEEE Software 1985)

(14)   G. Estrin, R. S Fenchel, R. R. Razouk and M. K. Vernon: "Modeling, analysis and simulation support for design of concurrent systems" (IEEE February 86)

TOWARDS A PERFORMANCE MODELLING ENVIRONMENT:

NEWS ON HIT

H. Beilner, J. Mäter, and N. Weißenberg

Informatik IV
Universität Dortmund

ABSTRACT

HIT is a comprehensive software tool supporting the model-based evaluation of computing system performance. HIT models exhibit a highly structured view of the systems to be assessed, based on (vertical) functional hierarchies and (horizontal) modularization as employed in modern software engineering and hardware architecture approaches. Analysis of HIT models is provided by analytic-algebraical, analytic-numerical, exact and approximate techniques and by discrete-event simulation. Both model description and model analysis utilize the model structure for convenient problem specification and efficient evaluation, respectively. Particular emphasis is placed on decomposition and aggregation options and on a mixed (heterogeneous) use of different analysis techniques. Great care is also employed with respect to tool handling aspects. This paper describes recent extensions of the HIT modelling environment and illustrates it by way of an extended office model example.

1. INTRODUCTION

In an age of continuously shrinking development and usage cycles of computing systems´ hardware and software, computer support during system design, realization and operations appears a must. The type of desirable support should (ideally) relate to all domains of requirements for these systems, to their functionality and correctness, their performance, their reliability and availability, etc. It seems that considerable effort will still have to be spent before such an ideal, integrated support can become operational: At present, a satisfactory level of (say: design-) support has not even been attained within the various, individual requirement domains (hardware and software correctness, performance, reliability), and sizeable R&D activities aiming at improved, domain-specific support are underway. On the other hand, it is certainly *not* too soon to acknowledge the integrated point of view as a major guideline and to try and move towards this target, from within the various requirement domains.

With these ideas in mind, and with the particular emphasis on performance modelling as one, necessary type of design support, a corresponding project was launched in Dortmund, in 1983, which has since focussed on the development of the modelling tool, HIT. HIT adheres to the sketched guideline by exhibiting a system/model description interface as tailored upon the prevalent structural view of computer architecture and software engineering (functional/virtual machine hierarchies, modularization, ADT/object-oriented fashions of thinking). The present status of HIT proves that the basic evaluation power of a performance modelling tool is not hampered by this approach: Simulative, analytic-algebraical, analytic-numerical, exact and approximate analysis techniques can in fact be fed from that structured description interface. Quite to the contrary, the description structure can be taken advantage of by structuring model evaluation processes accordingly, i.e. by using problem-specific description structures as the basis for decomposition/aggregation steps and corresponding structured (homogeneous or heterogeneous) evaluations displaying considerably improved, total evaluation efficiency.

HIT has of yet been made available in two major versions, a 0- and a 1-version, dated 1985 and 1987, respectively. Externally available references to HIT-0 include Beilner and Scholten (1985, in German), presenting the initial model world, and Wolf (1986, in French), concentrating in particular on the compilation techniques used. Special emphasis on simulative evaluation is placed in the HIT(-1) reference, Beilner and Stewing (1987, in English). The present contribution is intended to highlight recent progress in both model description and evaluation techniques incorporated in HIT, and to also focus on various handling aspects, which have been considerably enhanced by the implementation of an object management facility, OMA. The latter facility introduces systematic storage and retrieval options for (partial) model descriptions and results and eases automatic (total) model configuration.

Right at the beginning, acknowledgements are due to NIXDORF Computer and to the German Federal Department of Research and Technology, BMFT, without whose major support the development of HIT would not have been possible. Thanks are also extended to the whole HIT development team of which only a few members will be mentioned in the body of this paper. Finally, reference must be given to other performance modelling tools such as RESQ (Sauer and McNair, 1984), QNAP (Veran and Potier, 1984), MAOS (Jobmann, 1985), etc., which have not gone unnoticed while developing HIT. Also, the experience from our own, earlier tools, COPE (Beilner and Mäter, 1984) and NUMAS (Müller, 1984) has most certainly been exploited.

2. MODEL WORLD AND MODEL SPECIFICATION

For the purpose of describing a computing system, in other words: of specifying a corresponding model, HIT employs the familiar view of a hierarchy of functional levels and function-realizing layers. A level is characterized by a set of functions, called SERVICEs, which it PROVIDEs to its environment; the environment (a layer to be constructed on top of this level) may USE these functions within certain algorithmic patterns; naming these patterns, calling them services and providing them for use to some yet "higher" environment obviously establishes a next higher level (or a part of it). This scheme serves for constructing almost arbitrary *vertical* structures. To avoid misunderstandings: Levels are not necessarily system-wide; the hierarchy needs not be strict; recursion across the level structure is not allowed; the total structure is not necessarily a tree.

The sketched vertical level/layer structuring scheme is complemented in HIT by means for *horizontal* structuring, employing the equally familiar modularization view. A level (a set of services provided for use) is regarded as export interface of some machinery which is to realize this level´s services, is regarded as export interface of a "machine", in HIT terminology. That machine can be (horizontally) structured into a set of modules, called COMPONENTs, where every component is responsible for the realization of a subset of the machine-provided services, thereby partitioning the level-specific service set accordingly. Starting from the other end: Every component provides specific services; a machine includes some set of components and provides the union of services provided by these components.

Returning to the services (introduced above as patterns of using some lower "level"; recognizable now as patterns of using the services of a machine): A set of different services can, of course, be described for an individual machine interface, where such a service set is called a "load pattern", in HIT. Combining a machine with a machine-consistent load pattern and declaring particular services as provided (externally visible, exported) is equivalent with constructing a component, in the above sense. For this construction process, HIT insists on an explicit linking (REFERring) of names of USEd services (called upon in the load pattern) to names of PROVIDEd services (established by the machine) in order to introduce a certain naming independence and to thereby facilitate team efforts at constructing large models.

In total, the specification of a HIT model will consist of a series of more local, mutually fairly independent activities, each concerned with the declaration of a machine, with the programming of a load pattern and with referring that load pattern to that machine (for presumable execution). The total model will in the end (normally) include some "top" component (not providing any services and therefore independent of any environment), termed a MODEL. The bottom level, on the other hand, will (usually) consist of the interfaces of components which are to govern the "physical" resources, time and space. Some evaluation techniques (see sect. 4) depend upon employing the standard component types, SERVER (time consumption) and COUNTER (space consumption), for bottom levels.

The behaviour over time of the dynamic system/model to be described is governed by the instantiation of processes, where every process will obey by the pattern of a certain SERVICE. Instantiation of services is possible in a time-controlled and in an event-controlled mode: HIT allows to CREATE (an instance of) a service at a prescribed point in time, within every component; on the other hand, requesting the execution of a component-provided service, from within a "higher" service, constitutes an event- controlled instantiation (of a sub-process in the component providing this service). With respect to dynamics, a component behaves as an independent, autonomous dynamic entity: It can deny acceptance of a service request; if accepted, a service may be "scheduled" (or kept waiting), it may be caused to progress faster or slower, etc.

HIT model specification, mechanically speaking, employs a particular specification language, HI-SLANG. A partner tool, HIT-GRAFIX, supports graphics-based representations of model structures. HI-SLANG and HIT-GRAFIX representations build heavily on typing/instantiation schemes, achieving a considerable parsimony in model specification.

2.1 Illustration

A single, hypothetical example will be used throughout the paper to clarify most points to be made. The example goes as follows: Some company considers the introduction of computer support for her office work. Considerations start at supporting certain recurrent decisions and the preparations for them. Basically, one such decision activity is planned, per day per department. The company is, in a restructuring phase, moving from 5 towards 10 departments; eventually, 20 departments are to be catered for. The activities under consideration each consist of preparing 3 initial documents (dealt with sequentially, in the present environment) and subsequently joining these documents into some master report, which is later examined (with respect to any due decisions) and eventually finished off (filed away). In order to assess the office performance under heavy load, we assume for the moment that this activity pattern is continuously repeated, for every department (we are later going to relieve operations again towards the demanded "once per day"). The pattern can be easily encoded in (and understood from) the corresponding piece of HI-SLANG code (*Fig 2.1.1*).

```
LOOP                        {repeat forever}
    DO  3  TIMES  LOOP {repeat 3 times}
        prepare;
    END LOOP;

    join;
    examine;
    finish;
END LOOP;
```

Fig. 2.1.1. SERVICE body

Two further steps are now necessary: (i) The specified activity pattern is based upon sub-activities (prepare, join, examine, finish) to be dealt with by "somebody". In the present environment, two sub-offices, a secretaries´ office and a clerks´ office, exist which are responsible for editing and examination/archivation activities, respectively. Representing this structure unchanged, we introduce these two sub-offices as components assumed to provide the demanded services (more precisely: as instances of COMPONENT TYPEs, "handling" and "evaluation", to be specified later). (ii) We have to get one activity of *Fig. 2.1.1* going, per department. For this purpose, we make this pattern a proper SERVICE, "report", and CREATE (at time "0") as many report instances as there are departments. Looking ahead, where experiments with different numbers of departments can be expected, we immediately incorporate the whole scheme in a MODEL TYPE, "office", with (the number of) "departments" as parameter.

This verbal discussion is again easily transferred to HI-SLANG/HIT-GRAFIX notations; in particular, the way of referring used to provided services should be self-explanatory (*Fig´s 2.1.2a/b*):

```
TYPE office MODEL (departments:INTEGER);

    TYPE report SERVICE;
        USE SERVICE
            prepare; join; examine; finish;
        END USE;
    BEGIN {body of Fig. 2.1.1}
    END TYPE report;

    COMPONENT secretaries: handling;
              clerks:      evaluation;

    REFER report TO secretaries, clerks
    EQUATING
        report. prepare WITH secretaries. edit;
        {... cf. HIT-GRAFIX representation, Fig. 2.1.2b}
    END REFER;

BEGIN           {model body}
    CREATE departments PROCESS report;
        {i.e. one report activity per department}
END TYPE office;
```

Fig. 2.1.2a. MODEL TYPE, "office", HI-SLANG representation

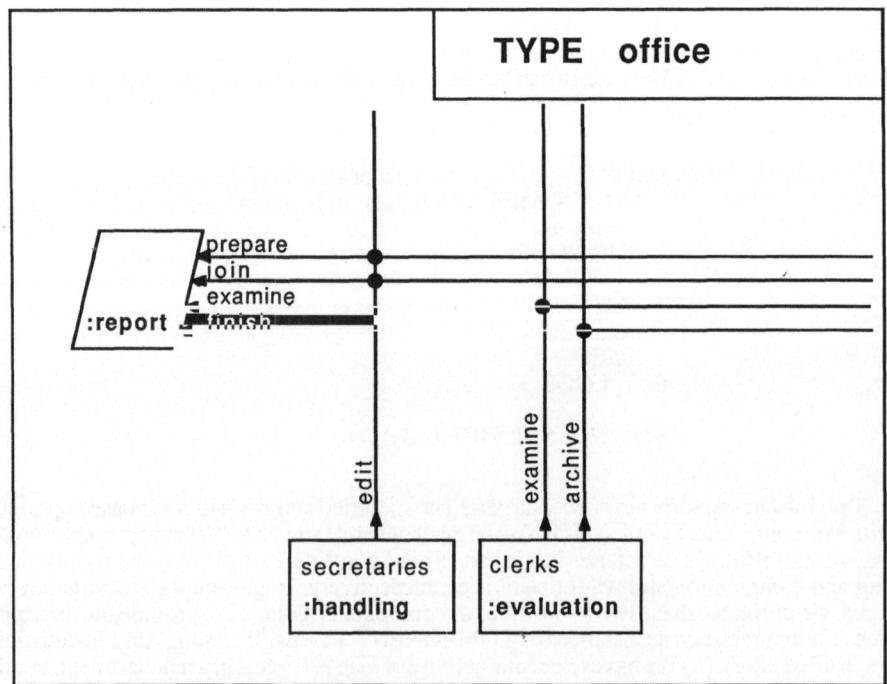

Fig. 2.1.2b. MODEL TYPE, "office", HIT-GRAFIX representation

```
TYPE edit SERVICE;                      TYPE handling COMPONENT;
    USE SERVICE                             PROVIDE SERVICE
        fetch    (time:REAL);                   edit;
        change   (time:REAL);               END PROVIDE;
        store    (time:REAL);
        think    (time:REAL);               TYPE edit SERVICE;
    END USE;                                    {...cf. Fig. 2.1.3}
                                            END TYPE edit;
BEGIN
    AVERAGE 10 TIMES LOOP               COMPONENT
    fetch (negexp(1/3));                    humans: server;
                                            sap:     server (LET dispatch
        AVERAGE 5 TIMES LOOP                                    :=shared);
        think (negexp(1/20));            ENCLOSE
                                            link:    server;
        BRANCH
           PROB 0.75: change(negexp(1/2));   REFER edit TO humans, sap, link
           PROB 0.25: change(negexp(1/10));      EQUATING {...cf. Fig. 2.1.4b}
        END BRANCH;                          END REFER;
    END LOOP;                               BEGIN {empty component body:
                                                    no internal processes}
                                            END TYPE handling;

        store (negexp(1/3));            COMPONENT link: server
    END LOOP;                                       (LET dispatch:=shared);
    END TYPE edit;
```

Fig. 2.1.3. HI-SLANG specification   *Fig. 2.1.4a.* component type, "handling",
of SERVICE, "edit"   HI-SLANG representation

As announced, the component types, "handling" and "evaluation", must now be specified, including the refinement of their provided services, "edit" and "examine/archive", respectively. As for the secretaries´ office (the "handling" type), it is known from actual operations that every editing activity is concerned with updating, on the average, 10 different pages of some document (of various documents, occasionally). Secretaries work page by page. They perform about 5 update actions per page, where these updates can be classified as either more complex (about 25% of this kind) or less complex (the remaining 75%). A decision for future, computer supported operations is, that single document pages will be transferred to the secretaries´ site on request (presumably from some central storage), be updated there and subsequently written back. With respect to modelling, an attempt is now made to relate all activities to "physical" resource consumptions. Necessary data are available: Having tried out some of the typical update actions on existing PC-type equipment, it is known that the less complex updates take about 2 sec (PC CPU-time, basically), the more complex ones 10 sec, on average. The volume of data to be moved per page transfer is estimated to about 3 KBytes; playing with the idea of utilising existing 10 Kbps lines, about 3 sec will be taken by a transfer. Finally, experience shows that about 20 sec of "secretarial thinking" must be considered, between any two individual update actions. The edit activity is (possibly more clearly than in its verbal form) specified in the "edit" SERVICE of *Fig 2.1.3*. Some additional explanations: All USEd services are parameterized with the time durations needed (time unit: 1 sec), with the forethought of REFERring them to bottom level server type components. The function calls, negexp (μ), render realizations of a negatively exponentially distributed random variable, with mean value $1/\mu$ (you can certainly guess why this choice is made here).

The requested component type, "handling", is in total depicted in *Fig´s 2.1.4a/b. Fig. 2.1.4a* also includes the "link" specification. Again some additional explanations: Instances of component type, "handling", will PROVIDE (export) a SERVICE, "edit". Services USEd by "edit" are REFERred to a machine consisting of 3 components, "humans", "sap" and "link", all of the server type. Different acceptance/scheduling/dispatching behaviours of instantiated component objects must be specified. The defaults (employed for "humans") indicate: accept unconditionally, schedule immediately, dispatch every service with full "speed" (1 service unit per time unit); this is the well-known Infinite Server scheme (the interpretation for "humans":

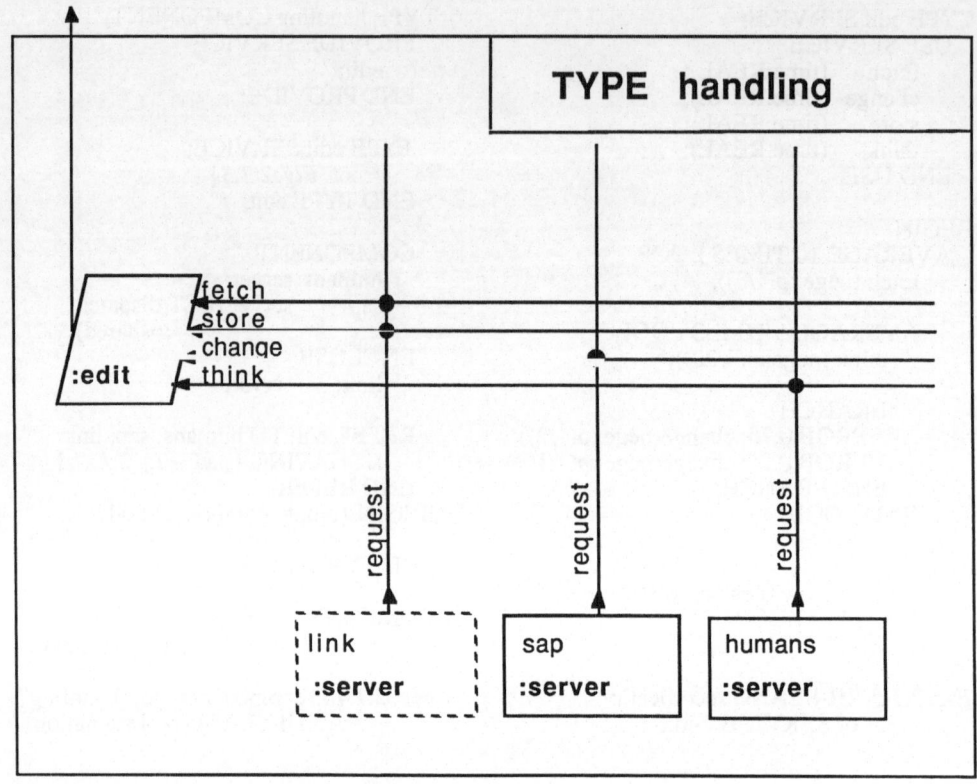

Fig. 2.1.4b. component type, "handling", HIT-GRAFIX representation

Arbitrarily many secretaries can concurrently be fully active). The dispatching behaviour, "shared" (prescribed for "sap"), shares the service capacity of 1 service unit per time unit equally amongst all present services - the well-known Processor Sharing case (interpretation for "sap": Just one unit of computing equipment is in time-shared use; never mind where the screens are, this is merely a first overview). One more point: The communication line, "link", is not owned by "handling", rather, it is ENCLOSEd, in HIT terminology, i.e. is in joint use with some other component(s) - see the "evaluation" type below. The specification (*Fig. 2.1.4a*) defines a Processor Sharing behaviour for "link".

Analogously to "handling", component type, "evaluation", has to be specified, mirroring the activities in the clerks´ office, which provides two services, "examine" and "archive". Based on similar kinds of observations as used for the former component type, *Fig´s 2.1.5a/b* describe the corresponding behaviour patterns.

```
TYPE examine SERVICE;
   USE ... END USE;
BEGIN
   AVERAGE 10 TIMES LOOP
      fetch(negexp(1/3));
      AVERAGE 3 TIMES LOOP
         think     (negexp(1/60));
         selecting(negexp(1/2));
      END LOOP;
   END LOOP;
END TYPE examine;
```

Fig. 2.1.5a. SERVICE, "examine"

```
TYPE archive SERVICE;
   USE ... END USE;
BEGIN

   AVERAGE 20 TIMES LOOP
      think(negexp(1/30));
      store(negexp(1/3));
   END LOOP;

END TYPE archive;
```

Fig. 2.1.5b. SERVICE, "archive"

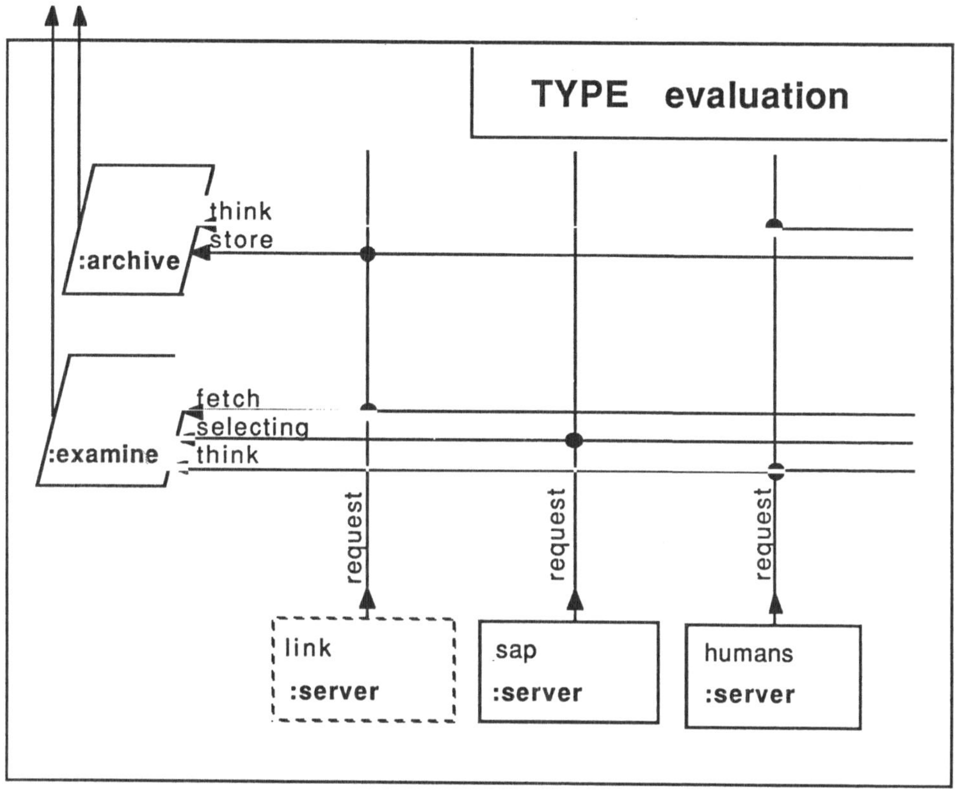

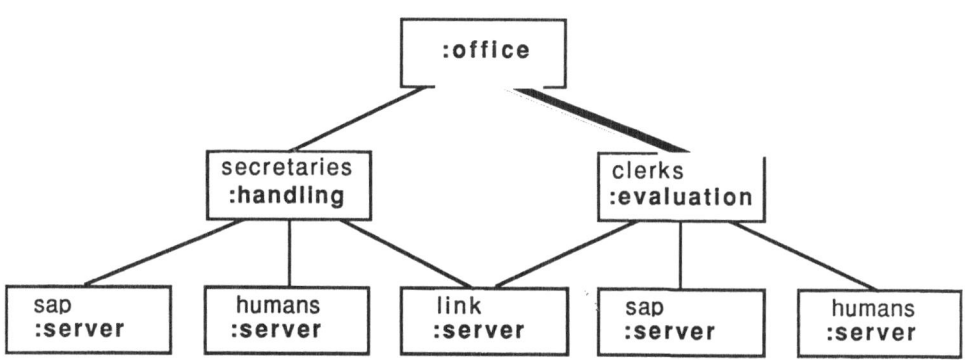

Fig. 2.1.6. COMPONENT TYPE, "evaluation", HIT-GRAFIX representation

Fig. 2.1.6 depicts the total "evaluation" type. *Fig. 2.1.7* exhibits the structure of the total model type, "office", specified so far.

Fig. 2.1.7. MODEL TYPE, "office", HIT-GRAFIX overview

63

3. HIT SYSTEM HANDLING

Specification of HIT models or model parts can obviously be prepared directly in HI-SLANG form using any normal text editor. Alternatively, the interactive HIT-GRAFIX user interface can be employed and component structures generated of an appearence as depicted in sect. 2.1. Frames of corresponding HI-SLANG component representations may then be generated automatically from these graphical representations, the algorithmic sections of the eventual, complete HI-SLANG form still to be manually inserted. HIT-GRAFIX will also supply a graphical representation of the total model structure, of an appearence as shown in sect. 2.1. Yet alternatively, or in combination with the sketched approaches, a control structure oriented editor, HIT-STAR, is available, which guides the user through the HI-SLANG syntax.

In all cases, a HI-SLANG model representation forms the basis for all following steps: The HI-SLANG compiler (see Müller and Weißenberg, 1986) translates the source code into SIMULA, which serves as host and target language for the HIT system; this compiler incorporates two different code generators, one of which will be employed depending upon the model evaluation technique selected (see sect. 4). Compilation of the SIMULA representation (inclusive of linking the selected evaluation module) and subsequent execution of the model follow, eventually furnishing all demanded analysis results in tabular and/or simple graphical forms.

A recent addition to the HIT toolbox is HIT-OMA, an object management facility, replacing an earlier used file management option. With OMA, all objects of a modelling and evaluation process such as model descriptions, listings and results, in all representation forms, can be stored in and retrieved from index sequential files called MOBASEs (modelling bases). The HI-SLANG compiler and all evaluation modules are capable of reading and writing mobase objects directly. OMA supports primarily the configuration process of HIT models and experiments with the help of particular objects called control files. OMA can, however, also be employed as proper user interface for the HIT system. An immediate value of a control file is its very existence as a single document describing precisely what a particular experiment was concerned with.

3.1 Illustration

We create a new mobase and enter our first configuration, employing OMA commands shown in *Fig. 3.1.1.* The first three ADDs concern the types of sect. 2.1, where the assumption is that all textual (HI- SLANG) objects had been created by some text editor and filed under their type names. All objects are given, as attributes, their representation, type and objectname. The experiment object will be described in 4.1. The control file named "configuration" is presented in *Fig. 3.1.2*, where allowed abbreviations are used due to lack of space.

The analysis of this model can be started by the OMA command, HIT, as displayed in *Fig. 3.1.3.* Listings and results are automatically written into the mobase under the objectname of the control file and can be displayed afterwards by SHOW.

More OMA commands exist for directory listing, for copying, selecting and erasing mobase objects, for changing object attributes, etc. The coding of OMA commands is greatly eased by flexible abbreviation options and default attribute values.

We are going to experiment with the model´s structure quite a bit. One of the configurations discussed in sect. 4.3 is depicted in *Fig. 3.1.4*: In comparison with *Fig. 2.1.7*, we will be

| NEWMOBASE | office.lib | | | creates a new mobase; |
| MOBASE | office.lib | | | this mobase is the actual mobase; |

	ADD office	TO	(HISLANG, MODEL,	office1)
	ADD handling	TO	(HISLANG, COMPONENT,	handling1)
	ADD evaluation	TO	(HISLANG, COMPONENT,	evaluation1)
	ADD experiment	TO	(HISLANG, EXPERIMENT,	expsep1)
	ADD configuration	TO	(CONTROL, CONTROL,	expsep1)

Fig. 3.1.1. Entering the first configuration into a new mobase

```
%COMMON ---------------- for compiler and analyzer------------------------------------
%MOBASE office.lib                               compiler and analyzer are to use
                                                 the same mobase;
%COMPILER ---------------configuration segment----------------------------------------
%BIND "this_office"        TO (HI, MOD, office1)   mobase object, office1, taken
                                                 as office of this model;
%BIND "this_handling"      TO (HI, COM, handling1)  analogously: handling,
%BIND "this_evaluation"    TO (HI, COM, evaluation1) evaluation
%BIND "this_experiment"    TO (HI, EXP , expsep1)   and expsep.

%ANALYZER --------------result "routing"----------------------------------------------
% comment: using defaults                        write all results (LISTING,
                                                 TABLE) to current mobase;
%END ----------------------model structure -------------------------------------------
%COPY "this_office"                              defining the modules
%COPY "this_handling"                            of this model
%COPY "this_evaluation"                          and their order of compilation;
%COPY "this_experiment"

%EOF ----------------------experiment description-------------------------------------
First experiment with the office model.          arbitrary comments;
```

Fig. 3.1.2. Control file for the first experiment

```
HIT       (CONTROL,  CONTROL,  expsep1)     start analysis;
SHOW      (DATA,     TABLE,    expsep1)     display results;
SHOW      (DATA,     LISTING,  expsep1)     display listing;
```

Fig. 3.1.3. Using OMA as HIT user interface

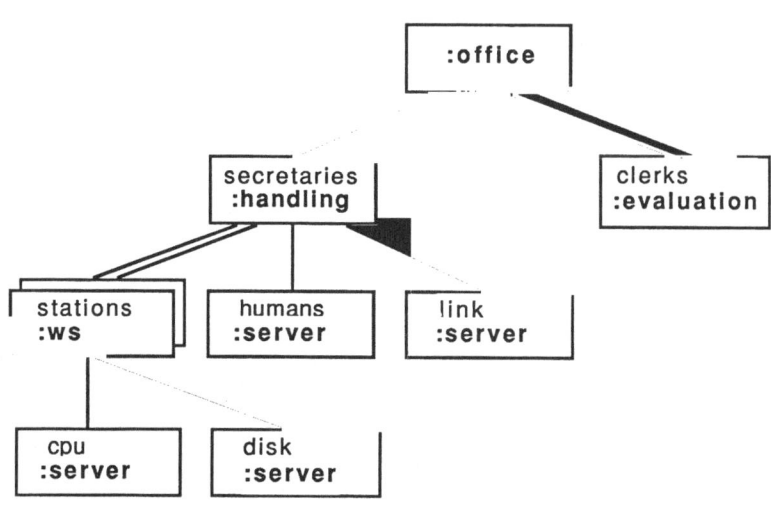

Fig. 3.1.4. Alternative office version: evaluation aggregated, sap substituted by two workstations.

dealing then with an aggregated representation of "evaluation", whereas refinements will take place in "handling", amounting to introducing, in the place of the formerly unstructured "sap" server, a vector of 2 workstations with their own "cpu"s and "disk"s. OMA supports the assembling of specified model parts in a new model configuration via the described "control files". Assuming the (refined) handling had been ADDed to the mobase under the name, "handling2", and the new (aggregated, PREANAlyzed) evaluation under "evaluation2", all that is necessary for a corresponding new experiment is to alter lines #5, 6 of *Fig. 3.1.2* to:

    %BIND "this_handling"   TO (HISLANG, COMPONENT, handling2)
    %BIND "this_evaluation" TO (PREANA , COMPONENT, evaluation2)

and to possibly adapt the experiment description to any new requirements.

4. MODEL EVALUATION AND EXPERIMENTS

Models are, of course, described to be analyzed. For this purpose, HIT incorporates a number of different evaluation techniques. At present, the following options are available:

* exact product-form solutions for "separable networks";
* approximate techniques for "large" separable networks;
* numerical evaluation of Markov-chain representations of general models;
* stochastic discrete-event simulation with appropriate statistical result estimation.

Additionally, emphasis is placed on sub-model analysis and subsequent aggregation with the objective of generating "equivalent" higher level representations, to be used in structured and/or heterogenous (total model) evaluation. Automatic aggregation and embedding is presently available for separable sub-models only. It must be stressed that HIT model specification (as described in section 2) is not directly influenced by the particular evaluation technique to be employed. There does, of course, exist an indirect influence whereby certain models will turn out not to be tractable by one or the other analysis technique, with simulation clearly offering the largest spectrum.

A so-called "experiment specification", separate from the model specification itself, must be furnished by the user to describe the results demanded from any particular model analysis. An experiment specification normally includes:

* an instantiation and parameterization of a model (of some specified model type);
* the specification of the model analysis technique to be applied;
* an indication of all "evaluation objects", i.e. of all model components to be assessed;
* indications of particular component characteristics ("performance indexes") to be evaluated for these evaluation objects.

Additional evaluation specifics may be necessary, such as (for simulation:) any rules for the start of data-gathering and for simulation termination. The employed separation of model and experiment specifications facilitates experimentation: One and the same model can be subjected to different experiments, with different kinds of results demanded. Finally, as not discussed above, the form of the results can be specified separately (tables of specifiable layouts, simple graphics, etc.).

4.1 Illustration

For the model type, "office", of sect. 2.1, we might be interested in performance values under different load conditions, say for 5,10 and 20 departments to be supported. The components to be evaluated are identified along the "contains"-hierarchy of the model; e.g., "off.secretaries.sap" is the "computer" within the secretaries´ office within the total office. Alias names (e.g. "s_sap") can be introduced for presentation purposes. The performance indexes to be calculated for these components can be picked from a standard set of indexes (this is mandatory for mathematical evaluation; simulation provides additional options, cf. sect. 4.5). A sample experiment specification is given in *Fig. 4.1.1*. This is the experiment description referred to in sect. 3.1.

EXPERIMENT office_analysis METHOD {...};	method depends on choice;
VARIABLE deps: INTEGER;	declarations for experiment block;
BEGIN	
FOR deps:= 5,10, 20 LOOP	different load situations;
EVALUATE MODEL off : office (deps);	instantiation of a particular model
EVALUATIONOBJECT	instance, "off", of type, "office";
s_off VIA off.secretaries,	identification of evaluation objects
s_sap VIA off.secretaries.sap,	and aliasing;
s_humans VIA off.secretaries.humans,	
{...c_off, c_sap, c_humans analogously}	
link VIA off.secretaries.link	also reachable by "off.clerks.link";
DEFAULT ESTIMATOR MEAN;	mean values demanded for the following, if not explicitly changed;
BEGIN	
MEASURE POPULATION	performance indexes to be
THROUGHPUT,	calculated;
TURNAROUNDTIME	
AT s_off DUE TO all;	DUE TO construct permits further
{...s_sap, s_humans, c_off, c_sap,	discrimination of measurements;
c_humans, link analogously}	such refinement is not employed,
END EVALUATE;	here;
END LOOP;	
END EXPERIMENT office_analysis;	

Fig. 4.1.1. Experiment specification for MODEL TYPE, "office"

4.2 Evaluation of product-form networks

A particular subclass of the models specifiable in HI-SLANG can be mapped onto the class of separable models (see Baskett et al., 1975). On user request, this mapping is performed automatically involving the corresponding code generator and evaluation module of the HIT system. The mapping is refused, should the model not meet the product form conditions. Covered is the full class of mixed, multi-chain/multi-class separable networks inclusive of all permitted state-dependencies of stations. The algorithm used for evaluation has evolved over the years, in Dortmund, guided by extensive practical application and experience. As it stands, it combines both convolution and mean value analysis types of ideas (see e.g. Reiser, 1979 and many follow-ups). An MVA-type algorithm, DOQ2 (Beilner, 1981), is first employed, aggregating all state-independent stations into a state-dependent substitute; DOQ2, although delivering not only the means of various performance indexes but also the normalization constants for all closed chain population vectors up to the requested limit vector, saves about a factor of 2 in time over "proper" MVA. The resulting substitute, together with the remaining state-dependent stations, is dealt with by a CONV-type algorithm, DOQ3 (Beilner and Noack). On top of the savings achieved by this (normally:) drastic reduction of the number of stations (from m=total nr. of stations to m'=1+nr. of state-dependent stations), DOQ3 saves an additional factor of approximately $m'/4$ over "proper" convolution, if performance indexes are requested for all stations. This is achieved by further exploitation of the decomposability properties of separable networks. DOQ3 will on demand also construct an aggregate of the total model in the form of a limited queue-dependent server with a state-dependency of the type discussed in Hong and Kim (1983). Relating this facility to the model specification domain, DOQ3 will in the aggregation case be confronted with a (more complex) COMPONENT and the task to aggregate this component into a (less complex) substitute component to be later embedded in a "larger" model. In this process, advantage is taken of the fact that a component provides well-specified services to its environment, that every (component-internal) service behaviour can be interpreted as a corresponding "chain" description and that, with the usual Norton-theorem based "shorting" procedure (see e.g. Chandy et al., 1975), the component can be analyzed for all "population" vectors (here: "nr. of services in progress"-vectors) up to some limit vector; with proper bookkeeping of intermediate results, the whole procedure boils, of course, down to just one DOQ3-execution.

4.3 Illustration

Models and experiment of sect´s 2.1, 4.1 conform with the separability conditions. Analysis can be demanded by setting ...METHOD ANALYTICAL "separable". *Table 4.3.1* shows the corresponding results of experiment #1 (for readability´s sake not copied from printer output).

The first conclusions are fairly obvious: Of the capacity-restricted servers (c_sap, s_sap, link), s_sap is clearly the bottleneck. What if it were not? Arbitrarily many s_sap units are introduced by changing (cf. *Fig.2.1.4a*: instantiation of "sap") the dispatch strategy of that server from "shared" to "equal" - the Infinite Server case. The new experiment #2 is easily configurated with the help of OMA. From the results of this experiment (another table like *Table 4.3.1*) we learn that "link" is now the bottleneck, being utilized to 79% at the 20 dep´s load, and showing correspondingly increased transmission times. This is hopeless - we have to move towards faster communication. An eventual LAN solution for allover office support is considered anyway, with a transmission rate of (at least) 1Mbps. Let us try that: Changing the dispatch strategy of "link" (cf. *Fig. 2.1.4a*) from "shared" to "shared(100)" gives it the 100-fold speed. The corresponding experiment #3 reveals that link utilization is now well below 1%. With a LAN solution, the overall system architecture will have to be changed. In particular, for the secretaries´ office (where we remember from exp. #1 a certain bottleneck problem), some number of workstation type units are considered with their own cpu´s and local disk units, and each serving a certain set of secretaries. In order to ease experimentation with various such configurations we undertake a few preparatory steps. First, as the LAN will obviously not be burdened solely by the load we are just investigating, and as we are not now in a position to predict overall LAN load, we leave the LAN utilization question for later, keeping (as a mere reminder) the transmission requests as simple time delays in the model (independent "equal(100)", i.e. IS-type with 100-fold speed, "link"s in both sub-offices). The same argument applies for a (not yet existing) "file server". Second, as the clerks´ office presents no performance problems at all (to be read off all 3 above experiments), we will not concern ourselves with its "interiour" any more and decide

Table 4.3.1. Results of experiment #1

At:	# dep´s	Population	Thr´put*sec	Turn´time/sec	Utilization
c_off	5	1,586	0,00124	1284	
	10	2,744	0,00212	1298	
	20	3,270	0,00250	1309	
c_humans	5	1,482	0,03090	48	
	10	2,538	0,05290	48	
	20	2,998	0,06250	48	
c_sap	5	0,038	0,01850	2,1	0,037
	10	0,067	0,03170	2,1	0,063
	20	0,081	0,03750	2,2	0,075
link	5	0,242	0,06790	3,6	0,204
	10	0,509	0,11600	4,4	0,349
	20	0,700	0,13700	5,1	0,412
s_off	5	3,414	0,00247	1382	
	10	7,256	0,00423	1716	
	20	16,730	0,00500	3348	
s_humans	5	2,470	0,12300	20	
	10	4,230	0,21100	20	
	20	4,996	0,25000	20	
s_sap	5	0,768	0,12300	6	0,494
	10	2,656	0,21100	13	0,846
	20	11,225	0,25000	45	0,999

			Thr´put*day	Turn´time/h	
report	5		17,86	2,25	
	10		30,53	2,63	
	20		36,00	4,45	

```
EXPERIMENT aggregate_evaluation METHOD ANALYTICAL "separable";
BEGIN
    AGGREGATE evaluation;
        CREATE 17 PROCESS archive;
        CREATE 17 PROCESS examine;
    END AGGREGATE;
END EXPERIMENT aggregate_evaluation;
```

Fig. 4.3.2. Experiment specification for aggregation of "evaluation"

to aggregate it. Experiment #4 (cf. *Fig. 4.3.2*) performs that aggregation, establishing for "evaluation" a substitute component type.

Let us have a look at the results needed for constructing this substitute, basically the throughput values of the two provided services (examine and archive) depending upon the pair of (#examine´s, #archive´s)-present, in all combinations. With a side-look on *Fig´s 2.1.5a/b* it comes as no surprise (unlimited # of clerks, totally underloaded link) that the two services do not impact upon each other, and that the archive throughput is linearly dependent on the #archive´s present:

archive.throughput=0.0017*#archive´s/sec.

The remaining dependency of the examine throughput on the #examine´s is depicted in *Fig. 4.3.3*. The dashed line depicts the linear case which is but slightly violated, confirming the "harmlessness" of the clerks´office.

We have now arrived at a structure as depicted in *Fig. 3.1.4*. If you inspect that figure closely, you see the "stations" of type "ws" (for: workstation) as a "thicker" box, indicating that we are prepared for an array of "ws"-instances, i.e. some set of stations. How many, will have to be determined now; incidentally also, how many screens (and humans) to be connected to a single workstation. The "interior" of the ws type must be specified for that. Just very shortly, because of space reasons: Every ws instance is designed to provide two services, a "long_update" and a "short_update" (compare with *Fig. 2.1.3*); both update services cycle through cpu and disk usage, the respective time durations determined from hardware and operating system characteristics of considered equipment (about twice as fast cpu´s as the PC originally considered as "sap", cf. *Fig´s 2.1.3/4*; about 40 msec access time for one disk track; about 20 cycles per up-

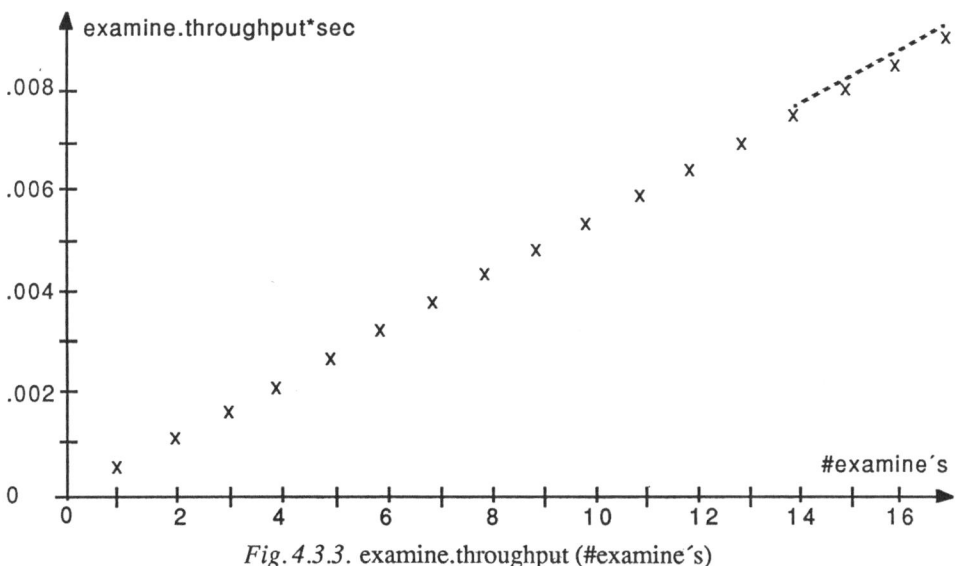

Fig. 4.3.3. examine.throughput (#examine´s)

Table 4.3.4. Results of experiment #6 (IS mode) and #7 (PS/FCFS mode)

At:	mode	Population	Thr´put*sec.	Turn´time/sec	Utilization
c_off	IS	7,029	0,0057	1236	
	PS/FCFS	5,669	0,0046	1235	
s_off	IS	12,971	0,0114	1141	
	PS/FCFS	14,331	0,0092	1561	
s_humans	IS	11,372	0,5686	20	
	PS/FCFS	9,180	0,4590	20	
s_sap	IS	1,592	0,5686	2,8	
	PS/FCFS	5,145	0,4590	11,2	
s_ws_cpu	IS	1,137	11,3720	0,10	
	PS/FCFS	4,578	9,1805	0,50	0,92
s_ws_disk	IS	0,455	11,3720	0,04	
	PS/FCFS	0,566	9,1805	0,06	0,37

At:	mode		Thr´put*day	Turn´time/h	
report	IS		81,94	1,95	
	PS/FCFS		66,10	2,42	

date). With these decisions we assess the two extreme situations, namely arbitrarily many work-stations (experiment # 6, both cpu and disk of IS type behaviours) and just one workstation (experiment #7, with the CPU of PS and the disk of FCFS type); we display some of the results in *Table 4.3.4*, the #dep´s kept at the maximum value of 20.

The interpretation: Although the throughput of reports is in both cases well over the re-quested 20/day, the utilization of the single s_ws_cpu is with 0.92 dangerously high. On the other hand, the population at s_ws_cpu is even at the "infinitely many" case with 1.14 just over 1. So, we decide for 2 workstations in the secretaries´office. Another conclusion: The population at s_off, in the modelled case of arbitrarily many screens/secretaries, just varies between 13 and 14+; so, 14 or even fewer screens should do, in any case.

4.4 Numerical evaluation of Markov-chains

Continuing from sect. 4.2, a further class of HI-SLANG-specifiable models can be inter-preted as generators of corresponding time-continuous Markov-chains. For such a model, the system of global balance equations can be set up automatically and solved for the stationary state distribution by numerical techniques (cf. e.g. Stewart, 1978). Analytic-numerical evalua-tion is possible in HIT for models which cover (most of) the separable class, extended by fea-tures for modelling synchronization aspects, general passive resources, restricted waiting rooms, priority and random multi-class service disciplines and a certain class of degradable multi-servers applicable for fault-tolerance problems.

The techniques employed in Dortmund for numerical evaluation have also grown over the years, and much of the experience with our earlier tool, NUMAS (Müller, 1984), has been port-ed to HIT. Next to the definition of a suitable model class, automatic set-up and storage of the generator matrix present major problems, which are dealt with by a follow-up module to one of the code-generators of the HI-SLANG compiler, and with extended use of sparse matrix tech-niques, respectively. For the evaluation of the stationary distribution, finally, three different al-gorithms are available, one of which is selected by HIT depending on the problem at hand. A di-rect algorithm based on Gaussian elimination is employed for smaller state spaces, whereas for larger state spaces an iterative, a Gauss-Seidel type algorithm is utilized. In the latter case a dras-tic speed-up of the evaluation is achieved for models with NCD properties by inserting, into the Gauss-Seidel iteration, occasional convergence-accelerating aggregation steps (cf. Müller, 1981).

We spend some lines on just one of the additional modelling features, the standard, bot-tom-level component type, "counter", applicable for various synchronization, restricted space and passive resource problems. A counter manages basically a vector of integers. It is instantiated (implicitly) with the vector´s length, say: n, and (explicitly) with an "init" vector (initial values), a "max" vector (upper limit values) and a "min" vector (lower limit values). A counter provides a service, "change (<n-vector of integers>)". From a certain internal "state", $(x[1], x[2], ..., x[n])$, the counter will upon the request, "change $(c[1], c[2], ..., c[n])$", perform the operation $(x[1], ..., x[n]) := (x[1], ..., x[n]) + (c[1], ..., c[n])$, iff the result falls within the (min,max) range, for all vector positions. If not, the operation is not performed and the request-issuing process (a service) halted. Eventual continuation of a halted process occurs only after the state vector has been suitably "changed" (by some other process). A particular scheduling rule (also specified explicitly upon counter instantiation) resolves any competition situations. The "counter" can quite obviously be employed as semaphore, token pool, etc. More application examples can be found in Müller-Clostermann and Rosentreter (1987).

4.5 Simulation

The broadest model class can, of course, be analyzed by simulation. HI-SLANG must in this respect be viewed as a full-fledged High-Level-Language, incorporating the usual data structures and data operations, providing the usual control structures enhanced by concurrency features and offering all performance modelling constructs described in the sections above. The concept of autonomous components is easily interpreted as one of operationalized Abstract Data Types, and the desired bridge between performance and correctness related issues becomes available by the possibility to assess performance *and* test code correctness of systems described in HI-SLANG.

The performance related analyses are based on the concept of STREAMs, sequential samples (time series, trajectories) of observed variables. Three different classes of streams are available, each necessitating a specific approach of statistical analysis:

* STREAMs of type EVENT serve for the serial recording of values;
  example: turnaround times (response times) of service executions at a (of a) component;
* STREAMs of type STATE encode the history of piecewise constant state variables;
  example: population (number of) service executions "present" in a component;
* STREAMs of type COUNT keep track of occurrences of events;
  example: throughput (of service executions) of a component.

Certain streams (response times, populations, utilizations, etc.) are provided as standards and fed automatically with data. The user can define his own, additional streams and feed them by purpose-tailored code.

Statistical stream analysis employs a time-series approach. The inevitable autocorrelation problem intrinsic to that approach is taken care of by adapting techniques for the identification and parameter estimation of autoregressive, statistical models (cf. e.g. Fishman, 1978). HIT uses an online-update version of these techniques (Litzba, 1985) which has also evolved over the years, in Dortmund, and now replaces the earlier used batch means and replication approaches (cf. COPE, Beilner and Mäter, 1984). The main advantage of the autoregressive approach can be seen in the fact that the user is not normally requested to supply any parameters for statistical estimation purposes and will still be provided with correct estimates of means, variances and confidence intervals. More precisely speaking, experience has shown that with a standard order of 20 for the autoregressive models a good compromise between result precision and estimation overhead is (almost) always attained. The latter is kept at a low level by a "self-adaptive" convergence planning scheme which reduces the number of (autoregressive model) parameter estimations.

Simulator execution, as a whole, can be controlled by specifying maximum model time, maximum execution (CPU) time, maximum number of particular events, maximum width of particular confidence intervals. A certain degree of interactive control of the simulator´s execution is possible by demanding the display of intermediate results, at regularly or irregularly spaced display instants, and by the possibility of consequently stopping or continuing the simulation.

4.6 Illustration

We continue from sect. 4.3. It has so far not concerned us that there is, amongst the documents dealt with in the office, one central document in joint use and allowing only exclusive access. It is known from actual operations that about 1 out of 10 accesses is to a page of that central document, which has to be locked in total during the corresponding ("edit") activity. For modelling that situation, we employ a 1-dimensional counter instance as binary "semaphore", i.e. with a state range of {0,1} and an initial state of 1. We then bracket that part of the edit activity which is concerned with an individual page (cf. *Fig. 2.1.3*: from just before "fetch" until just after "store") with the usual P/V-operations pair, a "change(-1)" before and a "change(+1)" after. More precisely, the brackets are only encountered with probability 0.1 ("every tenth time, on average"). The corresponding model is now outside the "separable" class, but without any further alterations of its specification amenable to both numerical evaluation and simulation.

We make a big step now: To be in a position of embedding the whole secretaries´office in a larger model and to efficiently continue experimenting, we attempt to aggregate that office, i.e. create a substitute component for it. HIT will not (yet) do that automatically for us, in the non-separable case at hand. We can, however, apply the "shorting" procedure "by hand" in a series of experiments determining the "edit" throughput through "secretaries", for 1, 2,... edit activities concurrently in progress. *Fig. 4.6.1* depicts the results obtained. For #edit´s up to 5, numerical evaluation has been used; for #edit´s above 5 it becomes more economical to employ simulation but with the price to be paid of obtaining only statistically "uncertain" results. (*Fig. 4.6.1* shows 95% confidence intervals for mean throughputs, the simulator being stopped when these intervals´ widths fall below 10% of the corresponding point estimates).

An additional, upper curve is marked in *Fig. 4.6.1* by the "+" signs: This is the throughput dependency for the "handling" version *without* data locks (received by automatic algebraic aggregation). You will notice that it is imperative to acknowledge the lock influence for higher "edit" populations.

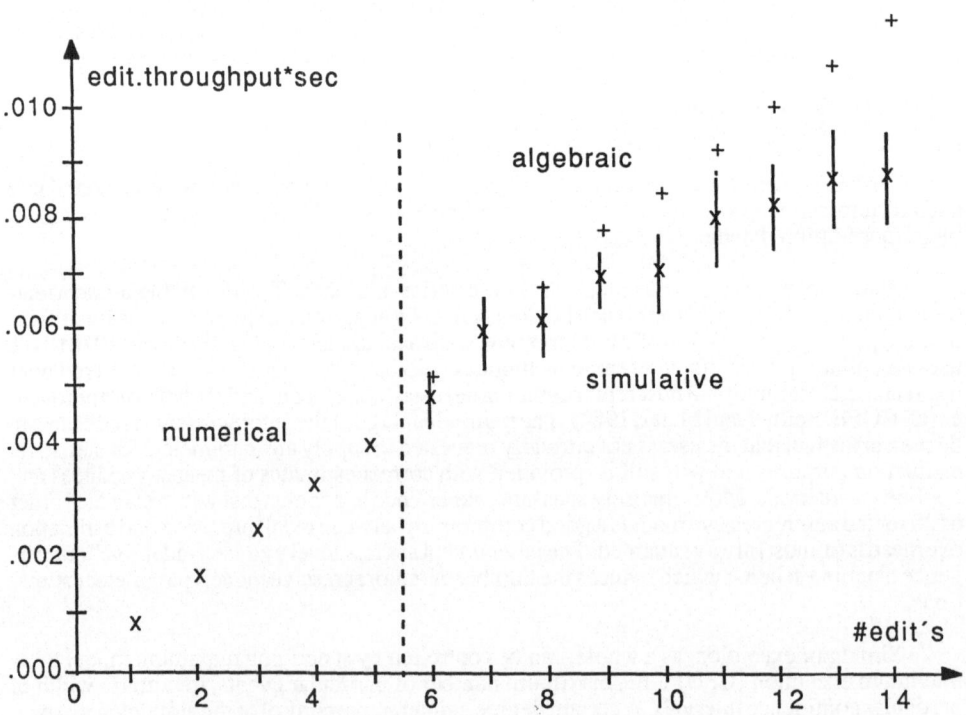

Fig. 4.6.1. edit.throughput(#edit´s), manual and automatic aggregation of 2 different "handling" versions

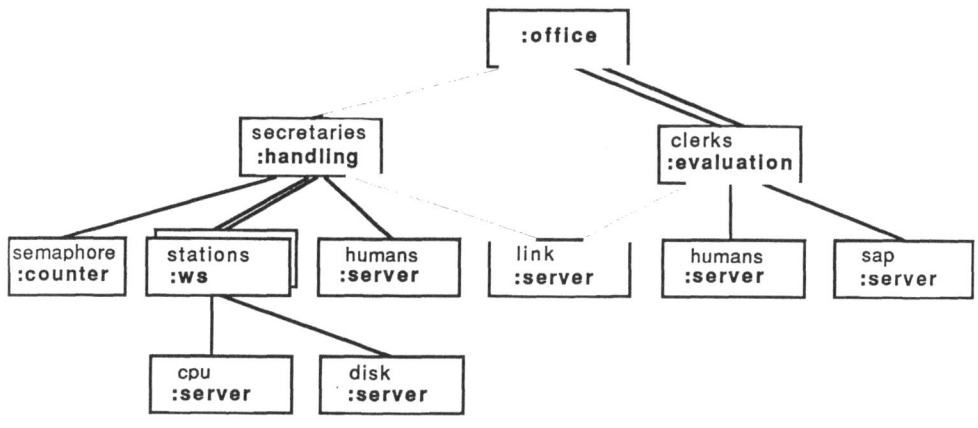

Fig. 4.6.2. Detailed office structure

Let us become very short now: Embedding the lock-including handling version in the upper office (a very small model, as the office now includes just one handling aggregate and one evaluation aggregate) renders a model which becomes again amenable to efficient algebraic evaluation. The results? A report throughput, for the 20 dep´s case, of 61.1/day with an average report turnaround time of 2.6 h (as opposed to, were the lock not considered, 77.2/day and 2.1 h). We should now, as promised right at the beginning of sect. 2.1, lower the load again to a realistic level. Step 1: Alter the "report" body (*Fig. 2.1.1*) by removing the outer (never-ending) LOOP. Step 2: Alter the "report" instantiation code (*Fig. 2.1.2a*) to

CREATE 1 PROCESS report EVERY negexp (departments/28800);

i.e. 1 report per work-day per department at random instants. Results at 20 dep´s: An average report turnaround time of 2.0 h with an average report population (# of report activities in progress) of 5.1. Looks allright, does it not?

We could obviously go on and, with relatively little effort, shift our center of concentration from one aspect to the next, actually *understanding*, where the performance problems are and what must be done to avoid them.

Incidentally, we might be asked why did we not always evaluate the total model in all detail. Well, the total structure is now as shown in *Fig. 4.6.2*. With the various characteristics discussed, the only evaluation technique left for that model is simulation. Simulating that model turns out no fun at all: After having simulated a model time of over 2 work-days (equivalent to about 2 h of CPU-time on a 1.2 MIPS processor) you find still some 95% confidence intervals, for performance indexes, of a width of over 20% - *and* you are left with comparatively little insight into the key problems of the system to be designed.

5. PRESENT STATUS AND FUTURE DEVELOPMENTS

Focussing on recent extensions of HIT in the direction of establishing an integrated performance modelling environment, we have not attempted to give an overview over this software system which is in any sense complete. A broader account of HIT features is provided in Müller-Clostermann (1988).

HIT has been developed under the Siemens BS2000 operating system and is also operational in IBM MVS environments. Portations are underway to UNIX installations with a particular emphasis on graphics based model specification and result representation facilities. On the evaluation side, a linearizer type algorithm (cf. e.g. Chandy and Neuse, 1982) has more recently been added supporting an efficient (approximate) solution of large separable models. Further in the approximation direction, algorithms covering priority stations and multiclass FCFS stations are in an extensive test stage. Inclusion of performance bounds approaches (cf. e.g. Eager and Sevcik, 1986) is also scheduled for this year. More fundamental research is concerned with broadening the aggregation capabilities of HIT. Last not least, there are "zillions" of smaller improvements constantly being achieved aiming at broader applicability and higher acceptability.

Recent "serious" applications by HIT users include studies of file catalog and lock managements, assessments of pipeline architectures and optical disk devices, evaluation of LAN controller designs and workstation cluster configurations, in total demonstrating the high versatility and flexibility of the HIT modelling environment.

6. REFERENCES

Baskett, F., Chandy, K. M., Muntz, R. R. and Palacious, F. G., 1975, Open, Closed and Mixed Networks of Queues with Different Classes of Customers, JACM, vol. 22, no. 2

Beilner, H., 1981, "Algorithms for Evaluating Separable, Mixed, State-Independent Queueing Networks or Improving (Slightly) on Mean Value Analysis", Forschungsbericht Fachbereich Informatik Universität Dortmund, Nr. 124

Beilner, H., ed., 1985, "Messung, Modellierung und Bewertung von Rechensystemen", Informatik-Fachberichte, vol. 110, Springer

Beilner, H. and Mäter, J., 1985, COPE: Past, Presence and Future, in: Potier (1985)

Beilner, H. and Noack, F., "DOQ3: Yet another algorithm for Mixed Separable Networks", in preparation

Beilner, H. and Scholten, H., 1985, Strukturierte Modellbeschreibung und strukturierte Modellanalyse: Konzepte des Modellierungswerkzeuges HIT, in: Beilner (1985)

Beilner, H. and Stewing, F. J., 1987, Concepts and Techniques of the Performance Modelling Tool, HIT, in: "Discrete Event Simulation and Operation Research", Adelsberger, H. H. and Broeckx, F. , ed´s., Simulation Councils

Chandy, K. M., Herzog, U. and Woo, L., 1975, Parametric Analysis of Queueing Networks, IBM Journal Res. Dev., vol. 19, no. 1

Chandy, K. M.and Neuse, D., 1982, Linearizer: A Heuristic Algorithm for Queueing Network Models of Computing Systems, CACM, vol. 25, no. 2

Eager, D. L. and Sevcik, K. C., 1986, Bound Hierarchies for Multiple Class Queueing Networks, JACM, vol. 33, no. 1

Fishman, G. S., 1978, "Principles of Discrete Event Simulation", John Wiley & Son

Hong, J. P. and Kim, G. , 1983, Class Dependent Queueing Disciplines with Product Form Solutions, in: "Performance ´83", Agrawala, A. K., Tripathi and S. K. , ed´s., North Holland

Jobmann, M. R., 1985, Modellbildung und -analyse von Rechensystemen mit Hilfe des Programmsystems MAOS, in: Beilner (1985)

Litzba, D., 1985, "Auswertung von Simulationsdaten mittels autoregressiver Modelle", Forschungsbericht Fachbereich Informatik Universität Dortmund, Nr. 203

Müller, B., 1982, Decomposition Methods in the Construction and Numerical Solution of Queuing Network Models, in: "Performance ´81", F. J. Kylstra, ed., Amsterdam, North Holland

Müller, B., 1985, NUMAS: A Tool for the Numerical Modelling of Computer Systems, in: Potier (1985)

Müller-Clostermann, B., 1988, " HIT - An Introduction", Projektbericht, Informatik IV, Universität Dortmund,

Müller-Clostermann, B. and Rosentreter, G., 1987, Synchronized Queueing Networks, Concepts, Examples and Evaluation Techniques, in: Herzog, U. and Paterok M., ed´s., "Informatik Fachberichte", vol.154, Springer

Müller, B. and Weißenberg, N., 1986, Using SIMULA 67 for the Implementation of a Hierarchical Tool for Modelling and Performance Evaluation of Computing Systems, in: "Proc. 14th SIMULA Users´Conference", Stockholm

Potier, D., ed., 1985, "Modelling Techniques and Tools for Performance Analysis", North Holland

Reiser, M., 1979, Mean Value Analysis of Queueing Networks - A New Look at an Old Problem, in: "Performance of Computer Systems", Arató, M., Butrimenko, A., Gelenbe, E., ed´s, North Holland

Sauer, C. H. and MacNair, E. A., 1985, The Evolution of the Research Queueing Package, in: Potier (1985)

Stewart, W. J., 1978, A comparison of numerical techniques in Markov modelling, CACM, vol.21, no. 2

Veran, M. and Potier, D., 1985, QNAP2: A Portable Environment for Queueing Systems Models, in: Potier (1985)

Wolf, H., 1986, Outil de Modélisation et d´Evaluation HIT, Journées d´Etudes Modélisation et Evaluation de Systèmes Informatique, Sophia Antipolis

... ...

LANSF – A MODULAR SYSTEM FOR MODELLING

LOW-LEVEL COMMUNICATION PROTOCOLS

Pawel Gburzynski[1] and Piotr Rudnicki[1]

Department of Computing Science
The University of Alberta
Edmonton, Alberta, Canada T6G 2H1

ABSTRACT: We present LANSF – a modular programming system for modeling communication protocols at the Medium Access Control level. The most interesting aspects of such protocols manifest themselves in Local Area Networks. LANSF is based on an exact model of communication channels which reflects all relevant elements of their temporal behaviour. The system offers a collection of tools for defining network architectures, specifying protocols, defining traffic conditions, modeling, and tracing the network behaviour on-line. Although originally designed for modeling Local Area Networks, LANSF was successfully used for investigating other distributed systems. LANSF runs under UNIX[2] and is available upon request from the authors.

1. Introduction

The software system presented in this paper was written after the authors had become stuck with never ending and increasingly burdensome modifications of a number of its specialised, individually hand-coded predecessors. Those programs, originally written as very efficient simulators of some specific MAC-level protocols, were adapted a number of times to model other protocols. In many cases the modifications were both painful and obscure; eventually, it became clear that some drastic solution must be sought. During those experiments we had noticed that all the simulators had many common features; however, they lacked a common denominator. Having abandoned the old solutions we have decided to start the work from scratch and ... write again a number of dedicated simulators, but at the least possible effort.

The solution consisted in creating a set of predefined modules (C files) which, after supplying some additional, protocol-dependent modules, can be configured into specific simulators. These standard modules offer tools for: defining network topologies, describing traffic conditions, modeling physical carriers, event-driven discrete simulation of the time flow, on-line monitoring of the network behaviour, and collecting performance statistics. The standard modules alone do not constitute a complete runnable program. The behaviour of stations (i.e. the protocol) must be defined in a separate module. Then a specific instance of the system can be created – a program which simulates the behaviour of a class of networks. This class is further parametrised by a set of input data which specify: the number of stations, the traffic conditions, the lengths of channels, etc.

---

[1] This work was supported in part by NSERC grants no. OGP9183 and OGP9107.

[2] UNIX is a trademark of AT&T Bell Laboratories.

The user-supplied protocol specification is contained in a C file. Protocols are programmed with the help of a number of primitive functions built into LANSF. The code of a protocol looks like a natural description of interrupt driven processes, although the coding is done entirely in C. Recently a similar approach was reported by Bagrodia et al. ([BCM87]) to message based discrete-event simulation.

An important feature of LANSF is the built-in accurate model of the communication channel. Modelling in LANSF is (or at least can be) exact, so that from the viewpoint of the communication phenomena the model emulates the underlying physical system. Certain expermental results obtained by the present authors (e.g. [GbR87]. [GbR88b], [GbR88c]) indicate that accurate modeling of MAC-level protocols often reveals hidden implementation problems. Due to these problems, some theoretical anticipations regarding the protocol performance may not hold in reality (cf. [GbR88b], [GbR88c]).

LANSF has been used to develop a number of new protocols and re-examine the performance of numerous known protocols for Local Area Networks. These include: some variations of Ethernet [GMW87], Virtual Token [GbR87], CSMA/CD-DP [KiK83], Hybrid Token-CSMA/CD [GoW85], Tree Collision Resolution [Mol85], Token Ring [Sta86], Hubnet [HTW86]. Although LANSF was originally intended as a tool for simulating LAN's, we have come up with a system in which wide-area networks can also be described and modeled. Recently we are experimenting with Blazenet [HaC87]. Some of our colleagues apply LANSF for modeling distributed data bases. Multiprocessor architectures (e.g. n-cube) are also suitable for modeling in LANSF.

The limited space of this paper does not allow us to present all technical details - they are contained in [GbR88]. Here we describe the key ideas and principles on which LANSF is based, and present a number of examples. The paper is organised as follows: In section 2 we introduce the basic terminology. Section 3 contains a brief description of the LANSF protocol definition language. In section 4 we give some hints on the user interface. Section 5 discusses four examples. Final remarks in section 6 conclude the paper.

2. Basic Terminology

2.1. Network Configuration: Links, Ports, Stations

By a communication system we understand a number of *stations* which exchange messages. The stations are interconnected via *links* which are the message passing media (communication channels). Stations are connected to links via *ports*. Each port connects a single station to a single link. Using separate ports, a station can be connected to more than one link, and more than once to a single link. If a station wants to pass a message to another station, it inserts an *activity* into one of its ports. The activity propagates along the corresponding link and reaches all ports connected to it. If both parties are connected to the same link, they can communicate directly; otherwise, their communication must involve other (relaying) stations.

For example, a bus-type network, e.g. *Ethernet* ([Sta86]), consists of a single link and a number of stations, each station having a single port to the link. A ring network, e.g. *Token Ring* ([Sta86]), is built of a number of stations and the same number of links. Each station is connected to exactly two links. In Hubnet [HTW86], there are $n+1$ stations and $n+1$ links. One of the links (the broadcast link) interconnects all stations. The central station (the hub) is connected to every other station via a dedicated (selection) link. Thus the hub has $n+1$ ports, while regular stations have two ports each.

2.2. Time units, bits, and distances

In LANSF time is discrete. Time instants are denoted by natural numbers. The interval between two consecutive time instants is called the *Indivisible Time Unit* (*ITU*). The experimenter is responsible for establishing the correspondence between *ITU* and an interval of real time. This correspondence is irrelevant from the viewpoint of LANSF. Practically, the granularity of the modeled time may be arbitrarily low (in the present implementation of LANSF, time instants are represented as integer binary numbers up to 155 bits long).

The information sent by stations through links is organised into finite sequences of *bits* called *packets*. With each port we associate its *transmission rate*, a positive natural number which says how many *ITU*'s are required to insert a single bit into the port. Different ports, even those connected to the same link, can have different transmission rates.

The geometry of a link is described by a distance matrix which specifies the distance between each pair of ports, expressed as the propagation time in *ITU*'s. The distance between two ports connected to different links is undefined. Note that *ITU* has to be chosen in such a way that the transmission rates of all ports and all distances are expressible as its multiples.

2.3. Activities, Servers and Events

The experimenter defines a collection of processes describing the behaviour of each station. These processes constitute the network protocol. From the viewpoint of the modeled system, all the processes run concurrently. More than one process can be associated with a station. Processes can generate various *activities* that result in *events*. The transformation of activities into events is done by the built-in handlers called *servers*. These are: the port servers, the *timer*, the *signaler*, and the *client*. Each server models a certain part of the station's environment. Processes communicate with servers by calling LANSF functions (see section 3).

For all ports connected to one link, the collection of their servers constitutes the link server which models a single communication channel. The link server is visible by station processes exclusively through port servers. The link server processes activities inserted by stations and predicts future events on ports. In the case when there is only one activity in the link, the link server simply simulates its propagation along the carrier and predicts when particular ports will hear it. When multiple activities are present in the link at the same time, the situation becomes more complex: the link server has to determine when two (or more) of such activities interfere. An interference of two or more activities is interpreted as a col-lision. The formal semantics of a link is given in [GbR88a].

Processes belonging to a single station may exchange internal signals (interrupts) which are not transmitted through links. The passing of signals among processes is controlled by the *signaler*. The purpose of signals is to provide synchronisation primitives for processes (see examples 5.2 and 5.3). The *timer* provides each process with a general purpose alarm clock (see 3.5). The network traffic is supplied by the so-called *client* server which is external to stations. The client can be viewed as a *daemon* interfacing the network with the outer world (see 3.3). The client generates messages and queues them at stations. A station can request to be interrupted by the client when a new message arrives.

3. Programming protocols in LANSF

LANSF is a collection of modules (C files) that can be configured into an event driven simulator. The modules defining the protocol have to be supplied by the experimenter. The configuration of the network and the parameters of the traffic to be investigated are read as input data (see 4).

3.1. Protocol module

The user-defined protocol is described by a collection of processes associated with stations. The code of a process is specified as a C function. The protocol definition must contain the following elements: the declaration of non-standard station attributes, the definition of processes to be run by stations, and the declarations of two functions in_protocol and out_protocol. The function in_protocol is called by LANSF at the beginning of simulation – to initialise variables, read the protocol-specific input, create, and then start the processes. The function out_protocol is invoked at the end of simulation and its purpose is to print out the protocol-specific results.

The number of processes at a station is arbitrary – usually a single process executes some logically separable set of protocol functions. For example, in the case of the Ethernet protocol, it is natural to have two processes at a station, namely the transmitter and the receiver (see 5.1). Similarly, for the token ring, there are two processes per station – each process servicing one port (see 5.2). For Hubnet, there are three processes at each regular station: transmitter, receiver, and acknowledger, and *n* processes at the hub, where *n* is the number of regular stations (see 5.3).

3.2. Processes

The code of a process (the process function) can be shared by a number of actual processes. In particular, some (or all) stations may obey the same protocol and share the same process functions (e.g. Ethernet). A process is created by the following function:

```
new_process (code, version)
int    (*code)(), version;
```

which takes the pointer to the C function representing the process body as the first argument, and the process version number as the second argument. The purpose of the process version is to tell apart multiple processes running the same code at the same station (cf. section 5.3). No two processes with the same `code` and `version` can be defined at one station at the same time. The function pointed to by `code` will be called whenever the execution of the process is resumed. Global integer variable `process_version` will then contain the value of `version`.

The environment of a process is described by the contents of the global variables `station`, `action`, `process_version`, `the_packet`, and `the_port`. Variable `station` is the pointer to a data structure representing the station to which the process belongs. Variable `action` is an integer value used to identify the entry point of the process. Immediately after a new process is created, it is started with the value of `action` equal `INITIALIZE`. This standard and protocol-independent entry point should contain the initialisation code of the process. The last two variables (`the_packet` and `the_port`) are used to pass additional information to the process. For example, if the process is restarted due to a packet being heard at one of the station's ports (see section 3.5), `the_packet` points to a data structure representing the packet and `the_port` identifies the port.

A process can be either active or suspended. An active process suspends itself by executing `return`. Before doing so, the process can specify a set of events that may wake it up in the future. When a process is active, it can tell the simulated time by looking into the global variable `current_time`. The simulated time does not flow when a process is active.

3.3. Messages and packets

The client server maintains a message queue at each station. The arrival of new messages (the traffic pattern) is described in the input data set as a collection of the so-called *message types*. A single message type can be viewed as the description of a single arrival process with specific distributions of the inter-arrival time and the message length. A message type can be declared as biased (not all stations contribute equally to the traffic) and/or bursty (messages arrive in bursts). Non-standard processes which generate messages can be programmed (LANSF offers tools for it), should the built-in means become insufficient.

Messages are split into packets according to the minimum and maximum packet length defined by the protocol. Whenever a station wants to acquire the next packet for transmission it calls the function:

```
int    get_next_packet (min, max, frm)
int    min, max, frm;
```

The three parameters of `get_next_packet` are the minimum packet length, the maximum packet length, and the length of the frame information respectively. All these lengths are specified in bits. If the value returned by the function is 0 (*false*), it means that the message queue is empty and there is nothing to transmit at this moment. In such a case, the station can wait for a message arrival from the client (see 3.5); otherwise, the next packet is put into the packet buffer (structure `current_packet`). The packet buffer is emptied by calling `release_current_packet ()`. The following function must be called by the receiver of a packet as soon as the packet is completely received.

```
accept_packet (packet, port_id)
PACKET  *packet;
int     port_id;
```

This function updates the performance measures of the network. A station can learn from the port server that it is receiving a packet (see 3.5).

3.4. Starting and terminating link activities

Each activity which exists in a link has been inserted into it by a station. There are two kinds of link activities: a packet transfer and a jamming signal. The following functions are used to start and terminate activities.

```
start_transfer (port_id, packet)
int      port_id;
PACKET   packet;
```

By calling start_transfer, a station starts transmitting a packet (which is described by the contents of structure packet) on port port_id. The transfer lasts until the station terminates it by either stop_transfer or abort_transfer.

```
stop_transfer  (port_id)
abort_transfer (port_id)
int      port_id;
```

Function stop_transfer is used when the entire packet has been successfully transmitted. The second function aborts the transfer of a partially sent packet, e.g. after a collision. The timer can be used to determine when the packet has been entirely transmitted (see 3.5). The following two functions control the emission of jamming signals.

```
start_jam (port_id)
stop_jam  (port_id)
int      port_id;
```

3.5. Wait requests

Before a process puts itself to sleep (by executing return) it can specify events which will wake it up in the future. It is done by calling the following function.

```
wait_event (s,e,a)
```

The parameters identify:

s - the server expected to generate the waking event; it can be CLIENT, TIMER, SIGNAL, or a port identifier.

e - an event type appropriate for server s.

a - a user defined integer value.

After the waking event e occurs at server s, the process is restarted (its function is called) and the value of a is passed to the process in global variable action. The variable action is meant to identify the entry point of the restarted process. Thus the most natural way of organising the process code is to make it a single switch instruction controlled by action (see examples in section 5).

A process may execute a number of wait requests before it eventually goes to sleep. The function wait_event returns to the process which is continued until it executes return. Then the process is suspended and will be resumed only when one of the awaited events takes place. Multiple wait requests executed before return are collected on a list. When the process is restarted due to the occurrence of one of the awaited events, its entire wait list is cleared.

The valid port events are listed below (their formal semantics is presented in [GbR88a]):

SILENCE   The event occurs at the beginning of the nearest silence period heard by the station. If no activity is heard on the port when the request is issued, the event occurs immediately.

ACTIVITY   The event occurs at the beginning of the nearest activity (of any type) preceded by a silence period. If an activity is being heard by

	the station on the specified port when the request is issued, the event occurs immediately.
COLLISION	The event occurs when the nearest collision is heard on the specified port.
BOJ	The event occurs when the station hears the beginning of the nearest jamming signal preceded by a silence period or by a transfer.
EOJ	The event occurs when the station hears the nearest end of a jamming signal (followed by a silence period or by a transfer attempt).
EOT	The event occurs when the station hears the end of a successful packet transmission.
MY_PACKET	The event occurs when the beginning of a packet is heard for which the requesting station is the receiver.
END_MY_PACKET	The event occurs when the end of a packet is heard for which the requesting station is the receiver.
ANY_EVENT	This event occurs whenever the station begins to hear a new activity or stops sensing some activity.

For all events generated by undisturbed packet transmissions, variable the_packet returns the pointer to the data structure describing the packet being transmitted. For all link events, variable the_port returns the number of the port on which the event has occurred.

A number of event types is associated with the client. The most relevant of them is MESSAGE_ARRIVAL indicating the arrival of a message (of any type) to the station. For an event of such a type, the global variables the_message and the_message_type return the pointer to a data structure representing the new message and the message type number, respectively.

For the signal server (SIGNAL), e denotes the signal number (which may be an arbitrary integer value). The event specified for a TIMER request is interpreted as an integer number representing a time interval (in *ITU*'s). The event occurs when the time interval elapses. It is legal to wait for the delay of 0 time units, in particular, the sequence:

```
wait_event (TIMER, 0, a);
return;
```

available as the macro:

```
continue_at (a);
```

can be viewed as a structural branch to action a.

The following macro for start_transfer sets up the timer for the time delay corresponding to the total length of the transmitted packet:

```
transmit_packet (port_id, packet, eot_action)
```

expanded as:

```
start_transfer (port_id, packet);
wait_event (TIMER, packet.total_length*rate[port_id],
                                    eot_action);
```

A similar alias can be used instead of start_jam — to set up the timer for the duration of the jamming signal:

```
emit_jam (port_id, jam_length, eoj_action)
```

expanded as:

```
start_jam (port_id);
wait_event (TIMER, jam_length, eoj_action);
```

3.6. Signaler

In general, signals can be sent between any two processes, not necessarily belonging to the same station. The following function is used to send a signal to a process run by the same station:

```
internal_signal (n)
int   n;
```

After the function is called by a process, any process at the same station can receive the signal, provided that the signal number n has been awaited by it.

3.7. Link inquiries

Besides awaiting various port events, a station is also able to perform port (link) inquiries. The station processes need not remember the history of past events: they can inquire the link servers. Functions performing port inquiries are listed below. The parameter port_id is of type int and identifies the station's port, and thus the link, to which the inquiry is addressed.

- inquiries about the beginning of the last collision:

```
TIME   last_collision_sensed (port_id)
```

- inquiries about the last beginning of any activity:

```
TIME   last_boa_sensed (port_id)
```

- inquiries about the beginning of the current silence period. A special value (constant TIME_INF) representing undefined time is returned if an activity is currently being heard.

```
TIME   last_eoa_sensed (port_id)
```

- inquiries about the end of the last successful transfer:

```
TIME   last_eot_sensed (port_id)
```

- inquiries about the beginning or the end of the last jamming signal heard:

```
TIME   last_boj_sensed (port_id)
TIME   last_eoj_sensed (port_id)
```

- inquires about the present configuration of activities perceived by the port:

```
activities_sensed (port_id, transfers, jams)
int    *transfers, *jams;
```

The last function returns (via the two integer parameters passed by pointers) the number of transfer attempts and the number of jamming signals currently heard at the port.

4. Input and Output

4.1. Input data

The standard system modules together with the user-supplied modules defining a specific protocol are compiled into a stand-alone simulator. The simulator requires a set of input data. Some data items are standard, and so:

− Topology parameters define the network backbone, i.e. the stations and the configuration of their ports. For each link, we describe the ports connected to the link and the link's part of the distance matrix.

− Client parameters declare the traffic conditions, i.e. the message types, and the associated traffic patterns.

– Termination conditions can be given by: the limit on the number of messages that are to be entirely transmitted and received, the simulation time limit as the number of *ITU*'s, or the CPU time limit. When any of the three limits is reached, the simulation terminates, and the output file is produced.

The protocol module may read additional input data. This has to be done by function in_protocol (see 3.1). Examples of protocol specific data items are: the minimum and maximum packet length, the length of the inter-packet space, etc.

4.2. Output data

The standard output file produced by LANSF contains a number of performance measures, e.g. the effective throughput, the statistics of the packet and message delays. These statistics are available separately for each link and message type, as well as for the entire network. The depth of the statistics generated by the simulator is definable by the user (e.g. central moments of arbitrary order are supported). The performance measuring tools can be extended in the protocol module – to gather additional, protocol-specific statistics. There exists a standard data type (STATISTICS) to represent random variables, and a number of standard operations are defined on the objects of that type.

4.3. User interface

A very convenient feature of LANSF's user interface is the window-oriented dynamic display toolbox. This collection of functions offers monitoring tools similar to sophisticated debugging systems. LANSF defines a collection of standard windows, any subset of which can be displayed on the terminal screen. It is possible to monitor the behaviour of each station as well as the global behaviour of the entire network. The most often used windows display:

- lengths of message queues at all stations (graphically),

- the status of selected stations,

- global dynamic parameters of the simulation (e.g. the simulated virtual time, the number of processed events, the number of queued and transmitted messages),

- the performance statistics, both global and specific (e.g. for a given link or message type),

- the contents of the event/action queue.

The simulator can be put into the step mode in which the contents of the screen are frozen after processing a single simulation event. Additional windows can be defined in the user-supplied protocol module.

5. Examples

5.1. Ethernet

In Ethernet (cf. [Sta86]), all stations execute the same protocol. In our model, this protocol is described by two processes, the transmitter and the receiver. The transmitter code is listed below.

```
transmitter () {
    switch (action) {
case INITIALIZE :
    wait_event (CLIENT, MESSAGE_ARRIVAL, NEXT_MESSAGE);
    return;
case NEXT_MESSAGE :
    if (! get_next_packet (mnl, mxl, f))
        continue_at (INITIALIZE);
    station->collision_counter = 0;
case RETRY :
    if (def (t = last_eoa_sensed (BUS))) {
            if ((t = current_time - t) >= packet_space) {
                transmit_packet (BUS, station->current_packet,
```

```
                    PACKET_TRANSMITTED);
            wait_event (BUS, COLLISION, COLLISION_HEARD);
        } else {
            wait_event (BUS, ACTIVITY, ACTIVITY_HEARD);
            wait_event (TIMER, packet_space-t, RETRY);
        }
    } else {
        wait_event (BUS, SILENCE, BUS_IDLE);
    }
    return;
case BUS_IDLE :
    wait_event (BUS, ACTIVITY, ACTIVITY_HEARD);
    wait_event (TIMER, packet_space, RETRY);
    return;
case ACTIVITY_HEARD :
    wait_event (BUS, SILENCE, BUS_IDLE);
    return;
case PACKET_TRANSMITTED :
    stop_transfer (BUS);
    release_current_packet ();
    continue_at (NEXT_MESSAGE);
case COLLISION_HEARD :
    station->collision_counter ++;
    abort_transfer (BUS);
    emit_jam (BUS, jam_length, JAM_SENT);
    return;
case JAM_SENT :
    stop_jam (BUS);
    wait_event (TIMER, backoff (), RETRY);
    return;
  } }
```

The structure of the transmitter reflects its interrupt-driven nature. As soon as the station acquires a packet to transmit, it obeys the inter-packet spacing rules and starts the transfer. Note that for a new packet, `collision_counter` (a user-defined station attribute) is reset to 0. This attribute is used for calculating the after-collision back-off. If the value returned by `last_eoa_sensed` is not defined (function `def` returns 0), which means that the station is currently hearing some activity, the transmitter waits until the activity disappears. Then it has to wait for `packet_space` time units. If an activity appears in the meantime, the waiting must be repeated. If the bus has been idle for some period of time, but that period is shorter than `packet_space`, the transmitter has to wait for the difference. Having started the transfer, the transmitter issues a wait request to the timer (this is done implicitly by `transmit_packet` - see 3.5) – to learn when the packet is entirely sent, and to the port – to detect a possible collision. If the packet is successfully transmitted, the station attempts to get the next packet from the client's message queue. If a collision has occurred, the transmitter updates `collision_counter`, aborts the transfer, sends a jamming signal, backs-off, and starts again. The simple function calculating the back-off delay has been omitted.

```
receiver ()    {
    switch (action) {
case     INITIALIZE :
    wait_event (BUS, END_MY_PACKET, END_OF_PACKET);
    return;
case     END_OF_PACKET :
    accept_packet (the_packet, BUS);
    wait_event (TIMER, min_packet_length, INITIALIZE);
    return;
  } }
```

Immediately after a packet is entirely received by the station (event END_MY_PACKET), the receiver calls `accept_packet` – to update the performance measures. Note that before the receiver starts waiting for the next packet, it sleeps for a while – to make sure that the end of the last packet has disappeared from the station's port. Without that delay the receiver would loop, as it would be immediately restarted by the end of the packet just received (no simulated time elapses while a process is active).

Below we present a sample standard output produced by LANSF for Ethernet:

```
Protocol: Commercial Ethernet, Mon Jun 13 15:14:27 1988

Configuration:   NStations          NLinks
                    50                 1
Message type 0: Interarrival time:   EXPONENTIAL Mean = 2e+03
                Length distribution: EXPONENTIAL Mean = 1e+03

Senders:   all stations (equal weights of 0.020000)
Receivers: all stations (equal weights of 0.020000)

Protocol specific parameters:
  PrpgtnDelay   MinPcktLength   MaxPcktLength   PcktHdrLength
        100           368           12000             208
  MinGapLength   MaxGapLength   MinJamLength   MaxJamLength
         96            101             32              36

Simulated virtual time:                            59701119

Message type 0:
                Absolute message delay:
Number of items:        30050      Minimum value:           578
Maximum value:         1.1e+06     Mean value:          2.26e+04
Variance:             4.16e+09     Standard deviation:  6.45e+04

                Absolute packet delay:
Number of items:        30050      Minimum value:           578
Maximum value:         1.1e+06     Mean value:          1.22e+04
Variance:             1.78e+09     Standard deviation:  4.21e+04

Link  0:   LRcvdBits     LTrnsmtdBits    Collisions    Throughput
           29912376        29912376        27427          0.501

93.033333 CP Seconds Execution Time
```

5.2. Token Ring

In a ring-type network, stations and links form a circular structure such that each station is directly connected with two immediate neighbours via two separate ports. Each station receives information on one (input) port and transmits on the other (output) port. A special packet (token) is circulated among the stations. If the station receiving the token does not have a data packet to be transmitted, it immediately passes the token on its output port. In the opposite case, the station stops the token and passes the data packet instead. Having completed the transmission, the station passes the token.

In the presented version of the protocol, a station may only transmit one data packet per each acquisition of the token. A station detecting a data packet addressed to itself receives the packet and removes it from the ring. Other data packets are passed around until they reach their proper destinations. In our model, each of the two station ports is serviced by a separate process. The processes communicate by exchanging signals. The input port is denoted by LEFT_PORT and the output port is denoted by RIGHT_PORT. The passing_delay says how much time elapses between the reception of the first bit of a packet and passing that bit on the output (right) port. Note that that time is generally non-zero as the station has to recognise at least a part of the packet header before it decides what to do with the packet. The two station processes are listed below.

```
left_port_process () {
  switch (action) {
  case    INITIALIZE :
    if (station->id != 0) {
        wait_event (LEFT_PORT, ACTIVITY, RECEIVING);
        return;
    }
    make_token ();
  case    HAVE_TOKEN :
    internal_signal (GOT_TOKEN);
    wait_event (LEFT_PORT, SILENCE, LEFT_PORT_IDLE);
    return;
  case    LEFT_PORT_IDLE :
    wait_event (LEFT_PORT, ACTIVITY, RECEIVING);
    return;
  case    RECEIVING :
    if (the_packet -> type == TOKEN_PACKET) {
        station->buffer = *the_packet;
        wait_event (TIMER, passing_delay, HAVE_TOKEN);
        return;
    }
    if (my_packet (the_packet)) {
        wait_event (LEFT_PORT, EOT, PACKET_RECEIVED);
        return;
    }
    station->buffer = *the_packet;
    wait_event (TIMER, passing_delay, READY_TO_PASS);
    return;
  case    READY_TO_PASS :
    internal_signal (GOT_OTHER_PACKET);
    wait_event (LEFT_PORT, SILENCE, LEFT_PORT_IDLE);
    return;
  case    PACKET_RECEIVED :
    accept_packet (the_packet, the_port);
    continue_at (LEFT_PORT_IDLE);
  } }

right_port_process ()  {
  switch (action) {
  case    INITIALIZE :
    wait_event (SIGNAL, GOT_TOKEN, TRANSMIT_OWN_PACKET);
    wait_event (SIGNAL, GOT_OTHER_PACKET, RELAY);
    return;
  case    TRANSMIT_OWN_PACKET :
    if (get_next_packet (min_pl, max_pl, frame)) {
        transmit_packet (RIGHT_PORT, station->current_packet,
                          PACKET_TRANSMITTED);
        return;
    }
  case RELAY :
    transmit_packet (RIGHT_PORT, station->buffer, RELAYED);
    return;
  case    RELAYED :
    stop_transfer (RIGHT_PORT);
    continue_at (INITIALIZE);
  case    PACKET_TRANSMITTED :
    stop_transfer (RIGHT_PORT);
    release_current_packet ();
    wait_event (TIMER, packet_space, RELAY);
    return;   } }
```

Station 0 is responsible for the initial creation of the token packet (function `make_token` is not listed here). Whenever an activity is sensed on the left port, the process determines what type of a packet is being received. If the packet is to be passed, i.e. it is either the token or a data packet addressed to another station, a local copy of the packet is made and put into `packet_buffer`. Then the process waits for `passing_delay` – to simulate the time spent on recognising the relevant part of the packet header. If the packet has reached its proper recipient (the standard function `my_packet` returns *true*), it is received similarly as for Ethernet; otherwise, the right-port process is signaled as soon as the packet destiny is determined. The right-port process is awakened by signals from the left-port process. Whenever the token is acquired (signal `GOT_TOKEN`), the right-port process checks whether there is a data packet awaiting transmission, and if so, it transmits the data packet and then passes the token preceded by a packet space. Packets addressed to other stations are relayed on the right port – in the same way as the token packet.

5.3. Hubnet

Hubnet consists of a number of stations connected to a central switching device – the so-called *hub*. Each station is connected to the hub via two channels: the input channel and the output (selection) channel. All the input channels are connected together and form a uniform broadcast medium (a single link). The selection channels are not connected: each selection channel forms a separate link. A station willing to transmit a packet sends it on the selection link. If the broadcast link is not busy, the hub propagates the transmission on the broadcast link, so that the packet will be heard by all stations in due time; otherwise the transmission is ignored. The transmitting station listens for the echo of its packet on the input channel. If the echo does not appear there after a certain amount of time, the station assumes that its transmission was unsuccessful and tries again.

The hub is a special station. Each regular station executes three processes: the transmitter, the receiver, and the acknowledger. Immediately after the transmitter initiates a transfer, it signals the acknowledger to start awaiting the echo of the transmission. At the same time the acknowledger sets up an alarm clock – to be awakened if the echo is not heard for the duration of `echo_delay`. An appropriate signal is sent back to the transmitter to indicate either the success or the failure of the transfer attempt.

The hub runs as many processes as there are regular stations connected to it. Each selection link connected to the hub is handled by a separate process. The process structure of the hub is initialised by the following sequence of instructions (in `in_protocol`):

```
station = stt [n_stations - 1];
hub_status = IDLE;
for (i = 0; i < n_stations - 1; i ++) {
        new_process (hub_selection_process, i);
}
```

Array `stt` transforms station identifiers (numbers) into pointers to the corresponding data structures. Numbers 0 ... n_stations–2 identify regular stations. Station n_stations–1 models the hub. The n_stations–1 processes of the hub share the same code. Each process recognises itself by the version number (see 3.2). The hub processes have been created in such a way that the version number of a process is equal to the number of the hub port serviced by the process. This number also identifies the corresponding (regular) station. The boolean variable `hub_status` tells whether the broadcast link is busy. Below we list the code of a hub process:

```
#define  SELECTION_PORT  process_version

hub_selection_process    () {
  switch (action) {
case    INITIALIZE :
    wait_event (SELECTION_PORT, ACTIVITY, PORT_ACTIVE);
    return;
case    PORT_ACTIVE :
    if (hub_status != IDLE) {
        wait_event (SELECTION_PORT, SILENCE, INITIALIZE);
```

```
         return;
    }
    hub_status = BUSY;
    station->packet_buffer = *the_packet;
    wait_event (TIMER, switch_delay, PORT_CONNECTED);
    return;
case    PORT_CONNECTED :
    transmit_packet (BROADCAST_PORT, station->packet_buffer,
                PACKET_SENT);
    return;
case    PACKET_SENT :
    stop_transfer (BROADCAST_PORT);
    hub_status = IDLE;
    continue_at (INITIALIZE);
} }
```

The hub (actually the broadcast channel) can be in one of two states: BUSY or IDLE. If the broadcast channel is busy, i.e. connected to one of the selection channels, the hub ignores transfer attempts incoming on other channels; otherwise, one of the incoming transmissions is relayed (after a switch_delay incurred by the hub's switch) along the broadcast channel which is immediately marked as busy and remains busy for the duration of the transfer. Note that variable hub_status is a semaphore guarding the broadcast channel. This semaphore is manipulated in an implicit critical section (since no active process can be interrupted before it goes to sleep).

The simplest of the three processes run by a regular station is the receiver which is identical to the Ethernet receiver (see 5.1). The remaining two processes co-operate by exchanging signals. Their code is listed below.

```
transmitter () {
  switch (action) {
case    INITIALIZE :
    wait_event (CLIENT, MESSAGE_ARRIVAL, NEXT_MESSAGE);
    return;
case    NEXT_MESSAGE :
    if (! get_next_packet (mnl, mxl, f))
        continue_at (INITIALIZE);
case RETRY :
    t = last_eoa_sensed (MY_SELECTION_PORT);
    if ((t = current_time - t) < (ps = packet_space)) {
        wait_event (TIMER, ps - t, SPACE_OBEYED);
        return;
    }
case    SPACE_OBEYED :
    transmit_packet (MY_SELECTION_PORT, station->current_packet,
                PACKET_TRANSMITTED);
    internal_signal (START_ECHO_WAIT);
    wait_event (SIGNAL, NEGATIVE_ACK, PACKET_UNACKNOWLEDGED);
    return;
case    PACKET_TRANSMITTED :
    stop_transfer (MY_SELECTION_PORT);
    wait_event (SIGNAL, NEGATIVE_ACK, LATE_NACK);
    wait_event (SIGNAL, POSITIVE_ACK, PACKET_ACKNOWLEDGED);
    return;
case    PACKET_UNACKNOWLEDGED :
    abort_transfer (MY_SELECTION_PORT);
case    LATE_NACK :
    continue_at (RETRY);
case    PACKET_ACKNOWLEDGED :
    release_current_packet ();
    continue_at     (NEXT_MESSAGE);
} }
```

```
acknowledger     () {
  switch (action)            {
case    INITIALIZE :
    wait_event (SIGNAL, START_ECHO_WAIT, WAIT_FOR_ECHO);
    return;
case    WAIT_FOR_ECHO :
    station->delay_to_ack = echo_delay;
    station->echo_wait_started = current_time;
case STILL_WAITING :
    wait_event (MY_BROADCAST_PORT, ACTIVITY, PACKET_ARRIVAL);
    wait_event (TIMER, station->delay_to_ack, NO_ECHO);
    return;
case    PACKET_ARRIVAL :
    station->delay_to_ack -= current_time -
                                        station->echo_wait_started;
    station->echo_wait_started = current_time;
    if (the_packet -> sender == station) {
      wait_event (TIMER, rec_delay, PACKET_RECOGNIZED);
      wait_event (TIMER, station->delay_to_ack, NO_ECHO);
      return;
    }
    wait_event (MY_BROADCAST_PORT, SILENCE, END_ACTIVITY);
    wait_event (TIMER, station->delay_to_ack, NO_ECHO);
    return;
case    PACKET_RECOGNIZED :
    internal_signal (POSITIVE_ACK);
    wait_event (MY_BROADCAST_PORT, SILENCE, INITIALIZE);
    return;
case    END_ACTIVITY :
    station->delay_to_ack -= current_time -
                                        station->echo_wait_started;
    station->echo_wait_started = current_time;
    continue_at (STILL_WAITING);
case    NO_ECHO :
    internal_signal (NEGATIVE_ACK);
    continue_at (INITIALIZE);
} }
```

The acknowledger is awakened by the START_ECHO_WAIT signal from the transmitter, immediately after the transmitter starts a transfer attempt. Then the acknowledger waits for echo_delay time units and, at the same time, monitors activities in the broadcast channel. If nothing happens for the echo delay interval, the acknowledger sends NEGATIVE_ACK to the transmitter – requesting retransmission of the last packet. If a packet transmitted by this station is heard and recognised before the echo delay elapses, the acknowledger sends POSITIVE_ACK – to inform the transmitter that the packet has been passed to the broadcast channel. Having sent the START_ECHO_WAIT signal to the acknowledger the transmitter knows that one of the signals POSITIVE_ACK or NEGATIVE_ACK will come back and so the transmitter will learn whether the packet gets through.

5.4. Single-queue server

Although originally designed to simulate MAC-level protocols for communication networks, LANSF can be used as a general-purpose simulation tool. Let us consider the classical single-queue server system. In such a system we have a process (the so-called *server*) which takes care of requests arriving from the outer world. At any moment the server can be in one of two states, namely, it can be either idle or busy, i.e. processing a request. If a request arrives while the server is idle, the request is immediately taken care of, i.e. the server starts processing it. Otherwise, the request is queued using the FIFO scheme. When the server completes servicing the current request, it examines the queue and, if the queue is non-empty, the front request is taken for processing and removed from the queue. Otherwise, the server becomes idle.

In the simplest implementation of the single-queue server, the requests can be generated by the standard client. These requests are represented as messages with the message length describing the request service time. The server is implemented as a process associated with station number 0 which is the only station of our simulated system. The code of the server process is listed below.

```
server () {
  if (get_next_packet (0, 0, 0)) {
     wait_event(DELAY,(station->current_packet).length, NONE);
     release_current_packet ();
  } else
     wait_event (CLIENT, MESSAGE_ARRIVAL, NONE);
}
```

The structure of the server is so simple that we need no "actions" to describe its behaviour). Immediately after it is created, the server is started and attempts to acquire a new packet representing a request to be serviced. Note that the maximum packet length is specified as 0 which means that a packet always consists of an entire message. If a packet is acquired, the server simulates its service by going to sleep for the amount of time corresponding to the packet length. If no packet can be acquired by the server, which means that the request queue is empty, the process waits for a message arrival from the client. Whenever it is restarted, which may happen due to a request service being completed or to a new message arriving from the client, the server looks at the beginning of the message queue and attempts to acquire a new request for processing. Note that the value of `action` is irrelevant as in both cases the server has to perform the same actual action.

One disadvantage of the simple system described above is that no measurements are performed by the queue server. The standard output of the simulator is not very interesting as it describes message and packet delays for received (accept'ed) packets. However, it would be relatively easy to extend our simulator to generate the statistics of the service time:

```
server () {
  switch (action) {
case END_OF_SERVICE :
     accept_packet (&(station->current_packet), NONE);
     release_current_packet ();
case NEW_REQUEST :
     if (get_next_packet (0, 0, 0)) {
        wait_event (DELAY, (station->current_packet).length,
                                           END_OF_SERVICE);
        return;
     }
case INITIALIZE :
     wait_event (CLIENT, MESSAGE_ARRIVAL, NEW_REQUEST);
  }
}
```

Now we have introduced two actions (symbolic constants NEW_REQUEST and END_OF_SERVICE). When the service of a request is completed, the packet is accepted and the standard performance measures are updated – as if the packet was received at some station. Note that the mean absolute message delay calculated this way corresponds to the mean waiting time for a request to be serviced.

Another typical parameter to investigate would be the average observed length of the request queue. Statistics of this type are not included in the standard output produced by LANSF and therefore we have to introduce a non-standard random variable (section 4.2) declared as follows:

```
STATISTICS queue_length_statistics;
```

Moreover, we will program our own non-standard client – to keep track of the message queue length. The client is run as a process at station 0.

```
client () {
  switch (action) {
```

```
case NEW_ARRIVAL :
   generate_message (0, station, NONE,
               l_uniform (mt[0].min_length, mt[0].max_length));
   update_queue_length (1);
case INITIALIZE :
   wait_event (TIMER, generate_inter_arrival_time (0),
                                            NEW_ARRIVAL);
   }
}
```

Immediately after it is created, the client generates a random time delay according to the distribution of the message inter-arrival time declared in the input data, and waits for that delay — to create and queue a message. The functions `generate_message` and `generate_inter_arrival_time` are standard. The first parameter (the only parameter for the second function) identifies the message type. We assume that one message type (number 0) is declared in the input data set. The global array `mt` defines details of each message type. The new message created at NEW_ARRIVAL is automatically queued at the current station Its receiver attribute is irrelevant. The message length is uniformly distributed according to the boundary values declared with the message type in the input file. Having queued the message, the client calls the function `update_queue_length` (see below) to say that the queue has been augmented by one item and its length statistics should be updated appropriately. Then the client goes to sleep to wait for another inter-arrival delay, and so on.

The new version of the server is identical to the previous one with the exception that now the server calls:

```
        update_queue_length (-1)
```

immediately after acquiring a new packet from the queue. The purpose of `update_queue_length` is to keep track of the number of messages in the queue and to update the contents of the statistics package whenever that number changes.

```
update_queue_length (n) int n; {
   update_statistics (queue_length_statistics,
       (double) queue_length, current_time - last_update_time);
   last_update_time = current_time;
   queue_length += n;
   }
```

The global variable `last_update_time` should be set to 0 before the simulation is started. The action of `update_statistics` can be viewed as adding n copies of value v to the random variable `queue_length_statistics`, where v and n are the second and the third parameters, respectively. LANSF provides tools for printing out the contents of statistics packages.

6. Conclusions

We have presented a collection of software tools for simulating communication networks. These tools are in fact procedures and data structures expressed in C, and they don't have the shape of a single program. Each time a new protocol is to be investigated, some new modules must be added to the system, and then it can be configured into a simulating program. However, if we look at the examples in section 5, we get an impression that LANSF offers some kind of a programming language. Indeed, the structure of the system is not directly visible: the process of creating a specific version of the simulator resembles translation of a program written in a high-level language.

The very day LANSF was finished, we managed to rewrite into the new formalism a dozen protocols, previously modeled by different programs. Amazingly enough, LANSF turned out to be not much slower than its highly specialised predecessors. It seems to be due to the fact that LANSF is not a single interpreter for a variety of protocols, but it configures itself for each particular case.

The way LANSF has been programmed leaves it open for many natural modifications and extensions. In particular, it is planned to create a version of LANSF in which the servers will be distributed among a number of actually concurrent processors. It is also intended to equip LANSF with tools for automating the validation and verification of protocols. Our work is aimed at implementing a system similar to Lotos [BoB87] or Estelle [BuD87], but specialised for the Medium Access Control level protocols.

References

[BCM87]   Bagrodia R.L., K. Mani Chandy and J. Misra, A Message Based Approach to Discrete-Event Simulation, IEEE Transactions on Software Engineering, vol. SE-13, No. 6, June 1987.

[BoB87]   Bolognesi T. and E. Brinksma, Introduction to the ISO Specification Language LOTOS, Computer Networks and ISDN Systems, vol. 14, no. 1, pp. 25-59, 1987.

[BuD87]   Budkowski S. and P. Dembinski, An Introduction to ESTELLE: A Specification Language for Distributed Systems, Computer Networks and ISDN Systems, vol. 14, no. 1, pp. 3-23, 1987.

[GMW87]   Gburzynski P., J.C. Majithia and T.C. Wilson, An Improved Backoff Algorithm for Ethernet-type Local Area Networks, TR 87-9, Dept. of Comp. Sci., The University of Alberta, Edmonton, 1987.

[GbR87]   Gburzynski P. and P. Rudnicki, A Better-than-Token Protocol with Bounded Packet Delay for Ethernet-type LAN's, Proceedings of the ACM/IEEE Symposium on the Simulation of Computer Networks, pp. 110-117, Colorado Springs, August 1987.

[GbR88]   Gburzynski P. and P. Rudnicki, LANSF - A Configurable System for Modeling Communication Networks, TR88-19, Dept. of Comp. Sci., The University of Alberta, Edmonton, 1988.

[GbR88a]   Gburzynski P. and P. Rudnicki, A Simulation Model of a Communication Channel, INFOCOM'89, to appear.

[GbR88b]   Gburzynski P. and P. Rudnicki, A Note on the Performance of ENET-II, IEEE Journal on Selected Topics in Communication, 1989, to appear.

[GbR88c]   Gburzynski P. and P. Rudnicki, Emulated Performance of Hymap, in preparation, 1988.

[GoW85]   Gopal P.M. and J.W. Wong, Analysis of a Hybrid Token-CSMA/CD Protocol for Bus Networks, Computer Networks and ISDN Systems 9, pp. 131-141, 1985.

[HaC87]   Haas Z. and D.R. Cheriton, A Case for Packet Switching in High-Performance Wide-Area Networks, Stanford University, unpublished, 1987.

[HTW86]   Hopper, A., Temple, S., Williamson, R.: Local Area Network Design. Addison-Wesley, 1986.

[KiK83]   Kiesel, W.M. and P.J. Kuehn, A New CSMA/CD Protocol for Local Area Networks with Dynamic Priorities and Low Collision Probability, IEEE Journal on Selected Areas in Communications, vol. SAC-1, no. 5, pp. 869-876, Nov. 1983.

[Mol85]   Molloy M.K., Collision Resolution on the CSMA/CD Bus, Computer Networks and ISDN Systems 9, pp. 209-214.

[Sta86]   Stallings W., A Tutorial on the IEEE 802 Local Network Standard, in: R.L. Pickholtz (ed.), Local Area and Multiple Access Networks, pp. 1-30, Computer Science Press, 1986.

IPWATCH: A TOOL FOR MONITORING NETWORK LOCALITY

Mark J. Lorence and
M. Satyanarayanan

Carnegie Mellon University
Pittsburgh, PA

1. Introduction

In the course of the last decade local area networks (LANs) have grown from simple single-segment Ethernet cables into multi-segment topologies composed of diverse physical media. Today, a LAN in a large organization is typically composed of a shared *Backbone* to which a number of semi-independent *Subnets* are attached via devices called *Routers* that perform packet switching. Multiple backbones may be present for enhanced reliability and performance. A variety of factors account for this increase in complexity. First, electrical considerations limit the lengths of individual LAN segments and the density of machines on them. Second, maintenance and fault isolation are simplified if a LAN is decomposable. Third, administrative functions such as the assignment of unique host addresses can be decentralized if a LAN can be partitioned. These considerations will increase in importance as distributed systems become more pervasive.

During the same period of time, distributed systems have been evolved to to provide *Network Transparency* for a variety of services such as remote file access [13], electronic mail [12] and remote program execution [6]. Network transparency masks underlying network complexity. Neither users nor application programs need be concerned with the details of the network traffic they generate. Unfortunately, performance inhomogeneities cannot be hidden even when a network is rendered functionally homogeneous. Routers, which introduce load-dependent transmission delays, are the primary source of performance inhomogeneity. Uneven loading of subnets is a secondary cause. Ignoring the effects of network topology can result in suboptimal use of a network by a distributed system. Nonuniform performance is already observed by users of large distributed systems such as Andrew [5]. Further growth will exacerbate the problem.

This paper describes the design, implementation and calibration of a tool called *IPwatch* that will assist implementors in building and maintaining distributed systems that make optimal use of the underlying network. Section 2 examines the nature of locality in distributed systems and explains why it is relevant to the concerns expressed in the preceding paragraph. Section 3 outlines the considerations that influenced the design of the tool and describes its design. Section 4 presents results from a series of experiments conducted to validate the tool and calibrate it. Section 5 concludes the paper with a discussion of work in progress.

2. Network Locality

2.1. Definition

We define *Logical Network Locality* as the property whereby a small fraction of many possible host pairs account for most end-to-end network traffic. It is influenced by the behavior of users and application programs and by the design of distributed systems. *Physical Network Locality*, on the other hand, is defined as the property whereby most network traffic traverses as few routers as possible, preferably none. It is influenced by logical network locality, network topology, and the placement of hosts. Since physical locality minimizes network delays, an optimal mapping of a distributed system on to a network will exhibit the highest possible physical locality.

Our primary goal is to understand and measure logical network locality. We are convinced that such knowledge is critical for tuning a distributed system for optimal performance. Information about logical network locality can be used to improve physical network locality by modifications to one or more of the following areas:

1. Network topology
2. Placement of hosts on the network
3. Design of distributed system software.

For brevity we use the term *Locality* to mean logical network locality in the rest of this paper. Physical network locality will always be referred to by its full name.

2.2. Origin

The origin of locality can be best understood by an example. The Andrew system, which motivated this work, consists of over 500 workstations accessing files from a small collection of file servers. Workstations cache copies of most-recently-used files to improve performance and minimize workstation-server interactions. Most communication between a workstation and servers is to fetch files missing from the cache or to write back a file that has been modified. Files are fetched and stored in their entirety, using a specialized bulk transfer protocol. Since Andrew provides true location transparency, a user at a workstation can use any file stored in the shared file system, totally unaware of the specific servers that he is interacting with.

At the next level of detail, however, the architecture of Andrew substantially complicates an understanding of the resulting network traffic patterns. First, system files that are read often but rarely modified can have read-only replicas at multiple servers. It is indeterminate which one of these replicas get used by a workstation. Second, since the files of a user are typically located on one server, this server is likely to participate in most of the traffic with the user's workstation. However, when a user at a public workstation logs out and a new user starts work, most of the workstation references will be to the file server that stores the files of the new user. Even users who have workstations dedicated to them may localize their references to different servers as they proceed with different aspects of their computing activities. Third, when a file is modified, all workstations with currently valid cache copies are notified by the server responsible for that file. Although write-sharing is rare for private

96

files, it is common for shared writable directories such as bulletin boards. The effect of this aspect of the design on locality is an open question. Finally, low-function machines such as the IBM-PC use the Andrew file system via surrogate workstations called *PCServers* [11]. PCServers are located on the same subnet as the PCs, but may access servers on other networks. Thus the logical simplicity of the Andrew file system at the user level does not carry over to the next level of detail. Although the existence of locality is undeniable, it is impossible to characterize this locality without observation and measurement.

Though we have used Andrew as an example, locality is not specific to it. Even in a network used only for terminal emulation and user-initiated file transfers, there will be locality arising from the fact that users deal with a small number of hosts at a time, typically one. In general, if we define a logical *Connection* as a source-destination pair, only a subset of possible connections will contribute significantly to traffic at any given time. How small this subset is, and how rapidly its membership changes are measures that characterize the locality of a network. A complete understanding of a distributed system requires data on its short, medium and long-term locality.

Locality in a network is analogous to locality of virtual memory references. If one views the concatenated source and destination addresses of a packet as defining an address space, only a small fraction of this address space is likely to be heavily referenced at any given time. But the analogy is imperfect. Virtual memory references exhibit both *Temporal* and *Spatial* locality. Networks do exhibit temporal locality, but not spatial locality. If a pair of machines communicate it is likely they will communicate again in the near future. However, there is no reason to believe that if two machines communicate, machines whose network addresses are close to theirs are also likely to communicate. Spatial locality is therefore not a meaningful concept here.

2.3. Measurement

Existing tools are inadequate for measuring locality. Simple tools [15] merely present network utilization, packet counts and byte counts. More sophisticated tools allow selective filtering of packets [2], but are not capable of dynamically modifying their behavior based on what connections seem "interesting" at any given time.

Early in our design of a tool to measure locality, it became clear that a brute force technique for monitoring all possible pairs of machines was inappropriate. First, such an approach may require excessive amounts of memory. On a large network of over 5000 machines, such a tool would have to keep track of over $\binom{5000}{2}$ connections, double this number if communication is expected to be asymmetric. Equally important, such a tool cannot track the shifts in locality that occur over time. What is needed is a tool that is adaptive to the current traffic patterns and can focus its attention on those pairwise communications that currently contribute to the bulk of the traffic.

3. Design of the Tool

3.1. Hardware

The hardware we used for IPwatch had to possess certain important characteristics. First, it had to be usable with Ethernet [3] as well the IBM token-ring [4] since both these technologies are prevalent in our environment. Second, it had to possess adequate memory and processing power to perform monitoring without any loss of information even during periods of intense network activity. Third, it had to be easily transportable so that it could be used anywhere on campus as well as at other sites.

As far as possible we wished to use off-the-shelf hardware that met our requirements. Fortunately such hardware is readily available. Our choice was an IBM AT with 640 Kbytes of memory, running at a clock speed of 6 Mhz. Besides meeting the criteria listed above, it also uses a lightweight operating system, MS-DOS, that provides us with easy access to all parts of the system. At the same time it has a rich collection of robust software development tools.

To interface the AT to the network we chose the Ungermann-Bass PC/NIC Ethernet adapter and the IBM 6100 token-ring adapter. These adaptors are fast and possess adequate buffering to handle bursts of traffic. They are capable of operating in *Promiscuous Mode*, which allows them to receive all packets on the network, not just packets specifically addressed to them. Our initial work has been entirely on the Ethernet. We intend to extend our implementation to the token ring shortly.

3.2. Software Overview

As defined in Section 2.2, a connection is a source-destination pair. IPwatch makes short-term locality visible by separating *Interesting* connections from *Uninteresting* ones. Each interesting connection has an associated entry in a *Long-Term Cache*. At present this entry is used to keep track of packet and byte counts. It would be simple to modify the tool to monitor other information such as interarrival time distributions or packet traces.

IPwatch uses a small *Short-Term Cache* to keep track of connections that it suspects may be interesting, but is not certain about. This cache is periodically swept and each entry is *Promoted* to the long-term cache or *Flushed*. The criteria for promotion is discussed in detail in Section 3.4. If a network exhibits significant short-term locality only a few of the connections in the short-term cache will be promoted. Further, the connections which are flushed will only account for a small fraction of the total traffic.

An interesting connection may become uninteresting over time. To maintain the invariant that the long-term cache contains only connections that are currently interesting, the long-term cache must also be swept periodically. The tool does not yet incorporate such a mechanism, but we are in the process of developing it. Fortunately, the long-term cache has never been completely filled in our limited use of the monitor.

When IPwatch receives a packet, it first checks the long-term cache to see if this connection is an interesting one. If not, it examines the short-term cache to to check if the connection is being considered for promotion. If a match is found in either cache, the corresponding entry is updated. Otherwise a new entry is created in the short-term cache, since the current packet could be the first of a long stream that renders this connection interesting.

3.3. Software Implementation

IPwatch consists of two modules: an interrupt handler written in assembler and a processing program written in C. When a packet arrives, the interrupt handler places it in a circular buffer. The processing program is triggered by the placement of packets in this buffer and by a timer that initiates sweeps of the short-term cache. The two modules are thus organized as a producer and a consumer, with the buffer allowing packets to be received even while the short-term cache is being swept or a previous packet is being processed.

Both short-term and long-term caches are organized as hash tables, indexed by connection. The short-term cache is 1024 entries long. This size has proved adequate for the range of two parameters that we have considered (10 to 45 seconds). In our experiments with IPwatch there has never been an occasion when the short-term cache has become full. The long-term cache consists of five independent tables, each containing 2000 entries. This organization is imposed by the addressing limitations of the IBM PC-AT that restrict the maximum size of contiguous data structures to 64 Kbytes. Although this restriction complicates programming it has not noticeably affected the performance of the tool. Entries in both caches are identical. Each entry is 22 bytes long and consists of the following fields:

```
struct STPD_entry
    {
    unsigned char ip_dest[4];    /* dest IP address */
    unsigned char ip_src[4];     /* src IP address */
    long pkts;                   /* no. pkts - this connection */
    long bytes;                  /* no. bytes - this connection */
    short front_ptr;             /* front ptr for chaining */
    short back_ptr;              /* back ptr for chaining */
    short table_no;              /* table number for chaining */
    short no_ticks_yet;          /* flag for new conns */
    short ticks_left;            /* counter - promotion/flushing */
    };
```

3.4. Promotion Algorithm

The promotion algorithm specifies the criteria for a connection to be considered interesting. The criterion we use is short-term traffic intensity, where the time period of observation is a few seconds or minutes. This criterion represents our personal bias, based on our experience of factors that affect performance in distributed systems. We believe that an event such as 10 packets being transmitted in one second between two machines is of greater significance than an event where those 10 packets are sent at the rate of one packet a day.

We measure traffic intensity on a connection using two parameters. The first parameter, *Time-to-Live* (τ), specifies the amount of time a connection spends in the short-term cache before being considered for promotion. The second parameter, *Packet Threshold* (π), specifies the minimum number of packets that must be seen on a connection during the time it is in the short-term cache. We ensure that each short-term entry lives at least τ seconds. If the first packet on an entry arrives just before a cache sweep (χ), the entry will have τ seconds before being considered for promotion; if it arrives just after a sweep it will have $\tau+\chi$ seconds. On the average, therefore, a connection must accumulate at least π packets in $\tau+0.5\chi$ seconds if it is to be promoted.

In assessing the effect of τ and π we need to consider their impact on two dependent variables. The first variable, *Packet Capture Ratio*, is defined as the ratio of the number of packets represented in the long-term cache to the total number of observed packets. If we view the packets corresponding to flushed connections as lost information, the packet capture ratio is a measure of the accuracy of the tool. With infinite resources we could keep a trace of all network traffic and not lose any information at all. The second dependent variable,

Promotion Ratio, is defined as the fraction of connections entering the short-term cache that get promoted. This is a direct measure of short-term locality. The number of connections promoted is a direct measure of resource usage. If many connections are promoted a large long-term cache will be necessary.

The qualitative relationship between the input parameters of IPwatch and its dependent variables is easy to establish. With τ fixed, lower values of π will cause more connections to be promoted. Fewer connections will be flushed, so the packet capture ratio will be higher. With π fixed, larger values of τ will cause more connections to be promoted, again increasing the packet capture ratio.

If our hypothesis about short-term locality is true, these relationships will not be linear, though they will be monotonic. We should find it initially easy to improve packet capture ratio by lowering π or increasing τ. Beyond a certain threshold, intuitively corresponding to the "working set" of connections, such improvement should become much more difficult. How sharp the discontinuity in behavior is and where it occurs in the parameter space cannot be analytically determined. We therefore performed a number of experiments with the tool to empirically determine this relationship. These experiments are described in the next section.

4. Experiments with the Tool

Our experimental work was motivated by a number of distinct goals. First, our intuition about the presence of short-term locality in real networks had to be validated. Second, we were curious to know the degree of short-term locality in our environment. Was 80% of the traffic accounted for by 20% of the connections, as the classic 80/20 rule would imply? Or was the distribution skewed differently? Third, we needed to calibrate IPwatch by observing its behavior with respect to its input parameters τ and π. This information is important for our future work using the tool. Finally, we wished to understand how sensitive our observations were to the specific network being observed.

The following sections present our experimental work on short-term locality. Section 4.1 describes the environment in which we conducted our work. Section 4.2 describes the experimental setup and procedure, Section 4.3 analyzes the data, and Section 4.4 analyzes the sensitivity of this data with respect to the network.

4.1. Environment

The LAN at Carnegie Mellon University, where this work was performed, spans an area of about 1 square mile and encompasses 42 buildings. Figure 0 shows the details of this network. The LAN is composed of three different kinds of media: Ethernet, IBM token-ring, and Appletalk [1]. About 42% of the machines on the LAN are on Ethernet, 55% on token-ring, and 3% on Appletalk. There are approximately 60 subnets, usually one subnet per building, and a single Ethernet backbone.

TCP/IP [8, 10] is the dominant protocol in use, accounting for over 85 percent of the packet traffic. The routers that connect subnets to the backbone support a homogeneous IP address space. IP packets can be sent between any pair of machines at CMU without explicit routing information. Of the non-IP traffic, about 8 percent is Decnet [16]. The remaining 7% is composed of a miscellany of other protocols such as ARP [7], ICMP [9] and proprietary Apple protocols. Since TCP/IP has become a *de facto* standard at CMU we anticipate that its

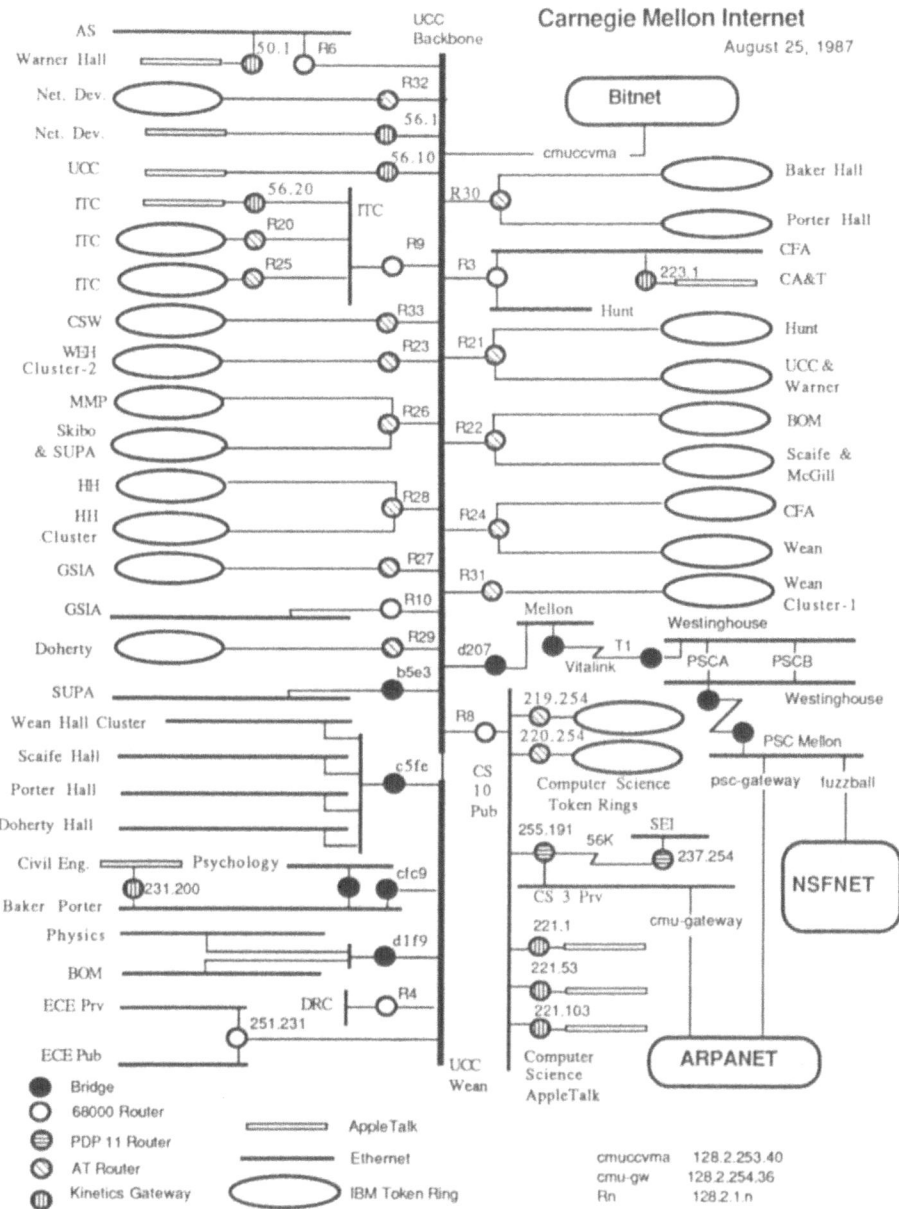

Figure 1. The CMU LAN

share of traffic will increase in the future. Consequently our tool only monitors IP traffic and ignores other packets.

There are approximately 2000 machines on the CMU LAN, spanning a diversity of types and using the network in a variety of ways. An approximate breakdown of these machines is as follows:

- 15 mainframes (IBM 3083, DEC20, etc.)
- about 70 minicomputers (VAX/780, PDP11/45, etc.)
- about 700 workstations (IBM PC-RT, DEC MicroVax, Sun-2, Sun-3, etc.)
- about 700 personal computers (IBM PC, Apple Macintosh, etc.)
- other miscellaneous machines, such as print servers and routers

Andrew workstations, of which there are over 500, interact primarily with file servers. The traffic they generate consists of machine-initiated file transfers using a non-TCP bulk transfer protocol, and remote procedure calls with relatively small arguments and results. Backups of Andrew file servers account for a large portion of the traffic. At night, 75 large disks from 17 file servers are backed up to tape, generating about a gigabyte of data.

The Computer Science Department (CSD) accounts for approximately 400 of the 2000 machines on campus. Few of these machines use Andrew. The workstations in CSD use the Software Update (SUP) protocol [14] to keep their files up to date. SUP traffic consists primarily of machine-initiated TCP-based file transfers from data servers. Paging traffic from diskless Sun workstations also contributes to traffic within the CSD subnet.

Human-initiated terminal emulation sessions, human-initiated file transfers, and electronic mail delivery are contributors to network traffic on the backbone and all subnets of the CMU LAN. On a few subnets , personal computers accessing PCServers (mentioned in Section 2.2) generate significant amounts of page-at-a-time file access traffic.

As one might expect, the backbone is the most heavily used network segment. It exhibited an average daily utilization of about 14% during the week when our experiments were performed. During the same period of time, the average daily backbone traffic amounted to over 44 million packets and 1.7 gigabytes.

4.2. Experiment Design

We first ran a number of preliminary experiments to debug our tool and to probe the parameter space for a range of interesting values for τ, the time-to-live and π, the packet threshold value. Based on the observations from these experiments we chose four values of π (2, 3, 5, and 30 packets) and four values of τ (10, 15, 30, and 45 seconds). This gave us sixteen different parameter combinations to investigate in detail.

We then set up a series of carefully controlled experiments on the CMU backbone, to observe the behavior of IPwatch for these parameter combinations. To achieve perfect experimental control we would have had to simultaneously run 16 instances of IPwatch, one for each parameter combination. To reduce the hardware requirements, we used four machines and ran four tests at a time, holding τ constant. Thus, with τ set to 10 seconds, we simultaneously ran the tests for π equal to 2, 3, 5, and 30 packets. This was then followed by the tests for τ set to 15 seconds, and so on. The short-term cache sweep time, χ, was constant at 5 seconds. Each test was run for 100 sweeps of the short-term cache.

IPwatch keeps counters of total packets, packets in promoted connections, total connections, connections promoted, and number of connections examined on each sweep of the short-term cache. From these counters we computed the following quantities:

- Packet capture ratio = packets in promoted connections / total packets
- Promotion ratio = connections promoted / total connections
- Memory usage = number of promoted connections + average number of entries in short-term cache

We express memory usage in terms of connections rather than bytes. Translating this value to bytes is trivial since a fixed amount of data is recorded for each connection.

We were interested in finding out whether short-term locality changes significantly from day to day and at different times of the day. Independent measurements of backbone utilization had indicated a peak at about 11am every day, a minimum around 7am, and a distinct period of activity around 2am when tape-backups were being performed. So we repeated the entire experiment at those three times every day, for a week that was representative of the academic year at CMU. A separate monitor was used to measure network utilization during our experiments. Since the data from our experiments was substantial (sixteen combinations run three times a day for seven days) we stored it in a relational database for convenient postprocessing.

An assumption implicit in our work is that the monitor is fast enough to observe every packet. Since traffic is bursty and there is limited buffering capacity in the network adaptors it is possible to miss packets during periods of intense network activity. Our adaptors have a status bit that is set whenever such an event occurs. IPwatch uses this status bit to keep track of the number of such events. Fortunately, there was no occasion when a packet was missed during our entire series of experiments.

4.3. Data Analysis

Initial analysis of the data showed that the variation between days was relatively small, particularly if we focused on weekdays. The weekends were similar to the weekdays in all respects except for lower utilization. We therefore focused on the weekdays and averaged the data for each time slot over 5 days. The resulting standard deviations are small relative to the mean, confirming that averaging across days is meaningful. This data is presented at the end of the paper in Tables 3, 4, and 5. For the convenience of the reader, a subset of the data from Table 5 is graphically displayed in Figures 2 through 5. The network utilization on the backbone during these experiments is shown in Table1.

The existence of short-term locality is made apparent by the presence of a sharp knee in Figure 2 and Figure 4. Figure 2, for instance, shows that a 90% capture ratio is attained with only a 15% promotion ratio. In other words, 90% of the packets are accounted for by 15% of the connections. Beyond this, small increases in the capture ratio require large increases in promotion ratio. Within the limits of statistical variation, this relationship is true for all the data presented in Tables 3 to 5. Coarsely summarizing the data in these tables it appears that less than 5% of the connections account for 75% of the traffic, less than 15% connections for 90% traffic, less than 60% connections for 98% traffic, and less than 85% connections for 99% traffic. This is a rough characterization of the short-term locality observed on the CMU backbone.

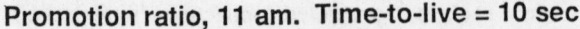

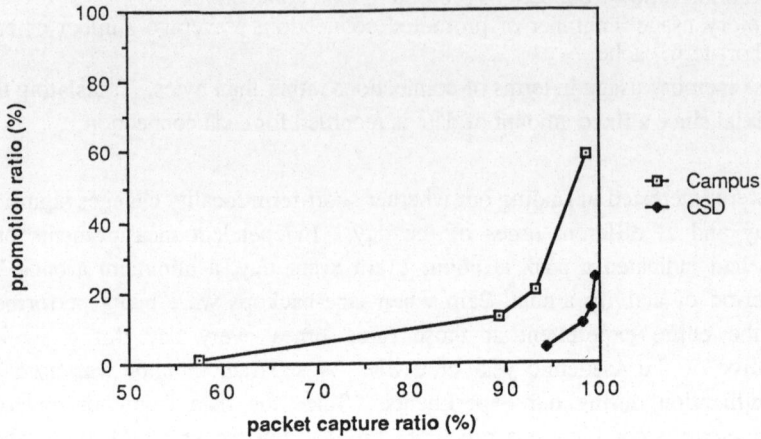

This data is obtained from Tables 5 and 8. Four data points are shown, corresponding to the four threshold values. The left-most point corresponds to a threshold value of 30 packets; the right-most point corresponds to a threshold value of 2 packets.

Figure 2. Promotion ratio versus packet capture ratio

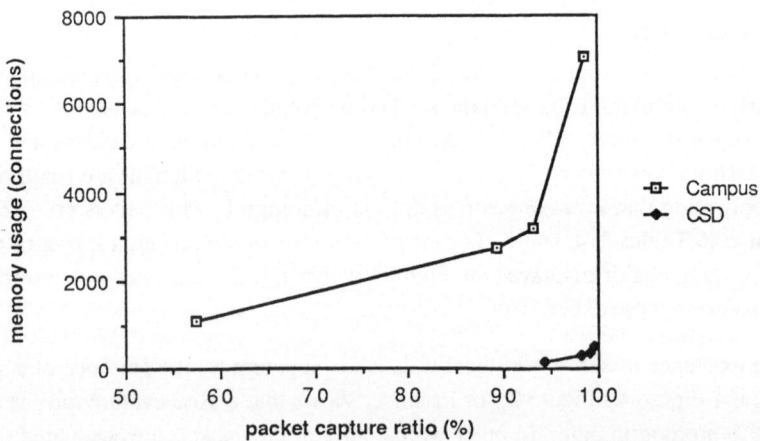

This data is obtained from Tables 5 and 8. Four data points are shown, corresponding to the four threshold values. The left-most point corresponds to a threshold value of 30 packets; the right-most point corresponds to a threshold value of 2 packets.

Figure 3. Memory usage versus packet capture ratio

Examination of Tables 3 to 5 indicates that for a given capture ratio there is little variation in promotion ratio between Tables 3, 4, and 5. However there is substantial difference in memory usage. In other words, the relative fraction of connections that are interesting does not vary significantly during the course of a day, although the total number of connections does. This is consistent with an interpretation that says that the factors contributing to short-term locality do not change even when the utilization of the network changes substantially.

This data also suggests the memory resources needed by IPwatch for medium-term monitoring of our LAN. For example, consider the data for 10 seconds in Table 5. As the threshold is increased from 2 to 3 packets, the packet capture ratio decreases from 98.6% to 93.1%. Memory usage, however, drops from 7041 entries to 3190. A relatively small sacrifice in accuracy thus leads to large savings in memory usage. The current implementation of IPwatch can have up to 10000 22-byte entries in its long-term cache. However, since the cache is organized as a hash table it should be operated well below capacity for good performance. It appears possible to operate it at about 30% capacity with an accuracy of over 90%. Alternatively we could double the amount of information maintained per connection and operate at the same accuracy using about 60% of the long-term cache capacity. The figures for memory utilization we have used here are an upper bound since they are obtained from Table 5, which corresponds to the most active part of the day. Medium-term monitoring at other times of the day will require less memory for the same accuracy.

For the set of parameter combinations we have studied, the tool is substantially more sensitive to the packet threshold π, than the time-to-live, τ. This observation holds quite strongly in all cases except for largest value of π (30 packets). Tables 3 to 5 show that a small change to π with τ fixed affects the capture ratio substantially. But changes to τ with π fixed barely change the capture ratio. The insensitivity to τ may be interpreted as meaning that a connection does not have to be monitored for long to determine if it is interesting.

For future work on our LAN we will probably use a value of 3 packets for π and 15 seconds for τ. This combination yields a capture ratio of over 90% with a promotion ratio of about 15% at all times of the day. The total memory utilization never exceeds 3000 entries, below a third of our long-term cache size.

4.4. Sensitivity of Data

Since locality is closely related to user and program behavior, it is necessary to observe a variety of networks to gain a comprehensive understanding of this property. We have taken an initial step in this direction by repeating the experiments described in Section 4.2 on the CSD subnet at CMU. As mentioned in Section 4.1, this subnet has software and usage patterns that differ significantly from the rest of CMU. It contributes little to the backbone traffic, since most traffic generated in it is addressed to hosts on the same subnet. To a first approximation, therefore, we may view the CSD subnet as an independent source of data.

The results of our experiments are shown in Tables 6, 7, and 8. As before, Figures 2 to 5 graphically depict a subset of this data. Table 2 presents the network utilization on the CSD subnet when these experiments were being run.

The presence of short-term locality is once again confirmed by the presence of a knee in Figures 2 and 3. In comparison to the backbone, the CSD subnet data shows significantly

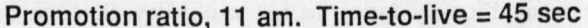

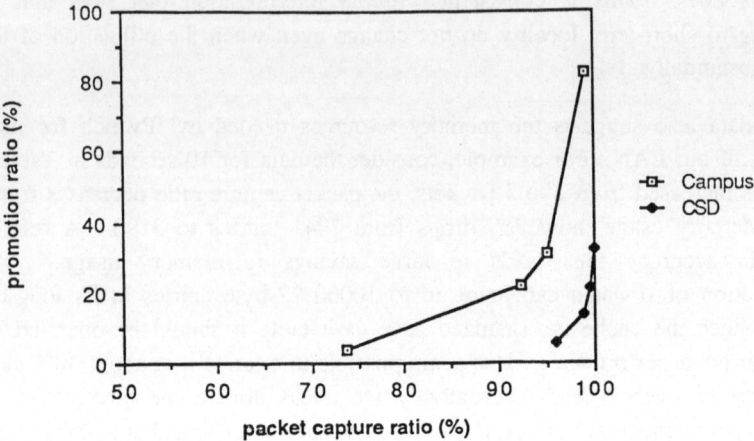

This data is obtained from Tables 5 and 8. Four data points are shown, corresponding to the four threshold values. The left-most point corresponds to a threshold value of 30 packets; the right-most point corresponds to a threshold value of 2 packets.

Figure 4. Promotion ratio versus packet capture ratio

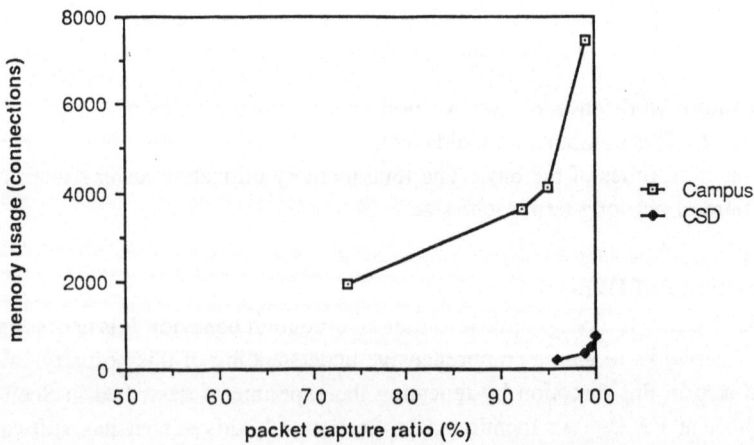

This data is obtained from Tables 5 and 8. Four data points are shown, corresponding to the four threshold values. The left-most point corresponds to a threshold value of 30 packets; the right-most point corresponds to a threshold value of 2 packets.

Figure 5. Memory usage versus packet capture ratio

Table 1. Utilization values for the campus backbone, Dec. 1 through Dec. 8, 1987

Value	Weekday	Weekend	Total
Avg. packets per day	44.4 million	28.3 million	39.8 million
Avg. bytes per day	1.7 gigabytes	1.1 gigabytes	1.5 gigabytes
Avg. utilization per day (24 hours)	15.5%	10.4%	14.1%
Avg. utilization at 2 am	12.9%	5.0%	10.7%
Avg. utilization at 7 am	10.8%	7.2%	9.7%
Avg. utilization at 11 am	14.8%	7.5%	12.7%

Table 2. Utilization values for the CSD subnet, Dec. 8 through Dec. 16, 1987

Value	Weekday	Weekend	Total
Avg. packets per day	20.2 million	10.8 million	17.5 million
Avg. bytes per day	1.1 gigabytes	0.4 gigabytes	1.0 gigabytes
Avg. utilization per day (24 hours)	11.4%	3.5%	9.1%
Avg. utilization at 2 am	8.2%	5.0%	7.3%
Avg. utilization at 7 am	5.8%	4.0%	5.3%
Avg. utilization at 11 am	21.6%	5.0%	16.9%

Table 3. Campus backbone results at 2 am

Threshold (pkts)	Time to live (sec)	Pkt Capture Ratio (%)	Promotion Ratio (%)	Memory Usage (conns)
2	10 seconds	98.0 (1.0)	53.8 (16.9)	6157 (1739)
3		92.1 (3.1)	16.5 (2.9)	2662 (398)
5		88.5 (4.8)	9.8 (1.5)	2057 (369)
30		64.1 (10.0)	1.1 (0.3)	861 (135)
2	15 seconds	98.1 (0.9)	56.9 (17.3)	5931 (1710)
3		92.8 (3.2)	13.7 (2.8)	2043 (328)
5		90.6 (4.0)	8.6 (1.9)	1536 (361)
30		71.1 (9.2)	1.6 (0.3)	913 (160)
2	30 seconds	98.8 (0.9)	66.9 (23.6)	6104 (1687)
3		93.2 (3.0)	16.0 (5.5)	2177 (527)
5		91.8 (3.4)	10.8 (4.2)	1776 (419)
30		76.8 (8.7)	2.3 (0.6)	1178 (166)
2	45 seconds	99.2 (0.9)	76.8 (24.5)	6639 (1929)
3		94.4 (2.2)	25.4 (4.0)	3321 (438)
5		91.3 (3.7)	15.8 (3.2)	2663 (595)
30		74.8 (11.8)	2.6 (0.6)	1451 (37)

Average network utilization during this period was 12.9 %. Each data point is the average of 5 weekday trials. Figures in parentheses are standard deviations. A memory connection is 22 bytes long.

Table 4. Campus backbone results at 7am

Threshold (pkts)	Time to live (sec)	Pkt Capture Ratio (%)	Promotion Ratio (%)	Memory Usage (conns)
2	10 seconds	98.0 (0.3)	57.8 (6.5)	5281 (1470)
3		90.7 (2.4)	15.1 (5.2)	1944 (608)
5		86.0 (2.8)	8.6 (1.3)	1486 (195)
30		61.4 (9.4)	0.6 (0.2)	563 (68)
2	15 seconds	98.1 (0.3)	57.0 (7.2)	5289 (1519)
3		91.5 (2.4)	10.9 (3.6)	1499 (363)
5		88.9 (2.8)	6.0 (2.6)	1063 (357)
30		71.4 (3.4)	1.1 (0.2)	604 (119)
2	30 seconds	99.3 (0.3)	70.6 (10.7)	5711 (1522)
3		93.1 (1.5)	15.0 (3.5)	1820 (446)
5		90.9 (1.9)	7.4 (2.5)	1257 (227)
30		80.8 (2.1)	1.7 (0.1)	830 (162)
2	45 seconds	99.6 (0.3)	79.5 (13.0)	6144 (1594)
3		94.8 (1.7)	23.8 (6.4)	2444 (281)
5		92.3 (1.9)	15.8 (3.2)	2078 (240)
30		78.1 (3.9)	1.8 (0.4)	1084 (179)

Average network utilization during this period was 10.8%. Each data point is the average of 5 weekday trials. Figures in parentheses are standard deviations. A memory connection is 22 bytes long.

Table 5. Campus backbone results at 11am

Threshold (pkts)	Time to live (sec)	Pkt Capture Ratio (%)	Promotion Ratio (%)	Memory Usage (conns)
2	10 seconds	98.6 (0.2)	58.7 (2.8)	7041 (769)
3		93.1 (1.6)	20.8 (2.7)	3190 (364)
5		89.3 (2.5)	13.3 (2.1)	2746 (183)
30		57.6 (4.2)	1.5 (0.1)	1080 (26)
2	15 seconds	98.5 (0.1)	59.6 (2.9)	6972 (697)
3		93.5 (0.8)	19.8 (2.8)	2868 (156)
5		90.9 (1.4)	13.2 (1.7)	2399 (156)
30		67.0 (2.2)	2.4 (0.2)	1233 (67)
2	30 seconds	99.1 (0.3)	74.4 (4.0)	7278 (1021)
3		94.1 (1.2)	23.2 (3.4)	3467 (444)
5		92.2 (1.0)	15.9 (1.5)	2664 (173)
30		73.6 (2.3)	3.7 (0.4)	1635 (112)
2	45 seconds	99.0 (0.9)	82.3 (5.5)	7459 (501)
3		94.9 (0.6)	31.3 (1.4)	4117 (150)
5		92.3 (0.8)	21.6 (1.0)	3604 (223)
30		73.7 (0.7)	4.0 (0.0)	1932 (110)

Average network utilization during this period was 14.9%. The data for 10 seconds is also presented in Figures 2 and 3. The data for 45 seconds is also presented in Figures 4 and 5. Each data point is the average of 5 weekday trials. Figures in parentheses are standard deviations. A memory connection is 22 bytes long.

Table 6. CSD subnet results at 2am

Threshold (pkts)	Time to live (sec)	Pkt Capture Ratio (%)	Promotion Ratio (%)	Memory Usage (conns)
2	10 seconds	99.5 (0.2)	20.7 (2.0)	449 (43)
3		98.9 (0.4)	16.0 (0.8)	365 (18)
5		97.0 (1.5)	12.9 (4.9)	339 (66)
30		86.3 (6.7)	2.9 (2.0)	150 (39)
2	15 seconds	99.5 (0.1)	24.4 (3.3)	527 (66)
3		98.6 (0.4)	15.6 (1.3)	355 (26)
5		97.6 (1.2)	12.8 (6.2)	303 (119)
30		94.7 (1.3)	4.6 (2.2)	134 (32)
2	30 seconds	99.5 (0.2)	22.1 (0.8)	499 (22)
3		99.3 (0.2)	19.3 (3.1)	446 (64)
5		98.3 (0.8)	13.8 (3.7)	343 (66)
30		94.7 (1.8)	5.5 (1.9)	194 (47)
2	45 seconds	99.7 (0.2)	32.1 (13.5)	702 (276)
3		99.4 (0.2)	20.4 (0.9)	478 (23)
5		98.7 (0.6)	17.4 (6.5)	424 (124)
30		96.4 (1.4)	6.6 (2.1)	228 (63)

Average network utilization during this period was 8.2%. Each data point is the average of 5 weekday trials. Figures in parentheses are standard deviations. A memory connection is 22 bytes long.

Table 7. CSD subnet results at 7am

Threshold (pkts)	Time to live (sec)	Pkt Capture Ratio (%)	Promotion Ratio (%)	Memory Usage (conns)
2	10 seconds	99.1 (0.2)	16.9 (0.7)	368 (14)
3		98.2 (0.4)	11.3 (1.5)	256 (29)
5		96.8 (1.0)	8.1 (0.9)	196 (16)
30		92.1 (2.4)	3.0 (0.7)	91 (17)
2	15 sections	99.2 (0.3)	17.9 (5.9)	391 (121)
3		98.3 (0.5)	11.5 (2.1)	266 (46)
5		97.2 (0.4)	10.6 (0.5)	258 (11)
30		92.4 (0.6)	3.1 (0.8)	105 (19)
2	30 seconds	99.5 (0.2)	22.0 (6.6)	497 (140)
3		99.1 (0.3)	16.8 (6.2)	389 (128)
5		97.7 (0.6)	9.5 (0.9)	248 (20)
30		93.0 (0.9)	3.3 (0.5)	124 (15)
2	45 seconds	99.9 (0.0)	30.9 (3.4)	676 (67)
3		99.4 (0.2)	22.7 (4.8)	521 (106)
5		98.5 (0.6)	13.9 (5.9)	359 (130)
30		94.3 (0.3)	3.8 (0.2)	152 (5)

Average network utilization during this period was 5.8%. Each data point is the average of 5 weekday trials. Figures in parentheses are standard deviations. A memory connection is 22 bytes long.

Table 8. CSD subnet results at 11am

Threshold (pkts)	Time to live (sec)	Pkt Capture Ratio (%)	Promotion Ratio (%)	Memory Usage (conns)
2	10 seconds	99.6 (0.1)	24.0 (2.0)	521 (41)
3		99.0 (0.5)	15.6 (1.5)	357 (28)
5		98.2 (0.8)	11.2 (1.6)	277 (31)
30		94.4 (2.2)	4.6 (0.1)	150 (0)
2	15 seconds	99.6 (0.1)	20.0 (1.9)	443 (39)
3		99.3 (0.2)	18.3 (1.5)	418 (28)
5		98.5 (0.5)	13.1 (0.8)	320 (14)
30		96.3 (1.3)	5.9 (0.3)	179 (14)
2	30 seconds	99.5 (0.1)	21.8 (3.5)	504 (70)
3		99.4 (0.2)	16.5 (0.6)	399 (14)
5		99.1 (0.4)	14.2 (1.6)	363 (34)
30		94.1 (2.0)	5.5 (0.7)	213 (0)
2	45 seconds	99.9 (0.0)	32.6 (4.5)	726 (95)
3		99.5 (0.2)	21.1 (2.2)	505 (43)
5		98.9 (0.4)	13.8 (1.0)	364 (20)
30		95.9 (0.7)	5.8 (0.8)	214 (13)

Average network utilization during this period was 21.6%. The data for 10 seconds is also presented in Figures 2 and 3. The data for 45 seconds is also presented in Figures 4 and 5. Each data point is the average of 5 weekday trials. Figures in parentheses are standard deviations. A memory connection is 22 bytes long.

lower memory usage and promotion ratios for a given capture ratio. The lower memory usage is attributable to the fact that there are fewer machines using the CSD subnet than the backbone. This corresponds to fewer total connections in the CSD subnet. But the lower promotion ratio indicates higher short-term locality. Less than 5% of the connections account for over 90% of the data. This is in contrast to the backbone where the top 5% of the connections accounted for only 75% of the data.

Our comparison indicates that there is indeed substantial difference in short-term locality between networks. We intend to pursue this issue further by monitoring networks outside CMU.

5. Conclusion

The work described in this paper is only the beginning of an effort to understand the nature and extent of locality in distributed systems. We view the tool described here as a common back end for a number of more specialized tools. For example, we intend to build a a real-time graphical monitor that allows operations personnel to easily keep track of those pairs of communicating hosts contributing most to network activity. The monitor would be a simple extension of the tool described here, with mechanisms for aging long-term cache entries and for displaying the most active entries. Abnormalities caused by defective software or incorrect actions by operations personnel can be detected at an early stage by the use of this monitor. Such abnormalities have seriously inconvenienced Andrew users in the past.

To understand medium-term locality, we will augment the tool described in this paper with an interface to a database system. Long-term cache entries will be entered in the database when they are flushed by an aging mechanism. The database of locality information can be used to model and improve physical network locality. As discussed in Section 2.2, such improvement may involve changes to network topology, placement of hosts, and modifications to software.

A recurring issue in empirical work is the specificity of results to the environment in which the work was done. How unique are the results presented here to CMU? Do other sites exhibit similar locality properties? To answer these questions we intend to repeat the experiments described in this paper at other organizations that use large LANs. The simplicity and portability of our tool are important virtues in this context.

In conclusion, we believe that measurement of locality is critical for tuning the performance of a distributed system. The goal of our work was to produce a tool to assist in this task. We are pleased that our implementation is accurate yet frugal, and look forward to using it to enhance our understanding of distributed systems.

References

1. *AppleBus Link Access Protocol Specification Version 1.0.* Apple Computer, Inc., 1984.

2. *LANalyzer EX 5000E Ethernet Network Analyzer User Manual.* Excelan Incorporated, San Jose, California, 1986.

3. Technical Committee Computer Communications of the IEEE Computer Society. *Carrier Sense Multiple Access Method and Physical Layer Specifications (CSMA/CD) ANSI/IEEE Std 802.3*. The Institute of Electrical and Electronic Engineers, 1985.

4. Technical Committee Computer Communications of the IEEE Computer Society. *Token-Ring Access Method and Physical Layer Specifications, ANSI/IEEE Std 802.5*. The Institute of Electrical and Electronic Engineers, 1985.

5. Morris, J. H., Satyanarayanan, M., Conner, M.H., Howard, J.H., Rosenthal, D.S. and Smith, F.D. "Andrew: A Distributed Personal Computing Environment". *Communications of the ACM 29*, 3 (March 1986).

6. Nichols, D.A. Using Idle Workstations in a Shared Computing Environment. Proceedings of the 11th ACM Symposium on Operating System Principles, November, 1987.

7. Plummer, David C. An Ethernet Address Resolution Protocol. Tech. Rept. RFC826, Network Working Group, 1982.

8. Postel, Jon, Editor. Internet Protocol DARPA Internet Program Protocol Specification. Tech. Rept. RFC791, DARPA, 1981.

9. Postel, Jon. Internet Control Message Protocol DARPA Internet Program Protocol Specification. Tech. Rept. RFC792, Network Working Group, 1981.

10. Postel, Jon, Editor. Transmission Control Protocol DARPA Internet Program Protocol Specification. Tech. Rept. RFC793, DARPA, 1981.

11. Raper, L.K. The CMU PC Server Project. Tech. Rept. CMU-ITC-051, Information Technology Center, Carnegie Mellon University, February, 1986.

12. Rosenberg, J., Everhart, C.F. and Borenstein, N.S. An Overview of the Andrew Message System. Proceedings of the ACM Sigcomm '87 Workshop, Stowe, Vermont, August, 1987.

13. Satyanarayanan, M., Howard, J.H., Nichols, D.N., Sidebotham, R.N., Spector, A.Z. and West, M.J. The ITC Distributed File System: Principles and Design. Proceedings of the 10th ACM Symposium on Operating System Principles, December, 1985.

14. Shafer, Steven. The SUP Software Upgrade Protocol. Carnegie Mellon University, Computer Science Department, 1985.

15. Striemer, Bryan L., Lorence, Mark J. Monitoring Local Area Networks at Carnegie-Mellon University: Tools for Network Planning. Tech. Rept. 07.885, IBM Corporation, 1988.

16. Wecker, S. "DNA: the Digital Network Architecture". *IEEE Transactions on Communications COM-28* (April 1980).

QUARTZ : A TOOL FOR PERFORMANCE EVALUATION OF DATA NETWORKS

Brigitte Delosme   and   Luc Coyette

CNET Paris A   SIMULOG
Issy les Moulineaux   Saint Quentin en Yvelines
France   France

ABSTRACT

We present a package developed to help data network designers and users by giving them means for estimating protocols performances. This tool provides an interactive data input and display with graphical facilities and a choice of models for algorithmic resolution. Quartz is an evolving tool; it can be easily completed as new protocols and evaluation methods appear.

INTRODUCTION

Faced with the complexity of data networks, a network service client or provider as well as a private network designer needs means to evaluate and compare the performances of different solutions.
Some of the main questions one needs to answer are for instance:
How to choose protocol parameters in order to achieve best network performances? How should a network evolve when the traffic characteristics change? What are the best network and the most suitable end to end protocol for an application's requirements?
These general questions cannot be answered easily. They require the experience and knowledge of skilled experts, and time. But the help of powerful computer tools may greatly alleviate these constraints.

Quartz has then be designed to allow everyone to carry out such various studies in a time reasonably short. It is intended to cover all the performance questions for which an answer or a good approximate solution can be obtained rapidly. These solutions are mostly based on analytic methods which are proposed in the literature.

The primary objective in developing Quartz software has been to provide a flexible environment for data network performance studies, which allows:
- to describe data networks protocols and topology easily;
- to define performance questions and to analyse and compare results quickly;
- to combine models freely;
- to implement new evaluation algorithms as simply as possible.

Apart the general purpose tools which require their user to learn a specific language or to describe a system according to a given modelling technique, a few dedicated tools[1,2] are available today for data network performance evaluation. These tools give means to describe a data network with its protocols by using the concepts and vocabulary generally used in this field. However all of them are simulation-oriented, and they do not take full advantage of the protocol analyses and evaluation methods which have been developed these last years.

In the following section we present the basic concepts which have led Quartz development and the resulting software features. The next section shows examples of study realizations. Some technical characteristics of Quartz implementation and performances are given next. Finally, we indicate the developments which are forecasted in a near future.

QUARTZ DESIGN

Layered Organization

All network architectures are structured in protocol layers and share a common set of basic functionalities. This layer or functionality division is widely used and has proved to be helpful for describing a data network. Network architecture is represented in Quartz by such a layered structure.

Most of the performance evaluation questions which are tackled in the literature concern the efficiency of a mechanism or the optimisation of a parameter. This corresponds with the protocol layer structure, the performance of a protocol or a procedure (associated with a layer) depending on characteristics of the two adjacent layers (see Fig. 1).

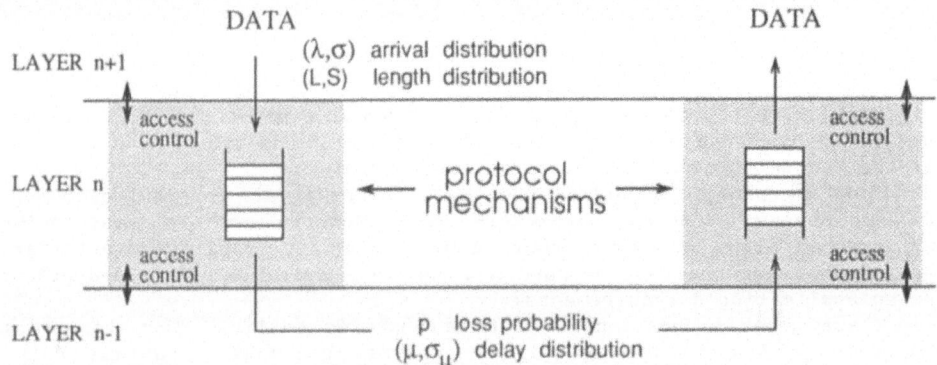

Fig. 1.   Protocol Layer Representation.
In order to provide a service to the layer above, protocols are defined at each layer, between peer entities; they use the service of the layer below for exchanging data. Control procedures, mechanisms, and parameters specify a protocol. The functionalities of a layer define the offered service, availability, loss probability and transfer delay characterize it.

"Study levels" are defined in Quartz, they have been associated with protocol layers according to an architecture such as that represented by the OSI reference model. At every study level Quartz proposes to solve a set of problems and to obtain selected performance measures, according to the existence of tractable computing methods. Currently, Quartz answers performance questions on the data transfer phase of protocols at the link, network and transport layers. A study level is also dedicated to end-to-end application services. Quartz also deals with other problems related to the network layer: node buffer allocation and blocking, and traffic routing.

Modelling Choice

To analyze the performance of a given protocol, several computation methods may be available through Quartz. Each method corresponds to a different model and requires a certain amount of data to be run. But the choice of a method depends mainly on the phenomenon and the parameters which are important to study or to take into account, in the user view.

Due to the layered organization of protocols, three points intervene in the model definition :
- the protocol modelling, it can take into account or neglect parameters and mechanisms;
- the arrival process of client data, it may correspond to different schemes and then calls for different models;
- the underlying data transfer service, which may also be represented by models which differ in their level of approximation.
Quartz solutions cover the classical models[3], based on queueing systems theory. Any numerical method can be implemented easily; this allows to introduce different models, to answer more questions, or to experiment new solutions.

The user can then build his own model by combining models at different study levels. For instance, when concerned by the network layer performances a user may choose to model the data links by M/G/1 queues[4]; the parameters of the general service time distribution can then be derived from different models of the link layer. For instance, the link protocol could be neglected if retransmissions are very rare; the link service time distribution may then be associated with the packet length distribution. On the other hand, for constant size packets, modelling the link error recovery procedure[5] provides the mean and variance of packet service time, which includes the possible retransmissions.

Adaptivity to User Knowledge

According to the layer based resolution, a user can study a protocol by giving only a simplified information on the service underneath and on the traffic input characteristics. He can thus concentrate his effort on the parameter analysis of the protocol he is concerned with.
However, if a user has a good knowledge of the network and of the protocols which intervene in the system under study, he can use this information to obtain more precise results by evaluating performance indices of underlying services.

Once the user has chosen his study level and the question he wants to answer, Quartz proposes different models to solve the problem. According to the user selection, the data which are needed to run the associated computation are displayed; they can be completed and modified by the user.
When needed data are lacking, the user can either get values through measurement campaigns or make use of Quartz set of default values or computation means. The default values of some variables -typical parameters of a protocol or a network- may be displayed on request. Other variables may be obtained by solving a problem at a lower layer; for this, the user can select one of the available models and associated computation method.
This possibility of performing a study with different degrees of detail on the system knowledge is one of the most important features of Quartz. It gives the user means to solve a problem at the best going more or less deeply in its modelling aspects.

Input/Output Interactivity

The user interaction needs are obviously not limited to the problem definition and the selection of solvers. The means for interactive input and output have also required a great attention for making Quartz a very practical tool.

The main care of Quartz about inputs is not to impose a sequence of entries when it is not necessary. Then, the user can start anywhere: he can describe a protocol, a network or a node, in any order, or he can go through model descriptions and define the overall system modelling. So, he may keyboard data before having precised both the problem he is interested in and the model defining the data needed for the computation. He can also focus on the problem solving and enter the data when asked by the solver.
Some data need to be entered at the keyboard but tedious keyboarding of data, such as the network topology input (nodes and links, and their type), may be avoided as graphical means can be used.

Graphics capabilities are largely used to display the results as they give a visual, immediate way of analysis. For instance, histograms and curves are the direct results of a user action: iteration on all the elements of a kind or parameter study through a step by step variation. The network topology representation is also a convenient medium to display various data. It is possible to highlight a route on the network representation, to show the links in a given area of load, to use a zoom, to display a subnetwork, to pick out an element and obtain detailed information on it, etc.

Information Storage Facilities

The last main point of Quartz is the additional means of storage and retrieval of data, results and study history according to the user will. When performing a study the user can store the data he modified and the results and statistics he obtained either on the current network files or on new files under a given network name. The environment of a user study, i.e. all the current files describing the data network, are saved on request under the selected network name. The file structure associated with a network is stored in the network directory, and the evolution of networks (or directories) is described in a history file.

Another kind of storage proposed by Quartz is the storage of what we call a scenario. When a user runs a Quartz session, he may move in Quartz menus, compute some variables at one level, some others at another level, and draw results. He may wish to repeat later on the same sequence of actions with slightly different data without going through all the steps leading to the expected result. Quartz allows the user to store under a given scenario name the series of computation routines which have been run during the ongoing session. The scenario can then be loaded for another run; parameters asked to the user (e.g. names of storage files may be needed) are reduced to minimum.

These storage facilities are completed with a graphical display of the existing network and scenario names. User comments and file or algorithm names which intervene are easily obtained from the diagram. They can be linked, moved, re-ordered, erased, on a graphical manner. For instance, in the case of a network deletion, the specific files which do not enter in another network combination will be destroyed. The way this information is managed depends on the user; this additional software offers means for drawing, modifying and storing a graph, and associating the directory organization.

120

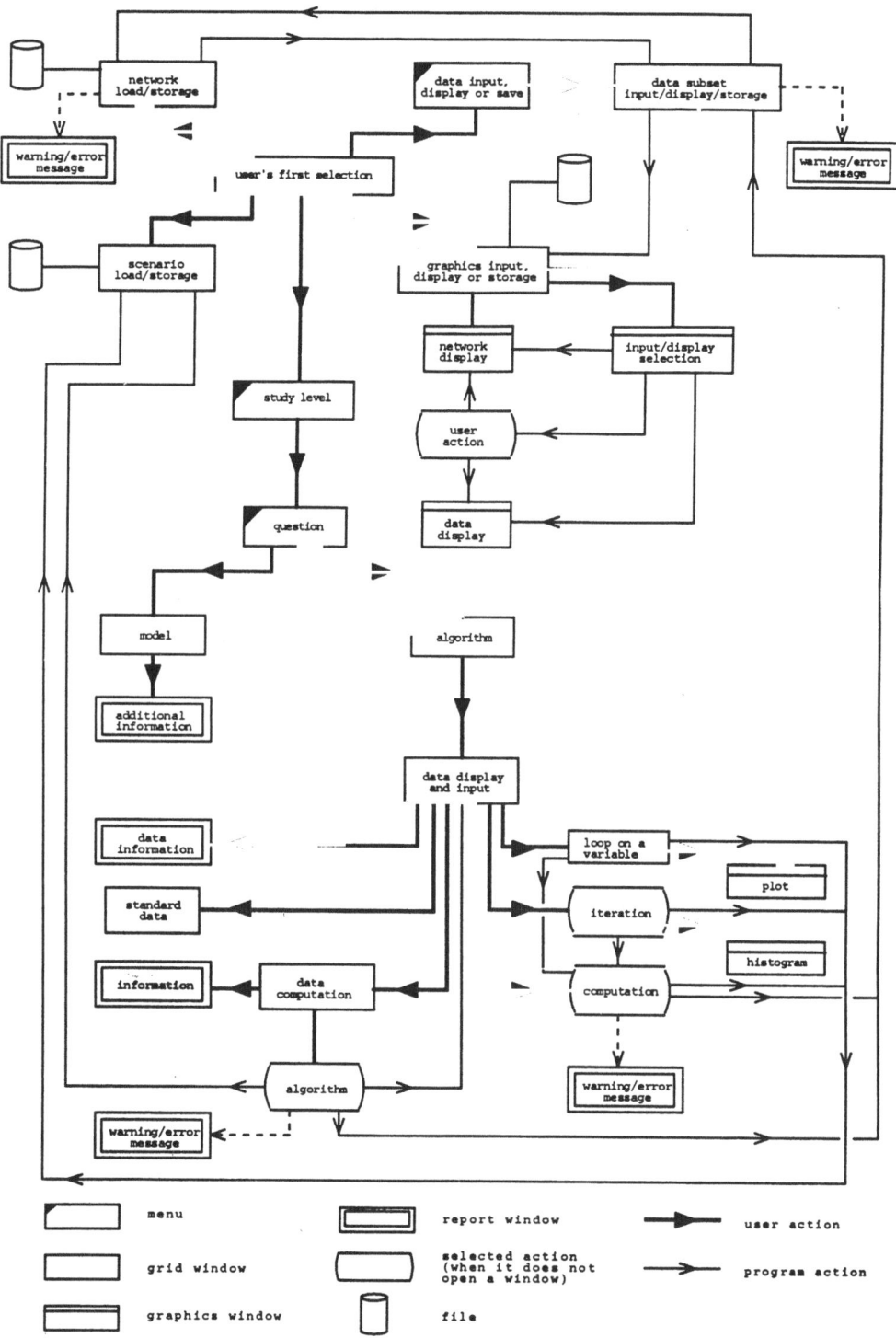

Fig. 2.   Quartz operation diagram.

Quartz Operation

Fig. 2 depicts the overall functionning of Quartz. It shows the possible series of steps in a Quartz session, and presents the links between software functions and user operations.

Quartz displays menus and windows under user actions through a mouse device. Walking in menus is permitted at any stage of a session, it allows to open several windows simultaneously. Open windows are correlated; any change in data due to user actions in a window causes their automatic update wherever they are displayed. But this does not mean that previous values are systematically lost. Quartz manages a current and a temporary value for each network variable. Modifying data in a window acts on temporary values. Controls available in the windows may update the current values (an algorithm run will not, a general computation will). The temporary values which are displayed become current ones if the user decides so for the session continuation. This provided flexibility may penalyze the overall consistency of data. The combination of models at different levels may also seem inconsistent. But this is what gives modelling study possibilities to the user. Some care has then to be taken when using Quartz. Data consistency checks can be run, a summary of modelling assumptions can be displayed; this should be done before interpreting the results of any study. However, Quartz can provide a consistent default model of the multi-layer architecture (in function of the network description and the performance question), which frees the user of the model combination process.

EXAMPLES OF STUDIES WITH QUARTZ

We present here two performance evaluation problems and we show how Quartz can be used to solve them. We assume that the user does not select a predefined scenario or a default option.

Link Level Procedure Optimization

Let us consider the design of a private network which will consist of dedicated data links. The network designer has selected to implement an HDLC type protocol on the links, but there exist many versions to choose among and several parameters to adjust. The study must result in giving the right configuration for the required performances as well as the minimum cost solution.

Entering in Quartz at the link level of study, the user selects the performance index he is interested in (throughput, delay). Then different models of protocol analysis are proposed to him together with explanations about their main differences. Models can take into account, or not, the occurence of errors or of window blocking, frames can be considered of constant or exponentially distributed length, etc.. The user may then ask for more detailed information on any of the proposed models and associated algorithm. Once the model has been selected, a grid of variables to be filled appears. Link characteristics (capacity, bit error rate, and propagation delay) must be entered as well as protocol parameter values. Link characteristics can be obtained from the data link provider. Protocol parameters (i.e., retransmission policy, window size, timeout, frame and header lengths) can be filled with default or standard values, some of them (e.g., the optimal timeout) may be computed by selecting a proposed calculation; typical values and computation formulas or algorithm names are displayed under the user's request.

In order to look at the effects of a variable or a parameter value, it is possible to make it vary by defining the loop parameters (bounds, step) and to draw automatically the resulting plot. The optimum value of the performance index can then be determined in a visual manner. This allows to choose, for instance, the frame length or the window size, for a given link.

Instead of doing a link per link analysis, the user may wish to act more globally. Then, another way to proceed is to first describe a network of links representing the characteristics of all the possible links. The user can define a protocol type and a link type which will be associated to each link; the associated parameters will not need to be entered for each link. The computation of the performance index can then be obtained by one action (iteration) which repeats the algorithm on all the network links. Results are displayed on request on an histogram. Changing a protocol parameter or a link characteristic (e.g., its capacity) will give another histogram to compare with the previous one. Further improvements may be achieved by analyzing the links which show the lowest performance.

Message Transfer Delay Evaluation

We consider now an interactive application where a user sends queries to an information system which sends back a message, e.g. a video-page. The data communication is established on a public packet network. One question of interest both for the user and the information service provider is : how long it will take between the sending of the user request and the display of the new page ?
The performance index of interest depends on the public network service characteristics and on the end to end layers which are implemented at both ends.
The response time we want to compute is a compound of the following delays :
a) the delay between the sending action of the user and the arrival of the generated packet in the network transmission queue;
b) the network transfer delay;
c) the packet delivery delay at the destination station;
d) the message (reply) generation delay;
e) the delay to put the first message packet in the transmission queue, and, if message packets do not arrive in one bulk, packet interarrival delays to this queue;
f) the time elapsed from the first packet emission to the last packet reception at the user station;
g) the delay between the message reassembly and the page display on the user's screen.
The delays b and f are directly related to the network performance indices. The delay d is a characteristic of the server information system performance. The other delays (a, c, e, and g) depend on the interlayer protocols response time and blocking features; they are very dependent on the protocol architecture implementation at both user and server stations.

Most of these delays cannot be obtained from computation methods in Quartz, they might be stored in the Quartz data base of standard values if the end station equipment configuration is a common one. These end delays can be entered by Quartz users as average delays or parametric functions which are obtained from measurements, simulations or specific models.
But the derivation of delays such as b or f (packet or message transfer time on the network) is a typical issue to be handled with Quartz.

These delays depend on whether or not there is a flow control mechanism and, if so, what type of flow control is implemented (point to point or end to end). They depend also on the network routing mode (datagram or virtual circuit). According to the given situation, the user can select a model where all the existing mechanisms are taken into account. But he may have then to modify some assumptions (or to restrict some parameters to given values) in order to get a result, as there may not exist any method to solve the modelled system he has in mind. On the other hand, the user may decide to ignore some of the existing mechanisms, as being of minor importance, in order to stay closer to the modelling assumptions he wishes to examine.

In order to make up his mind, the user can scan the different models proposed by Quartz, reading explanation messages, looking at the variables which are requested for running an algorithm and at the ways (and underlying models) to get them. However, if the user does not want to analyze closely the modelling aspects of the problem, Quartz will select the method which fits the best with what is known on the user's problem.

For instance, if we are concerned with a virtual circuit on an X25 network with end to end flow control, there exist network models taking into account the size of the end to end window. They allow the computation of the network mean transfer delay of a packet. These models vary as does the model of service for the data link transmission queue; the service time of a packet on a link being depicted by a negative exponential, a constant or a general distribution. In the latter case, the coefficient of variation of the general distribution can be given by the user, or the first two moments can be obtained from Quartz (by taking a model of HDLC protocol at the link level and computing the virtual service time of a packet). When these values are available, they are automatically used in the calculation of the network transfer delay if no contrary indication is received from the user.

The derivation of the message mean transfer delay relies on somewhat different modelling assumptions. However, it is possible to make different combinations of models in order to take into account various parameters. Models considering both message reassembling and window flow control are very simplified. Regarding the former problem, there are several realistic models; results are either exact (for a simple model), approximate or given only by bounds (when models are more general). For instance, there is a model[6] which gives the exact mean interpacket gap when the queues are assumed M/D/1, from which is derived the message mean reassembly time and its mean transfer time. Another model[7] bounds the mean reassembly time with very general assumptions both on the arrival process (which does not need to be Poisson) and on the service time distribution. Models taking into account the blocking due to the end-to-end window are derived by adjusting the initial gap between consecutive packets in function of the window blocking duration.

IMPLEMENTATION AND PERFORMANCE FEATURES

Current Implementation Characteristics

Quartz runs on a Sun 3 workstation under the Unix operating system. It uses Sunview, the Sun window and menu system which handles also keyboard and mouse inputs. Graphics are implemented over SunCore and SunGKS. Quartz software has been developed with an extensive use of the Sun facilities, in a view of rapidity. However, the software has been designed in order to ease its transfer on other Unix machines. Quartz is written in C and uses Fortran graphics libraries : Marc (by Simulog) for plots and statistics, and Flore (over GKS, by Cnet) for network representation and handling. Quartz does not use a database system but the file and directory management provided by Unix.

The compiled version of Quartz software takes less than 3 Megabytes of memory, and requires about 4 Megabytes of local memory.

The current prototype includes almost all the functions which have been described in the previous sections. Only the programming of a few isolated functions has been left aside, in this first version. They concern some additional facilities which enhance the management of Quartz sessions (such as network history). But their feasibility does not pose problems. As far as the performance evaluation process is concerned, some important studies have yet to be completed. They concern the validity of the multi-layer combination of existing models, and the definition of the standard modelling associated to the most common protocol architectures.

Examples of Quartz Displays

Figs. 3, 4 and 5 show a screen display obtained by Quartz (colors have been converted in black and white or grey scale for printing purpose). Fig. 3 presents grid windows and a histogram associated to a link level study. Fig. 4 presents graphical windows showing a network and the network drawing menu. Fig. 5 shows the graphical representation of a flow routing.

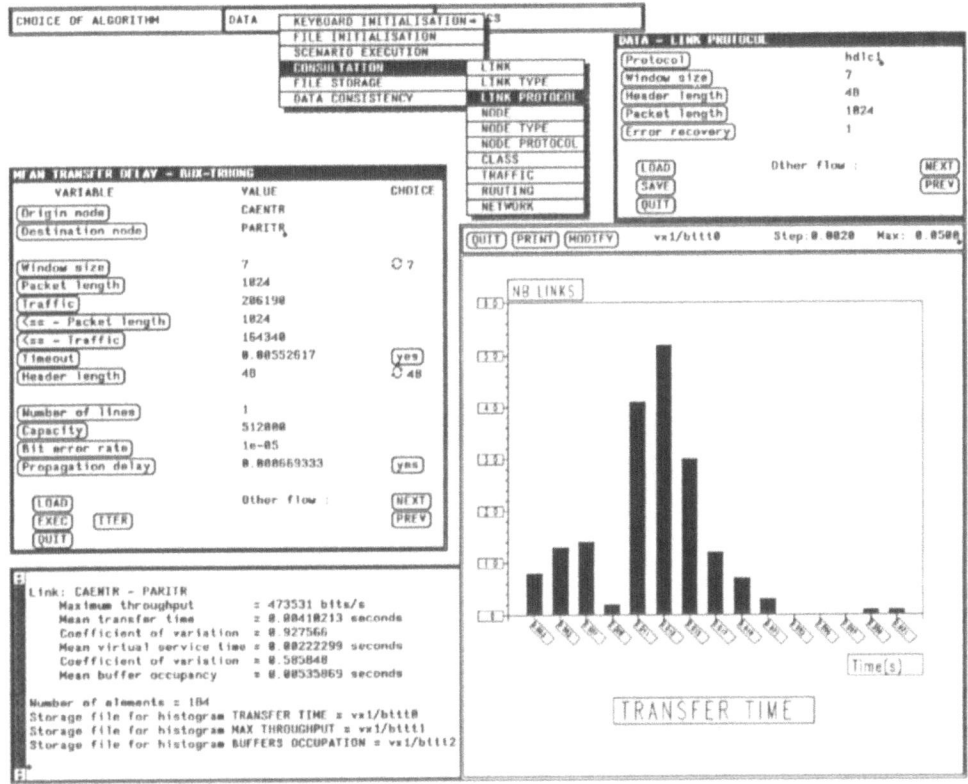

Fig. 3.   A screen display of Quartz menus, windows and statistics.
          A configuration of the general menu and a menu walk, leading
          to the visualization of a data subset, are displayed at the
          top of the screen. The latter selection opens the window
          presented in the upper right corner.
          A grid window has been opened when the algorithm was selected
          (on the middle left). The first rows are used to identify the
          element to study, the next ones define the protocol parameters
          and the input traffic, the last set of variables shows the
          element's characteristics.
          In the lower left corner, the report window gives the result
          of the algorithm when applied on the selected link. This run
          was followed by the computation iteration over the whole
          network and by the display of the corresponding histogram (in
          the lower right window).

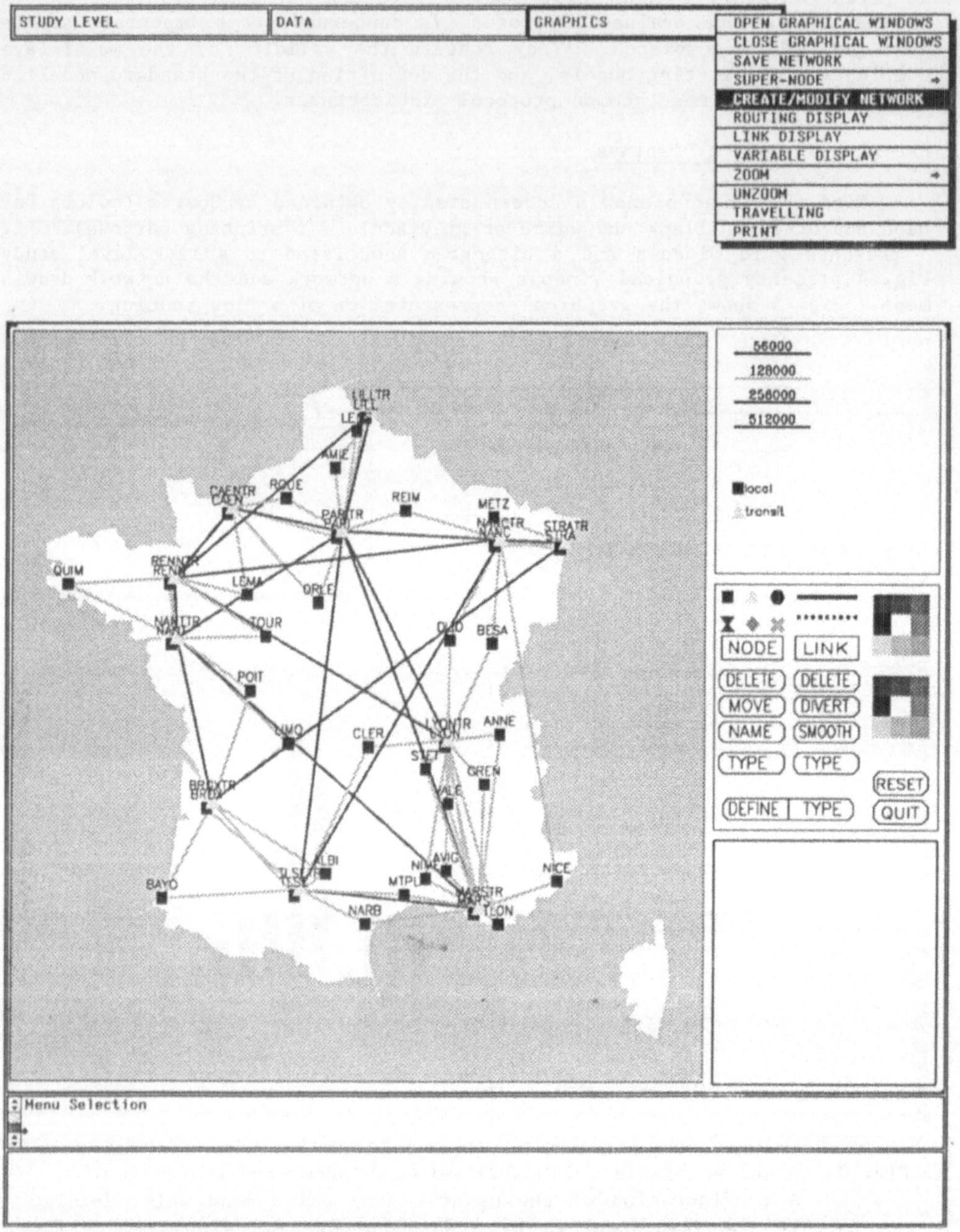

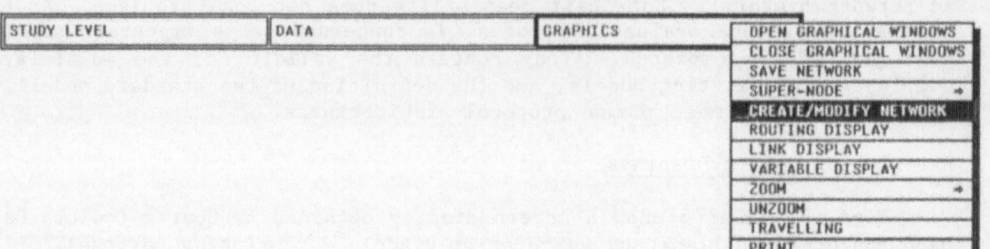

Fig. 4. A screen display of Quartz graphics windows.
The large window is used to display the whole network (or part of it, when zooming). The small window at the middle right displays icons, selection buttons, and color grids. Here, according to the menu selection, this window allows network drawing and modification. Actions are initiated by clicking the mouse on an icon, a color, or a button. Icons and colors are used to differentiate the nodes and the links in function of their type. The top right window shows the link and node types which have been already defined.

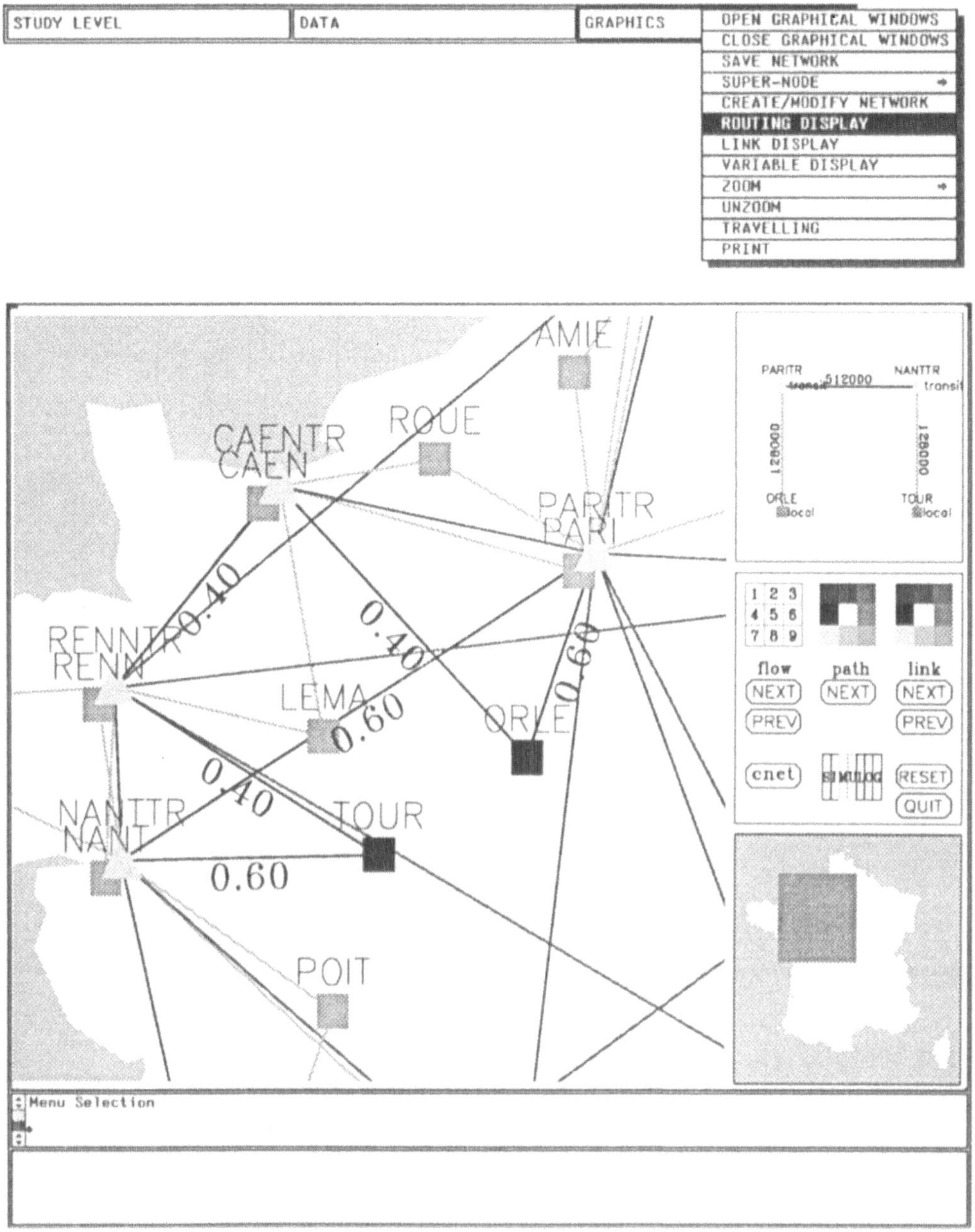

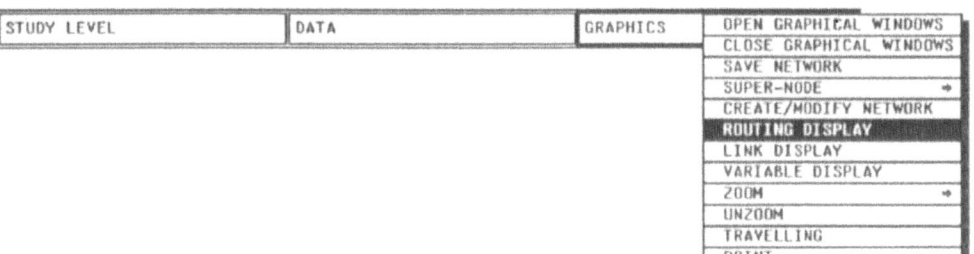

Fig. 5. Graphical display of a network routing.
          The large window presents a part of the network obtained by
          zooming.   The small window at the lower right shows the
          location of this part. The middle right window displays text
          and buttons which are used to visualize the routing paths used
          by a flow and link characteristics.
          The routes are highlighted on the large window, the proportion
          of traffic routed on each path is displayed on the links. The
          top right window shows successively the links and nodes along
          each routing path.

In order to give an idea of Quartz performances, as seen by a user, some time measurements are displayed in Table 1. These measurements have been taken on a Sun 3/260 in a network with several users; the version which was running did not use a floating point accelerator card, nor a graphical processor card.

Table 1. Performance measurements on a 49 nodes-184 links network

user action result	network loading	graphics display				
		initial display[a]	re-display[b]	zoom phys.	logi.	modifi-cations[c]
time duration	25s	25s	5s	5s	20s	25s

[a] includes graphics initialization (GKS and Flore)
[b] when there is no change in the graphical attributes of the elements on display
[c] when there is some change in the graphical attributes

user action result	algorithm iteration		
	link transfer delay (184)	network transfer delay (1728 VCs)	message transfer delay (1728 VCs)
time duration	3s	$5s^d$ 10 to $30s^{e,g}$ $300s^f$	6 to $8s^{d,g}$

[d] without flow control
[e] with end to end flow control (window = 2)
[f] with point to point flow control (window = 1)
[g] depending on the selected algorithm

CONCLUSION

Quartz software architecture has been completely realized today, however it is a never ending task to provide performance evaluation models and computation methods as new results and new protocols are developed everyday. The selection of algorithms to be implemented is time-consuming as they have first to be tested in order to check their validity domain. Numerical methods need also to be efficient. Considering both modelling and time requirements, problem analysis has often led us to develop new algorithms.

Currently we have implemented several algorithms at the link, network and transport levels (as defined by OSI) for meshed networks. Algorithms for node buffer sharing and traffic routing are also available. Next implementations will concern local area networks and internetworking issues.

Quartz now enters a phase of trials by potential users. This will point out both the main needs for algorithms, and the improvements of the user interface which are required.

ACKNOWLEDGEMENTS

We would like to mention all the persons who have participated in Quartz development: Yvon Coadou and Bernard Dao for graphics and algorithm programming respectively, Patrick Brown for his expertise in queueing network analysis, Andrzej Pach and Alain Simonian for their work on developing new algorithms.

REFERENCES

1. L. Coyette, D. Duong, B. Delosme, and P. Brown, Evolution of Performance Evaluation Packages, in "Proceedings of the International Workshop on Modelling Techniques and Performance Evaluation," G. Pujolle, ed., North-Holland (1987).
2. K. Barath-Kumar, and P.Kermani, Performance Evaluation Tool (PET): An Analysis Tool for Computer Communication Networks, IEEE J. on Sel. Areas in Comm., vol. SAC-2, n°1 (1984).
3. M. Reiser, Communication-System Models Embedded in the OSI-Reference Model, A Survey, in "Computer Networking and Performance Evaluation : Proceedings of the IFIP WG7.3," Hasegawa, Takagi, Takahashi, ed., North-Holland (1985).
4. M. Dao, Etude du contrôle de flux par fenêtre dans un réseau à circuits virtuels, CNET Int. Rep., NT/PAA/ATR/SST/911 (1983).
5. W. Bux, K. Kummerle, and H.L. Truong, Balanced HDLC Procedures: A Performance Analysis, IEEE Trans. on Comm., COM-28, n°11 (1980).
6. P. Brown, and A. Simonian, Evaluation of Inter-Packet Delay in a Packet-Switched Network, in "Proceedings of the Third International Conference on Data Communication Systems and their Performance," (1987).
7. P. Brown, B. Delosme, and A. Pach, Bounds on the average message reassembly time in a packet data network, CNET Int. Rep., DE/ATR/63.87 (1987), to be published.

TEL - A VERSATILE TOOL
FOR EMULATING SYSTEM LOAD

Maria Calzarossa
Dipartimento di Informatica e Sistemistica
Università di Pavia
27100 Pavia, Italy

Giuseppe Serazzi
Dipartimento di Scienze dell'Informazione
Università di Milano
20133 Milano, Italy
Ist. Analisi Numerica–CNR, Pavia, Italy

ABSTRACT

The evolution of computer system architectures, from isolated workstations to supercomputers and distributed systems, yields the development of new evaluation techniques. Benchmarking, i.e., one of the most popular methodology used to establish the system performance, has been deeply influenced. Sequence of timed–tests, like the original benchmarks, showed serious short–comings that have severely limited their applications on new computational environments (e.g., multiprocessors, local area and wide area networks, distributed systems). The tool for emulating system load, described in this paper, is designed with two basic objectives: to generate a repeatable workload on a system under test, and to easily modify the produced workload in order to tune its composition to match that of the real load to be emulated.

This work was partially supported by "Ministero della Pubblica Istruzione", Project 40%.

1. INTRODUCTION

Evaluation techniques have evolved with the continuous development of knowledge in the field of computer systems performance and of computer system technologies and architectures. Among the most popular methods, one can mention benchmarking and modelling.

In the computer field, the term *benchmark* means a point of reference, for other hardware or software products, which may be used for comparative evaluation purposes. Benchmarking is a direct measurement approach. An executable model of the real workload is input into the system to be evaluated (referred to as the System Under Test, or SUT), and the values of the various performance indices are measured during the run. In its simplest form, a benchmark is a set of individual application programs that are directly executable on the various systems analyzed. In these cases, benchmarking can be considered as a sequence of timed test performed on the computing environment under evaluation. Such tests have been extensively used in competitive procurement studies of batch systems (see e.g., [Stra72]). In some cases, benchmarks are purposely built for the particular problem at hand, e.g., [Wood71, Kern73], whereas in other cases preexisting programs are utilized, e.g., [Buch69, Gibs70].

Timed tests are recently used to evaluate the computational power of supercomputers through the execution of kernels, i.e., sequences of instructions characterizing the computational aspect of the applications, [Bail85, Lube85. Dong86].

One of the major drawbacks of timed tests is that they are not adequate to simulate the behavior of the load submitted by interactive users. Indeed, it has been recognized that the performance of interactive systems is strongly dependent on the types of command submitted as well as on the characteristics of their traffic.

Therefore, to avoid this short–coming, the technique of emulation has been incorporated into benchmarking. This has been done by constructing programs, i.e., drivers, that generate "user commands" according to prespecified parameters. Drivers intercept the messages directed from SUT to each user and submit the next command prescribed by the script they are following after an amount of time that accounts for the output, think, and type–in times. When the drivers run directly on the SUT, they are called Local Terminal Emulators; if they run on another system properly connected to the SUT, they are Remote Terminal Emulators.

Both types of driver have been employed in a large number of studies. e.g.,

[Gree69, Salt70, Foge72, Stra87]. It is important to observe that remote emulators do not appreciably influence the load they generate on the SUT, whereas local emulators perturb this load by superimposing on it the overhead they produce.

The primary objective of a driver is to provide a means of applying a repeatable user workload on the SUT. The type of load to be generated is a function of the objective of the study and of the characteristic of the considered SUT. In the analyses dealing with performance of an isolated interactive system the driver emulates the terminal user workload. The SUT must not be able to detect the difference between interactions with real users and with the driver.

When a SUT consists of a computer network or a distributed system, the driver must generate a controlled traffic of messages in the network [Shoc80, Bux84], and a controlled load on the various nodes of the system.

Depending on the characteristics of the study and of the SUT considered, various kinds of script are employed. Scripts used as interactive terminal emulators are sequences of commands sent from a terminal (the driver) and of the think times that are to elapse between any two consecutive commands in the stream. The commands may be executed locally or remotely depending on whether the SUT consists of one or more interconnected systems. When the performance of distributed and parallel systems is to be investigated, the scripts are constituted by a sequence of processes that are executed on the various CPUs (local or remote) and the problem of synchronization must also be taken into account.

A critical aspect in every benchmarking study is the representativeness of the scripts generated by the driver to emulate the real load. Indeed, these scripts must be constructed or selected among the real ones using appropriate techniques, [Ferr83]. Figure 1 illustrates several typical application environments corresponding to the various types of study that can be performed.

As already seen, the application of benchmarking technique encompasses all the most common types of performance study ranging from tuning, sizing, capacity planning, bottleneck identification, and competitive procurement.

The main objective of the Tool for Emulating system Load (TEL) described in this paper is to provide a versatile and general purpose tool for benchmarking different SUTs. Depending on their characteristics and on the objective of the study, suitable representative scripts must be considered and a particular methodology must be applied.

The operations performed by TEL are partitioned into three groups (modules), according to their characteristics, namely an Input Definition Module (IDM), a

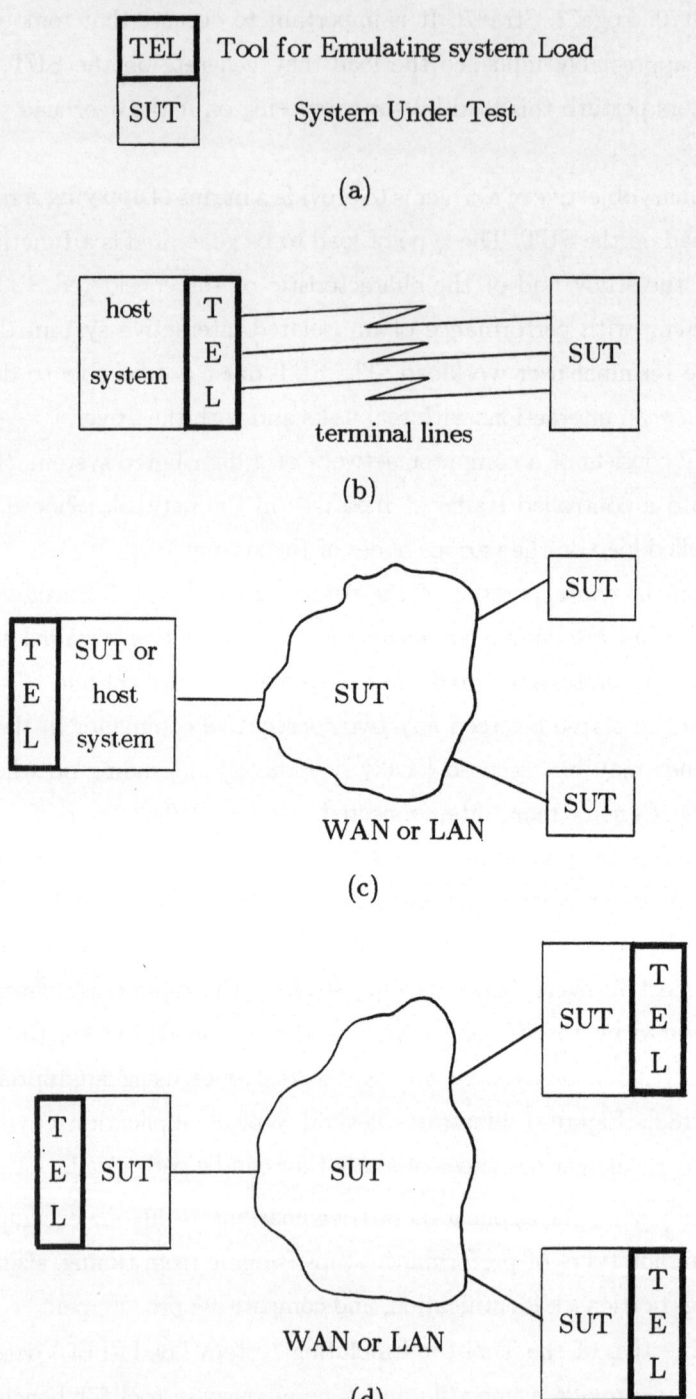

Figure 1 - Typical application environments of TEL (Tool for Emulating system Load) corresponding to various types of SUT: (a) and (b) isolated systems or workstations, (c) and (d) a local area and wide area network together with one or more systems or workstations.

Processing Module (PM), and a Data Analysis Module (DAM). The functional structure of the tool is presented in Section 2. A detailed analysis of each of its three components is given in Sections 3, 4, and 5, respectively. Final remarks and future developments are described in Section 6.

2. THE FUNCTIONAL STRUCTURE OF THE TOOL

According to its main objectives, the Tool for Emulating system Load (TEL) has been implemented with a highly flexible structure. The resulting tool is general purpose and can be easily adapted to the different environments to be tested.

TEL can run in several ways:

- resident on the SUT (Fig. 1a);

- stand–alone on its own system driving a separate SUT (Fig. 1b);

- as an application on one or more systems driving a network and several SUTs in distributed environments (Figs. 1c, 1d); the systems where TEL is resident can be the SUTs themselves.

To increase its portability and the reproducibility of the experiments, the tool is self–contained. A pseudo–random number generator, measurement instrumentation, report generator and statistical routines are provided. To perform a complete benchmarking experiment, users do not need to learn and employ a specific command language since TEL is interactive and menu–driven in all its phases.

Since the subject of this paper is the description of the tool, input and output are always defined from the TEL viewpoint. The files generated by TEL, consisting of a sequence of commands, are the input to the SUT.

The operations performed by the TEL can be subdivided into three functional modules: an *input definition* module, an execution or *processing* module, and a *data analysis* module (see Fig. 2).

Main operations performed by the input module are related to the setup of the experimental environment and to the load description. This module consists of an interactive program which runs prior to the execution of the experiment. The user is allowed to describe the proper physical and logical configuration required in the study (e.g., number of terminals emulated, locations of the SUTs) and how the communications between the tool and the SUT take place (e.g., via terminal lines, via network). The load to be executed is defined by the experimenter by means of the scripts. In principle, the scripts can be representative of either real or hypothetical (when no data are available) workloads to be

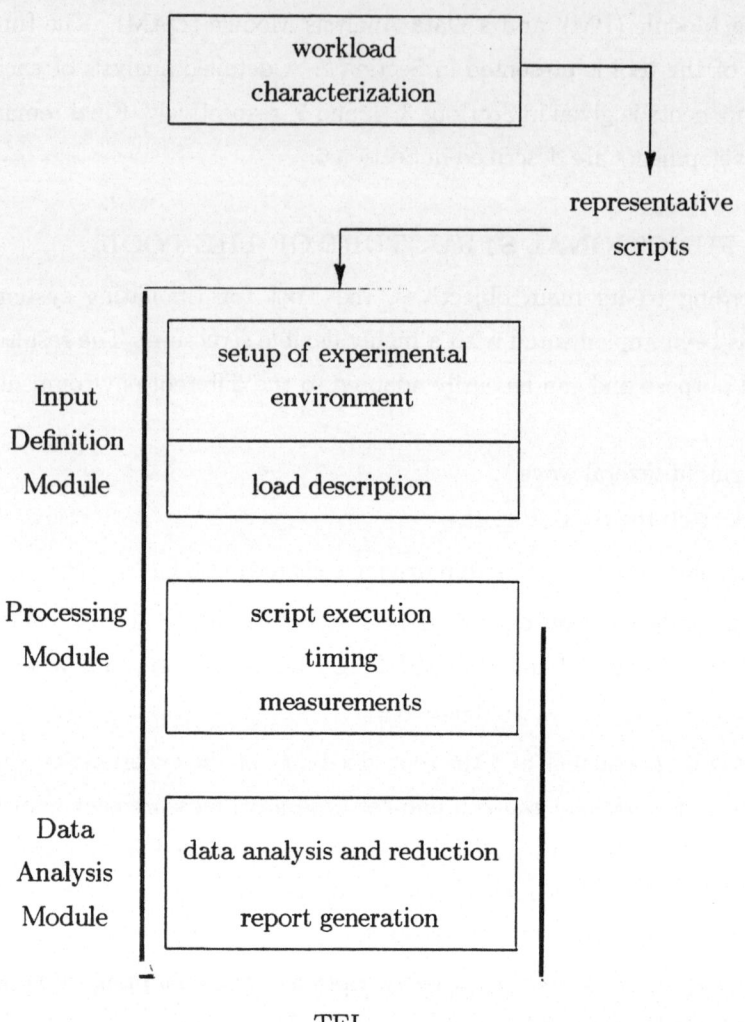

Figure 2 - Functional modules of the Tool for Emulating system Load (TEL).

emulated. The load description is a very critical operation for the success of an experiment and it must always follow a workload characterization study.

The level of detail adopted for the scripts which describe the workload (e.g., instructions, commands, kernels, processes) is related to the objective of the study and to the characteristic of the processing environment. Depending on these factors, a script may contain commands to be executed locally and commands whose execution must be performed on remote machines.

The load to be emulated can be flexibly defined choosing run–time the types of command (and therefore script) and also their time characteristics. Intra– and inter–script think time distributions of the emulated load must be similar to the ones in the real workload. To keep the overhead of the tool on the SUT on minimum values, timing information are collected only at the beginning and at the end of a script.

The processing module starts the experiment clock and executes on the SUT the scripts, i.e., the files of commands generated by the input module. It also produces several traces which record the time information concerning the experiment.

It is possible to control the progress of the execution of each emulated user through diagnostic messages whose frequency is defined in the input module. Several controls on the types of operation executed in each script are performed to assure repeatability of experiments. For example, all the commands are executed on copies of the original files.

Statistical analysis of data from log files and report generation are the main functions of the data analysis module. Several types of report are produced. The performance indices considered refer to the throughput rates, duration and overlap of user sessions, response time distributions (per script type and per interactive user). Statistical descriptors of variables useful to present the results of the experiment, e.g., think times, overhead parameters, are also shown.

3. INPUT DEFINITION MODULE

The Input Definition Module (IDM) is a fundamental step for the setup of all the experiments. Indeed, the validity of the results produced strongly relies on this phase. What has to be specified in the IDM are the various components typical of a terminal session and the related parameters. All these definitions must have as a main goal the exact reproduction of the behavior of the interactive users and therefore of the load conditions on the SUT.

Let us try to identify the input parameters for the TEL by analyzing the typical operations of a user working at a terminal. Each user starts typing a command and at the end he (or she) waits for the output from the computer. Then, he examines the results as soon as they come in, and, usually, types in a new command. This sequence can be repeated till the end of the session, or, at some point, the user may decide to start a new task, i.e., a different set of command types. This distinction is particularly important because it takes into account the possible differences that characterize the various activities. For example, the time spent looking at a list of a directory is substantially less than the time spent looking at a complex output produced by a compiler.

All the operations described above must be expressed, in the input definition module, in terms of suitable parameters. An initial set of variables, concerning load description, that can be identified from the above analysis, is:

1) *interactive command type:* this parameter refers to the "actual" command (e.g., dir, copy, ed) submitted by the user to be processed by the SUT. A set of one or more commands constitutes a *script;*

2) *intra-script think time:* the time spent typing a command, waiting for the response and thinking what command should be input next;

3) *inter-script think time:* the time spent between the end of a task (i.e., a script) and the beginning of the next one.

Bearing in mind these three parameters, we have to measure or, alternatively, to estimate their values. As already mentioned in the previous sections, before each evaluation study, it is necessary (or at least convenient) to characterize the workload, i.e., to determine which command types should be considered as representative of the load and how they "behave" with respect to each other [Calz85]. All these analyses are a preliminary step of the IDM.

A good and accurate source of workload data is represented by the information collected for accounting purposes. Whenever these files are not available or the objectives of the study require different parameters, some hypotheses on their possible values must be made.

Let us recall that all the operations of the input definition module (and of the data analysis module) are performed interactively by means of a user–friendly menu–driven interface. The first phase of the IDM requires the load definition, i.e., the number of different script types and their description must be specified. The scripts can be defined run–time or are selected from a library con–sisting of a set of scripts subdivided according to the applications performed and to the type of environment reproduced (e.g., scientific, commercial). It is impor–tant to point out that the scripts consist of a variable number of real commands which will be executed by the SUT during the emulation phase.

For sake of conciseness and clarity, in what follows we refer our notations and examples to a Unix environment. However, the TEL, which is coded in C language, can be executed on all the systems provided of a C compiler and of a command interpreter.

A session consists of sequence of different command types grouped together according to some predefined criterion, i.e., it can be seen as a sequence of script types. This is just a practical representation of the fact that the user performs various tasks during the day.

For example, he can start in the morning reading and sending electronic mail. After that, he does his standard job, writing, compiling and executing several programs. Sometimes, during the day, he can check again the mail. This situation is reproduced in the benchmark using two script types: the first one (script (a)) for the mailing and the second one (b)) for the programming activities, respectively, with different frequencies of occurrence. Figure 3 shows an example of these two scripts.

The maximum number of script types supported in the first version of IDM is equal to 9.

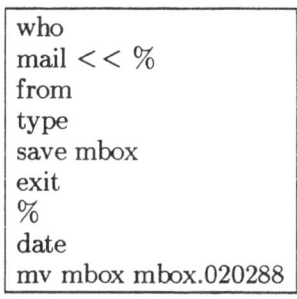

(a)

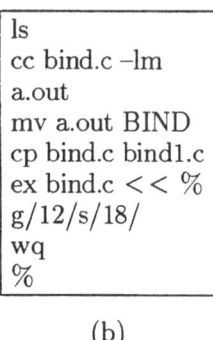

(b)

Figure 3 - Example of two script types: (a) for mailing activity and (b) for programming activity.

The setup of the experiment requires the specification of the number of scripts submitted by each user (whose maximum value is equal to 1000) and the percentage of each script type. Their mix, that is, their sequence of execution, will be determined by sampling the cumulative distribution constructed according to these percentages. To assure a high portability of the tool, making it completely independent of the system where it is executed, a function for random number generation has been included.

Figure 4 (a) shows a portion of the file, named *mix1*, containing the sequence of script types (in general, denoted by a letter from a to i) produced by the input module for one user (i.e., user1).

The inter–script think times, added next, are specified in terms of mean values. Furthermore, in order to take into account the variability and the dispersion of their values, the coefficient of variation cv, that is, the ratio between standard deviation and mean value, has been considered. In such a way, the distribution, which best fits the original data, i.e., exponential $(cv=1)$, hyperexponential $(cv>1)$, hypoexponential $(cv<1)$, or constant $(cv=0)$, can be represented. Think times are simulated by means of the command *sleep* which forces the execution to be suspended for a certain amount of time specified as a parameter (number of seconds). The file *mixt1* is illustrated in Fig. 4 (b). The inter–script think times have been inserted between a script and the next one.

Finally, it is necessary to add the intra–script think times, which in general are different from the inter–script components. Indeed, the times spent between a command and the next one are typical of each script and command types. Hence, since their values can vary from one script to another, they must be expressed, as in the case of the inter–script times, in terms of mean values and coefficients of variation.

Figure 4 (c) presents a portion of the file *user1* produced at the end of the IDM, that will be processed by the SUT during the experiment. The identifiers of the script types have been substituted with the commands they consist of. Further-more, some additional commands (see below), which take care of the control and of the reproducibility of the experiment, have been inserted. A command inter-preter, in our case the Unix shell, will read all the lines and process the com-mands listed in the file.

Let us remark that the IDM can be executed on the SUT itself or on a different machine, while the emulation phase (Processing Module) must be, obviously, performed on the SUT (see Fig. 1).

In order for the TEL to be able to reproduce the real load of an interactive sys-tem, it is necessary to emulate several users. This requires the definition of the workload processed by each of them in terms of the parameters above intro-

(a)	(b)	(c)
b	sleep 0	cd WorkDir1
a	b	copy 1
b	sleep 3	sleep 0
b	a	message 1 1
b	sleep 5	timem 1 2
b	b	ls
b	sleep 0	sleep 2
b	b	cc bind.c –lm
b	sleep 2	sleep 0
b	b	a.out
b	sleep 10	sleep 4
b	b	mv a.out BIND
b	sleep 1	sleep 2
b	b	rm garbage
b	sleep 0	cp bind.c bind1.c
b	b	sleep 0
a	sleep 0	ex bind.c << %
a	b	g/12/s/18/
a	sleep 1	w garbage
b	b	q
a	sleep 4	%
	b	timem 1 2
	sleep 0	sleep 3
	b	message 1 2
	sleep 1	timem 1 1
	b	who
	sleep 5	sleep 1
	b	mail << %
	sleep 0	from
	b	type
	sleep 5	save mbox
	a	exit
	sleep 5	%
	a	date
	sleep 1	sleep 0
	a	mv mbox mbox.020288
	sleep 0	sleep 0
	b	timem 1 1
	sleep 0	sleep 5
	a	message 1 3
	sleep 1	timem 1 2
		ls
		sleep 0

Figure 4 - Portions of the three files generated for one interactive user by the Input Definition Module; (a) after the sampling of the cumulative distribution of the percentages (file *mix* 1); (b) after the insertion of the inter–script think times (file *mixt* 1); and (c) at the end of the IDM execution (file *user* 1).

duced. Hence, from the IDM view point, each user will be characterized by a set of three files (see Fig. 4).

The working environment used by TEL consists of a general directory, named UserDir, which contains all the files required during the experiment, and several private directories, one for each interactive user, called WorkDir$j$, where j denotes the user number. In our case $1 \leqslant j \leqslant 8$. Before starting the emulation phase all user files are duplicated, by means of the function *copy* (see Fig. 4 (c)), and copied into the appropriate working directory. To assure the exact reproducibility of each script execution, the integrity of the files manipulated during the experiment is preserved by means of a "garbage" file. At the beginning and at the end of each script a routine, namely *timem*, is called for the measurement activities. For each user it records the values of the clock and the types of script.

It is possible to follow the evolution of the emulation, by printing some diagnostic messages (through the function *message*). This is particularly useful in the case of long experiments with many users.

The various terminal sessions can start at the same instant of time or some of them can be delayed. The option, which is specified in the IDM, corresponds to the value of the parameters of the first sleep in the files *user$j$*. In our case, the user number 1, starts working at time 0 (see sleep 0 in the file *user* 1).

Figure 5 summarizes the main steps of the IDM which produce, for each interactive user, two intermediate files (*mix$j$* and *mixt$j$*) and a global file (*user$j$*) containing the expansion (i.e., the real commands) of all the script types (denoted by a letter in the previous files). The Processing Module will read its input from *user$j$* and execute all the commands found there.

4. PROCESSING MODULE

As already mentioned in the previous section, the environment reproduced by the TEL consists of n directories which correspond to the user working directories. In such a way, there is a complete adherence to the real world, where every interactive user has his own account with his private files. The Processing Module (PM) deals with the execution of all the commands listed in each of the n files (*user$j$*) generated by the IDM. In order for the results to be completely accurate and depending on the types of study, it is usually necessary to run the experiments on a dedicated machine (SUT). Indeed, the users different from those generated by the IDM influence the performance of the SUT in some

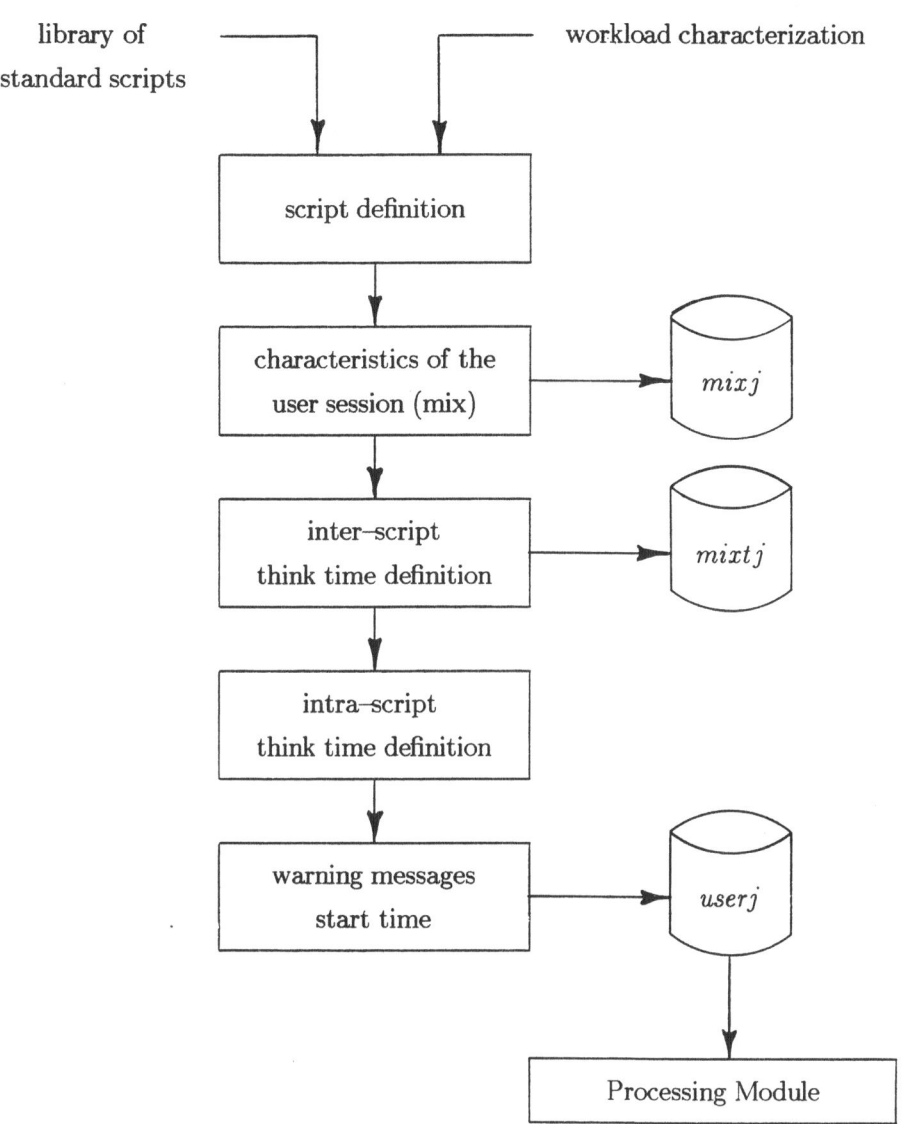

Figure 5 - Main steps performed by the Input Definition Module. The file names refer to user j .

unpredictable ways and therefore, can invalidate the experiments.

To keep the overhead produced by the tool as low as possible, the measurements performed in the PM are limited to the starting and stopping times of each script. However, since the commands are executed on real SUTs, it is possible to collect all the data recorded by the accounting routines and to obtain more detailed information concerning the load of the system and the utilizations of its resources (e.g., CPU utilization, number of I/O operations, average memory usage).

Figure 6 illustrates the structure of the processing module.

The files *user* 1, *user* 2, $\cdots$, *user* 8 are the input to the SUT which, by means of a command interpreter, executes simultaneously all the sequences of commands listed there. It is a representation of a multi–user environment. This means that the mix of commands in the system belongs to different users.

The output of the PM consists of several files containing the measured data, that are processed by the Data Analysis Module to obtain reports and statistical summaries of some performance indices useful to describe the experiment.

5. DATA ANALYSIS MODULE

The Data Analysis Module (DAM) deals with the problem of summarizing and organizing the results of the experiment. The output files of the PM, which contain for each script the times collected during the experiment, are taken as input by the DAM. Some graphical representations and reports of the main per–formance indices are produced. In particular, the cumulative frequency distribu–tions of the response time, computed for each script type within every user ses–sion, are presented. From these kinds of graph, it is possible to have a visual description of the data, and to see at a glance their pattern. An example of such a graph is shown in Figure 7. The times, expressed in seconds, are plotted on the y–axis, while the frequencies are on the x–axis. The exact values of both the relative and the cumulative frequency distributions are also reported.

A descriptive analysis of the data related to response times is also performed. Indeed, the main statistical measures, i.e., mean, minimum, maximum, standard deviation, variance, coefficient of variation, skewness and kurtosis, can give a deeper insight in the data. Table 1 presents a report containing, for user1, the statistical values for each script type. The throughput rates, i.e., the number of script types performed in a time unit, are shown in Table 2, which presents also a final summary of the experiment.

All these performance indices can be used as absolute figures of merit (e.g., to estimate the computing power of a SUT) or as relative measures (e.g., for comparison purposes).

6. CONCLUSIONS

The performance evaluation of centralized systems, as well as distributed ones, requires the construction of executable workload models. The versatility of

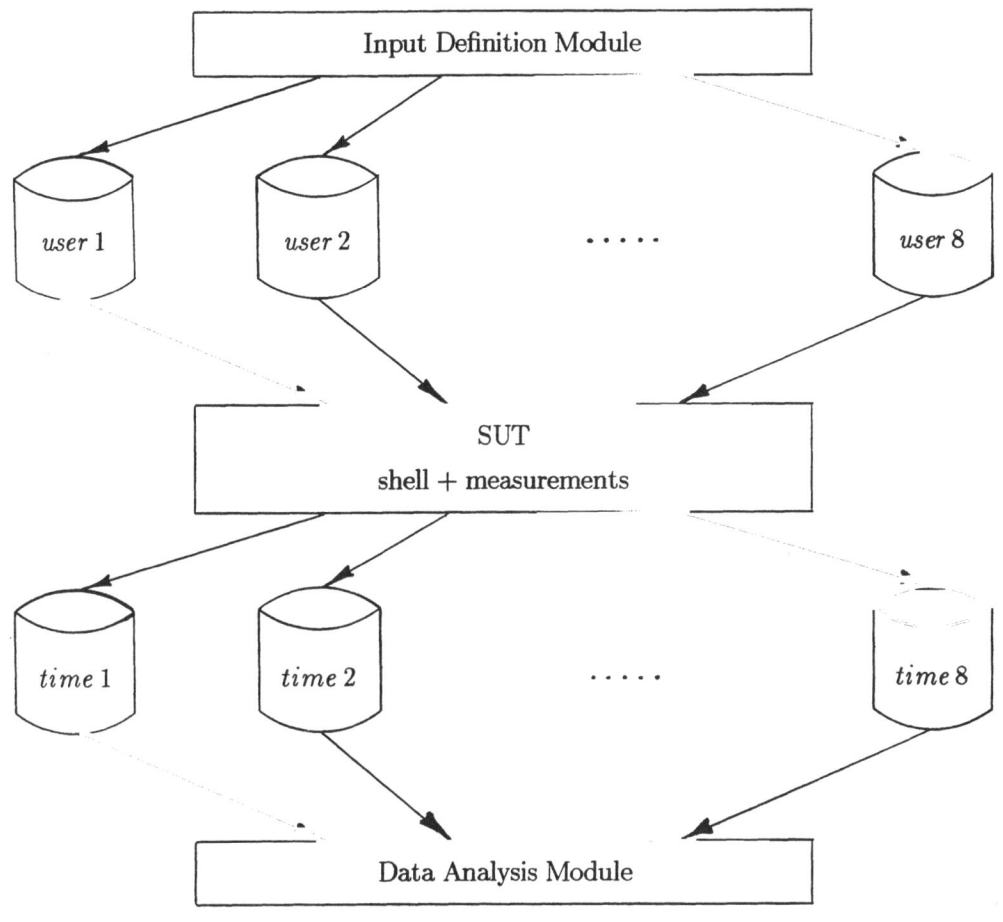

Figure 6 - Structure of the Processing Module (PM).

Table 1 - Statistical measures of the response time (in seconds) of the various script types submitted by user1. The last row of the table contains the global values.

| Script | Response Time | | | | | | | |
| | User 1 | | | | | | | |
Type	Mean	Variance	Std.Dev	C.Var	Min	Max	Skew	Kurt
a	4.6	0.3	0.5477	0.1191	4.	5.	−0.29	−2.3
b	17.8	1.2	1.095	0.0615	17.	19.	0.29	−2.3
c	1.6	1.8	1.342	0.8385	1.	4.	1.1	−0.92
d	6.	0.5	0.7071	0.1179	5.	7.	0.	−1.4
Global	7.5	41.	6.378	0.8505	1.	19.	0.83	−0.97

```
                        USER1 Script Type b
                                                    frequency  percentage
                                                    rel. cum.  rel.  cum.
20.   *                                              4    4    2.3   2.3
22.83***                                             7   11    4     6.2
25.67*****                                           7   18    4    10
28.5 *********                                       20   38   11    21
31.33****************                                23   61   13    34
34.17********************                            15   76   8.5   43
37. *************************                        20   96   11    54
39.83***************************                     13  109   7.3   62
42.67*******************************                 12  121   6.8   68
45.5 *********************************                8  129   4.5   73
48.33***********************************              9  138   5.1   78
51.17***********************************              8  146   4.5   82
54. ***********************************               5  151   2.8   85
56.83**************************************          10  161   5.6   91
59.67*****************************************         4  165   2.3   93
62.5 *****************************************         6  171   3.4   97
65.33*****************************************         2  173   1.1   98
68.17***************************************           0  173   0     98
71. ****************************************           1  174   0.56  98
73.83***************************************           0  174   0     98
76.67**************************************            0  174   0     98
79.5 **************************************            0  174   0     98
82.33**************************************            1  175   0.56  99
85.17**************************************            1  176   0.56  99
88. **************************************             0  176   0     99
90.83**************************************            0  176   0     99
93.67**************************************            0  176   0     99
96.5 **************************************            0  176   0     99
99.33**************************************            0  176   0     99
102.2 **************************************           0  176   0     99
105. **************************************            1  177   0.56 100
```

Figure 7 - Cumulative frequency distribution of the response time (in seconds) for the 177 scripts of type b executed by user1.

Table 2 - Final summary of the experiment.

User	Start Time	Stop Time	Throughput [script/sec]	Response Time [sec]	No. Scripts
User1	0	10272	0.01947	50.55	200
User2	0	10402	0.01923	51.05	200
User3	1	10454	0.01913	51.25	200
User4	0	10493	0.01906	51.56	200
User5	2	10522	0.01901	51.74	200
Global	0	10522	0.09504		1000

the tool described in this paper allows the definition of many kinds of experiment which may involve networks (LANs and WANs), supercomputers, and distributed systems. Furthermore, due to the flexibility of the Input Definition Module it is possible to reproduce different working environments which completely adhere to the real situations we want to represent.

For the moment, the implementation of TEL is limited to systems running under Unix. However, it will be extended to other systems. We plan to test the tool on computers with different operating systems (VM/CMS, VMS, MVS, and so on). Future developments also deal with the problem of constructing an Input Definition Module able to reproduce the behavior of parallel algorithms specified in terms of precedence graphs. Other extensions are related to distributed environments.

REFERENCES

[Bail85]   Bailey, D.H. NAS kernel benchmarks results, *Proc. IEEE*, pp. 341–345, 1985.

[Buch69]   Buchholz, W. A synthetic job fo measuring system performance, *IBM System Journal*, **8**, 4, pp. 309–318, 1969.

[Bux84]   Bux, W. Performance issues in local–area networks, *IBM Systems Journal*, **23**, 4, pp. 351–374, 1984.

[Calz85]   Calzarossa, M. and Serazzi, G. WORKSER: a user–friendly WORKload analySER tool, in: *Modeling Techniques and Tools for Performance Analysis*, N. Abu El Ata, Ed., pp. 171–186, North–Holland, 1985.

[Dong86]   Dongarra, J.J. Performance of various computers using standard linear equations software in Fortran environment, *Technical Memo*, No. 23, Mathematics and Computer Science Div., Argonne National Laboratory, 1986.

[Ferr83]   Ferrari, D., Serazzi, G., and Zeigner, A. *Measurement and Tuning of Computer Systems*. Prentice–Hall, 1983.

[Foge72]   Fogel, M., and Winograd, J. Einstein: an internal driver in a time–sharing environment, *Operating Systems Rev.*, **6**, 3, pp. 6–14, 1972.

[Gibs70]   Gibson, J.C. The Gibson mix, *IBM Technical Report*, No. 002043, 1970.

[Gree69]   Greenbaum, H.J. A simulator of multiple interactive users to drive a time–shared computer system, *Project MAC TR-58*, MIT, Cambridge, January, 1969.

[Kern73]   Kernighan, B.W., and Hamilton, P.A. Synthetically generated performance test loads for operating systems, *Proc. 1st ACM-SIGME Symp. on Measurement and Evaluation*, pp. 121–126, 1973.

[Lube85]   Lubeck, O., Moore, J., and Mendez, R. A benchmark comparison of three supercomputers: Fujitsu VP–200, Hitachi S810/20 and Cray X–MP/2, *Computer*, **18**, pp. 10–23, 1985.

[Salt70]   Saltzer, J.H., and Gintell, J.W. The instrumentation of Multics, *Comm. of the ACM*, **13**, 8, pp. 495–500, 1970.

[Shoc80]   Shoch, J.F., and Hupp, J.A. Measured performance of an Ethernet local network, *Comm. of the ACM*, **23**, 12, pp. 711–721, 1980.

[Stra72]   Strauss, J.C. A benchmark study, *Proc. AFIPS FJCC*, **41**, pp. 1225–1233, 1972.

[Stra87]   Straathof, J.F., Thareja, A.K., and Agrawala, A.K. Methodology and results of performance measurements for a new Unix scheduler, *Usenix Conf. Proc.*, Washington D.C., pp. 165–180, Winter 1987.

[Wood71]   Wood, D.C., and Forman E.H. Throughput measurement using a synthetic job stream, *Proc. AFIPS FJCC*, **39**, pp. 51–56, 1971.

A TOOL FOR PERFORMANCE-DRIVEN DESIGN OF PARALLEL

SYSTEMS

Ellen Boughter,
William Alexander, and
Tom Keller

MCC
3500 West Balcones Center Drive
Austin, Texas, USA 78759

ABSTRACT

Performance–driven design is systems design focused on performance prediction. It demands heavy use of performance models throughout the design process, and the consequent blurring of the distinction between the roles "performance analyst" and "systems architect". Large parallel systems performance prediction places its own extreme demands upon performance models. No monolithic model, utilizing one solution technique, can meet these demands. Thus a set of submodels, utilizing different solution techniques, is usually employed. This paper presents as a case study the modeling of a performance–driven, large, parallel database machine design. We have found that a "pipelined" system of submodels appears suitable to both the requirements of the design process and modeling large parallel systems. Examples illustrating the use of the pipelined modeling tool in our performance–driven environment are given.

1 INTRODUCTION

Large parallel systems performance prediction places extreme demands upon performance models. No monolithic model, utilizing one solution technique, can meet these demands. Thus a set of submodels, utilizing different solution techniques, is usually employed.

This paper presents as a case study the modeling requirements of a performance–driven, large, parallel database machine design. We have found that a "pipelined" system of submodels appears well suited to both the requirements of the performance–driven process and modeling large parallel systems. We also give two examples that illustrate the use of the pipelined modeling tool in our performance–driven design project. Section 2 describes the goals of the highly parallel database machine design and the requirements of its performance prediction models. Section 3 describes the "pipelined" approach to model construction and its first instantiation. The strengths and weaknesses of this instantiation are discussed. Section 4 gives two example studies, each of which led to substantial design changes. Near–term extensions to the pipelined model and its immediate, synergistic contribution to the software design effort are presented in Section 5. Conclusions regarding our approach are given in the last section.

2 THE DESIGN PROJECT

The Database Systems Architecture project at MCC is designing a database machine, which we call "Bubba", for the "knowledgebase" workloads expected in the mid–1990's [Alex88b] [Alex88c] [Bora88] [Cope88]. Bubba is a highly–parallel machine for data–intensive applications. It is designed to be scalable from 50 to 1,000 **intelligent repositories (IRs)**. Each IR has a main processor, a disk controller, a communications processor, a large main memory, and a disk. Its design philosophy is shared–nothing [Tera85] [Ston86] [DeWi86] [Tan87]; neither memory nor disks are shared between IRs. Bubba also has several **interface processors (IPs)** to handle interaction with users and some centralized functions. The IRs and IPs are connected by an interconnect, so that any IR or IP may send messages to any other IR or IP. This interconnect is the only shared resource; it makes a network out of the set of IRs and IPs. This network is a single machine; the IRs and IPs are physically close and message delays are small. The high–level architecture is illustrated in Figure 2.1.

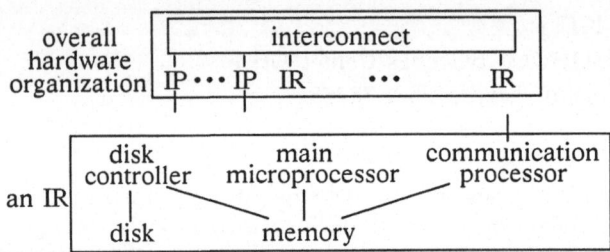

Figure 2.1. High–Level Hardware Organization

The performance objective is to deliver knowledgebase management functionality with cost and performance improvements between one and two orders of magnitude relative to conventional, general purpose computers of the mid–1990's. The target architecture permits scalability from 50 to 1000 nodes, where each node has its own complement of processors, fast buffer memory, and disk memory. Some of the important design issues being faced are: the interconnection scheme to use, how to distribute data optimally amongst the nodes, strategies for providing distributed transaction management, and new techniques for "non–stop" operation.

An experimental database system is being implemented using a commercially available parallel computer as a hardware platform for software design experiments.

The requirements for performance modeling in this design effort are formidable, particularly when high performance is a principal design objective. The principal requirements of the performance prediction models are:

- The models must be generalizable across different parallel hardware and software architectures. In addition, they must be capable of modeling the large number of physical resources in the design and must be capable of modeling the complex workload inherent in any large distributed system.

- The models must embrace different degrees of accuracy. Early in the design process order–of–magnitude accuracy is sufficient, as many design options are eliminated in the "disaster avoidance" phase. Late in the design process, the "tuning" phase, accuracy must be within 10 or 20 percent. Architectural design and workload characteristics must become increasingly detailed during the design process [Sevc81].

- Model turnaround must be fast. Results requiring weeks instead of days per instance in the design space usually don't make it into the design process.

• The models must have good, easy–to–use, external interfaces.

2.2 The Workloads

We use database application programs based on a conventional order–entry system as our workload. Five transactions comprise our workload: **Payment, Order–Shipped, New–Order, Suggested–Order** and **Store–Layout**, plus a mix of the five transactions, **Mixed**, forming a composite workload. These transactions and their workload characterizations are described in [Alex87]. The order–entry database consists of 36 relations; 8 of these relations are unnormalized, conceptual relations; the remainder are inverted copies of those 8 relations. The total size of the database is 320 Gbytes. The five transactions may be summarized as follows:

1) New_Order records a customer's order for an average of 10 different items after the customer's new outstanding balance is checked against his credit limit.

2) Order_Shipped generates an invoice for the customer after an order is filled.

3) Payment retrieves and updates the date–paid for an order and adjusts the associated customer, salesman, district and company sales totals.

4) Suggested_Order infers the number of items to order from suppliers in order to keep a warehouse sufficiently well–stocked.

5) Store_Layout assists a customer in configuring the layout of items on the shelves in the store in an attempt to maximize customer profit.

New_Order, Order_Shipped and Payment represent conventional database transactions, whereas Suggested_Order and Store_Layout represent knowledgebase queries. These transactions require roughly from 2x to 1,000x the work involved in the DebitCredit transaction [Anon85]. We think that workloads having a mix of simple and complex transactions as in Order_Entry will gradually replace simpler workloads like DebitCredit, largely because of the availability of reasonably priced systems with the performance needed to support them [Samm87].

3 THE MODEL PIPELINE AND INTERFACES

The modeling tool extends the workload characterization pipeline that is described in [Alex87]. The model pipeline, *FIRM,* its components, and its interface are described in this section. FIRM consists of a pipeline of various modules as shown in Figure 3.1. Workloads and architecture descriptions are input at various stages, and transaction throughput rates and other measures are output. Workloads are represented to FIRM as dataflow graphs.

FIRM consists of four C programs that communicate via data files. In addition, a prototype implementation of Bubba, the *Experimental Vehicle,* uses some of the data files that are produced by FIRM. Results can either be viewed through an interactive graphical interface or be printed or plotted. The important predictions that are produced are:

• maximum practical throughput sustainable for Bubba,
• average utilizations for every disk and CPU in Bubba,
• message traffic rate at each node, and
• average transaction response times and response time distributions.

3.1 Dataflow in FIRM

The *structure* of each transaction in the workload is characterized to FIRM as a dataflow graph of the Bubba transaction, which is programmed in a language called FAD [Banc87], the interface to Bubba. Each operation in the dataflow graph is called a *component*. A component is instantiated as processes on one or more nodes

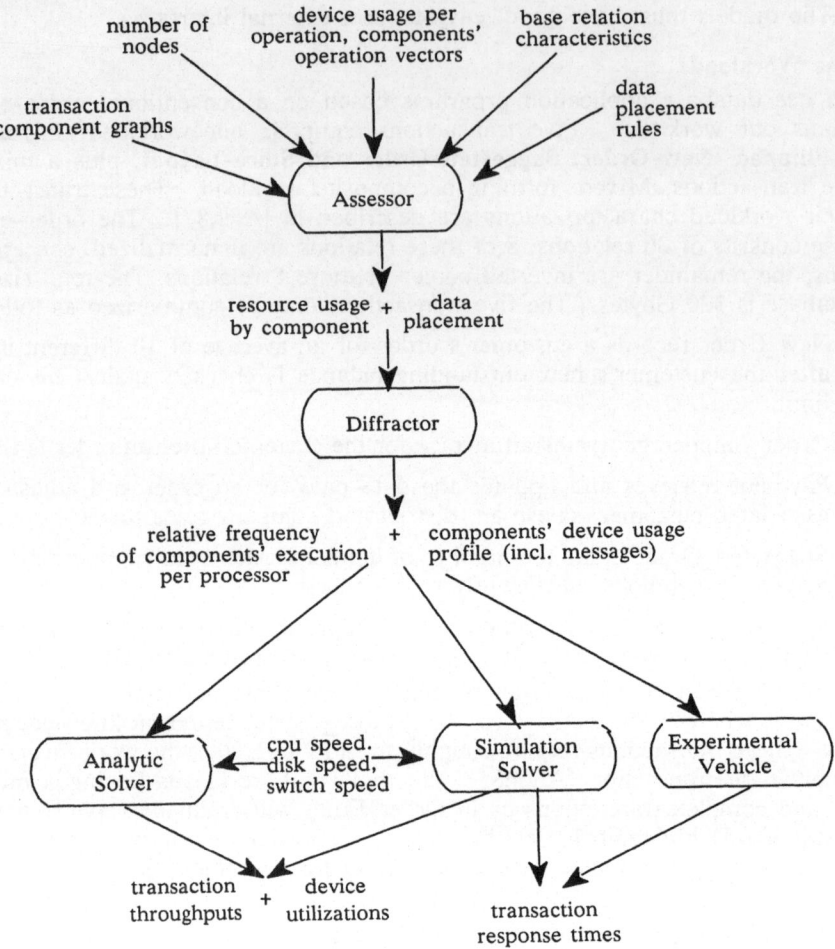

Figure 3.1. The FIRM Pipeline

of Bubba. The dataflow graph is a detailed and accurate representation of the FAD program, and is prepared manually by inspection of the FAD program.

The placement of the data across the nodes is computed by a program, *Assessor*, that, knowing the size of every relation, attempts to evenly distribute the load across the multiple nodes according to a set of rules. These rules are formed from placement heuristics thought to achieve better load balancing as well as constraints imposed by other design decisions [Cope88]. Once the data placement is determined, the costs of operations (such as a join) can be determined from the number of nodes expected to participate in the operation. These costs are:

1) the average number of CPU instructions,

2) the average number of data accesses,

3) the number of disk I/O's, and

4) counts of the total messages received and the total messages sent.

The placement information and the operation cost information are then used by a program, *Diffractor*, that maps the component graphs onto the multiple nodes. A traffic rate for each component type by each node in Bubba is calculated and fed to the *Analytic Solver* and to the *Simulation Solver*. The analytic solver is an open queueing network model; the simulation solver uses CSIM, a process oriented simulation language [Schw85].

The analytic solver accepts the relative traffic rates by component type, scales them by the transaction(s) arrival rate(s) and determines the performance measures described above for a configuration with CPUs and disks rated at specific speeds. The analytic solver uses simple operational analysis techniques [Denn78], as presented in [Lazo84], to determine these measures.

The simulation solver recognizes a more accurate representation of the execution of component graphs, including data dependencies and locking conflicts. Transaction response time distributions are an important measure obtained from the simulation solver that are unavailable from the queueing network model.

3.2 FIRMVIEW

FIRM's interactive, graphical user interface, *FIRMVIEW*, runs on a SUN workstation using the SUN windowing tools. With FIRMVIEW, a user varies the input parameters, runs FIRM, and views the results. Results include statistical reports and graphical utilization plots.

The parameters that can be varied using FIRMVIEW include the total number of nodes in the system, the size of the node groupings used in data placement, the speed of the processors at each node, and the disk access rates. Parameters are changed and executions initiated by toggling "buttons" or entering text. Figure 3.2 displays a sample FIRMVIEW screen.

3.3 Reality Vs. the Model Requirements

In Section 2.1 we listed four qualitative requirements for the modeling tool: generality across architectures, adjustable accuracy, speed, and interface. The present tool satisfies these requirements to different degrees.

Generality over Architectures

The modeling tool has proven quite flexible over a range of parameter values for a given design. It has accommodated some changes in hardware configuration and system software design. It has accommodated major changes in workload definition. All this has been possible because of its modular, pipelined, design and because, to a certain extent, the design changes we were asked to track were not too different from those we anticipated. The tool is, however, very specific to distributed systems, and to a lesser extent specific to the shared–nothing philosophy [Ston86] that was chosen by the design team early in the design process.

Adjustable Accuracy

Our main contributions to the design process to date have been made with a simple open queueing model that gives approximate throughput and capacity predictions. The first major use of FIRM involved data placement across the nodes in Bubba; this experiment is described in Section 4. The throughput and capacity predictions produced by FIRM aided the Bubba design team in revising their initial data placement algorithms.

We have also fed the node–by–node message traffic rates output by the diffractor directly into a detailed simulation of possible interconnect architectures. The results of this simulation were used to determine the type of interconnect that Bubba will use [Alex88a].

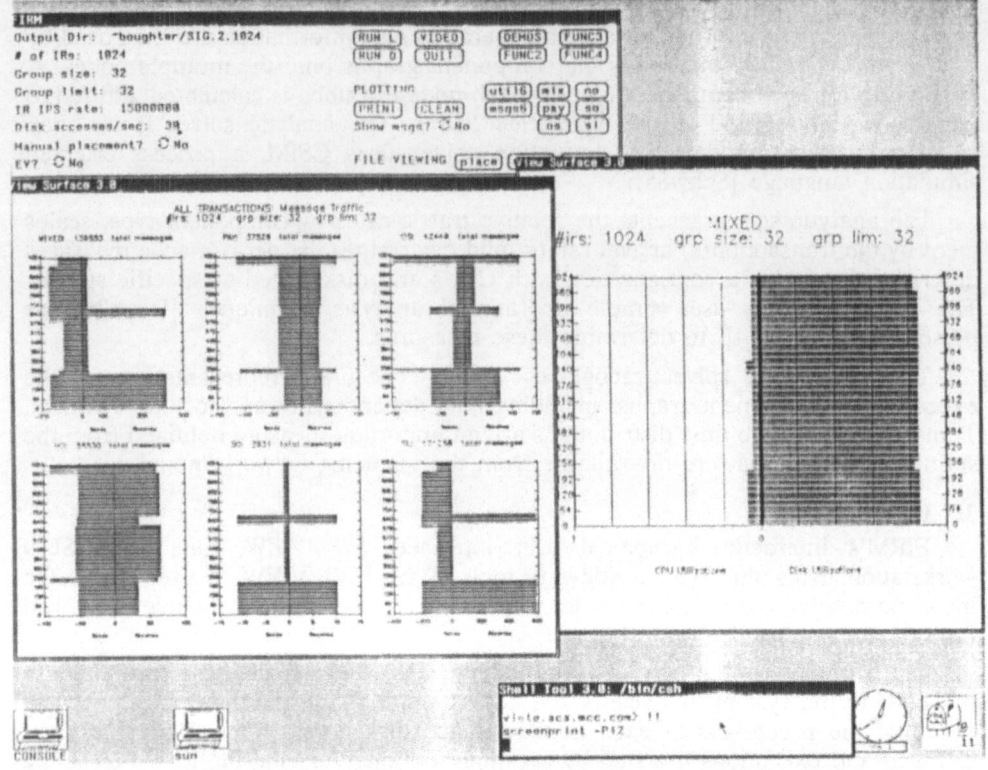

Figure 3.2. FIRMVIEW Screen

Recently, we added the simulation solver to FIRM; we inserted this simulation model directly into the pipeline, augmenting the analytic model, and we have encountered no serious interface problems. The first major use of the simulation solver has been a study of various types of concurrency control algorithms; the results of this study will help the Bubba design team to determine the type of concurrency control that Bubba will support.

We use the analytic solver to produce "ball-park" throughput estimates very quickly. We can then refine our experiments and continue to use the analytic solver. When we are satisfied with the design of our experiment, we can then use the longer-running simulation solver to produce more accurate results.

Speed

The open queueing model produces answers very quickly, even for 1000-node configurations. A complete trip through the pipeline from reading in the workload characterization and specifying system parameters to tabular output from the analytic solver takes about 3 minutes on a SUN 3 workstation. Graphical output on the screen takes about 3 additional minutes. The simulation solver, of course, runs much more slowly; a simulation of a 1000-node configuration may take more than 12 hours on a Sun 3.

Interface

We have found the FIRMVIEW interface described in Section 3.2 very useful. We emphasize that plots and other graphical output are indispensable to the kind of interactive exploration of the design space that the tool is intended to promote. Designers can run the pipeline for different settings and compare plots of CPU or disk utilizations or message traffic, by node, for two runs side-by-side on their workstation screen, all in minutes.

4 EXAMPLE STUDIES

One of the design goals of our model pipeline was to provide fast turnaround to the system architects. This section presents two example studies, each of which required some change in the input to FIRM, and each of which led to changes in the architecture of Bubba. The first study involves data placement, which is partitioning the base data among the nodes in Bubba. The second study determines the data cache size that results in the least expensive Bubba configuration. [1]

4.1 Data Placement

In a highly parallel architecture like Bubba, load balancing is critical. Parallel architectures on the scale of 50–1000 nodes cannot be cost/performance competitive without substantial aggregate processor utilization. In our design, processing is done where the data resides; the primary tool for load balancing is effective distribution of the data resident in the processors. "Declustering", the partitioning of a base relation's residence among multiple processing nodes, is one method of partitioning data among the nodes. Declustering has been shown to take good advantage of the parallelism inherent in these types of architectures [Livn87]. Thus, data placement includes two related decisions: the number of nodes over which to decluster a relation and which nodes to place the relation in.

We assume that the frequency of access to each base relation is known *a priori*, i.e. that simple measurements of the Bubba workloads have been made over time and hold as predictors. The frequency of access can be measured directly or calculated from the frequency of execution of transactions and knowledge of their references to base relations. Our detailed workload characterization allows us to make this calculation based on the assumed frequency of execution of the transactions.

The Bubba designers adopted the shorthand nomenclature *heat* for frequency of access, and we will use *heat* throughout this report. We next describe two experiments using different data placement strategies, each using heat. In these experiments the following assumptions hold:

1) The number of nodes is 1024.

2) Each node has 15 MIPs processing capacity.

3) Each node has unlimited disk storage capacity.

4) The average disk access capacity is 30 accesses per second.

5) Two copies of all data exist in the forms of a conceptual, base relation and the set of its inverted attributes.

4.1.1 Simple Placement

In the first of our placement experiments, the available nodes were divided into *groups* of size 32, giving a total of 32 groups. A proposed recovery and availability strategy imposed two constraints: first, each relation could occupy at most one group of 32 nodes and second, a conceptual relation and its inverted copies could not share a node. Each relation, whether conceptual or inverted, occupies an entire group unless it is so small that less than one block of data can be placed on a node. In that case, the relation occupies a number of nodes equal to the number of blocks required to store the relation. In this experiment there is no permanent caching of data.

---

[1] Both examples are drawn from many actual studies performed with FIRM. The values for system parameters and component costs presented in this paper, while reasonable, are not necessarily those used on the Bubba project.

A relation's heat was used to determine in which group a relation resided. Relations were ranked by their heats, then sequentially placed, "hottest" first, in the coolest available group that met the constraint that conceptual and inverted copies of a relation could not share nodes. If a relation occupied less than an entire group, the coolest nodes in the coolest group were selected. After placing a relation in a group, the cumulative heat values for the nodes in the group were incremented, and the next hottest relation was similarly placed. Placing relations in cool groups attempts to balance the disk load while satisfying the placement constraints.

Figure 4.1 shows the CPU and disk utilizations that FIRM predicted based on this data placement scheme; the practical disk saturation level is set in this example at 85%.[2] Table 4.1 shows the throughput rates that FIRM predicted.

Table 4.1. Saturation Throughput Rates

Workload	Trans/Sec	Saturated Resource
Payment	38	Disk
Order_Shipped	23	Disk
New_Order	8	Disk
Suggested_Order	.1	Disk
Store_Layout	.01	Disk
Mixed	4	Disk

Both throughputs and utilizations were very disappointing; the distribution of work across the 1024 nodes was extremely uneven, as seen in Figure 4.1. The results of this first experiment led the Bubba design team to consider developing different recovery and availability strategies which would relax some of the constraints, but only if performance could dramatically be improved. The following experiment was proposed.

4.1.2 Declustering by Heat

In this experiment, we removed the constraint that a relation could occupy at most one group of nodes; instead, we decided that a relation would occupy *at least* one group of nodes. Thus, the first constraint was removed. However, the second constraint, that a relation and its inverted copies could not share nodes, still held. To simplify implementation of a new recovery strategy, all of the inverted copies of a conceptual relation were forced to share exactly the same groups of nodes. In this experiment, we used *heat* to determine the number of groups over which a relation would be declustered. Since all of the groups, in this case, 32 groups of 32 nodes, were available for use by a conceptual relation and its inverted copies, we divided the groups between the two based on the ratio of their heats. For example, if the heat of conceptual relation A is 10, and the total heat of its inverted copies, A', is 20, A will be declustered over 1/3 of the groups, and A' will be declustered over 2/3 of the groups. As in the first experiment, heat was also used to determine which of the groups would hold a given relation; the coolest groups that met the recovery/availability constraints were the first chosen.

Because FIRM is modular, we were able to make these changes rapidly (in Assessor) and report our new throughput results and utilizations quickly. Table 4.2 shows the throughput values that FIRM predicted. The throughput rates predicted by FIRM have increased dramatically over the first experiment, and the CPU and disk utilizations, as shown in Figure 4.2, are well-balanced, which was the goal. The predicted improvement was so dramatic that the original recovery/availability strategy was dropped, and research began on one that did not impose the first constraint. (Data placement is further described in [Cope88].)

---

[2] This is much higher than the practical saturation level in today's shared disk mainframe systems.

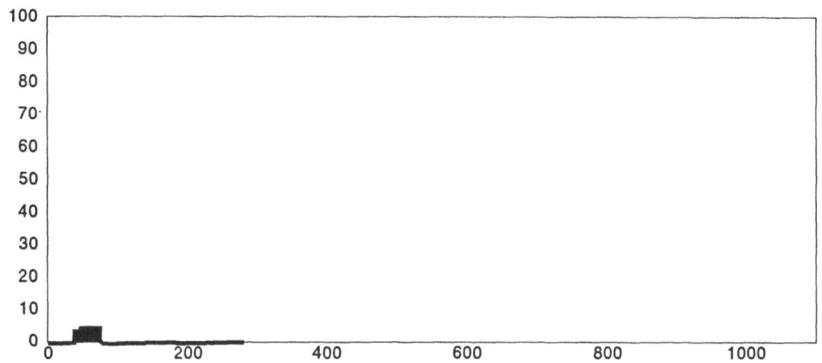

Figure 4.1a. CPU Utilization at Saturation

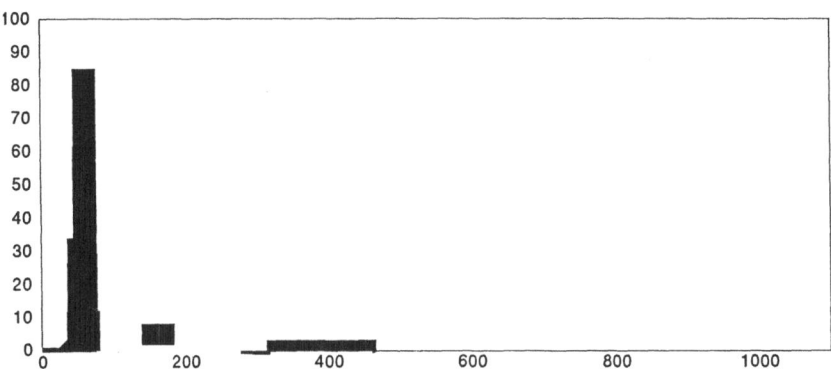

Figure 4.1b. Disk Utilization at Saturation

Table 4.2: Saturation Throughput Rates

Workload	Trans/Sec	Saturated Resource
Payment	647	Disk
Order_Shipped	511	Disk
New_Order	73	Disk
Suggested_Order	3	Disk
Store_Layout	4	Disk
Mixed	80	Disk

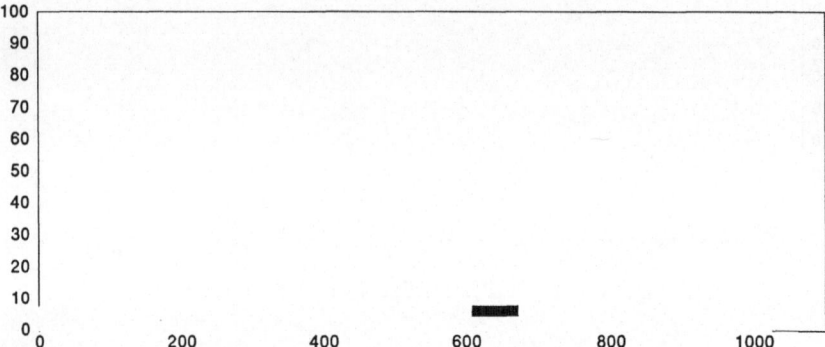

Figure 4.2a. CPU Utilization at Saturation

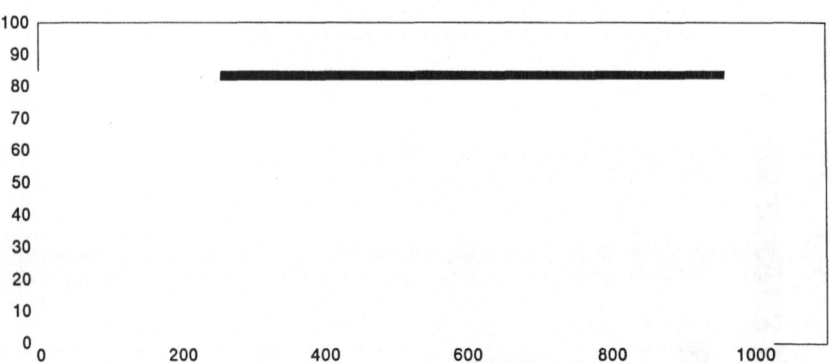

Figure 4.2b. Disk Utilization at Saturation

4.2 Cache Size/Cost

Another design issue was to consider using permanent data cache storage at every node in the system; this cache would be used to hold relations that were very "hot", thus minimizing physical I/Os to those relations. The experiment described in this section shows the use of FIRM as a tool to determine the number of nodes and the amount of permanent cache per node for the most cost-effective Bubba configuration that meets a specific throughput goal.

A number of trial runs were made to explore the modeling space for this experiment. We discovered that the total amount of permanent cache required was quite small, due to the high degree of locality exhibited by our workloads. However, increasing the cache size per node can result in a decrease in the total number of nodes required in the configuration, at an increase in cost per node, of course. In this example, we assume a performance goal of 400 composite transactions per second, where a composite is a weighted fraction of the five transaction types. We assume a simple cost of $5000 per node, which includes processor, memory, and disk subsystem, plus $50 per megabyte of memory to be used as a permanent data cache.

Figure 4.3 plots the number of nodes necessary to achieve the performance goal, given a fixed amount of data cache per node. Each point is annotated with a tuple displaying the dollar cost per node, the dollar cost for the machine, and the bottlenecking resource type. For example, the least expensive machine configuration that meets the above performance goal has a total cost of $3,168,000, reflecting a cost of $5500 per node with 10 Mbytes of data cache. Disks are the bottlenecking resource.

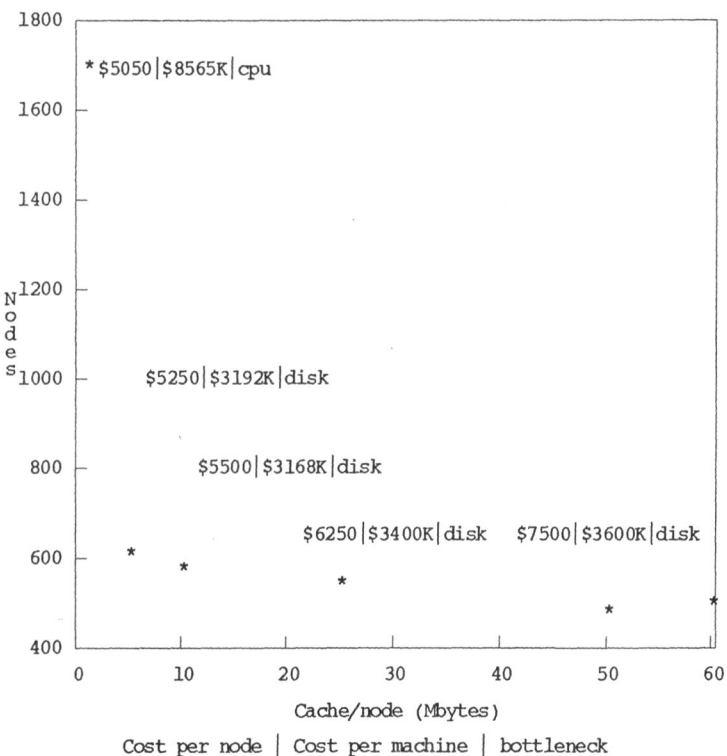

Figure 4.3. COSTS FOR VARIOUS CONFIGURATIONS

5 NEAR–TERM EXTENSIONS AND SYNERGISM

An experimental database system, denoted "EV" for "experimental vehicle", is being implemented by the Bubba design teams on a commercially available, 40 node parallel computer. A series of experiments testing different software design alternatives is scheduled for the EV. The EV serves as another performance model with a complementary (and, we will argue, synergistic) role with FIRM and the simulation pipeline model. As a performance model, the EV has the principal advantage of good fidelity to the software design but poor hardware fidelity and the additional disadvantage of small scale parallelism, less than 40 nodes. The simulation pipeline model has the principal advantage of large scale parallelism, with the limitation of a very coarse characterization of behavior.

This complementarity is exploited. The set of experiments now being performed on the EV provide high resolution behavior measures, such as component instruction counts and holding time distributions, to be used as input parameters to the simulation pipeline. Likewise, measures from the FIRM pipeline have been used to parameterize the EV for characteristics of software not yet implemented on the EV. In fact, more than measures are being provided to the EV from FIRM: code from FIRM has been ported to the EV. Assessor has been ported to the EV Software System in order to obtain the data placement mapping. The identical transaction component graphs used by FIRM are used to drive the EV.

Since both the model components and the EV software are implemented in C, there is more than simple sharing of algorithms: there is a synergistic sharing of data structures, component graph files, and code.

Of course, the simulation solver will be validated for small degrees of parallelism against the EV. Since the operational analysis assumptions used by the FIRM analytic solver hold for the EV, it is expected that comparisons of mean utilizations and mean traffic rates between the EV and FIRM will provide insight into EV software implementation mistakes, i.e., "It works, but not like we assumed from the documentation."

A thorough measurement system has been implemented in the EV to provide a detailed event trace, from which the EV measures are reduced. While the motivation for the detailed measures is providing parameters to the pipelined simulation, an important secondary use of the event trace and trace analyzer is in debugging the distributed system. Coding bugs, not merely performance bugs, have already been uncovered by the trace.

6 CONCLUSION

System design is a heuristic and dynamic process of exploring points in a large space of possibilities. The level of detail being considered changes frequently, tending to finer detail as the design progresses. If a performance model is to be an integral part of the design process, it must be able to model a wide range of points in the relevant space, it must accommodate differing level of detail, and it must provide timely and usable results.

We have built a design tool with these properties and used it to aid the design of a highly parallel database system. The tool is a pipeline of modules that process characterizations of the workload and system, model some aspect of the system's behavior, and present model output in a variety of forms. The results so far have been very gratifying. The tool, while not perfect, has enabled a performance team to have a significant impact on the system design. In this paper we recounted the use of the tool on two design decisions.

However, the design is not yet complete. Toward the end of the design process, less flexibility but more detail and accuracy are required from the performance model. Accordingly, we are shifting from an analytic to a simulation model in the model–solving module of the pipeline. We have also managed to incorporate an actual experimental implementation of the system under design directly into our pipeline, and have already begun comparing experimental and modeling results.

Acknowledgment

Chris Buckalew designed and produced FIRMVIEW; he also coded many of the modifications to FIRM. His assistance is greatly appreciated.

REFERENCES

[Alex87] Alexander, W., Keller, T., and Boughter, E., "A Workload Characterization Pipeline for Models of Parallel Systems", *Proc. 1987 ACM Sigmetrics Conference on Measurement and Modeling of Computer Systems, Performance Evaluation Review*, Vol. 15, No. 1, May 1987, pp 186–194.

[Alex88] Alexander, W. and Kim, D., "Dynamic vs. Static Routing in Hypercubes", MCC Technical Report Number ACA–ST–146–88, April, 1988.

[Alex88b] Alexander, W. and Copeland, G., "Process and Dataflow Control in Distributed Data–Intensive Systems", *Proc. 1988 ACM Sigmod International Conference on Management of Data*, June, 1988.

[Alex88c] Alexander, W. and Copeland, G., "Comparisons of Dataflow Control Techniques in Distributed Data–Intensive Systems", *Proc. 1988 ACM Sigmetrics Conference on Measurement and Modeling of Computer Systems, Performance Evaluation Review*, May, 1988.

[Anon85] Anon el al, "A Measure Of Transaction Processing Power," *Datamation*, Vol. 31.7 (April 1985).

[Banc87] Bancilhon, F., Briggs, T., Khoshafian, S., and Valduriez, P., "FAD, A Simple and Powerful Database Language", *Proc. of Int. Conf. on VLDB*, Brighton, September 1987.

[Bora88] Boral, H., "Parallelism and Data Management", *Proceedings of the 3rd International Conference on Data and Knowledge Bases*, June, 1988.

[Cope88] Copeland, G., Alexander, W., Boughter, E., and Keller, T., "Data Placement in Bubba", *Proc. 1988 ACM Sigmod International Conference on Management of Data*, June, 1988.

[Denn78] Denning, P., Buzen, J., "The Operational Analysis of Queuing Network Models", *Computing Surveys 10,3*, September, 1978.

[DeWi86] DeWitt, D.J., Gerber, R.H., Graefe, G., Heytens, M.H., Kumar, K.B., and Muralikrishna, M., "GAMMA--A High Performance Dataflow Database Machine," *VLDB Conference*, Japan (August 1986).

[Lazo84] Lazowska, E., Zahorjan, J., Graham, G., Sevcik, K., *Quantitative System Performance*, Prentice–Hall, Inc., 1984.

[Livn87] Livny, M., Khoshafian, S., Boral, H.,"Multi–Disk Management Algorithms", *Proceedings of the 1987 SIGMETRICS Conference on Measurement and Modeling of Computer Systems"*, (May, 1987).

[Samm87] Sammer, H.W., "Online Stock Trading Systems: Study Of An Application," *IEEE COMPCON*, San Francisco (February 1987).

[Schw85] Schwetman, H., "CSIM: A C–Based, Process–Oriented Simulation Language", MCC Parallel Processing Report No. PP–080–85, September 1985.

[Sevc81] Sevcik, K. C., "Data Base System Performance Prediction Using an Analytical Model", *Proceedings of 7th VLDB conf.*, 1981, pp 182–189.

[Ston86] Stonebraker, M.,"The Case for Shared Nothing", *Database Engineering*, Vol. 9, No. 1, 1986.

[Tan87] The Tandem Database Group, "NonStop SQL, A Distributed, High–Performance, High–Availability Implementation of SQL," *Workshop on High Performance Transaction Systems*, Asilomar, CA (September 1987).

[Tera85] "DBC/1012 Data Base Computer System Manual, Release 1.3," C10-0001-01, Teradata Corp., Los Angeles (February 1985).

PERFORMANCE ANALYSIS OF A BUFFER UNDER LOCKING PROTOCOLS

E. G. Coffman, Jr. and Leopold Flatto

AT&T Bell Laboratories
Murray Hill, New Jersey 07974

D. P. Gaver, Jr.

Department of Operations Research
Naval Postgraduate School
Monterey, California 93940

ABSTRACT

This paper formulates and analyzes stochastic models of process communication in computer systems. Messages are entered in a buffer (mailbox) by a source, and removed by a sink, at rates that are allowed to differ. The source, following message entry, and the sink, following buffer depletion, leave the buffer for independent exponentially distributed periods of absence, with rate parameters λ and μ, respectively. Locking protocols are in effect, i.e., message entry and removal can not occur simultaneously. The decision of the source or sink arriving to find the buffer active can be to wait until it is free, or to leave on another period of absence. We apply the analysis to both the "wait" and "no wait" options.

A study of the fluid-approximation model shows that renewal theory forms the proper basis of the analysis; the important relevant results are briefly reviewed. These results along with renewal-theoretic arguments, especially those exploiting regenerative properties, are then applied to derivations of basic performance measures, e.g., transforms or expectations of busy periods and steady-state buffer levels. In particular, the formulas bring out the dependence of the expectations on the variance of message lengths. Desirable extensions of the models are sketched.

1. INTRODUCTION

We examine the behavior of a buffer system that acts as an intermediate storage facility in a computer system. We speak of inputs from a *source* and outputs to a *sink* as being *messages* consisting of data. The function of the buffer is to hold temporary accumulations of messages that arise because of irregular or randomly occurring input and output.

The source alternates between states when it is at the buffer entering a message at rate r^+, and when it is away from the buffer. The loading of messages requires random time periods denoted generically by T. After a message is entered, the source leaves the buffer for a random *rest period*, R, before returning. Symmetrically, the sink alternates between states when it is away from the buffer and when it is at the buffer removing data at rate r^-. The sink always completely empties the buffer before leaving; it returns following a rest period S.

The sink immediately leaves on another rest period whenever it encounters an empty buffer.

We assume that there is no limit to the amount of storage that can be made available to the buffer. However, several styles of interaction between the source and sink will be considered. Styles in the class of interest in this paper are called *locking protocols*. According to such protocols, source and sink activities can not occur simultaneously; one activity locks out the other. Within this class of protocols, variants are determined by the reaction of the source or sink wishing to enter or remove data when it encounters the buffer in use. The taxonomy of models to be studied is denoted by (NW, NW), (NW, W), (W, NW), and (W, W). W and NW denote "wait" and "no wait," respectively, and the first and second elements of a pair refer to the source and sink, respectively. Under the no-wait options an arriving source or sink encountering a buffer in use is assumed to leave the buffer for another source or sink rest period that is stochastically identical to and independent of the previous one. Under the wait options an arriving source or sink simply waits for the start of the other's next rest period, at which time it immediately begins entering or removing data, respectively. Depending on the application, it may be assumed that the message of a source turned away from a busy buffer is lost, and a new message is generated in the next rest period, or it may be assumed that the source attempts to enter the same message after the next rest period. The wait/no-wait options are also known as blocking/non-blocking options.

In a primary (NW, NW) application motivating this paper, the source and sink are taken as autonomous processes. The buffer may be thought of as a mailbox where from time to time the source deposits mail and the sink collects mail. Message-based operating systems provide an important example. The computer system may be centralized or distributed, with the degree of coupling arbitrary; the coupling influences parameter values rather than model structures. The assumption $r^+ = r^-$ would frequently apply; the source and sink operate on identical machines. This assumption usually simplifies formulas without affecting the underlying analytical approach.

In a (NW, W) or (W, W) application, the source messages may be viewed as the intermediate products of a complex computation being passed on from one sub-process to another. In general, applications requiring one or both wait options imply a greater input or output dependence between source and sink; synchronization may be one of the functions being performed, along with message passing.

This paper contributes to a substantial literature on the analysis of buffer models. While there appears to be no recent survey, the extensive reference lists in a book by Aven, Coffman and Kogan (1987) and a recent paper by Mitra (1987) will be useful to the interested reader. We remark that this literature focuses chiefly on systems in which the sink is a slave process; the sink is always at the buffer either removing data or ready to do so. A notable exception is the recent work of Mitra (1987), where a multiple-source multiple-sink system without locking is analyzed; each source alternates between rest states and states when it is entering data into the buffer along with any other sources currently at the buffer. Each sink visits the buffer after successive rest periods until it finds a non-empty buffer, at which point it remains at the buffer removing data, along with any other sinks currently at the buffer, until the buffer is empty.

The following questions concerning buffer behavior are of interest, and are addressed in later sections:

- What is the characteristic occupancy level, e.g., the mean, or the probability distribution, of the buffer contents $X(t)$ as $t \to \infty$?

- What is the mean, or probability distribution, of the time of first passage from an idle state $(X(t) = 0)$ to a state $x > 0$, or from a busy state, $x > 0$ to idleness? In particular, what is a busy period duration?

It appears that such questions are often answered conveniently by thinking of the buffer process as alternating between idle periods of generic duration I, and busy periods of duration B. In fact, it is often possible to proceed by restricting the analysis to the *busy-period process*, $\{X_b(t), t \geqslant 0\}$, where the latter refers to the content process $\{X(t), t \geqslant 0\}$ over periods during which the latter is positive. Under convenient and natural initial assumptions the sequences of idle periods and busy periods are composed of mutually independent random variables, and are themselves independently and identically distributed, and so renewal-theoretic arguments and theorems (particularly the *key renewal theorem*) can be applied; see Smith (1955, 1958), Feller (1971) or Karlin and Taylor (1975). A number of the basic results are reviewed in the next section in preparation for the subsequent analysis.

First-passage time results can be found by exploiting the ideas of terminating renewal processes and large deviations; see Feller (1971), and also Gaver and Jacobs (1986) in a different context. Similar and complementary results can often be obtained, and quite intuitively, by application of renewal-reward theorems derived from the strong law of large numbers; see Ross (1983). Results of this type are planned for a forthcoming paper.

2. THE MODEL

We present below a standard probabilistic formulation, but specialize it in later sections in order to obtain explicit solutions.

Message loading periods form a sequence of independent, identically distributed (i.i.d.) random variables $\{T_i, i = 1, 2, ...\}$ with distribution function (d.f.) $F(t)$ and density $f(t)$. Between-message rest times, or message interarrival times $\{R_i; i = 1, 2, ...\}$ are also i.i.d. random variables with d.f. $G(t)$ and density $g(t)$. Idle times, $\{I_i\}$, form a sequence of i.i.d. random variables, although often it is natural to think of them as being the same as source rest times. Sink interarrival times are i.i.d. with d.f. $K(t)$ and density $k(t)$. All processes are assumed independent.

In later sections, the above model, with $G(t)$ and $K(t)$ exponential, gives rise to simple formulas that promise insights. The phase-type formulations, *cf* Neuts (1981), among others, should also provide explicit, although awkward formulas in terms of elementary functions; we do not consider such elaborations here.

In what follows we adopt the following notational conventions. $F^*(\theta)$ denotes the Laplace-Stieltjes transform of the d.f. $F(t)$, $F^{(n)}(t)$ denotes the d.f. of a sum of n i.i.d. random variables with d.f. $F(t)$, and $\bar{F}(t) = 1 - F(t)$ denotes tail probabilities.

Regenerative Structure and Renewal-Theoretic Results — Let $X(t) \geqslant 0$ denote the state of the buffer process (e.g., the number of bits stored) at time t. The state space is $\mathscr{R}^+$, so we deal in the usual fluid approximation. The process $\{X(t), t \geqslant 0\}$ has a regenerative property, describable in terms of a *cycle* sequence $\{C_i\}$, made up of i.i.d. random variables, $C_i = I_i + B_i$, I_i being the ith idle period and B_i the ensuing busy period, during which the buffer contents are positive. The sequence $\{C_i\}$ comprises a renewal process. Let $\{N(t), t \geqslant 0\}$ be the number of cycle completions in $(0, t]$, and let the renewal function of $\{N(t)\}$ (the expected number of complete cycles in $(0, t]$) be denoted by

$$n(t) = \sum_{j=1}^{\infty} \Pr\left[\sum_{i=1}^{j} C_i \leqslant t\right] = \sum_{j=1}^{\infty} F_c^{(j)}(t),$$

where $F_c^{(j)}(t)$ denotes the d.f. of the sum of j cycles. Let $H(t)$ be the d.f. of idle periods.

For $x > 0$,

$$p_b((dx), t) = \Pr\{x \leqslant X_b(t) \leqslant x+dx \mid X_b(0) = 0\}$$

(2.1)

$$= \Pr\{x \leqslant X(t) \leqslant x+dx, \ X(\tau) > 0 \ \forall \tau : 0 < \tau \leqslant t \mid X(0) = 0\}$$

provides the probability element for the busy period process. It is convenient to say, informally, that $p_b((dx), t)$ gives the probability that $X(t)$ is at x. Then we can express the probability that $X(t)$ is at x at any time, given $X(0) = 0$ and an idle period just beginning, as

(2.2)
$$p((dx), t) = p_c((dx), t) + \int_0^t p((dx), t-\tau) F_c(d\tau),$$

where

(2.3)
$$p_c((dx), t) = \begin{cases} 1 - H(t), & x = 0, \\ \int_0^t p_b((dx), t-\tau) \, H(d\tau), & x > 0, \end{cases}$$

which represents the probability that $X(t)$ is at x during the first cycle. Note that (2.2) is formally solved in terms of the renewal function as

(2.4)
$$p((dx), t) = p_c((dx), t) + \int_0^t p_c((dx), t-\tau) \, n(d\tau),$$

the first term being the probability that $X(t)$ is at x and t belongs to the first cycle, and the second being the probability that $X(t)$ is at x and t belongs to some later cycle. For the point mass at $x = 0$, we write

(2.5)
$$p_0(t) = \Pr\{X(t) = 0 \mid X(0) = 0\} = \overline{H}(t) + \int_0^t \overline{H}(t-\tau) n(d\tau).$$

In terms of Laplace transforms on t, with $n^*(s) = \int_0^\infty e^{-st} n(dt)$,

(2.6)
$$p^*((dx), s) = \int_0^\infty e^{-st} p((dx), t) dt = \frac{H^*(s) p_b^*((dx), s)}{1 - n^*(s)}$$

(2.7)
$$p_0^*(s) = \int_0^\infty e^{-st} p_0(t) dt = \frac{[1 - H^*(s)]/s}{1 - n^*(s)},$$

which can occasionally be inverted explicitly, given a nice form of the busy-period transform $p_b^*((dx), s)$. One can also interpret $sp^*((dx), s)$ as the probability that $X(z) = x$, with z having the density se^{-sz}, i.e., the probability of state x when viewing the system at a random (exponential) instant.

Long-run $(t \to \infty)$ information is often available from the key renewal theorem, or from Tauberian/Abelian theorems for Laplace transforms; see Feller (1971) or Widder (1946). For example, if $p_b((dx), t)$ is directly Riemann integrable, then

(2.8)
$$p(dx) = \lim_{t \to \infty} p((dx), t) = \frac{1}{E[C]} \int_0^\infty p_b((dx), t) dt.$$

For $p_b((dx), t)$ to be directly Riemann integrable, it is sufficient that it be positive, non-increasing and integrable; see Ross (1983). These conditions will be verifiable in particular cases. For another useful result let $\psi(x)$ be any function such that

(2.9)
$$\psi_b(t) = \int_0^\infty \psi(x) p_b((dx), t)$$

is directly Riemann integrable. Then

(2.10)
$$\lim_{t \to \infty} E[\psi(X(t))] = \frac{\psi(0) \cdot E[I] + \int_0^\infty \psi_b(t) dt}{E[C]}.$$

In particular, the long-run expected buffer content is

(2.11)
$$\lim_{t \to \infty} E[X(t)] = \frac{\int_0^\infty \left[\int_0^\infty x p_b((dx), t) \right] dt}{E[C]} = \frac{\int_0^\infty E[X_b(t)] dt}{E[C]}.$$

Because of positivity (Fubini's theorem),

$$\int_0^\infty E[X_b(t)] \mid X_b(0) dt = E\left\{ \int_0^B X_b(t) dt \right\},$$

B being the length of a busy period, so to calculate the long-run expected buffer contents it is enough to calculate the expected area under the random function $X_b(t)$, $0 \leqslant t \leqslant B$. As will be seen, such expectations are often straightforward for specific buffer models. In addition,

(2.12)
$$\lim_{t \to \infty} \Pr\{X(t) \leqslant x\} = \int_0^\infty \frac{\Pr\{X_b(t) \leqslant x\} dt}{E[C]}$$

$$= \frac{E\left\{ \int_0^B \chi(X_b(t), x) dt \right\}}{E[C]},$$

where the indicator function $\chi(X_b, x) = 1$ if $X_b \leqslant x$, and $\chi(X_b, x) = 0$ otherwise. Interpret the numerator as the expected time in a cycle during which buffer contents do not exceed x.

3. THE BUFFER WITH NO SOURCE OR SINK WAITING

We analyze the (NW, NW) system under exponential assumptions for the source and sink rest periods:

(3.1)
$$g(t) = \lambda e^{-\lambda t}, \quad t \geqslant 0$$

(3.2)
$$k(t) = \mu e^{-\mu t}, \quad t \geqslant 0.$$

The process of buffer contents, $\{X(t)\}$, evolves as follows. Suppose $X(0) = 0$; then after an idle period of duration I, a busy period begins; buffer contents at time t following the beginning of the busy period, and before it ends, are $X_b(t)$. At some time after the beginning of the busy period, the sink arrives. If it arrives while the source is at rest, it is said to be *effective* and immediately begins depleting the buffer; otherwise, the sink

167

commences a new (i.i.d.) rest period. We let L denote the time from the start of the busy period to the moment buffer emptying begins, and we let $S(L)$ denote the time required to empty the buffer, once emptying begins. A message arrival during $S(L)$ is turned away; the source commences a new (i.i.d.) rest period, at the end of which it returns with the message. (Observe that L is not simply a sink interarrival time, i.e., it does not have the density (3.2), but must be derived from scratch.) At busy period termination a new idle period of duration I begins, and so the process continues. For this model, I has the distribution of a rest period, i.e., it has the density (3.1).

We now discuss various random quantities characterizing the above processes; see Fig. 1. The ultimate aim of the analysis is an expression for the expected long-run buffer contents (see (3.24)-(3.26)).

(a)   For the time from the beginning of a busy period to an effective sink arrival (SA), we write

(3.3) $$L = T_1 + R_1' + T_2 + R_2' + \cdots + T_{M-1} + R_{M-1}' + T_M + R_{M-1}'' ,$$

where M denotes the number of messages in the buffer at the time of an effective sink arrival, and R' (respectively, R'') is a rest period that is not (respectively, is) interrupted by an SA. By the exponential assumptions R' and R'' are equal in distribution. We look upon these modified source-rest periods as i.i.d. exponentials with parameter $\lambda+\mu$; at the end of such a period, depletion begins with probability $\mu/(\lambda+\mu)$, and a new message begins entering with probability $\lambda/(\lambda+\mu)$. Since M is geometrically distributed,

$$\Pr\{M=m\} = \left(\frac{\lambda}{\lambda+\mu}\right)^{m-1} \left(\frac{\mu}{\lambda+\mu}\right), \quad m \geqslant 1 ,$$

we can represent L as

(3.4) $$L = \begin{cases} T_1 + R_1'', & \text{when } M=1 \text{ (first SA effective),} \\ & \text{i.e. with probability } \mu/(\lambda+\mu), \\ \\ T_1 + R_1' + L^\# & \text{when } M>1 \text{ (first SA ineffective),} \\ & \text{i.e. with probability } \lambda/(\lambda+\mu), \end{cases}$$

with $L^\#$ independent of L and having the same d.f. Now introduce transforms to find

$$\phi_L(\theta) = E[e^{-\theta L}] = F^*(\theta) \int_0^\infty (\lambda+\mu)e^{-(\lambda+\mu+\theta)t} dt \left[\frac{\mu}{\lambda+\mu} + \frac{\lambda}{\lambda+\mu}\phi_L(\theta)\right] ,$$

so that

(3.5) $$\phi_L(\theta) = \frac{\mu F^*(\theta)}{\mu+\theta+\lambda[1-F^*(\theta)]} .$$

From (3.5), we obtain

(3.6) $$E[L] = \mu^{-1}[1 + (\lambda+\mu)E(T)] ,$$

and

$$\mu E[L] \sim \frac{E[T]+E[R]}{E[R]} \quad as \quad \mu \to 0 ,$$

as is intuitive. It is possible to show that $\hat{L} = L/E[L]$ will tend weakly to the unit exponential d.f. as $\mu \to 0$.

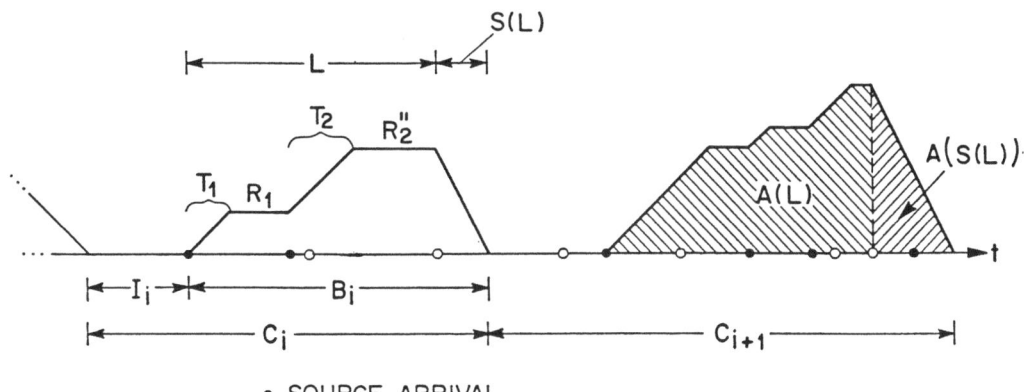

BUFFER PROCESS: X(t)

- SOURCE ARRIVAL
○ SINK ARRIVAL (SA)

FIGURE 1. THE (NW, NW) BUFFER PROCESS $(r^+ = \frac{1}{2} r^-)$

(b)   Next, consider the maximum level reached during a busy period

(3.7)
$$X(L) = r^+(T_1 + T_2 + \cdots + T_M).$$

In terms of transforms again, $\phi_{X(L)}(\theta) = E[e^{-\theta X(L)}]$ is given by

(3.8)
$$\phi_{X(L)}(\theta) = E[\{F^*(r^+\theta)\}^M] = \frac{\mu F^*(r^+\theta)}{\mu + \lambda[1 - F^*(r^+\theta)]},$$

from which

(3.9)
$$E[X(L)] = \mu^{-1}(\lambda + \mu) r^+ E[T],$$

and

(3.10)
$$\mu E[X(L)] \sim r^+ \lambda E[T] \quad as \quad \mu \to 0.$$

For μ small, we correctly anticipate

(3.11)
$$E[X(L)] \approx r^+ \frac{E[T]}{E[T] + E[R]} E[L].$$

These results are applied trivially to the buffer emptying time, by means of

(3.12)
$$S(L) = X(L)/r^-.$$

(c)   For an analysis of busy periods,

(3.13)
$$B = S(L) + L,$$

we first refer to (3.3)-(3.7) and (3.12) to see that

$$E[e^{-\theta_S S(L) - \theta_L L} \mid M, R_1', ..., R_{M-1}', R_M'']$$

(3.14)
$$= \left[E[e^{-(\theta_S(r^+/r^-) + \theta_L)T}] \right]^M e^{-\theta_L(R_1' + \cdots + R_{M-1}' + R_M'')}.$$

Removing the rest-period conditions (recall R' and R'' are i.i.d.), we obtain

(3.15)
$$E[e^{-\theta_S S(L) - \theta_L L} \mid M] = [F^*(\theta_S(r^+/r^-) + \theta_L)]^M \left(\frac{\lambda + \mu}{\lambda + \mu + \theta_L} \right)^M.$$

Then, we remove the condition on M,

$$\phi_{S(L),L}(\theta_S, \theta_L) = \sum_{m \geq 1} E[e^{-\theta_S S(L) - \theta_L L} \mid M = m] \left(\frac{\lambda}{\lambda + \mu} \right)^{m-1} \frac{\mu}{\lambda + \mu},$$

to find a result similar in form to (3.5) and (3.8)

$$\phi_{S(L),L}(\theta_S, \theta_L) = \frac{\mu F^*(\theta_S(r^+/r^-) + \theta_L)}{\mu + \theta_L + \lambda[1 - F^*(\theta_S(r^+/r^-) + \theta_L)]}.$$

By (3.13), we have $\phi_B(\theta) = E[e^{-\theta B}] = \phi_{S(L),L}(\theta, \theta)$, and hence

(3.16)
$$\phi_B(\theta) = \frac{\mu F^*((r^+/r^- + 1)\theta)}{\mu + \theta + \lambda[1 - F^*((r^+/r^- + 1)\theta)]},$$

with

(3.17)
$$E[B] = \frac{1}{\mu} \left[1 + \left[\frac{r^+}{r^-} + 1 \right] (\lambda + \mu) E[T] \right].$$

(d) In order to evaluate the long-run expectation of buffer contents we proceed to find the expected area under $X(t)$ during a busy period. Begin with the filling portion; a glance at Fig. 1 shows that the area of random triangles and rectangles is

$$A(L) = \frac{r^+}{2}(T_1^2 + T_2^2 + \cdots + T_M^2)$$

(3.18)
$$+ r^+[T_1 R_1' + \cdots + (T_1 + T_2 + \cdots + T_{M-1})R_{M-1}' + (T_1 + \cdots + T_M)R_M''],$$

but a closer look provides the more convenient form

(3.19)
$$A(L) = \begin{cases} r^+(T_1^2/2 + T_1 R_1'') & \text{when } M = 1 \text{ (first SA effective)} \\ r^+(T_1^2/2 + T_1 R_1') + A(L)^\# + (r^+ T_1)L^\# & \text{when } M > 1 \text{ (first SA ineffective)}, \end{cases}$$

where the regenerative properties of $\{X(t)\}$ have been fully exploited; i.e., both $A(L)^\#$ and $L^\#$ have the same distributions as $A(L)$ and L, respectively.

Now take expectations in (3.19),

$$E[A(L)] = r^+ \left\{ \frac{1}{2} E[T^2] + E[T]E[R'] \right\}$$

(3.20)

$$+ \Pr\{M > 1\}\{E[A(L)] + r^+ E[T]E[L]\},$$

then substitute (3.6), $E[R'] = \dfrac{1}{\lambda + \mu}$, and $\Pr\{M > 1\} = \dfrac{\lambda}{\lambda + \mu}$ to obtain

(3.21)
$$E[A(L)] = r^+ \left[\frac{\lambda + \mu}{\mu} \right] \left\{ \frac{1}{2} E[T^2] + \frac{1}{\mu} E[T](1 + \lambda E[T]) \right\}.$$

Turning now to the area under the emptying portion of a busy period, we have

(3.22)
$$A(S(L)) = \frac{1}{2} X(L)S(L) = \frac{1}{2r^-} X^2(L) = \frac{(r^+)^2}{2r^-} (T_1 + \cdots + T_M)^2.$$

Focusing on $Y = T_1 + \cdots + T_M$, we write conditionally

$$Y = \begin{cases} T_1, & \text{if } M = 1 \\ T_1 + Y^{\#}, & \text{if } M > 1, \end{cases}$$

so

$$Y^2 = \begin{cases} T_1^2, & \text{if } M = 1 \\ T_1^2 + 2T_1 Y^{\#} + (Y^{\#})^2, & \text{if } M > 1, \end{cases}$$

where Y and $Y^{\#}$ are independent and equal in distribution. Remove conditions to find

$$E[Y] = E[T] + \frac{\lambda}{\lambda + \mu} E[Y] = \frac{\lambda + \mu}{\mu} E[T],$$

$$E[Y^2] = E[T^2] + \frac{\lambda}{\lambda + \mu}(2E[T]E[Y] + E[Y^2])$$

$$= \frac{\lambda + \mu}{\mu} \left\{ E[T^2] + \frac{2\lambda}{\mu} (E[T])^2 \right\},$$

and hence

(3.23)
$$E[A(S(L))] = \frac{(r^+)^2}{r^-} \frac{\lambda + \mu}{\mu} \left\{ \frac{E[T^2]}{2} + \frac{\lambda}{\mu} (E[T])^2 \right\}.$$

We assemble previous results and deduce expected long-run buffer constants from the key renewal theorem or the strong law of large numbers (cf (2.11)):

(3.24)
$$E[X] = \lim_{t \to \infty} E[X(t)] = \frac{E[A(L)] + E[A(S(L))]}{E[C]},$$

where $E[C] = \dfrac{1}{\lambda} + E[B]$. Substitution of (3.17), (3.21) and (3.23) yields

171

(3.25)

$$E[X] = \left(\frac{\lambda+\mu}{\mu}r^+\right) \cdot \frac{\dfrac{E[T^2]}{2}\left[\dfrac{r^+}{r^-}+1\right]+\dfrac{1}{\mu}E[T]\left[1+\lambda\left[\dfrac{r^+}{r^-}+1\right]E[T]\right]}{E[C]}$$

with

(3.26)

$$E[C] = \frac{1}{\lambda} + \frac{1}{\mu}\left\{1+\left[\frac{r^+}{r^-}+1\right](\lambda+\mu)E[T]\right\}.$$

4. RESULTS ON WAIT PROTOCOLS

In general, wait protocols complicate matters; however, the principles of the analysis remain the same. This can be seen in the following treatment of the source no-wait, sink wait protocol. Because of its similarity with section 3, the analysis is somewhat condensed.

Figure 2 illustrates the two types of busy-period sample functions that can arise in the (NW, W) model; the peaked ones occur when an SA encounters an active source, and waits until it finishes, while the remainder occur when an SA encounters a source rest period. The analysis of the random variables in the preceding section proceeds as follows.

(a) We can express the time until emptying begins, measured from the start of a busy period, as

(4.1)

$$L = \begin{cases} T'; & M=1, \text{ SA during first loading period} \\ T''; & M=1, \text{ SA during first source-rest period} \\ T''+R'+L^\#; & M>1, \end{cases}$$

where $L^\#$ is independently distributed as L,

(4.2)

$$\Pr\{t \leqslant T' \leqslant t+dt\} = (1-e^{-\mu t})F(dt)/[1-F^*(\mu)]$$

$$\Pr\{t \leqslant T'' \leqslant t+dt\} = e^{-\mu t}F(dt)/F^*(\mu),$$

R' has the same distribution as in section 3, and M has the geometric distribution

(4.3)

$$\Pr\{M=m\} = \left[\frac{\lambda F^*(\mu)}{\lambda+\mu}\right]^{m-1}\left[1-\frac{\lambda F^*(\mu)}{\lambda+\mu}\right].$$

Note that $F^*(\mu)=E[e^{-\mu T}]$ is the probability of no SA during a message entry. Then the transform becomes

$$\phi_L(\theta) = \int_0^\infty e^{-\theta t}(1-e^{-\mu t})F(dt)$$

(4.4)

$$+ \int_0^\infty e^{-(\mu+\theta)t}F(dt)\left\{\int_0^\infty \mu e^{-(\mu+\theta)t}[1-e^{-\lambda t}]dt + \phi_L(\theta)\int_0^\infty \lambda e^{-(\lambda+\mu+\theta)t}dt\right\},$$

172

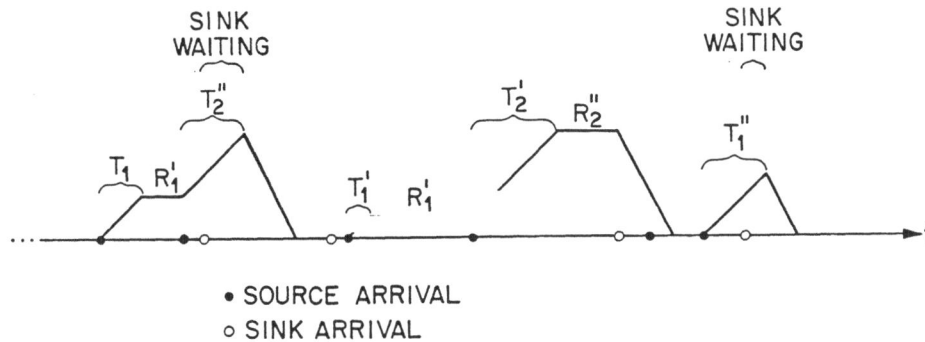

BUFFER PROCESS: X(t)

SINK
WAITING

SINK
WAITING

• SOURCE ARRIVAL
○ SINK ARRIVAL

FIGURE 2. THE (NW, W) BUFFER PROCESS $(r^+ = \frac{1}{2} r^-)$

so after simplification,

(4.5)
$$\phi_L(\theta) = \frac{(\lambda+\mu+\theta)F^*(\theta) - (\lambda+\theta)F^*(\mu+\theta)}{\mu+(\lambda+\theta)[1-F^*(\mu+\theta)]}.$$

For the expected value we find

(4.6)
$$E[L] = \frac{(\lambda+\mu)E[T]+F^*(\mu)}{\mu+\lambda[1-F^*(\mu)]},$$

and $\mu E[L] \sim 1$ as $\mu \to 0$, for there are no re-tries, and the time to begin emptying after an SA is asymptotically the exponential SA time. In fact, expansion of (4.6) shows that, as $\mu \to 0$,

$$E[L] \sim \frac{1}{\mu} + \frac{E[T^2]}{2E[T]} \left[\frac{E[T]}{E[T]+E[R]} \right],$$

which is intuitively appealing (note that $E[T^2]/(2E[T])$ is an expected residual message loading time and $E[T]/(E[T]+E[R])$ is asymptotically the fraction of L spent loading messages).

(b)   For the maximum level reached in a busy period, we have in agreement with (3.7)

$$X(L) = r^+(T_1 + \cdots + T_M),$$

and consequently,

$$E[S(L)] = E[X(L)]/r^- = \frac{r^+}{r^-} E[T]E[M]$$

or

(4.7)
$$E[S(L)] = \frac{r^+}{r^-} \frac{(\lambda+\mu)E[T]}{\mu+\lambda[1-F^*(\mu)]}.$$

This together with (4.6) yields for $E[B] = E[L] + E[S(L)]$,

(4.8)
$$E[B] = \frac{(\lambda+\mu)\left[\frac{r^+}{r^-}+1\right]E[T]+F^*(\mu)}{\mu+\lambda[1-F^*(\mu)]}$$

and, as $\mu \to 0$,

(4.9)
$$E[B] \sim E[L]\left\{1 + \left[\frac{r^+}{r^-}\right] \frac{E[T]}{E[T]+E[R]}\right\},$$

as would be anticipated for rare SA's.

(c) To obtain $E[X]$, we start, in close analogy with (3.19), by expressing $A(L)$ as

$$A(L) = \begin{cases} r^+(T''^2/2; & M=1, \quad \text{SA during first loading period} \\ r^+[(T_1')^2/2 + T_1'R_1'']; & M=1, \quad \text{SA during first source-rest period} \\ r^+[(T_1')^2/2 + T_1'R_1'] + A(L^{\#}) + (r^+T_1')L^{\#}; & M>1. \end{cases}$$

Taking expectations, a calculation shows that

(4.10) $E[A(L)] = r^+(\lambda+\mu)\left\{\dfrac{E[T^2]/2}{\mu+\lambda[1-F^*(\mu)]} + \dfrac{E[Te^{-\mu T}][1+\lambda(E[T]+F^*(\mu)/(\lambda+\mu))]}{\{\mu+\lambda[1-F^*(\mu)]\}^2}\right\},$

and that as $\mu \to 0$,

$$\mu E[A(L)] \sim r^+(E[L])^2 \frac{E[T]}{E[T]+E[R]}.$$

Next, write

$$A(S(L)) = \frac{1}{2} \frac{(r^+)^2}{r^-} S_M^2,$$

where

$$S_M = \begin{cases} T_1''; & M=1, \quad \text{first SA during first loading period} \\ T_1'; & M=1, \quad \text{first SA during first source-rest period} \\ T_1' + S_M^{\#}; & M>1. \end{cases}$$

A straightforward calculation leads to

174

$$E[S_M] = \frac{(\lambda+\mu)E[T]}{\mu+\lambda[1-F^*(\mu)]},$$

$$E[S_M^2] = (\lambda+\mu)\left\{\frac{E[T^2]}{\mu+\lambda[1-F^*(\mu)]} + \frac{2\lambda E[Te^{-\mu T}]E[T]F^*(\mu)}{\{\mu+\lambda[1-F^*(\mu)]\}^2}\right\},$$

so that

(4.11) $\quad E[A(S(L))] = \dfrac{(r^+)^2}{r^-}(\lambda+\mu)\left\{\dfrac{E[T^2]/2}{\mu+\lambda[1-F^*(\mu)]} + \dfrac{\lambda E[Te^{-\mu T}]E[T]F^*(\mu)}{\{\mu+\lambda[1-F^*(\mu)]\}^2}\right\},$

whereupon $E[X] = E[A(L)] + E[A(S(L))]$ follows by substitution of (4.10) and (4.11).

We conclude with brief observations on the source-wait models. The burden added to the analysis of these models results from a new idle period d.f., which now has an atom at 0 (see Fig. 3). Clearly, $\Pr\{I=0\}$ is the probability that the source arrives with a message during $S(L)$. To preserve regenerative structure, it is convenient to deal with *composite busy periods*, and idle periods that are residual source rest periods, as in Section 3. A composite busy period, $\tilde{B}$, consists (with probability 1) of a sequence of busy periods $B_i, B_{i+1}, ..., B_{i+j}$, where B_{l+1} begins when B_l ends, $i \leqslant l \leqslant j-1$, and B_i and B_{i+j} are preceded and followed, respectively, by idle periods of positive duration (in particular, with density $\lambda e^{-\lambda t}$); see Fig. 3. The statistics of composite busy periods are easily derived. For example, write

(4.12) $\qquad\qquad \tilde{B} = \begin{cases} B, & \text{with probability } e^{-\lambda S(L)} \\ B + \tilde{B}^{\#}, & \text{with probability } 1-e^{-\lambda S(L)}, \end{cases}$

where $\tilde{B}$ and $\tilde{B}^{\#}$ are independent and equal in distribution. Then,

$$E[\tilde{B}] = E[B] + E[\tilde{B}]E[1-e^{-\lambda S(L)}]$$

and

(4.13) $\qquad\qquad E[\tilde{B}] = \dfrac{E[B]}{E[e^{-\lambda S(L)}]}.$

By lines already well established, an analysis of the (W, NW) system leads to an expression for $E[e^{-\lambda S(L)}]$ having a familiar form:

(4.14) $\qquad\qquad E[e^{-\lambda S(L)}] = \dfrac{\mu F^*(\lambda)}{\mu+\lambda[1-F^*(\lambda)]}.$

Then $E[\tilde{B}]$ is determined from (3.17) (with $r^+ = r^- = 1$), (4.13), and (4.14). The analysis of the renewal process $C_i = \tilde{B}_i + I_i$, $i = 1, 2, ...$, continues in analogy with Section 3.

5. CONCLUSIONS AND EXTENSIONS

The models presented and analyzed represent in a simple way many situations encountered in computer/communication systems. Of course, there are many extensions to be considered, an important one being to recognize the finiteness of the buffer, i.e. there is a capacity b so that $X(t) \leqslant b < \infty$. This means that protocols must be established to deal with message inputs colliding with the capacity b. Possibilities include: (i) split such messages, sending the overflow and all subsequent messages before the next SA to an effectively unlimited secondary buffer, or (ii) reject such messages and close the buffer until the sink reappears; see Gaver and Jacobs (1980) for some partial but relevant results. Design questions concern the determination of b, as a function of source and sink rates and message statistics, so as to achieve a suitably small probability of overflow.

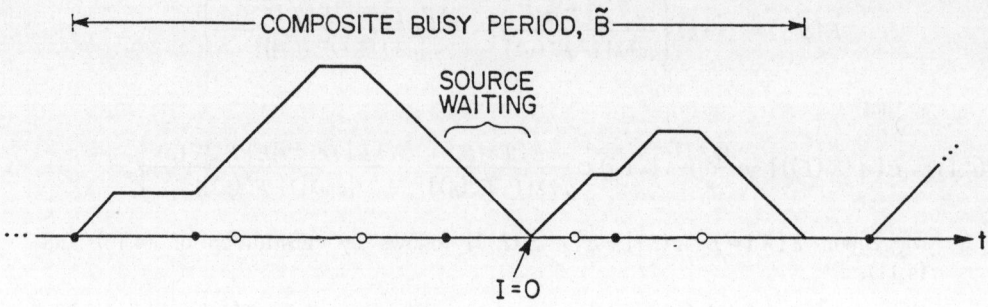

BUFFER PROCESS: X(t)

|←——————— COMPOSITE BUSY PERIOD, B̃ ———————→|

SOURCE
WAITING

I = O

• SOURCE ARRIVAL
○ SINK ARRIVAL

FIGURE 3. THE (W, NW) BUFFER PROCESS ($r^+ = r^-$)

More complete information than the simple expectations exhibited here is desirable. Transforms of the time-dependent distributions of buffer contents are available, from which the tail behavior and its dependence on $F(t)$ can frequently be derived; the tool is large deviation theory. The present analysis can also be extended to multiple sources. Results have been obtained and will be reported in a forthcoming paper.

REFERENCES

Aven, O., Coffman, E. G., Jr. and Kogan, Y., 1987, *Stochastic Models of Computer Storage*, Reidel Publ. (Note: see Chap. 2, *Buffer Storage*.)

Feller, W., Vol. I, 1950; Vol. II (2nd ed.) 1971, *An Introduction to Probability Theory and Its Applications*, John Wiley, New York. (Note: see Chap. XI of Vol. II, *Renewal Theory*.)

Gaver, D. P. and Jacobs, P. A., 1980, "Storage problems when demand is 'all or nothing'," *Naval Res. Log. Quart.*, 27:529.

Gaver, D. P., and Jacobs P. A., 1986, "On inference and transient response for M/G/1 models," *Proc. Conference on Teletraffic Analysis and Computer Performance Evaluation*; O. J. Boxma, J. W. Cohen, H. C. Tijms (eds.), Elsevier Science Pubs., B. V. (North Holland), 163.

Gaver, D. P., and Lehoczky, J. P., 1982, "Channels that cooperatively service a data stream and voice messages," *IEEE Trans. on Communications*, 30:1153.

Karlin, S., and Taylor, H. M., 1975, *A First Course in Stochastic Processes*, Academic Press, New York.

Mitra, D., 1988, "Stochastic Theory of a Fluid Model of Producers and Consumers Coupled by a Buffer," *Adv. Appl. Prob.*, 20:646.

Neuts, M., 1981, *Matrix-Geometric Solution in Stochastic Models: An Algorithmic Approach*, Johns Hopkins Univ. Press. (Note: see Chap. 2: *Probability Distribution of Phase Type.*)

Ross, S. M., 1983, *Stochastic Processes*, John Wiley, New York.

Smith, W. L., 1955, "Regenerative stochastic processes," *Proc. Royal Statistical Soc., A*, 232:6.

Smith, W. L., 1958, "Renewal Theory and its ramifications," *J. of the Royal Statistical Soc., B*, 20:243.

Widder, D. V., 1946, *The Laplace Transform*, Princeton Univ. Press, Princeton, NJ.

AVERAGE MESSAGE DELAY OF AN ASYMMETRIC SINGLE-BUFFER POLLING SYSTEM WITH ROUND-ROBIN SCHEDULING OF SERVICES

Tetsuya Takine, Yutaka Takahashi and Toshiharu Hasegawa

Department of Applied Mathematics and Physics
Faculty of Engineering, Kyoto University
Kyoto 606, Japan

Abstract

An asymmetric polling system with single-message buffers is considered. Each message consists of multiple packets and only one packet is transmitted when polled. For a symmetric system with constant length of a packet and switchover time, the average performance measures, including the average message delay, have been explicitly derived in the recent paper [Taka87c]. The main result of this paper is the exact derivation of the average message delay for an asymmetric system, where transmission time of a packet and switchover time are assumed to be distributed according to general probability distribution functions which are different among stations.

1   Introduction

Polling system is considered as a system of multiple queues with cyclic service. Analysis of polling system has been studied for about 30 years, and is still one of the most active fields in performance analysis of computer communication systems because the result is directly applicable to the performance evaluation of Token-Passing local area networks. There are many variations in polling systems and most of them are assumed to have buffers of an infinite capacity. Takagi provides extensive surveys on analytical results [Taka86], [Taka87b].

Single buffer polling system has been studied in several papers, including the oldest works in polling systems [Mack57a], [Mack57b]. Explicit expression of the probability distribution of message delay is derived only for a symmetric system with constant transmission time and switchover time [Kaye72], [Taka86]. Takagi provides an exact analysis of the average message delay for a general symmetric system, where general probability distribution functions (PDF's) of transmission time and switchover time are assumed [Taka85]. This approach needs the solution of $O(2^M)$ linear simultaneous equations, where M denotes the number of stations in the system, and cannot be applied to asymmetric systems. Also Takine, Takahashi and Hasegawa study the interdeparture process in a general symmetric system [Taki86]. Ibe and Cheng show the exact result of the average message delay for a general asymmetric system with two stations [Ibe86]. Recently Takine, Takahashi and Hasegawa develop the unified approach to derive the *Laplace-Stieltjes* transform (LST) of the PDF of message delay for general asymmetric systems [Taki88a,b]. This approach needs to solve $O(2^M)$ linear simultaneous equations for each station in asymmetric systems.

In all of the models in the above-mentioned works, it is assumed that each station transmits a whole message when polled. In this paper, we consider a more general model with single-message buffers. Messages arriving at stations are divided into several packets and only one packet is transmitted at each polling instant. The number of packets in a message is geometrically distributed. This model is first introduced by Wu and Chen [Wu75], where the average message delay is approximately derived in the symmetric case with constant transmission time of a packet and constant switchover time. Recently, for the same model as in [Wu75], Takagi provides the exact and explicit expression of the average message delay [Taka87c] according to the approach in [Taka86]. Takagi also proposes a similar polling model with feedback, where each station has a buffer of infinite capacity, and exactly derives the average message delay [Taka87b]. It is noted that there are several applications of these models [Taka87a–c]:

1. Long file transmission by segments in Token-Passing local area networks: we may be interested in the total delay until the whole file is transmitted.

2. Error-prone transmission channel: each message is transmitted successfully with probability $1 - p$ (and leaves the system) or erroneously with probability p (and remains in the system).

3. Time sharing system with M multi-programming level: the processor serves each process in a round-robin fashion.

Other areas in applications may be found. It is also noted that the conventional models, where a whole message is completely transmitted at the polling instant, can be viewed as the special case of the above models under consideration.

The main result of this paper is the derivation of the average message delay for an asymmetric single buffer polling system with round-robin scheduling of services. Our model is rather general in the following points. Arrival process of messages is Poisson whose mean may be *different* among stations. Each message may consist of multiple packets and the number of packets in a message is geometrically distributed with *different* means among stations. Transmission time of a packet and switchover time are distributed according to *general* probability distribution functions which may also be *different* among stations. The analytical approach is similar to [Taki88a,b], where the LST of the PDF of message delay is derived for the conventional model. With the analysis in [Taki88a,b], the average message delay can be numerically obtained through the solution of $O(2^M)$ linear simultaneous equations for *each* station. On the other hand, the analysis in this paper only needs to solve $O(2^M)$ linear simultaneous equations to derive the average message delay for *all* stations. Therefore even in the conventional model, the approach presented here is rather efficient compared with the previous method.

In Section 2, the mathematical model is described. In Section 3, the exact analysis of the model is provided and the average performance measures are derived. Finally the summary and the conclusion are given in Section 4.

2 Model

The polling system under consideration consists of M stations with indices 1 to M. Each station has a single-message buffer, so that a new message cannot be generated while an outstanding one is there. It is assumed here that each message at station i $(i = 1, \ldots, M)$ is divided into several packets and that the number of packets in a message at station i is geometrically distributed with parameter p_i. Then the probability that a message at station i consists of j packets is $(1 - p_i)p_i{}^{j-1}$ $(j = 1, 2, \ldots)$. Each station is polled in cyclic order. If station i has outstanding packets when polled, only one packet is transmitted and its transmission time, h_i, is assumed to be independently distributed according to a general PDF, $H_i(t)$. $H_i^*(s)$ and $\overline{H}_i$ denote the LST and the mean of $H_i(t)$ respectively. It is assumed that a new message is generated at station i after an interval exponentially distributed with parameter λ_i since completion of the previous message's transmission (that is, the completion of the last packet in the previous message). If station i has no outstanding packet when polled or if a packet has been completely transmitted, the next station is polled. Switchover time, u_i, from station $i - 1$ to i (from station M to 1 for $i = 1$) independently obeys a general PDF, $U_i(t)$. Let $U_i^*(s)$ and $\overline{U}_i$ be the LST and the mean of $U_i(t)$ respectively.

3 Analysis

We first define station time at station i as the time interval between consecutive polling departure instants from station $i - 1$ and from station i (from station M and from station 1 for $i = 1$). Let $t_i^{(n)}$ be station time at station i in the n-th cycle $(n = 1, 2, \ldots)$ and $\boldsymbol{t}^{(n)}$ be $(t_1^{(n)}, \ldots, t_M^{(n)})$. Moreover we introduce a state vector, $\boldsymbol{v}^{(n)} = (v_1^{(n)}, \ldots, v_M^{(n)})$, where $v_i^{(n)}$ $(i = 1, \ldots, M)$ takes 1 if station i transmits a packet in the n-th cycle or 0 otherwise. It is noted that the stochastic processes of $\boldsymbol{t}^{(n)}$ and of $\boldsymbol{v}^{(n)}$ are mutually dependent. Then we define the random vector $(\boldsymbol{t}^{(n)}, \boldsymbol{v}^{(n)})$ as,

$$(\boldsymbol{t}^{(n)}, \boldsymbol{v}^{(n)}) = (t_1^{(n)}, \ldots, t_M^{(n)}, v_1^{(n)}, \ldots, v_M^{(n)}) \tag{1}$$

and a pair of its component, $(t_i^{(n+1)}, v_i^{(n+1)})$, is given by,

$$
(t_i^{(n+1)}, v_i^{(n+1)})
$$
$$
= \begin{cases} (u_i^{(n+1)}, 0) & \text{with prob. } (1 - p_i v_i^{(n)})e^{-\lambda_i(\tau_i^{(n+1)} + u_i^{(n+1)})} \\ (u_i^{(n+1)} + h_i^{(n+1)}, 1) & \text{otherwise} \end{cases} \tag{2}
$$

where

$$\tau_i^{(n+1)} = t_{i+1}^{(n)} + \cdots + t_M^{(n)} + t_1^{(n+1)} + \cdots + t_{i-1}^{(n+1)}.$$

We note that the stochastic process of $(\boldsymbol{t}^{(n)}, \boldsymbol{v}^{(n)})$ is an imbedded Markov process. In the following subsection, the transform of the joint probability distribution of station times, $\boldsymbol{t}^{(n)}$, and of state vector, $\boldsymbol{v}^{(n)}$, is derived.

3.1 Joint Probability Distribution of Station Times and State Vector

Let J_k be the transform of the joint probability distribution of $t_i^{(n)}$ and of $v_i^{(n)}$ ($i = k, \ldots, M$), which is defined as,

$$
J_k = E\left[e^{-s_k t_k^{(n+1)}} \ldots e^{-s_M t_M^{(n+1)}} z_k^{v_k^{(n+1)}} \ldots z_M^{v_M^{(n+1)}} \right.
$$
$$
\left. \mid t^{(n)}, t_1^{(n+1)}, \ldots, t_{k-1}^{(n+1)}, v^{(n)}, v_1^{(n+1)}, \ldots, v_{k-1}^{(n+1)} \right] \quad (k = 2, \ldots, M)
$$
$$
J_1 = E\left[e^{-s_1 t_1^{(n+1)}} \ldots e^{-s_M t_M^{(n+1)}} z_1^{v_1^{(n+1)}} \ldots z_M^{v_M^{(n+1)}} \mid t^{(n)}, v^{(n)} \right]. \tag{3}
$$

It is noted that J_1 is the transform of the joint probability distribution of $t^{(n+1)}$ and $v^{(n+1)}$ when $t^{(n)}$ and $v^{(n)}$ are given. J_k's ($k = 1, \ldots, M-1$) satisfy the following recursive equations.

$$
J_k = E\left[e^{-s_k t_k^{(n+1)}} z_k^{v_k^{(n+1)}} J_{k+1} \right.
$$
$$
\left. \mid t^{(n)}, t_1^{(n+1)}, \ldots, t_{k-1}^{(n+1)}, v^{(n)}, v_1^{(n+1)}, \ldots, v_{k-1}^{(n+1)} \right] \quad (k = 2, \ldots, M-1)
$$
$$
J_1 = E\left[e^{-s_1 t_1^{(n+1)}} z_1^{v_1^{(n+1)}} J_2 \mid t^{(n)}, v^{(n)} \right]. \tag{4}
$$

We note here that,

$$
E\left[e^{-s_k t_k^{(n+1)}} z_k^{v_k^{(n+1)}} \mid t^{(n)}, t_1^{(n+1)}, \ldots, t_{k-1}^{(n+1)}, v^{(n)}, v_1^{(n+1)}, \ldots, v_{k-1}^{(n+1)} \right]
$$
$$
= E\left[e^{-(s_k + \lambda_k) u_k^{(n+1)}} \right](1 - p_k v_k^{(n)}) e^{-\lambda_k \tau_k^{(n+1)}} + E\left[e^{-s_k (u_k^{(n+1)} + h_k^{(n+1)})} z_k \right]
$$
$$
\quad - E\left[e^{-(s_k + \lambda_k) u_k^{(n+1)}} e^{-s_k h_k^{(n+1)}} z_k \right](1 - p_k v_k^{(n)}) e^{-\lambda_k \tau_k^{(n+1)}}
$$
$$
= U_k^*(s_k) H_k^*(s_k) z_k + U_k^*(s_k + \lambda_k)(1 - H_k^*(s_k) z_k)(1 - p_k v_k^{(n)}) e^{-\lambda_k \tau_k^{(n+1)}}
$$
$$
= \sum_{X_k=0}^{1} \left((1 - X_k) U_k^*(s_k) H_k^*(s_k) z_k \right.
$$
$$
\left. + X_k U_k^*(s_k + \lambda_k)(1 - H_k^*(s_k) z_k)(1 - p_k v_k^{(n)}) e^{-\lambda_k \tau_k^{(n+1)}} \right)
$$
$$
= \sum_{X_k=0}^{1} U_k^*(s_k + X_k \lambda_k)(X_k + (1 - 2X_k) H_k^*(s_k) z_k)(1 - X_k p_k)^{v_k^{(n)}} e^{-X_k \lambda_k \tau_k^{(n+1)}}. \tag{5}
$$

Using the expression of eq.(5), we can calculate the recursive equations in eq.(4). Successive algebraic manipulations yield,

$$
J_k = \sum_{X_k=0}^{1} \cdots \sum_{X_M=0}^{1} \left(\prod_{j=k}^{M} U_j^*(s_j + \sum_{i=j}^{M} X_i \lambda_i)(X_j + (1 - 2X_j) H_j^*(s_j + \sum_{i=j+1}^{M} X_i \lambda_i) z_j) \right.
$$
$$
\left. \cdot \prod_{j=k}^{M} (1 - X_j p_j)^{v_j^{(n)}} \prod_{j=k+1}^{M} e^{-(\sum_{i=k}^{j-1} X_i \lambda_i) t_j^{(n)}} \prod_{j=1}^{k-1} e^{-(\sum_{i=k}^{M} X_i \lambda_i) t_j^{(n+1)}} \right) \tag{6}
$$

and we finally get,

$$
J_1 = \sum_{X_1=0}^{1} \cdots \sum_{X_M=0}^{1} \left(\prod_{j=1}^{M} U_j^*(s_j + \sum_{i=j}^{M} X_i \lambda_i)(X_j + (1 - 2X_j) H_j^*(s_j + \sum_{i=j+1}^{M} X_i \lambda_i) z_j) \right.
$$
$$
\left. \cdot \prod_{j=1}^{M} (1 - X_j p_j)^{v_j^{(n)}} \prod_{j=2}^{M} e^{-(\sum_{i=1}^{j-1} X_i \lambda_i) t_j^{(n)}} \right). \tag{7}
$$

In the above and following equations, the summation and the product taken in decreasing order are defined to be zero and one respectively. We define $P^{(n)}(s, z)$ as the transform of the joint probability distribution of $t^{(n)}$ and $v^{(n)}$,

$$P^{(n)}(s, z) = E\left[e^{-s_1 t_1^{(n)}} e^{-s_2 t_2^{(n)}} \quad \cdots \quad e^{-s_M t_M^{(n)}} z_1^{v_1^{(n)}} \quad \cdots \quad z_M^{v_M^{(n)}}\right] \tag{8}$$

where

$$s = (s_1, \quad \cdots \quad , s_M)$$
$$z = (z_1, \quad \cdots \quad , z_M).$$

Then we have,

$$P^{(n+1)}(s, z) = \sum_{X_1=0}^{1} \cdots \sum_{X_M=0}^{1} \left(\prod_{j=1}^{M} U_j^*(s_j + \sum_{i=j}^{M} X_i \lambda_i)\right.$$
$$\left. \cdot \left(X_j + (1 - 2X_j)H_j^*(s_j + \sum_{i=j+1}^{M} X_i \lambda_i)z_j\right) P^{(n)}(a(X), p(X))\right) \tag{9}$$

where

$$a(X) = (0, X_1\lambda_1, X_1\lambda_1 + X_2\lambda_2, \quad \cdots \quad , X_1\lambda_1 + \ldots + X_{M-1}\lambda_{M-1})$$
$$p(X) = (1 - X_1 p_1, \quad \cdots \quad , 1 - X_M p_M).$$

As n tends to infinity, the system approaches to the steady state, which is assumed to exist. Then we define,

$$P(s, z) = \lim_{n \to \infty} P^{(n)}(s, z). \tag{10}$$

Thus we obtain the transform of the joint probability distribution of $t^{(n)}$ and $v^{(n)}$ in the equilibrium state.

$$P(s, z) = \sum_X G_X(s, z) P(a(X), p(X))$$
$$= \sum_{X \neq 0} G_X(s, z) P(a(X), p(X)) + G_0(s, z) \tag{11}$$

where

$$X = (X_1, \quad \cdots \quad , X_M)$$

$$0 = (\underbrace{0, \quad \cdots \quad , 0}_{M})$$

$$G_X(s, z) = \prod_{j=1}^{M} U_j^*(s_j + \sum_{i=j}^{M} X_i \lambda_i)\left(X_j + (1 - 2X_j)H_j^*(s_j + \sum_{i=j+1}^{M} X_i \lambda_i)z_j\right).$$

It is noted that eq.(11) contains $2^M - 1$ unknown values, namely, $P(a(X), p(X))$'s ($X \neq 0$). In the Appendix, we provide a system of linear simultaneous equations in matrix form to compute these unknown values.

3.2 Average Performance Measures

In this subsection, we derive various performance measures. First we define f_k as the probability of no outstanding packet at station k when polled. Then we have,

$$f_k = P(0, \underbrace{1, \quad \cdots \quad , 1}_{k-1}, 0, 1, \quad \cdots \quad , 1). \tag{12}$$

Main performance measures in a single buffer polling system are throughput, which is the number of messages transmitted in a unit of time, and the average message delay, which is the average length of the interval from the arrival instant of a message to the completion instant of the last packet's transmission. Let θ_k and $\overline{D}_k$ be throughput and the average message delay at station k respectively. Then the following equations hold.

$$
\begin{aligned}
\theta_k &= \frac{1}{\overline{D}_k + 1/\lambda_k} \\
&= \frac{(1 - p_k)(1 - f_k)}{\overline{C}}
\end{aligned}
\tag{13}
$$

where $\overline{C}$ is the average length of cycle time, which is defined as the time interval between consecutive polling instants at a station, and is given by,

$$\overline{C} = \sum_{k=1}^{M} \left(\overline{U}_k + (1 - f_k)\overline{H}_k \right).$$

With eqs.(12) and (13), the average message delay and throughput for each station can be numerically obtained through the solution of $O(2^M)$ linear simultaneous equations given in the Appendix.

Now we investigate the average message delay more precisely. It is noted that $\overline{D}_k$ consists of three factors as follows,

$$\overline{D}_k = \overline{W}_k + \overline{H}_k + \left(\frac{1}{1 - p_k} \right) \overline{C1}_k \tag{14}$$

where $\overline{W}_k$ is the average waiting time from the arrival instant of a message to the instant just before the first packet's transmission at station k and $\overline{C1}_k$ is the average length of cycle time beginning with station k which transmits a packet. To derive $\overline{W}_k$ and $\overline{C1}_k$, we define intervisit time at station k, I_k, as the time interval from the departure instant to the next arrival instant of the poll at station k. Let $I_k^*(s)$ be the LST of the PDF of I_k. Then we have,

$$
\begin{aligned}
I_1^*(s) &= \lim_{n \to \infty} E\left[e^{-st_2^{(n)}} \quad \cdots \quad e^{-st_M^{(n)}} e^{-su_1^{(n+1)}} \right] \\
&= P(0, s, \quad \cdots \quad , s, 1)U_1^*(s)
\end{aligned}
\tag{15}
$$

where

$$1 = (\underbrace{1, \quad \cdots \quad , 1}_{M}).$$

In the analysis of $P(\mathbf{s}, \mathbf{z})$, each cycle starts at station 1. Therefore $I_1^*(s)$ can be derived from $P(\mathbf{s}, \mathbf{z})$. However $I_k^*(s)$ $(k \neq 1)$ cannot be derived from $P(\mathbf{s}, \mathbf{z})$ because of the spiral nature of dependency among station times. In order to derive $I_k^*(s)$ $(k \neq 1)$, we should choose station k as the starting station of the cycle, that is, perform the cyclic shift operation of station index i to $\mathrm{mod}(i - k, M)+1$, and reproduce the analysis. In the following, we are only concerned with station 1.

We consider two types of intervisit time: type A is for the case when the poll leaves station 1 without transmission and type B is for the case when the poll leaves station 1 after transmission of a packet. We denote the above two types of intervisit time by I_1' and I_1'' respectively. Then,

$$
\begin{aligned}
I_1^*(s) &= E\left[e^{-sI_1} \mid v_1 = 0\right]\mathrm{Prob}\{v_1 = 0\} + E\left[e^{-sI_1} \mid v_1 = 1\right]\mathrm{Prob}\{v_1 = 1\} \\
&= I_1'(s)f_1 + I_1''(s)(1 - f_1)
\end{aligned}
\tag{16}
$$

where $I_1'(s)$ and $I_1''(s)$ are the LST's of the PDF of I_1' and I_1'' respectively. With eqs.(11) and (12), $I_1'(s)$ is given by,

$$
I_1'(s) = P(0, \underbrace{s, \quad \cdots \quad , s}_{M-1}, 0, \underbrace{1, \quad \cdots \quad , 1}_{M-1})U_1^*(s)/f_1.
\tag{17}
$$

Also with eqs.(16) and (17), we have,

$$
I_1''(s) = \left(I_1^*(s) - I_1'(s)\right)/(1 - f_1).
\tag{18}
$$

Station 1 can generate a new message during intervisit time of type A, and additionally during that of type B when the last packet is transmitted at station 1. Therefore the LST of the PDF of intervisit time in which station 1 can generate a new message, $I1_1^*(s)$, is given by,

$$
I1_1^*(s) = \frac{I_1'(s)f_1 + I_1''(s)(1 - f_1)(1 - p_1)}{f_1 + (1 - f_1)(1 - p_1)}.
\tag{19}
$$

With eq.(19), we can obtain the LST of the PDF of waiting time at station 1, $W_1^*(s)$, as follows,

$$
W_1^*(s) = \frac{\lambda_1}{s - \lambda_1}\frac{I1_1^*(\lambda_1) - I1_1^*(s)}{1 - I1_1^*(\lambda_1)}
\tag{20}
$$

from which we have,

$$
\overline{W}_1 = \frac{1}{1 - I1_1^*(\lambda_1)}\frac{E[I_1']f_1 + E[I_1''](1 - f_1)(1 - p_1)}{f_1 + (1 - f_1)(1 - p_1)} - \frac{1}{\lambda_1}.
\tag{21}
$$

In the following, $E[I_1']$ and $E[I_1'']$ are derived. We define $f_{1,i}$ as the joint probability of no outstanding packet at stations 1 and i ($i \neq 1$) in a cycle. Then we have,

$$
f_{1,i} = P(\mathbf{0}, 0, 1, \quad \cdots \quad , 1, \underset{i\text{-th}}{0}, 1, \quad \cdots \quad , 1).
\tag{22}
$$

$E[I_1']$ is given by,

$$
E[I_1'] = \sum_{i=1}^{M}\overline{U}_i + \sum_{i=2}^{M}\left(1 - \frac{f_{1,i}}{f_1}\right)\overline{H}_i.
\tag{23}
$$

Also we have the following relationship from eq.(16),

$$
\begin{aligned}
E[I_1] &= \sum_{i=1}^{M}\overline{U}_i + \sum_{i=2}^{M}(1 - f_i)\overline{H}_i \\
&= E[I_1']f_1 + E[I_1''](1 - f_1).
\end{aligned}
\tag{24}
$$

Therefore $E[I_1'']$ is obtained by eq.(24), and as a result, we have $\overline{W}_1$ in eq.(21). Also we can easily obtain,

$$\overline{C1}_1 = E[I_1^r] + \overline{H}_1. \tag{25}$$

Finally the average delay of a message consisting of j packets at station 1, $\overline{D}_{1|j}$, is given by,

$$\overline{D}_{1|j} = \overline{W}_1 + \overline{H}_1 + (j-1)\overline{C1}_1. \tag{26}$$

4 Conclusion

In this paper, an asymmetric single-message buffer polling system with round-robin scheduling of services was considered. Compared to previous work, our model is rather general and has high applicability. We derived the average message delay through the solution of $O(2^M)$ linear simultaneous equations. In the previous analysis for the single packet model, we need to solve $O(2^M)$ linear equations to derive the average message delay for *each* station. With the analysis in this paper, we can obtain the average message delay for *all* stations by solving $O(2^M)$ linear equations.

We also derived the LST's of the PDF of waiting time and of intervisit time. Unfortunately, the LST of the PDF of message delay cannot be obtained because successive cycle times are dependent.

Appendix   (Matrix Representation of Simultaneous Equations)

Eq.(11) contains all the information to compute unknown values involved in itself. The substitution of each $a(X)$ and $p(X)$ for s and z of eq.(11) yields the following system of equations,

$$P = AP + B \tag{27}$$

where

$$Y = (Y_1, \quad \cdots \quad , Y_M), \qquad Y_i = 0 \text{ or } 1 \qquad (i = 1, \ldots, M)$$

$$i(X) = \sum_{k=1}^{M} X_k 2^{k-1}$$

and

$$[P]_{i(Y)} = P(a(Y), p(Y)) \qquad (Y \neq 0)$$

$$[A]_{i(Y), i(X)} = G_X(a(Y), p(Y)) \quad (X, Y \neq 0)$$

$$[B]_{i(Y)} = G_0(a(Y), p(Y)) \qquad (Y \neq 0).$$

References

[Ibe86]   O.C. Ibe and X. Cheng, "Analysis of Polling Systems with Single-Message Buffers," *Proceedings of IEEE GLOBECOM '86*, pp.939–943, Houston, TX, 1986.

[Kaye72]   A.R. Kaye, "Analysis of a Distributed Control Loop for Data Transmission," *Proceedings of 22nd International Symposium on Computer-Communication Networks and Teletraffic*, pp.47–58, Polytechnic Institute of Brooklyn, NY, 1972.

[Mack57a] C. Mack, T. Murphy and N.L. Webb, "The Efficiency of N Machines Uni-Directionally Patrolled by One Operative when Walking Time and Repair Times are Constant," *Journal of the Royal Statistical Society*, Series B, Vol.19, No.1, pp.166–172, 1957.

[Mack57b] C. Mack, "The Efficiency of N Machines Uni-Directionally Patrolled by One Operative when Walking Time and Repair Times are Variable," *Journal of the Royal Statistical Society*, Series B, Vol.19, No.1, pp.173–178, 1957.

[Taka85]   H. Takagi, "On the Analysis of a Symmetric Polling System with Single-Message Buffers," *Performance Evaluation*, Vol.5, No.3, pp.149–157, 1985.

[Taka86]   H. Takagi, *Analysis of Polling Systems*, The MIT Press, Cambridge, MA, 1986.

[Taka87a] H. Takagi, "Analysis and Applications of a Multiqueue Cyclic Service System with Feedback," *IEEE Transactions on Communications*, Vol.COM-35, No.2, pp.248–250, 1987.

[Taka87b] H. Takagi, "A Survey of Queueing Analysis of Polling Models," *Proceedings of 3rd International Conference on Data Communication Systems and Their Performance*, pp.277–296, Rio de Janeiro, Brazil, 1987.

[Taka87c] H. Takagi, "Exact Analysis of Round-Robin Scheduling of Services," *IBM Journal of Research and Development*, Vol. 31, No. 4, pp.484–488, 1987.

[Taki86]   T. Takine, Y. Takahashi and T. Hasegawa, "Performance Analysis of a Polling System with Single Buffers and Its Application to Interconnected Networks," *IEEE Journal on Selected Areas in Communications*, Vol.SAC-4, No.6, pp.802–812, 1986.

[Taki88a] T. Takine, Y. Takahashi and T. Hasegawa, "Analysis of an Asymmetric Polling System with Single Buffers," *Performance '87*, P.-J. Courtois and G. Latouche (eds.), pp.241–251, North-Holland, Amsterdam, 1988.

[Taka88b] T. Takine, Y. Takahashi and T. Hasegawa, "Exact Analysis of Asymmetric Polling Systems with Single Buffers," *IEEE Transactions on Communications*, Vol.COM-36, No.10, pp.1119–1127, 1988.

[Wu75]   R.M. Wu and Y-B. Chen, "Analysis of a Loop Transmission System with Round-Robin Scheduling of Services," *IBM Journal of Research and Development*, Vol.19, No.5, pp.486–493, 1975.

ON A MULTICLASS QUEUE WITH CLASS DEPENDENT WINDOW-FLOW CONTROL[*]

Raif O. Onvural
H.G. Perros
Computer Science Department
Center for Communications and Signal Processing
North Carolina State University
Raleigh, NC 27695-8206, USA

U. Koerner
Department of Communication Systems
Lund University
Box 118, S-22100 Lund, SWEDEN

Abstract: We consider a single server queue shared by N different classes of jobs. Class i jobs arrive at the queue in a Poisson fashion with a class dependent rate. The total number of class i jobs allowed to wait in the queue is w_i, the window size of this class. A class i job that arrives to find w_i class i jobs in the shared queue is forced to wait in an input queue. There is one input queue for each class. All classes receive the same service at the shared queue, which is exponentially distributed. We analyze the two-class model numerically. For more than two classes, we obtain an approximate decomposition algorithm that utilizes the two-class numerical procedure. Validation tests showed that the approximation procedure is fairly accurate.

I. Introduction

One of the resource management tasks which critically affects the performance of computer communication networks is the flow control, i.e. the regulation of accepted traffic such that the network is not overloaded. Unless proper flow control is enacted, throughput of the network may significantly degrade below its optimum value. The principle of flow control is to shift congestion from the interior of the network to the points of admittance. The most widely known protocol to control the flow in a network is the window-flow control. The idea is simply to refuse admittance of new traffic when a certain number of messages in a region of the network is unacknowledged. The permissible upper bound of unacknowledged messages is called the window size (cf. Reiser [6]).

---

[*]Supported in part by a grant from AIRMICS through the Center for Communications and Signal Processing, NC State University, and by the National Science Foundation under grant no. CCR-87-02258

In this paper, we consider the case where multiple connections use the same resource, depicted by a single server queue. The traffic along each connection is regulated with a window-flow mechanism. In general, most of studies reported in the literature on window-flow control deal with a single connection (see Fdida, Perros and Wilk [1] for a literature review). Reiser [5] modeled a computer communication network consisting of many virtual routes with end-to-end window flow control as a closed multi-chain queueing network. Each chain represented a different virtual route under the assumptions of a loss system. That is, he assumed that packets that arrive to find a full window are discarded. He proposed a computationally efficient approximation procedure based on mean value analysis for evaluating large closed multi-chain networks. The model is used to obtain transit delays and blocking delays. Lam [3] extended the class of multi-chain queueing networks of the product type to include mechanisms of state dependent loss and triggered arrivals.

The problem of analyzing multiple window flow control mechanisms can be formulated as a single or multi-class closed queueing network with population constraints. The population constraint is imposed as follows: In the single class case, it is assumed that a subnetwork is subject to a population constraint. That is, only upto a predefined number of customers are allowed in the subnetwork. The remaining customers are queued in an input queue. In the multi-class case, for a particular subnetwork, each class (or a group of classes) has its own population constraint. These models have been analyzed approximately as closed queueing networks by several authors. A review of these approximations can be found in Thomasian and Bay [7]. The reader is also referred to Krzesinski and Teunissen [2] for a more recent approximation algorithm. We note that these models were originally developed for multiprogramming systems, and they may not be suitable for modeling window-flow control mechanisms, which naturally give rise to open queueing networks. It is necessary, therefore, to develop solution techniques for open multi-class queueing networks with population constraints.

In this paper, we study a queueing model consisting of a single server multi-class queue as shown in figure 1 (hereafter referred to as the shared queue). The total number of class i jobs allowed to wait in this queue may not exceed a finite number, w_i (hereafter referred to as the window size), i=1,...,N, where N is the number of classes. A class i job that arrives to the network at a time that there are w_i jobs in the shared queue is forced to wait in an input queue. Let C_i be the capacity of the input queue. C_i can be finite or infinite. A class i job waiting in the input queue is allowed to enter the shared queue only when a class i job departs from the network. There is one input queue per class.

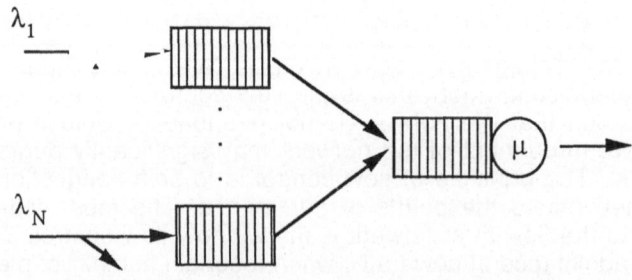

Figure 1. A multi-class open queueing model

Let λ_i, $1/\mu$ be respectively the rate of arrivals of class i jobs and the mean service time of a job in the shared queue. All interarrival times and service times are assumed to be exponentially distributed. Jobs at each input queue move into the shared queue in a FIFO manner. The service discipline at the shared queue is assumed to be processor sharing. We note that the marginal probabilities of each class are the same whether the service discipline at the shared queue is processor sharing, service in random order, or FIFO. This can be easily verified by comparing the steady state equations for each discipline.

Exact analysis of this model is rather difficult. In this paper, we analyze this queueing model numerically and approximately. In particular, the two-class model is analyzed numerically. For more than two classes, we analyze the model using an approximate decomposition technique which utilizes the two class numerical procedure. In the following section, we describe the numerical procedure. In section III, we present the approximation procedure and its validation. In section IV, we analyze the behavior of some performance metrics with respect to the arrival rates and window sizes. Finally, the conclusions are given in section V.

II. The Queueing Model with Two Classes

Let us consider the queuing model described in section I with two classes. Let (n_1,n_2) denote its state where n_i is the number of class i jobs in the network, i=1,2. We have $0 \le n_i \le w_i + C_i$. Furthermore, let $P(n_1,n_2)$ be the steady state probability of being in state (n_1,n_2). Seeing that the system under study is Markovian we have the following steady state equations:

for $w_1 \le n_1 \le w_1 + C_1$, $w_2 \le n_2 \le w_2 + C_2$

$$(\lambda_1+\lambda_2+\mu)P(n_1,n_2) = \lambda_1 P(n_1-1,n_2) + \lambda_2 P(n_1,n_2-1) + \{w_1/(w_1+w_2)\}\mu P(n_1+1,n_2) + \{w_2/(w_1+w_2)\}\mu P(n_1,n_2+1))$$

for $0 \le n_1 < w_1$, $w_2 \le n_2 \le w_2 + C_2$

$$(\lambda_1+\lambda_2+\mu)P(n_1,n_2) = \lambda_1 P(n_1-1,n_2) + \lambda_2 P(n_1,n_2-1) + \{(n_1+1)/(n_1+1+w_2)\}\mu P(n_1+1,n_2) + \{w_2/(n_1+w_2)\}\mu P(n_1,n_2+1))$$

for $w_1 \le n_1 \le w_1 + C_1$, $0 \le n_2 < w_2$

$$(\lambda_1+\lambda_2+\mu)P(n_1,n_2)=\lambda_1 P(n_1-1,n_2) + \lambda_2 P(n_1,n_2-1) + \{(n_2+1)/(n_2+1+w_1)\}\mu P(n_1,n_2+1)) + \{w_1/(n_2+w_1)\}\mu P(n_1+1,n_2)$$

for $0 < n_1 < w_1$, $0 < n_2 < w_2$

$$(\lambda_1+\lambda_2+\mu)P(n_1,n_2)= \lambda_1 P(n_1-1,n_2) + \lambda_2 P(n_1,n_2-1) + \{(n_2+1)/(n_2+1+n_1)\}\mu P(n_1,n_2+1)) + \{(n_1+1)/(n_2+n_1+1)\}\mu P(n_1+1,n_2)$$

and, $(\lambda_1+\lambda_2) P(0,0)=\mu\{P(1,0)+P(0,1)\}$

we note that in these equations, the probability of being in an unfeasible state, i.e. $n_i > C_i + w_i$ or $n_i < 0$, is equal to zero.

The above system of equations does not possess a product form solution. Furthermore, it is very difficult to obtain an analytical solution. In view of this, we analyze this model numerically. This involves the following three step procedure: i) Generation of states; ii) Creating the rate matrix Q and iii) Numerical solution of the system $Q^T P(n_1,n_2)=0$. The states can be generated easily as follows:

```
    ind:=0;
    for i:=0 to w₁+C₁ do
        for j:=0 to w₂+C₂ do
            begin
                ind:=ind+1;
                states(ind):=(i,j);
            end;
```

The generation of the rate matrix can be accomplished easily by going through the list of states and generating all feasible transitions for each state. In general, from an arbitrary state (n_1,n_2) there are four feasible transitions to states (n_1-1,n_2), (n_1+1,n_2), (n_1,n_2-1), and (n_1,n_2+1). The order of the rate matrix is:

$$(w_1+C_1+1)*(w_2+C_2+1)$$

Once the rate matrix is set up, the steady-state queue length distribution can be obtained using a numerical technique such as power method, Gauss-Seidel method, etc.

A numerical procedure using the power method was implemented on a VAX-11/785 to calculate the joint queue length distributions for upto four classes. As expected, the CPU time required to generate the states and to generate the rate matrix was observed to be negligible. However, the numerical solution of the system $Q^TP(n_1,n_2)=0$ required a considerable amount of CPU time even for the two-class case. Clearly, the numerical approach becomes infeasible as the number of classes increases (see section III.3).

III. The Approximation Procedure

In this section, we present a decomposition procedure for the approximate analysis of the N-class queueing system shown in figure 1. Below, we first consider the case of finite capacity input queues, i.e. $C_i < \infty$, i=1,...,N. The algorithm is then extended to the case of infinite capacity input queues in section III.2. Finally, in section III.3, both cases are validated and the time complexity of the algorithm is given.

III.1. Finite Capacity Input Queues
Let us consider the N class queueing model shown in figure 1 with parameters λ_i, w_i, μ, and $C_i<\infty$, i=1,...,N, with N≥3. We decompose the N-class system into N two-class systems, the first class of which is the class under consideration and the second class which is the aggregation of all other classes.

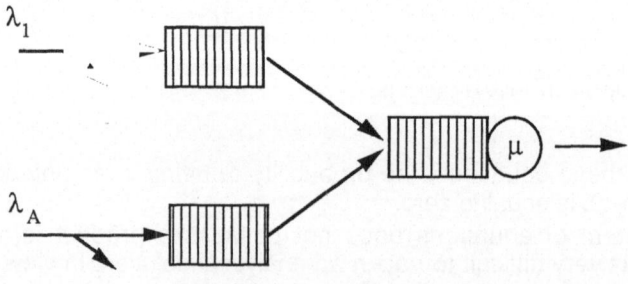

Figure 2. A Two-class Model

Without loss of generality, consider class 1 as the class under consideration. The second class is then the aggregation of classes 2 to N (hereafter referred to as class A) as shown in figure 2. The accuracy of the approximation clearly depends on how well the parameters of the aggregate class are specified. Let λ_A, w_A, and C_A be respectively the arrival rate, window size and the capacity of the input queue of the aggregated class. In the original model, the total number of class A jobs in the shared queue varies between zero and the sum of the window capacities of classes 2 to N. Therefore, we set:

$$w_A = \sum_{i=2}^{N} w_i$$

We also set the arrival rate of class A jobs equal to the sum of the arrival rates of the individual classes, i.e.

$$\lambda_A = \sum_{i=2}^{N} \lambda_i$$

Setting the values of w_A and λ_A as above results in an overestimation of the number of class A jobs in the shared queue. The total arrival rate is equal to $\sum_{i=2}^{N} \lambda_i$ as long as the total number of class A jobs in the shared queue is less than $\min\{w_j, j=1,...,N\}$. Once this limit is reached, then in the real system, jobs belonging to the class with the smallest window size may not enter the shared queue. Clearly, this is not considered in the aggregate class with $\lambda_A = \sum_{i=2}^{N} \lambda_i$ and $w_A = \sum_{i=2}^{N} w_i$. We reduce the effect of overestimating the number of class A jobs in the shared queue by fixing appropriately the capacity of the input queue of the aggregate class. The size of this input queue can be anything between zero and $\sum_{i=2}^{N} C_i$. For a given arrival rate λ_A, the probability of having k jobs in the shared queue increases as C_A increases where $0 \leq k \leq w_A$. Therefore, in order to counter balance the overestimation of the shared queue, C_A should be small. Accordingly, we studied the following problem numerically: Given the parameters of class 1, $\lambda_A = \sum_{i=2}^{N} \lambda_i$ and $w_A = \sum_{i=2}^{N} w_i$ what is the value of C_A such that the marginal probabilities of class 1 jobs are approximated with minimum error. Rather surprisingly, this numerical study suggested that $C_A = 0, 1$ or 2. Although these values of C_A does not always give the best approximate values, they are observed to be the best in most cases and they are never too far from the value of C_A which results in the best approximate values. This is true for a range of different values of the parameters of the queueing model.

Once we fix the parameters of the aggregate class, the resulting two-class model is solved numerically using the procedure given in section II. The steps of the algorithm are summarized as follows:

Step 1: Without loss of generality, consider class 1 as the class under consideration. Let the parameters of the aggregate class be as follows:

$$w_A = \sum_{i=2}^{N} w_i \,, \; \lambda_A = \sum_{i=2}^{N} \lambda_i, \; \rho = \sum_{i=1}^{N} \lambda_i/\mu \text{ and } C_A = \begin{cases} 2 \text{ if } \rho < 0.8 \\ 1 \text{ if } 0.8 \leq \rho \end{cases}.$$

Step 2: Solve the two-class network numerically to calculate the marginal queue length distribution of class 1.

By renumbering classes, the algorithm is readily applicable to any other class.

III.2. Infinite Capacity Input Queues

We will now consider the N-class model with $C_i=\infty$, i=1,...,N, and N$\geq$3. Let $\pi(n)$ be the total number of jobs in the network without distinguishing between classes. Then, the following lemma is immediate by appealing directly to the steady-state equations.

Lemma: Consider an N-class queueing model as shown in figure 1 with parameters λ_i, w_i, C_i, μ and with $C_i=\infty$, i=1,...,N. Furthermore, let $\pi(n)$ be the probability that the total number of jobs in the network is n. Then:

$$\pi(n-1)\sum_{i=1}^{N}\lambda_i = \mu\,\pi(n), \quad \text{where } \pi(0)=1-\sum_{i=1}^{N}\lambda_i/\mu \text{ with } \sum_{i=1}^{N}\lambda_i < \mu.$$

Hence, the system behaves like an M/M/1 queue if we do not distinguish between classes. In order to use the numerical procedure developed in section II, we should know the total capacity for each class, i.e. w_i+C_i. In the case of infinite capacity input queues, we obtain these values by first determining the total finite capacity, C^*, such that $\sum_{n=0}^{C^*}\pi(n)$ is approximately equal to one, where t

$\sum_{n=0}^{C^*}\pi(n)=1-\rho^{C^*+1}$. In particular, we use the following procedure to calculate C^*.

Step 1: Let $\rho=\sum_{i=1}^{N}\lambda_i/\mu$ with $\rho<1$, and let $C^*=1$.

Step 2: while $1-\rho^{C^*+1}<0.99999$ do
$$C^*=C^*+1$$

Once C^* is calculated, we apply the algorithm presented above for finite capacity input queues assuming $C_i=C^*$ for all i.

III.3. Time Complexity and Accuracy of the Procedure

The approximation procedure presented above decomposes the N-class queueing system into N two-class systems. The number of states in each two-class system is $B_i=(C_i+w_i)(2+w_A)$. Hence, the total time complexity of the algorithm to calculate the marginal probabilities of all classes is $O\left(\sum_{i=1}^{N}B_i^3\right)$. We note that the time complexity of the exact numerical procedure is $O\left(\left(\prod_{i=1}^{N}C_i+w_i\right)^3\right)$.

Hence, the approximation is considerably faster than solving the entire queueing system numerically. In table 1, we give CPU times of the exact numerical and the approximation procedures for nine different examples.

Table 1. CPU times of the exact and the approximate procedures

N	$\lambda_1,...,\lambda_N$	μ	$C_1,...,C_N$	$w_1,...,w_N$	Numerical Proc. (sec)	Approximate Proc. (sec)
3	(1,2,3)	12	$(\infty,\infty,\infty),9$	(3,2,4)	73.3	9.6
3	(1,3,2)	9	$(\infty,\infty,\infty),11$	(2,3,4)	389.9	19.2
3	(1,1,1)	5	(4,4,4)	(2,2,2)	6.1	5.3
3	(1,1,1)	5	(8,8,8)	(2,2,2)	93.4	9.1
3	(1,2,3)	7	(8,8,8)	(2,2,2)	120.2	12.5
3	(1,2,3)	12	$(\infty,\infty,\infty),8$	(3,3,3)	73.3	11.4
3	(1,1,1)	7	$(\infty,\infty,\infty),9$	(2,2,2)	113.2	6.3
4	(1,2,5,4)	18	(6,6,6,6)	(2,2,2,2)	719.5	12.1
4	(1,2,1,4)	15	(6,6,6,6)	(2,3,5,4)	656.4	21.1

The algorithm was applied to the N-class model, where the number of classes was varied from 3 to 4. The validation tests show that the relative error percentage (i.e. 100* (exact value-approximate value)/exact value) was fairly low. The numerical results were obtained using the numerical procedure described in section II. A representative set of examples are given in figures 12 to 20, where Prob(0), mql-shared and mql-total are respectively the probability of having zero class i jobs in the shared queue, mean number of class i jobs in the shared queue and mean number of class i jobs in the system. The parameters of these examples are summarized in table 2.

IV. Performance Metrics

The performance metrics used in this analysis are defined as follows: Let $\pi_i(n_i)$ be the marginal probability of having n_i class i jobs in the network, MQL-S_i be the mean number of class i jobs in the shared queue, where

$$MQL\text{-}S_i = \sum_{n_i}^{C_i+w_i} \min(n_i,w_i)\pi_i(n_i)$$

MQL-I_i be the mean number of class i jobs in the queue, where:

$$MQL\text{-}I_i = \sum_{n_i=w_i+1}^{C_i+w_i} (n_i-w_i)\pi_i(n_i)$$

and T_i be the throughput of class i jobs, where

$$T_i = \begin{cases} \lambda_i & \text{if } C_i=\infty \\ \lambda_i(1-\pi_i(C_i+w_i)) & \text{otherwise} \end{cases}$$

For the two-class model, we study the behavior of MQL-S_i, MQL-I_i, and T_i as i) the arrival rate of a class varies and ii) the window size of a class varies while all the other parameters are kept the same. The values of these performance metrics are calculated numerically using the procedure described in section II.

Consider now the two class model with parameters $C_2=11$, $\lambda_1=2$, $\lambda_2=1$, $w_2=2$, and $\mu=4$. In figures 3 to 5, w_1 is varied from 2 to 11 while $C_1=11-w_1$. We observe that both MQL-S_1 and MQL-S_2 increases as w_1 increases. As w_1 increases, there are more class 1 jobs in the shared queue. This in turn reduces the rate at which class 2 jobs depart from the shared queue, thus increasing MQL-S_2. As w_1 increases, there are less class 1 jobs in the input queue hence MQL-I_1 decreases. However, as the departure rate of class 2 jobs decreases, MQL-I_2 increases seeing that more jobs arrive to find w_2 jobs in the shared queue. For

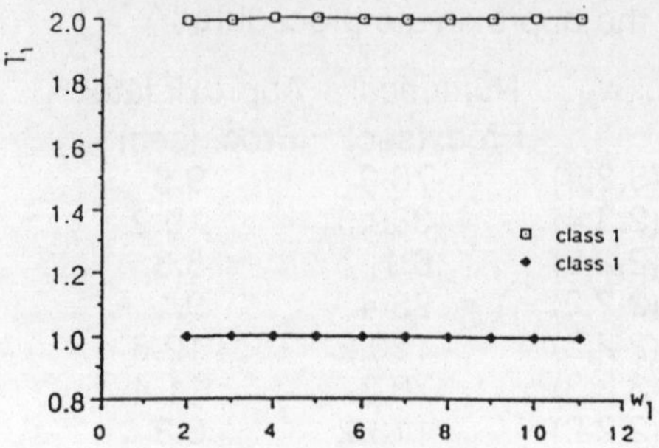

Fig 3. Throughput of class i jobs vs w_1

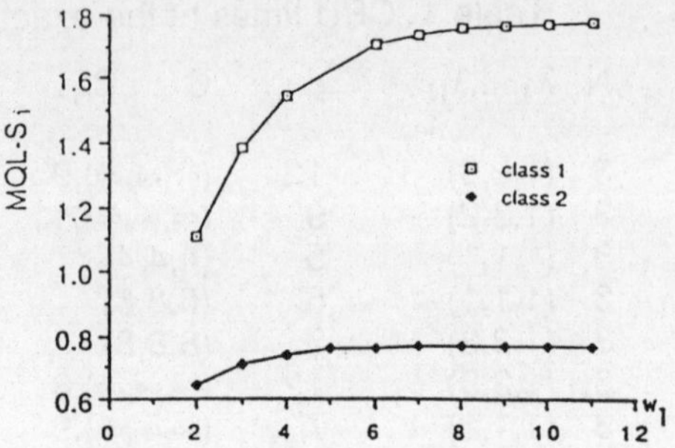

Fig 4. Mean no of class i jobs in the shared queue vs w_1

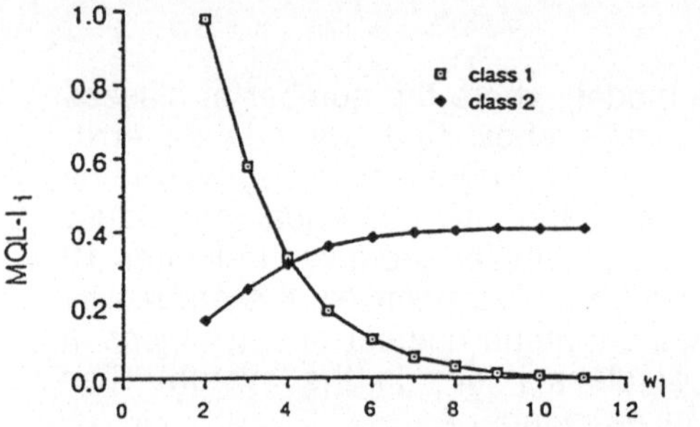

Fig 5. Mean no of class i jobs in the input queue vs w_1

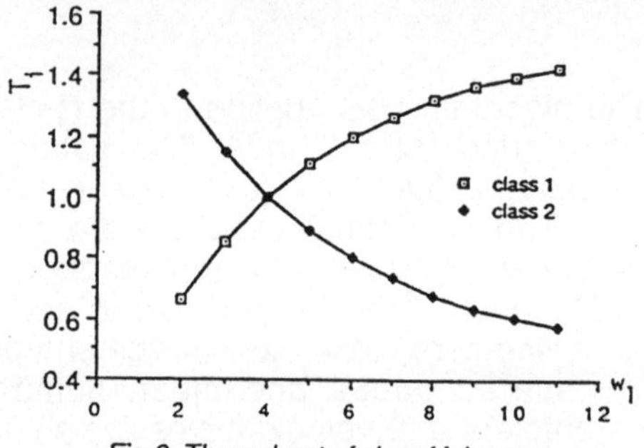

Fig 6. Throughput of class i jobs vs w_1

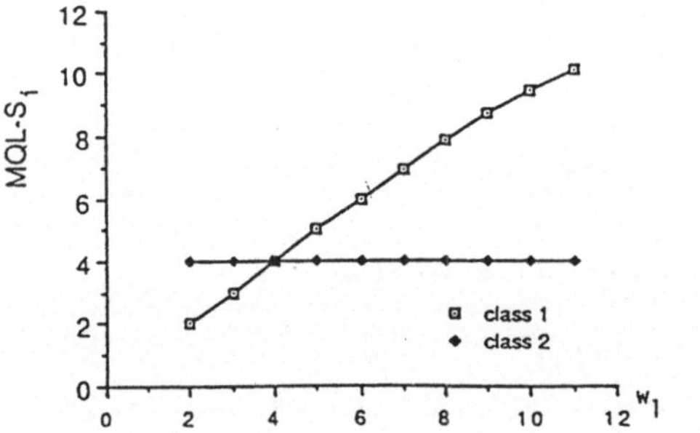

Fig 7. Mean no of class i jobs in the shared queue vs w_1

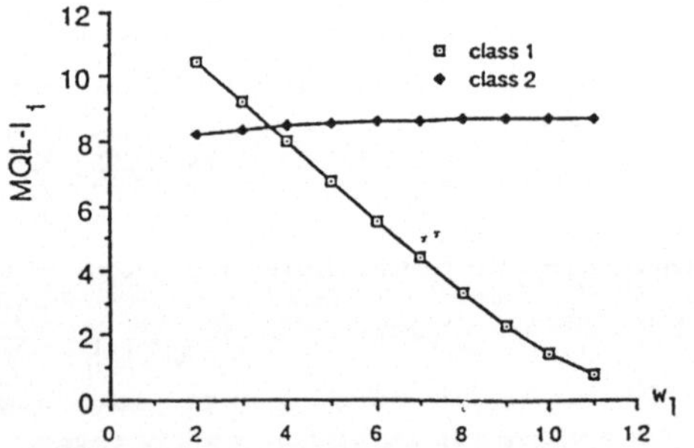

Fig 8. Mean no of class i jobs in the input queue vs w_1

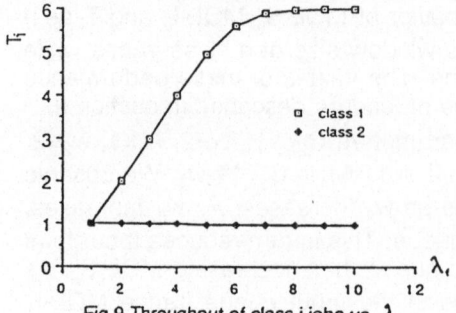

Fig 9. Throughput of class i jobs vs λ_t

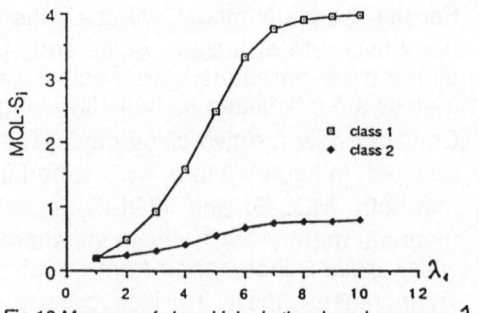

Fig 10. Mean no of class i jobs in the shared queue vs λ_t

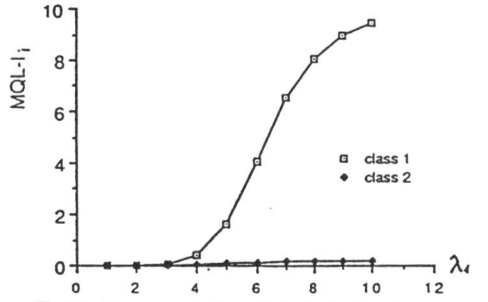

Fig 11. Mean no of class i jobs in the input queue vs λ_i

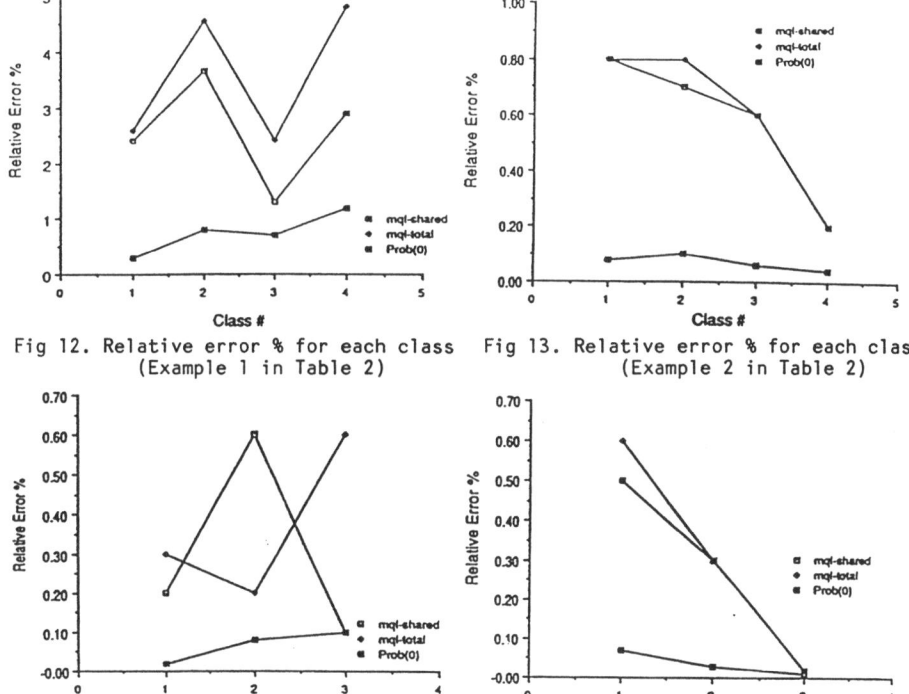

Fig 12. Relative error % for each class
(Example 1 in Table 2)

Fig 13. Relative error % for each class
(Example 2 in Table 2)

Fig 14. Relative error % for each class
(Example 3 in Table 2)

Fig 15. Relative error % for each class
(Example 4 in Table 2)

Table 2. Data for the examples in figures 12 to 20.

Ex #	$(\lambda_1,\lambda_2,\lambda_3,\lambda_4)$	C_1,C_2,C_3,C_4	(w_1,w_2,w_3,w_4)	μ
1	(1,2,5,4)	(4,4,4,4)	(2,2,2,2)	18
2	(1,2,1,4)	(4,3,1,2)	(2,3,5,4)	15
3	(1,2,3)	(5,5,5)	(3,3,3)	12
4	(3,2,3,4)	(4,3,4,3)	(2,3,2,3)	16
5	(3,2,4,1)	(5,4,5,5)	(2,3,2,2)	7
6	(3,2,4,1)	(5,4,5,5)	(2,3,2,2)	10
7	(3,2,3,4)	(4,3,4,3)	(2,3,2,3)	16
8	(3,2,3,4)	(4,3,4,3)	(2,3,2,3)	10
9	(1,3,2)	(9,8,7)	(2,3,4)	9

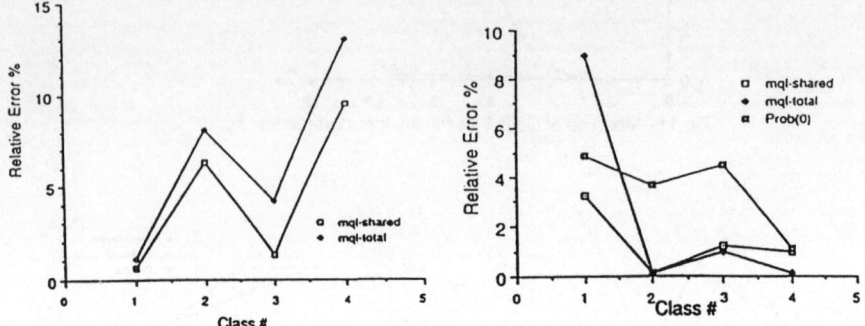

Fig 16. Relative error % for each class (Example 5 in Table 2)

Fig 17. Relative error % for each class (Example 6 in Table 2)

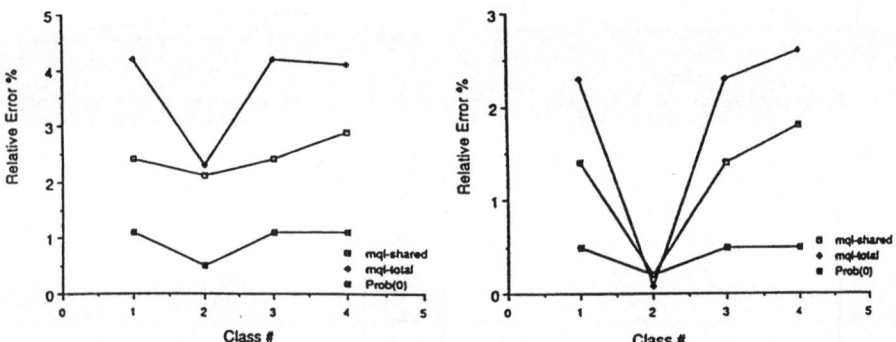

Fig 18. Relative error % for each class (Example 7 in Table 2)

Fig 19. Relative error % for each class (Example 8 in Table 2)

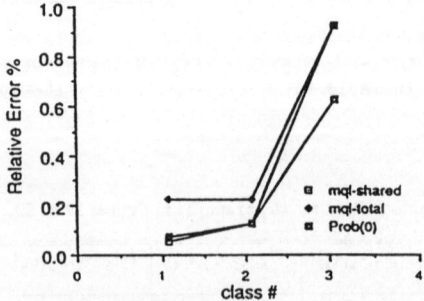

Fig 20. Relative error % for each class (Example 9 in Table 2)

this example, both T_i's stay about the same as w_1 increases. Seeing that their values are very close to their respective arrival rates, we conclude that the capacities of the input queues are as if they were infinite. We note that in this example $\lambda_1+\lambda_2<\mu$. Now, let us consider another example where $\lambda_1+\lambda_2>\mu$. Let $C_2=9$, $\lambda_1=2$, $\lambda_2=3$, $w_2=4$, and $\mu=2$. In figures 6 to 8, w_1 is varied from 2 to 11 while $C_1=13-w_1$. In this case, all performance metrics are pushed to their limits, i.e. MQL-$S_i\approx w_i$, $T_1+T_2\approx\mu$, MQL--$I_1\approx 13-w_1$, and MQL-$I_2\approx 9$. Finally, we give an example to show the effect of varying the mean arrival time of a class while all the other parameters are kept the same. In particular, consider the two-class model with parameters $C_1=11$, $C_2=13$, $w_1=4$, $w_2=2$, $\mu=7$, and $\lambda_2=1$. In figures 9 to 11, λ_1 is varied from 1 to 10. Increasing λ_1 causes both MQL-S_1 and MQL-I_1 to increase, as expected. As MQL-S_1 increases, the departure rate of class 2 jobs decreases, causing MQL-S_2 to increase slightly. This in turn causes MQL-I_2 to increase.

V. Conclusions

We presented a model for the case where multiple connections use the same resource, depicted by a single server queue. A numerical procedure was implemented to calculate the steady state joint queue length distributions. The number of states grows rapidly with the number of classes. In view of this, the numerical approach becomes infeasible even with a few classes. This necessitated the development of an approximation algorithm for more than two classes. The procedure decomposes the model to N two-class models, one for each class. Each two-class model is then analyzed numerically. Validation tests show that the results are fairly accurate.
In real situations, more than one node may be required to represent a virtual route. Furthermore, although the approximate procedure saves considerable amount of CPU time in the case of more than two classes, an accurate approximation procedure for the two-class model may result in even more time savings. We are currently working on these two problems as an extension of the ideas presented in this paper.

REFERENCES

[1] S. Fdida, H.G. Perros and A. Wilks, Semaphore Queues: Modeling Multilayered Window Flow Control Mechanisms, Tech. Rep., Computer Science, 1988, North Carolina State University
[2] A. Krzesinski and P. Teunissen, Multiclass Queueing Networks with Population Constrained Subnetworks, Proc. ACM SIGMETRICS Conf. on Measurement and Modeling of Computer Systems, Austin TX, August 1985, 128-139
[3] S.S. Lam, Queueing Networks with Population Size Constraints, IBM J. Res. Dev., 370-378, July 1977
[4] E.D. Lazowska and J. Zahorjan, Multiple Class Memory Constrained Queueing Networks, Proc. ACM SIGMETRICS Conf. Measurement and Modeling of Computer Systems, Seattle WA, August 1982, 130-140
[5] M. Reiser, A Queueing Network Analysis of Computer Communications Network with Window Flow Control, IEEE Trans. Comm., COM 27, 1199-1209, 1979
[6] M. Reiser, Performance Evaluation of Data Communications Systems, Proc. IEEE, 70, 171-196, 1982
[7] A. Thomasian and P. Bay, Analysis of Queueing Network Models with Population Size Constraints and Delayed Blocked Customers, Proc. ACM SIGMETRICS Conf. Measurement and Modeling of Computer Systems, Cambridge, 202-216, 1984

SOLVING SOME PRACTICAL PROBLEMS OF COMPUTING SYSTEM
CONFIGURATION AND DESIGN BY THROUGHPUT CONTROL
IN CLOSED SEPARABLE QUEUEING NETWORKS

Günter Totzauer
Nixdorf Computer AG
Pontanusstr. 55
D - 4790 Paderborn

Abstract: Typical requirements that are to be accomplished during system
configuration and design are given transaction rates to be processed by the
computing system. The task may be to choose a fitting configuration or to
develop a certain system component, the use of which will guarantee the
requirements to be met. By means of throughput control this problem can be
solved. We show how to incorporate throughput control in closed separable
queueing networks and derive explicit formulae for the necessary parameters. The application of the results is demonstrated at hand of two practical problems.

1. Introduction

In practice we often have to deal with problems of the following type. A
customer wants to know how a certain computer system will behave when it
has to process different transaction types with given frequencies. A similar problem has to be solved when a new component for a subsystem will be
developed which is intended to enable the whole system to process transactions with given rates. Either an answer is wanted whether the planned component is able to guarantee this throughput rates or the requirements that
have to be fullfilled by the component to meet the goal are to be determined.

In our plant this kind of task appears much more frequently than others.
This is the reason why in an often used simulation model it is possible to
fix the throughput according to a given parameter though the network is
closed.

Thus, the throughputs are given and an open network should be used to model
the system. On the other hand in real systems there may not be arbitrarily
many customers. If the maximum number of tasks in a system is small a closed
network should be chosen for modelling. To combine these two needs, it
is useful to have a mechanism that allows throughput control in closed
queueing networks.

We present such a mechanism in this paper. The computer system is modelled
by a closed separable queueing network without state-dependent service
rates. The load to be processed is representd by closed chains. Adjusting
the throughputs is accomplished via a chain specific delay of the tasks in
a delay queue. For that purpose the queueing network is extended by an

infinite servers station. This simple mechanism allows throughput control in a wide range. The idea of job delay was presented by Gelenbe and Kurinckx in connection with another problem, namely the prevention of overload situations in virtual memory (GeKu76).

In this paper we first describe the mechanism of throughput control by a delay station followed by the calculation of the required delay times which is based on the Bard/Schweitzer approximation (Bard79,Schw79). This calculation is direct and not iterative. It is shown how this approach can be used to determine the necessary speed up of some station to make the whole network able to process customers of different chains with given throughputs. An interesting conformity of this formulae and those for open queueing networks is pointed out. Finally the practical application of the derived results is demonstrated at hand of the sketch of two case studies.

2. Throughput Control using a Delay Station

In separable networks a customer's way is modelled by chains. Stations be numbered from 1 to M and chains from 1 to C. We want to adjust given chain throughputs $T(1)$, $T(2)$,...,$T(c)$,...,$T(C)$. This is done delaying each customer a chain specific period of time. Therefore an additional infinite servers station is incorporated into the network. In our model we call it station 0. It is visited by each chain and without loss of generality the mean number of visits at it is set to 1 for all chains.

3. Computation of the Control Variables

In this section we present formulae to calculate the desired delay times. The followwing symbols are used:

M	number of service stations
type(m)	type of service station m, FCFS, PS, LCFS, or IS
C	number of chains
S(m,c)	mean total service time of a chain c customer at station m per task
W(m,c)	mean total waiting time of a chain c customer at station m per task
T(c)	throughput of chain c tasks
n(m,c)	mean number of chain c customers at station m
N(c)	mean number of customrs of chain c
u(m,c)	= T(c) S(m,c) utilization of station m by chain c
U(m)	utilization of station m

We start from the waiting time approximation formula of the Bard/Schweitzer algorithm.

$$W(m,c) = \begin{cases} S(m,c) & \text{for type}(m) = IS \\[2em] S(m,c) \left(1 + \sum_{k<>c} n(m,k) + \dfrac{N(c)-1}{N(c)} n(m,c) \right) & \text{else} \end{cases} \quad (1)$$

$$(1<=m<=M, \ 1<=c<=C)$$

202

Further only the nontrivial case where type(m) <> IS is of interest. n(m,k) is replaced according to Little's theorem by T(c) W(m,c) yielding

$$W(m,c) = S(m,c) \left(1 + \sum_{k<>c} T(k) W(m,k) + \frac{N(c)-1}{N(c)} T(c) W(m,c) \right) \quad (2)$$

For every station m (1<=m<=M) this is a system of linear equations in the variables W(m,c) (1<=c<=C).

Using the exact MVA formula for W(m,c) instead of formula (1) would not yield a linear system of equation. A solution for W(m,c) for given through-puts could not be derived directly. This is the reason why we base our method on the Bard/Schweitzer approximation.

In (ScTo85) equation (2) is already derived but not yet solved analytically as we do here. Some simple transformation yields:

$$\sum_{k<>c} - T(k) W(m,k) + \left(\frac{1}{S(m,c)} - \frac{N(c)-1}{N(c)} T(c) \right) W(m,c) = 1 \quad (3)$$

Substituting

$$x(c) = W(m,c) \qquad\qquad (1<=c<=C)$$

$$a(c) = \frac{1}{S(m,c)} + \frac{T(c)}{N(c)}$$

$$\qquad\qquad\qquad\qquad (1<=c<=C) \qquad\qquad (4)$$

$$= \frac{N(c) + T(c) S(m,c)}{S(m,c) N(c)}$$

$$b(c) = - T(c) \qquad\qquad (1<=c<=C)$$

we get

$$\sum_{k<>c} b(k) x(k) + (a(c) + b(c)) x(c) = 1 \quad (5)$$

In the appendix the solution of this system of equations is derived as

$$x(c) = \frac{1}{a(c) \left(1 + \sum_{i=1}^{C} \frac{b(i)}{a(i)} \right)} \quad (6)$$

Replacing a(.), b(.), x(.) yields

$$W(m,c) = \frac{\dfrac{S(m,c) N(c)}{N(c) + T(c) S(m,c)}}{1 - \displaystyle\sum_{i=1}^{C} \dfrac{N(i) + T(i) S(m,i)}{S(m,i) N(i)}} \quad (7)$$

This formula allows the calculation of· W(m,c) (1<=c<=C, 1<=m<=M) if type(m)<>IS in the closed queueing network where the throughputs are given as T(c) (1<=c<=C).

The denominator in (7) must be positive. If it is 0, W(m,c) is undefined. If it is negative W(m,c) would become negative. This has no interpretation in a real system. It can easily be shown, that U(m)<1 implies the denominator to be positive. So no restrictions are imposed on the allowed model class by the form of the solution formula.

The delay times W(0,c) (1<=c<=C) have still to be calculated. Applying Little's theorem for the extended network yields:

$$\sum_{m=0}^{M} W(m,c) = \frac{N(c)}{T(c)} \qquad (1<=c<=C) \qquad (8)$$

This can be solved for the unknown control variables W(m,0).

$$W(0,c) = \frac{N(c)}{T(c)} - \sum_{m=1}^{M} W(m,c) \qquad (1<=c<=C) \qquad (9)$$

All W(0,c) (1<=c<=C) must not be negative. If one value is negative this indicates that the desired throughputs cannot be adjusted.

Formula (7) has an interesting form.

Substituting

$$SS(m,c) = S(m,c) \, / \, (\, 1 + \frac{T(c) \, S(m,c)}{N(c)} \,) \qquad (10)$$

yields

$$W(m,c) = \frac{SS(m,c)}{1 - \sum_{i=1}^{C} T(i) \, SS(m,i)} \qquad (11)$$

This is the same formula as that for an open queueing network with service times SS(m,c) (1<=m<=M,1<=c<=C). That means that after a service time transformation (8) waiting times in a closed queueing network with given throughputs may be calculated like for an according open queueing network.

That means that even for closed queueing networks the waiting time can be computed directly using (11). No iteration is needed. Using exact MVA the necessary delay times to adjust the wanted throughputs have to be determined iteratively and each MVA computation consists of the recursive computation of characteristics for many populations. Depending on the kind of tested networks, the mean error of our approximation formula is about 5% and thus lies in the same range as that of the Bard/Schweitzer algorithm compared to exact MVA reported by Neuse and Chandy (NeCh81).

If the requirements for a new component have to be derived, the service times have to be calculated. The component under consideration is omitted from the original network and throughput control is performed for the remaining network. If the resulting waiting times can be adopted at the new component, the desired throughputs are accomplished. The only remainig task is to calculate the necessary service times from the delay times. Formula (2) is merely solved for $S(0,c)$.

$$S(0,c) = \frac{W(0,c)}{1 + \sum\limits_{k<>c} T(k)\ W(0,k) + \frac{N(c)-1}{N(c)}\ T(c)\ W(0,c)} \qquad (12)$$

4. An Application in System Design

The computing power of the Nixdorf 8860 system family had to be extended to allow customers a further upgrade without system change. A throughput factor 4 should be realized. The availability of communication software especially the remote file access and the growing importance of computer networks created the idea to connect several computers to increase computing power. Common data is administrated by one or several file servers and the applications are served by socalled application servers. This proposal has the advantage that the existing systems can be used and the main effort consists of creating software that makes many computers look like a single system.

It was our task to evaluate this concept within two months. The questions to be answered were:

- Can the throughput factor 4 be realized?

- How long are the response times?

- How large are the utilizations of the different CPUs and the disks?

- Which alternate solutions exist?

Fortunately during the life of the 8860-family many measurements have been performed. Manifold results exist concerning run times of system routines, the composition of overhead depending on the kind of configuration and even about many applications covering a wide range of different loads.

Models of the existing system as well as of the Multi Computer (MC) had to be constructed. A configuration with up to 20 terminals connected to a 8864-CPU and 4 disks (Figure 1) was chosen as a base for the performance study. The application is described by a scheme (figure 2), where many param... can be influenced to describe loads from I/O-intensive to CPU-orient...

The functions beginnig with "std" are operations on sequential files and those beginning with "skam" work on index sequential files (Sequential Keyed Access Method). As an example skam_read is explained in detail. The CPU-time is dependent on the depth of the index tree and the hit ratio of index and data accesses in the buffer. If a block is in the buffer the block access is finished else the physical disk I/O is performed. This is followed by an additional CPU phase to put the block into the buffer. The other operations are described in a similar manner. The parameters envoluted are system or load specific and are obtained from measurements.

The model of this basic configuration can be constructed straight forward as a closed separable queueing network. Results are the throughput and response times.

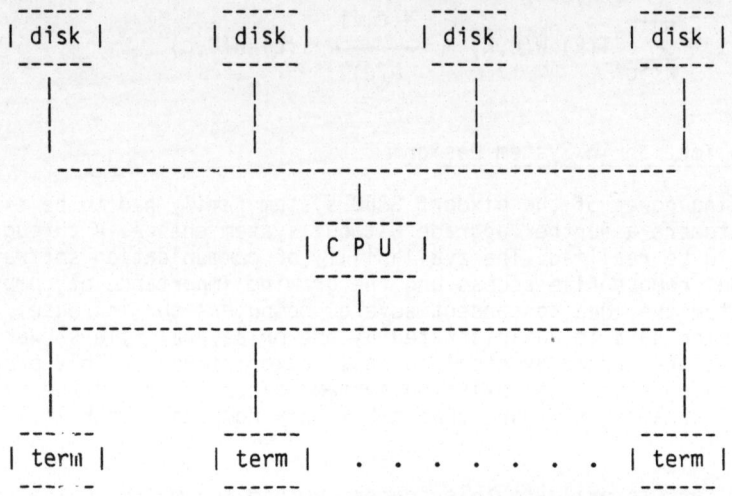

Figure 1. Configuration of a single Nixdorf 8864-system

```
while true do
{
    think time at terminal       time1 ms
    8864 CPU time                time2 ms
    for i:= 1 to n1 do                          n1 : mean number of logical
                                                     disk accesses per
    {                                                terminal input
        8864 CPU time            time3 ms
        branch with probability
        {
            p1:  std_get;
            p2:  std_read;
            p3:  std_put;
            p4:  std_write;
            p5:  skam_get;
            p6:  skam_read;
            p7:  skam_write;
        }
        8864 CPU time            time4 ms
    }
}
```

Figure 2. Scheme of the system load

This model has been calibrated by adjusting the hit-ratios for STD and SKAM file accesses and the think time at the terminals. Validation experiments were not performed explicitly. The results for I/O- and CPU-bound load models were consistent with the experience of system experts.

Starting from the single system model the Multi Computer model had to be constructed. The MC consists of several CPUs used as application servers (AS) or file servers (FS) each of which serves 4 disks. A configuration example is shown in figure 3.

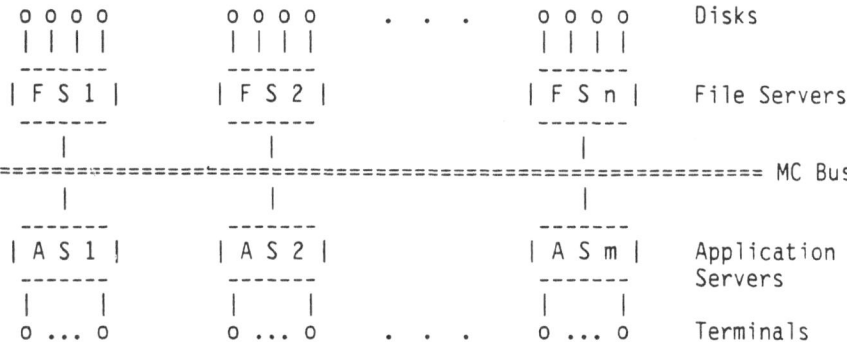

Figure 3. Nixdorf Multi Computer 8864

The same kind of transaction than on the single system has to be executed. The difference is that for each file access a message has to be send to a file server and the data block has to be transmitted from/to the application server. This results in additional load.

Sending a message from an application to a file server needs processing time on that server, a delay time on the bus and a further CPU phase at the FS-CPU. The parameter values again are obtained from measurements and some by estimation. This message sending has to be taken into account for every file access.

The MC8860-model consists of several times the stations of a single system where a communication media is added and its use is expressed in holding times and additional CPU times to control its access. In this model it is helpful to use throughput control to define the throughput 4 times as high as in the first model. MC-configurations with different numbers of AS and FS are considered to find the one which deals best with the desired throughput, that means with acceptable response times and e.g. disk utilizations.

The results showed in which range of load parameters the goal could be reached and in which it was not possible. Figures 4 and 5 display the predicted throughput factors for a CPU-bound load and an I/O-bound load. These are the limit throughputs where the response times are the same as for the single system. Each column indicates the possible throughput factor for a certain configuration characterized below the columns. The numbers of terminals, disks and application and file servers as well as the utilizations of the AS, FS and disks are given. For CPU intensive loads the throughput factor 4 could be realized with better response times in the single system. For I/O oriented loads this was not possible which can be explained by the additional communication overhead neccessary for every disk access.

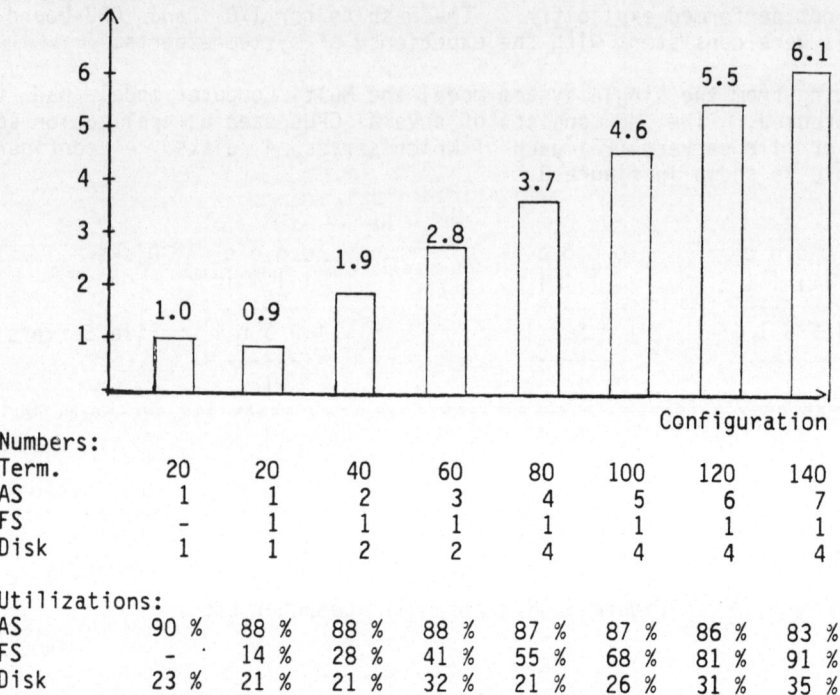

Figure 4. Feasible Throughput Factors for CPU-bound Load

Numbers:								
Term.	20	20	40	60	80	100	120	140
AS	1	1	2	3	4	5	6	7
FS	-	1	1	1	1	1	1	1
Disk	1	1	2	2	4	4	4	4

Utilizations:								
AS	90 %	88 %	88 %	88 %	87 %	87 %	86 %	83 %
FS	-	14 %	28 %	41 %	55 %	68 %	81 %	91 %
Disk	23 %	21 %	21 %	32 %	21 %	26 %	31 %	35 %

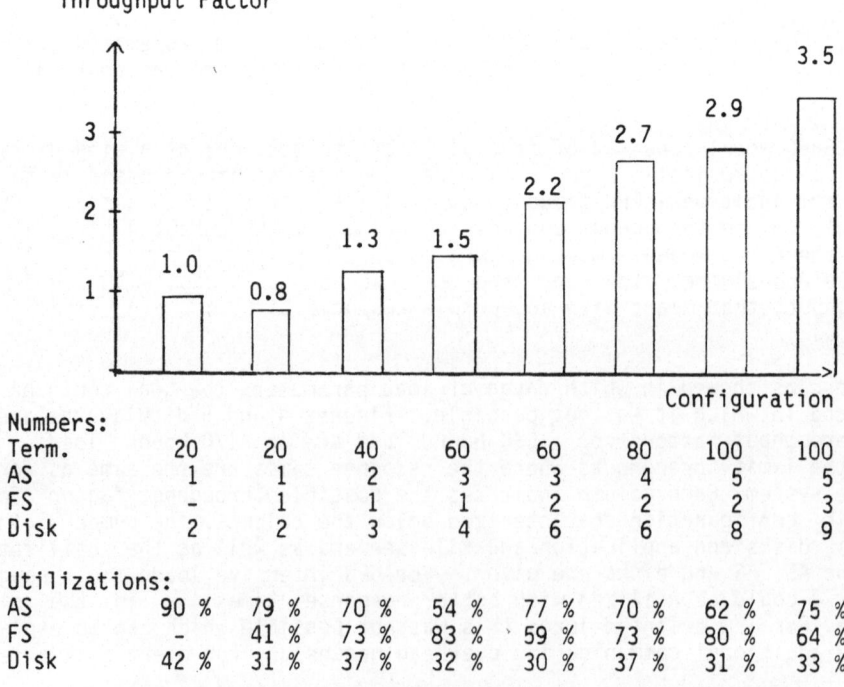

Figure 5. Feasible Throughput Factors for I/O-bound Load

Numbers:								
Term.	20	20	40	60	60	80	100	100
AS	1	1	2	3	3	4	5	5
FS	-	1	1	1	2	2	2	3
Disk	2	2	3	4	6	6	8	9

Utilizations:								
AS	90 %	79 %	70 %	54 %	77 %	70 %	62 %	75 %
FS	-	41 %	73 %	83 %	59 %	73 %	80 %	64 %
Disk	42 %	31 %	37 %	32 %	30 %	37 %	31 %	33 %

At the time of the study a validation of the MC-model could not be performed because neither the system nor measurement data about it did exist.
When the system had been built one I/O-intensive application program was
analyzed on the single system and the behaviour was measured on the MC. It
was found that instead of the predicted throughput factor 3.2 even 3.4
could be realized.

Because of the very short computing times of about 0.1 CPU seconds on a
Targon /35 per model, evaluation parameters and configurations were varied
systematically in a wide range. About 5000 evaluations have been performed.

5. Evaluation of a Planned HW-Component

In another study a system had to be examined in which the disk I/O was
often found to be the bottleneck. The goal was to change the system in a
way to make it possible to serve twice as many terminals as actually with
the same response times and doubled throughput compared with the former
system. It was planned to develop a 1 MB disk cache to render that goal
possible.

Our task was to check if the disk cache would be able to speed up the
system in the intended way. The answer had to be given within 4 weeks.
Under this circumstances an extensive simulation study could not be taken
into account. Only a rather rough model could be built.

At hand of two applications from the field the mean number of disk accesses
per transaction was found to be 800 and even the number of tracks to be
crossed per access had been measured. It was 40 tracks. Only a single disk
had to be served by the controller. So in the model controller and disk
were modelled as a single station. The time for one disk access is the sum
of controller time, seek time, latency and transfer time which add up to 25
ms. The total disk service time per transaction is 800*25 ms = 20000 ms =
20 s.

From the mask sizes the times needed for terminal I/O could be estimated.
Mean input from the keyboard were 600 characters and mean output to the
display were 900 characters. The input scan for each of the terminals takes
66 μs (micro seconds) of computing power of the terminal controller whether
there are input characters or not. Thus the input from a certain terminal
takes 600*32*66 μs = 1267 ms per transaction because 32 terminal connec-
tionsare to be checked. The output of a character takes 66 μs which yields
a total output time of 900*66 μs = 60 ms per transaction. This time influences the possible input speed. The load caused by other peripheral devices
is negligible and needs not be modelled.

The available data did not contain any data about used CPU-times. So CPU
service times were roughly estimated from some available data about some
other transaction. Additionally CPU times were varied from two to eleven
seconds to estimate the sensitivity of the buffer cache depending on different loads.

The simple separable model for the existing system consisted of the CPU, a
disk and the terminals with its visit counts and mean service times.

For this basic model the number of terminals was varied from 1 to 16 with
growing steps. The interesting results of this closed separable queueing
network were the throughputs and the response times. These throughputs
multiplied by two are the throughputs to be adjusted in the model representing the system with the new disk cache.

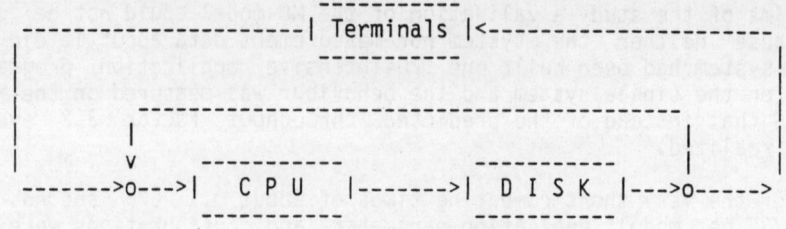

Figure 6. Simple system model

Because the calculation of hit ratios in the disk cache needs detailed
information about the locality of accesses which was not available we decided to construct a model which allows to calculate the necessary hit ratio
in the cache which makes it possible to get twice the throughput as in the
original network.

Therefore a model was constructed without the disk subsystem. Throughput
control allowed the computation of the waiting time at the delay server
which guarantees twice the throughput of the basic system calculated by the
first model. This is the waiting time which must not be exceeded by the new
disk subsystem consisting of the cache and the disk. The corresponding maximum service time of the subsystem can be calculated according to formula
(12). The result is shown in figure 7.

The response times of the second model were compared with those of the
first. They did not exceed them in any case.

So far in a top down approach the required service time of the buffer/disk
subsystem has been calculated. In the second step it has to be evaluated

disk/buffer service time

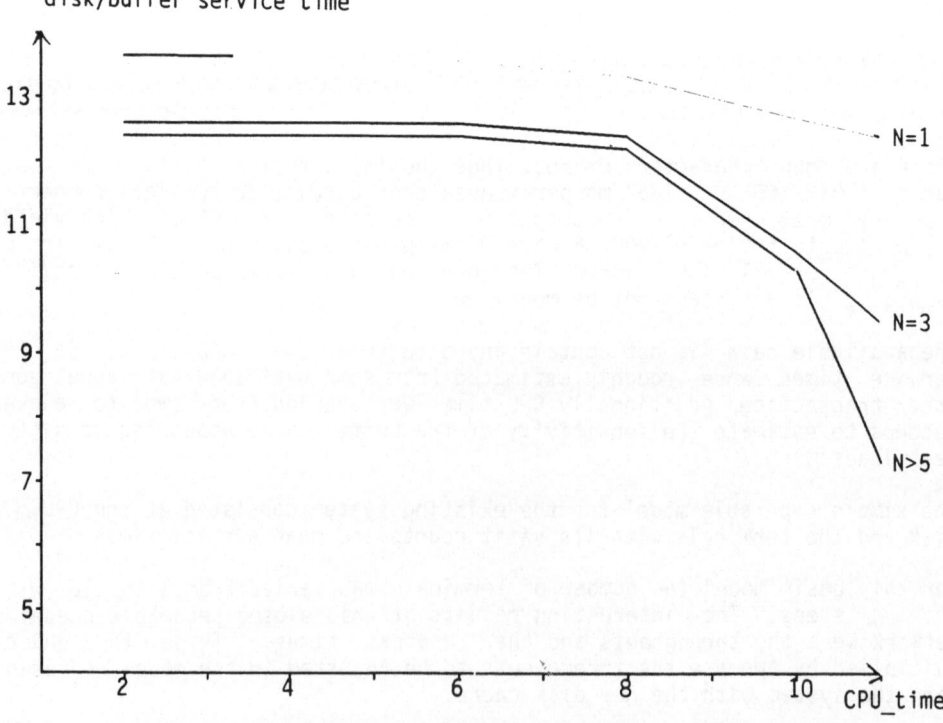

Figure 7. Maximum Service Time dependent on CPU-load

which times can be reached by the planned hardware dependent on the hit ratio p in the buffer.

As this part has nothing to do with throughput control it will be kept rather short.

From the hardware development data was available to calculate the buffer service time as 0.2 ms if the block is in the buffer and 0.55 ms else. Taking into consideration that in the case of a mismatch a physical disk access is necessary the service time of the buffer/disk subsystem dependent on p is

$$S(p) = p * 0.2 \text{ ms} + (1 - p) * 25.55 \text{ ms}$$

$$= 25.55 \text{ ms} - p * 25.35 \text{ ms} \tag{13}$$

From figure 7 it can be seen, that up to a cpu service time of 10 seconds, even more than 5 customers a service time of 10 ms for the buffer/disk subsystem will do. (11) yields a necessary hit ratio of 60 percent.

Without a detailed analysis of program locality it cannot definitely be stated that this hit ratio will be reached. But the comparison with meared hit ratios of buffer mechanism in other system families makes it nearly sure that this hit ratio of at least 60 percent is realistic. Some often used system parts are intended to be fixed in the buffer. Finally it can be said with a very small risk that the buffer will be able to achieve the desired throughput goal.

6. Conclusions

Formulae for throughput control in closed separable queueing networks have been derived. Theirhelpful use in typical studies during system configuration and development has been demonstrated especially for cases where an answer has to be given quickly and there is no time to put more details in a model that extends the class of separable networks.

7. Appendix

The solution of the following system of equations is derived.

$$\sum_{i<>c} b(i) \, x(i) + (a(c) + b(c)) \, x(c) = 1 \quad (1<=c<=C) \quad (A1)$$

It can be written in matrix form.

$$
\begin{bmatrix}
a(1)+b(1) & b(2) & & b(C) \\
b(1) & a(2)+b(2) & & \cdot \\
\cdot & b(2) & & \cdot \\
\cdot & \cdot & & \cdot \\
\cdot & \cdot & & \cdot \\
b(1) & b(2) & & a(C)+b(C)
\end{bmatrix}
\begin{bmatrix}
x(1) \\
x(2) \\
\cdot \\
\cdot \\
\cdot \\
x(C)
\end{bmatrix}
=
\begin{bmatrix}
1 \\
1 \\
\cdot \\
\cdot \\
\cdot \\
1
\end{bmatrix}
$$

$$A \, x = b \tag{A2}$$

The system of equations will be solved via Cramers rule. A is the same matrix as in /ToSc87/. Some transformations which do not change det(A) are performed.

- subtract row C from every row i $\quad\quad\quad\quad$ (1<=i<=C-1)
- add row i multiplied by -b(i)/a(i) to row C (1<=i<=C-1)

det(A) can than be computed as the product of the diagonal elements and is:

$$det(A) = \prod_{c=1}^{C} a(c) \left(1 + \sum_{c=1}^{C} \frac{b(c)}{a(c)} \right) \quad\quad (A3)$$

To apply Cramer's rule some more determinants have to be computed. A(c) (1<=c<=C) can be formed by replacing column c of matrix A by <1,1,...,1>. The calculation of det(A(c)) is the same as for det(A) with b(c)=1 and a(c)=0. This yields

$$det\,(A(c)) = \prod_{\substack{i=1 \\ i<>c}}^{C} a(i)$$

This finally yields:

$$x(c) = \frac{det(A(c))}{det(A)} = \frac{1}{a(c) \left(1 + \sum_{i=1}^{C} \frac{b(i)}{a(i)} \right)} \quad\quad (A4)$$

$$q.e.d.$$

8. Literature

Bard79 $\quad$ Y. Bard
$\quad\quad\quad\quad$ Some Extensions to Multiclass Queueing Network Analysis
$\quad\quad\quad\quad$ in Performance of Computer Systems
$\quad\quad\quad\quad$ M. Arato, A. Butrimenko, E. Gelenbe
$\quad\quad\quad\quad$ IIASA, North - Holland Publishing Company (1979)

GeKu76 $\quad$ E. Gelenbe, A. Kurinckx
$\quad\quad\quad\quad$ Random Injection Control of Multiprogramming in
$\quad\quad\quad\quad$ Virtual Memory
$\quad\quad\quad\quad$ in Modelling and Performance Evaluation of Computer Systems
$\quad\quad\quad\quad$ Gelenbe (ed.)
$\quad\quad\quad\quad$ North Holland Publishing Company (1976)

NeCh81 $\quad$ D. Neuse, K. Chandy
$\quad\quad\quad\quad$ SCAT: A Heuristic Algorithm for Queueing Network
$\quad\quad\quad\quad$ Models of Computing Systems
$\quad\quad\quad\quad$ ACM Sigmetrics Vol. 10 No. 3 Fall 81 (1981)

Schw79 $\quad$ P. Schweitzer
$\quad\quad\quad\quad$ Approximate Analysis of Multichain Closed
$\quad\quad\quad\quad$ Queueing Networks
$\quad\quad\quad\quad$ Int. Conf. Stochastic Control and Optimization
$\quad\quad\quad\quad$ Amsterdam 1979

ScTo85   A. Schätter, G. Totzauer
          Sharing Computer Capacity by Controlling Throughputs
          (in German)
          Proceedings Messung, Modellierung und Bewertung von
          Rechensystemen, Dortmund (FRG) 1985
          Inf. Fachbericht 110, Springer Verlag

MODELLING DASD CONFIGURATIONS WITH
MULTIPATHING AND MULTIPLE BLOCKING POINTS

Gilbert E. Houtekamer

Delft University of Technology
Faculty of Electrical Engineering
Mekelweg 4 Delft, The Netherlands

ABSTRACT

A method is described to model the reconnect blocking probability in I/O subsystems. The model handles systems with multiple blocking points, multipathing, and dynamic reconnect. A few restrictions are imposed on the I/O configurations to be modelled, but they do not conflict with real life systems. The restrictions enable us to compute all controller and path utilizations without the need for iteration. A consistent set of conditional controller busy probabilities and a generalized multipathing operator are introduced to compute blocking probabilities. The model proposed pairs accuracy with an intuitively appealing approach. Extensive validation results are presented for the model, showing its accuracy.

1. Introduction

In the past, quite a few papers have been written on disk I/O subsystem modelling. Here, we present an efficient approximative method to determine the blocking probabilities in the disk I/O subsystem. The paper concentrates on the computation of the probability that all available paths are busy when a reconnection attempt is made. The modelling method can be applied to any disk system with shared controllers, although the discussion concentrates on the IBM System/370 XA architecture.

The model presented is an open model, where the I/O throughput for all disks in known in advance. In that sense, the approach is similar to [Brandwajn 1983].

Previously, [Bard 1980] and [Lazowska 1984] described methods to obtain the utilizations of the disk controllers. In a system with multipathing, a known throughput at the device level does not necessarily imply a known throughput at the controller or internal path level, since the I/O requests may be routed through different controllers. They assume that I/O requests are handled by the controllers that can be reached most easily, i.e. the probability that a path or controller is selected for reconnection is proportional with the probability that it is free. [Bard 1980] then solves the problem with the maximum entropy method. [Lazowska 1984] uses iteration to compute the path selection probabilities, assuming convergence. The problem with both methods is that they require iteration, making them computationally less attractive.

Brandwajn uses decomposition in the models he presented [Brandwajn 1981] [Brandwajn 1983] [Brandwajn 1986]. The I/O subsystem model is decomposed into a number of small closed queueing network models, each representing a "bottleneck" in the system. This approach yields accurate results and is reasonably efficient, since each submodel can use a simple loss system model to predict the probability that all available paths (servers) are busy at each level. The problem with this approach is that it requires the solution of a large number of related submodels, and that the submodel structure depends on the system configuration.

In our model, the controller utilizations are derived directly from the disk loads, assuming a controller load which is balanced over the controllers that are used to drive the disk. This assumption is valid for most DASD configurations that use some form of load balancing in either the controller hardware, or the software that drives it. Brandwajn uses similar assumptions in his models.

Based on the utilizations thus obtained, conditional blocking probabilities can be computed for the internal path, storage director and channel level. Once all blocking probabilities are known, the probability that all available paths are busy (the RPS miss probability) is approximated using a *multipathing operator*. >From this miss probability, the average number of RPS misses can be computed.

The average pending time is computed using a similar approach, combining the all path busy probability with the average channel connect time.

Since the method involves no iteration, it is numerically efficient. With a proper definition of the multipathing operator, very accurate results are obtained, as will be shown in the validation study. The model can be used in closed queueing system models using the iterative scheme proposed in [Lazowska 1984].

In the terminology of the System/370 XA architecture, the model handles blocking at the internal path, string controller, storage director and channel level for systems with the dynamic reconnect capability. It supports the device level select (DLS) and device level select enhanced (DLSE) DASD protocols for internal path selection [IBM 1983a] [IBM 1983b] [IBM 1985b] [IBM 1987].

The structure of the paper is as follows. Section 1 is this introduction. The topology for the I/O subsystems studied is described in section 2 in more detail. The modelling approach is introduced in section 3, and section 4 defines the symbols used. Section 5 and 6 describe the multipathing operator and the model for the RPS miss probability respectively. Validation results for the RPS model for balanced and non-balanced load are presented in section 7. Section 8 describes the model used for the pending delay, with validation results in section 9. Section 10 summarizes the results.

2. I/O Subsystem Configurations Studied

Most implementations of the System/370 architecture use an I/O subsystem with several controller levels. The disks themselves are connected to (up to four) internal paths, each internal path is connected to (up to two) string controllers, the string controllers are connected to storage directors, and the storage directors are connected to (up to eight) channels.

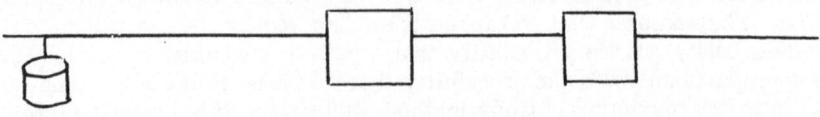

disk   internal path   string controller   storage director   channel

Figure 1. Controller topology.

Figure 1 depicts the controller structure graphically. The exact configuration depends on the disk and controller types used. In most modern systems, each disk can be reached via two to four different internal paths. Each storage director usually has one string controller connection, and a channel connection for each system it is attached to.

When an I/O request is issued, a connection must be established to initiate the I/O action. The connection from channel to disk may use any available storage director and internal path. Such a connection is referred to as a *path*. When no path is available, the request remains *pending* until a path becomes available. Once the I/O request has been started, the disk will *disconnect* from the channel and storage director. It will then seek to the cylinder specified, and wait until the requested angular position is reached. The angular position of the disk surface is sensed with the Rotational Position Sensing (RPS) mechanism. As soon as the specified angular position is reached, the disk will try to *reconnect* to the storage director and channel. The reconnection will fail when no proper path is available, i.e. when no internal path-storage director-channel connection can be made. Such a failure is called an *RPS miss*. If it occurs, the disk will have to wait for a full rotation until the same angular position is reached again. A new reconnection request will then be issued. The process is repeated until a successful reconnection is made. Finally, the data transfer can take place.

For the purpose of our discussion, some simplifying restrictions are imposed on the controller structure, as described below.

1. Each disk may have one or more connections to internal paths, and the disk's load is assumed to be balanced over all paths connected.

2. Each internal path may have one or more connections to string controllers, and the internal path load is assumed to be balanced over all string controllers connected.

3. Each string controller has one connection to a storage director. Storage directors can be shared between different string controllers.

4. Each storage director may be connected to many systems, but it may have only one channel connection per system.

5. More than one storage director may be connected to one channel, but the resulting configuration must be symmetric in the sense that all storage directors that can be used to access a particular device see the same channel utilization. Figure 2 illustrates this constraint: the top configuration is symmetric, because the channels 1 and 2, and 3 and 4 respectively, have the same utilization. In the bottom configuration, the utilization will be different for each channel.

Within these restrictions, blocking may occur at the internal path (devices share internal paths), storage director (internal paths share storage directors), and channel level.

Of these restrictions, the requirement for a balanced channel path and controller load is probably the most severe one. In the IBM System/370 XA architecture channel path load balancing is accomplished by the channel subsystem microcode. In non-XA systems running the MVS operating system, MVS will attempt to balance load at the channel level. In most configurations, this implies balanced storage director, string controller and internal path load. In non-XA systems running the VM operating system, channel and storage director load balancing is not guaranteed by the operating system nor hardware.

The restriction that string controllers are connected to only one storage director fits with the current implementations of the IBM 3380 disk drives and the associated 3880 and 3990 controllers. They allow us to disregard the string controllers from the model, since a string controller is only busy when the storage director to which it is connected is busy. In the discussions below, and in the model, the string controllers are thought to be included in the storage directors.

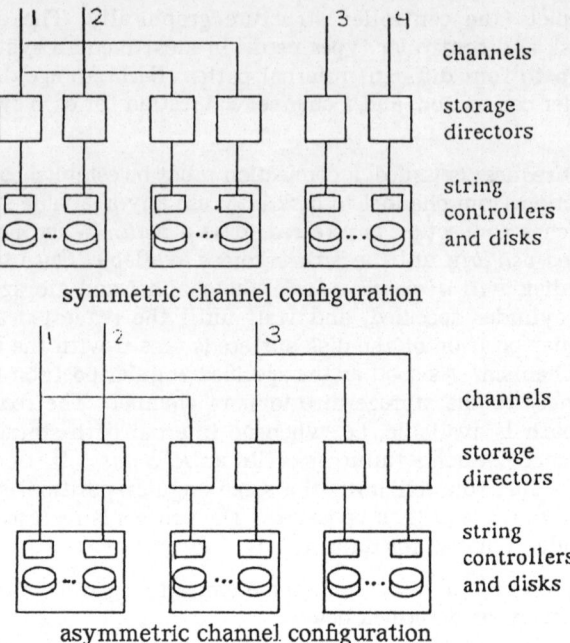

symmetric channel configuration

asymmetric channel configuration

Figure 2. Example of a symmetric channel configuration that can be modelled, and an asymmetric one that cannot.

In this paper we will only consider systems with dynamic reconnect capability, i.e. an I/O request that has been started using a particular controller path may reconnect to any available controller path on the same system. The dynamic reconnect capability is provided in the hardware of the IBM System/370 XA system [IBM 1983b][IBM 1985b].

Many different controller topologies can be realized within the constraints described above. The six configurations used to validate our model are shown in Figure 3.

— Configuration A consists of 8 disks connected to one non-shared controller path. This configuration corresponds to a single IBM 3350 string with one storage director.

— Configuration B consists of 16 disks, each connected to one internal path. The four internal paths in the configuration are connected to two string controllers, and the string controllers are directly connected to the storage directors. This configuration corresponds to a system with 16 3380As with two 3880 storage directors.

— Configuration C consists of 32 disks, in two independent groups of 16. The groups have the same configuration as in B, but they share a common pair of channels.

— Configuration D consists of 16 disks, each connected to two internal paths. Each internal path is connected to one string controller. This configuration corresponds to a system with 16 3380D/Es with two 3880 type storage directors.

— Configuration E consists of 32 disks, in two groups of 16. The groups have the same configuration as in D, but they share a common pair of channels.

— Configuration F consists of 32 disks, each connected to four internal paths. Each internal path is connected to one string controller. This configuration corresponds to a system with 32 3380J/Ks with four 3990 type storage directors [IBM 1987].

218

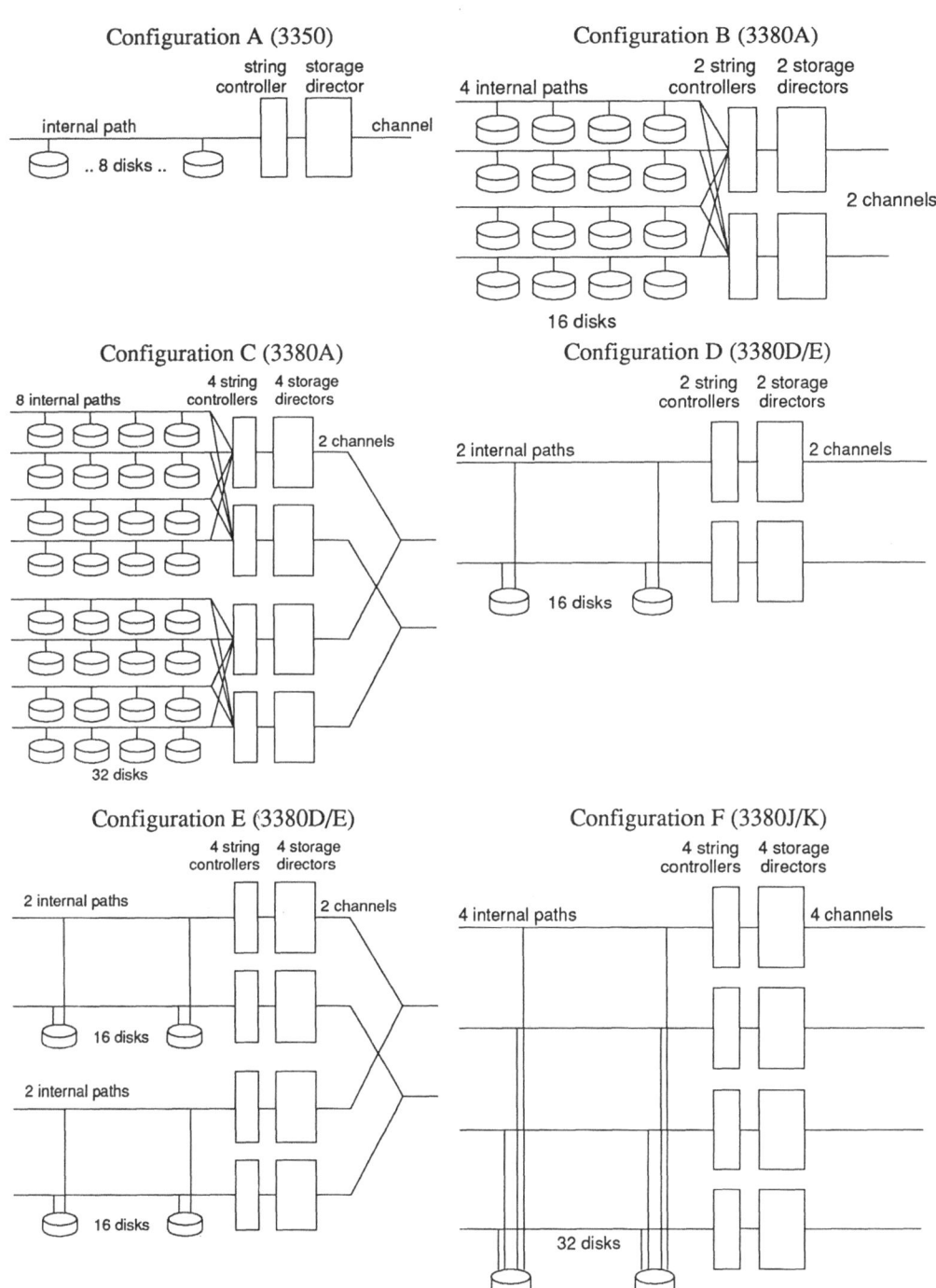

Figure 3. Six standard configurations used for model validation.

3. Modelling Approach

The disk service time consists of several components. The components considered in our model are

Pending Time The average pending time $s_{pending}$ is the average wait time for a controller path to a disk drive to become available. A pending delay occurs if all controller paths to a disk are busy with transfers to other disks, when an I/O request is started. The average pending time obviously depends on the system load, and in particular on the device and controller utilizations. Section 8 describes a method to estimate the pending delay.

Seek Time The seek time s_{seek} is the average time needed to position the disk head on the cylinder requested. The seek time depends on the type of workload, but not on the device or controller utilizations (assuming that no seek optimization is performed).

Latency The latency $s_{latency}$ is the time needed to reach the rotational position specified. On the average, this delay will be half the rotation time $T_{rotation}$. The average latency does not depend on the device or controller load (assuming that no optimization with regard to the angular position is done).

RPS miss delay The RPS miss delay s_{RPS} results from failed RPS reconnection attempts. A reconnection attempt will fail if no controller path is available for reconnection. This component depends on the controller load.

Connect Time The connected search time, the controller command decoding time and the data transfer time are collectively referred to as the connect time $s_{connect}$. Like the seek time, the connect time depends on the workload characteristics only.

While not part of the service time, the controller cleanup time after completion of the I/O request ($s_{cleanup}$) has to be taken into account also, since it causes additional internal path and storage director load.

Of the disk service time components, only the pending time and RPS miss delay have to be computed by our model. The average seek time, latency and connect time are assumed to be known from the disk workload. These workload parameters can be estimated from data collected by the Resource Measurement Facility (RMF) [IBM 1985a] [Hunter 1982] or, more accurately, from traces made with the Generalized Trace Facility [IBM 1981] [Houtekamer 1986, 1988].

In a real system not all transfers will use the RPS protocol for reconnection. The model can be changed to reflect this workload property, in a way similar to [Houtekamer 1986].

The complete model accepts the disk workload characteristics s_{seek}, $s_{latency}$, $s_{connect}$, $s_{cleanup}$ and the arrival rate λ for each disk drive. It uses these values to compute the load dependent components: the pending delay $s_{pending}$ and RPS miss delay s_{RPS}. The RPS miss delay is derived from the probability P_{miss} that all paths are busy when a reconnection attempt is made. Assuming that consecutive reconnection miss probabilities are independent, the number of missed reconnections has a geometric distribution. The probability that i misses occur is thus

$$P[N_{miss}=i] = P_{miss}^i (1-P_{miss})$$

The average number of RPS reconnection failures is then found as

$$N_{miss} = \sum_{i=0}^{\infty} iP_{miss}^i (1-P_{miss}) = \frac{P_{miss}}{1-P_{miss}}$$

The RPS delay thus equals

$$s_{RPS} = T_{rotation} \frac{P_{miss}}{1 - P_{miss}}$$

The disk service time $s_{service}$ is found as the total of the individual components $s_{pending}$, s_{seek}, $s_{latency}$, s_{RPS}, and $s_{connect}$. Finally, the disk utilization ρ_{disk} is found as

$$\rho_{disk} = \lambda s_{service}$$

4. Notation used for Controller and Path Utilizations

The notation to be used in this paper is introduced here, along with some definitions for utilizations.

The individual components in the system are referred to with the five letters defined below

d for disks,

i for internal paths,

s for storage directors,

c for channels,

p for systems (processor complexes).

The disk workload, and the model outputs for the disk drives are denoted with the symbols defined below. Note that the model does not require a balanced disk load; the workload parameters can be specified independently for each disk and system. Some of the formulas below use the device index only (i.e. $s[d]$ instead of $s[d,p]$) to denote the average value over all systems.

$\lambda[d,p]$ The I/O arrival rate for disk d caused by the system p workload.

$s_{pending}[d,p]$ The average pending time for disk d, as observed by system p.

$s_{seek}[d,p]$ The average seek time for disk d for the workload form system p.

$s_{latency}[d]$ The average latency (rotational delay) for disk d.

$s_{RPS}[d,p]$ The average RPS miss delay for disk d, as observed by system p.

$s_{connect}[d,p]$ The average connect time for disk d for the workload from system p.

$s_{cleanup}[d]$ The average cleanup time after I/O completion for disk d.

The path and controller utilizations are computed from the controller connect and cleanup load for the individual disk drives, using the balanced load assumptions described in section 2.

The controller configuration is described with sets. Sets are used to denote all connections to a particular disk, internal path or storage director. The set of all disks connected to internal path i is denoted with D[i], and defined as

D[i] = {$d \mid d$ is connected to internal path i}

Similarly, the set of internal paths connected to storage director s is denoted with I[s], and the set of storage directors connected to channel c is referred to as S[c]. Finally, the channel used to connect storage director s with system p is written as C[s,p]. In our model, the set C[s,p] will contain at most one entry, since we assume that each storage director can be connected to only one channel per system.

The number of connections to a type b component for component a is indicated with $N_b[a]$, e.g. $N_i[d]=2$ indicates that disk d is connected to two internal paths, and $N_s[i]=4$ indicates that internal path i is connected to four storage directors (string controllers).

The utilizations are now defined as

$\rho_d[d]$ the total utilization caused by disk d on the internal paths. This utilization is obtained from the arrival rate, and the connect time components from the individual systems. Note that the cleanup component is included, since it causes device, internal path and controller load.

$$\rho_d[d]=\sum_p \lambda[d,p](s_{connect}[d,p]+s_{cleanup}[d])$$

$\rho_i[i]$ the internal path utilization for path i caused by all disks connected to it. It is defined as

$$\rho_i[i]=\sum_{d \in D[i]} \frac{\rho_d[d]}{N_i[d]}$$

$\rho_s[s]$ the storage director utilization for storage director s, for the load from all internal paths connected to it. It includes all cleanup and overhead components.

$$\rho_s[s]=\sum_{i \in I[s]} \frac{\rho_i[i]}{N_s[i]}$$

$\rho_s^c[s,p]$ the contribution of storage director s to the channel c load. It denotes the part of the channel c load that is caused by s. The controller cleanup time is excluded since during it no channel connection is required. In the definition below, the inner summation refers to the internal path load, and the outer summation refers to the storage director load.

$$\rho_s^c[s,p]=\sum_{i \in I[s]} \frac{1}{N_s[i]} \sum_{d \in D[i]} \frac{\lambda[d,p]s_{connect}[d,p]}{N_i[d]}$$

$\rho_c[c,p]$ the utilization for a particular channel on one of the systems

$$\rho_c[c,p]=\sum_{s \in S[c]} \rho_s^c[s,p]$$

Since our assumptions are such that each storage director can have only one channel connection per system, there is no need to divide $\rho_s^c[s,p]$ by the number of channel connections.

Obviously the model is feasible only when all utilizations are less than 1. If one of the utilizations exceeds one, the system cannot handle the load.

5. Multipathing Operator

With systems using dynamic reconnect, a reconnection fails only when all eligible paths have been found to be busy. This *all path busy* probability is a function of the probability that the reconnect for an individual path will fail, the number of paths and the configuration. In this section three versions of a *multipathing operator* will be defined to describe the *all path busy* function. The multipathing operator as defined computes the all path busy probability from the probability that the reconnect for an individual path will fail, and from the number of paths that can be selected. Because of the restrictions imposed on the configuration, the probability that a particular internal path will block a disk's reconnection is the same for all paths connected to the disk. In a particular configuration, it may be necessary to apply the multipathing operator at several blocking points.

The probability $P_{all\ busy}$ that *all* paths are busy when a reconnection attempt is made, is now written with the multipathing operator $\mathbf{M}$ as

$$P_{all\ busy} \equiv \underset{N}{\mathbf{M}}\ P_{path}$$

with P_{path} the probability that the reconnect on an individual path p will fail, and N the number of paths.

If the P_{path} probabilities are assumed to be independent, the $\mathbf{M}$ operator is equivalent to the product of the P_{path} values, i.e.

$$\underset{N}{\mathbf{M}}\ P_{path} \equiv P_{path}{}^{N}$$

with N the number of paths that can be tried for a reconnection. This product approximation is recommended by [Lazowska 1984].

More accurate estimates for the *all path busy* probability can be obtained by using the results for an open M/M/N system or an M/M/N/N loss system. The N parallel servers in these systems can be compared with the N paths that can be selected in our multipathing problem. Arrivals to the M/M/N and M/M/N/N systems are equivalent to reconnections in the disk system.

This analogy is based on the assumption that the server utilization ρ in the M/M/N and M/M/N/N systems is similar to the probability P_{path} that a reconnection attempt to a path fails in the disk system. Assuming the equivalence, the probability that all servers are busy can be used to approximate the *all path busy* probability.

The probability that an arriving customer has to wait in the M/M/N system is known as the Erlang's C formula, written as $C(N,u)$. The traffic intensity u is found easily from the server utilization as $u = N\rho$. The Erlang C formula reads

$$C(N,u) = \cfrac{u^N/N!}{(1-\rho)\left\{\left[\displaystyle\sum_{n=0}^{N-1}\frac{u^n}{n!}\right]+\frac{u^N}{N!(1-\rho)}\right\}}$$

with N the number of servers and the traffic intensity [Allen 1978]. This formula applies to a queueing system with N parallel servers, which take their customers from a single queue. The interarrival and service time have an exponential distribution, and the average service time is the same for all customers.

In our disk system, the latter assumption need not be true, since the average connect periods can be different for each disk drive. Furthermore, the probability that a customer must wait is *not* the same as the probability that the controller path is found busy, since in the M/M/N system the customer will wait until a path becomes available, while a reconnection attempt is lost. This means that substituting the average controller path busy P_{path} for the server utilization ρ in the Erlang C formula is just an approximation. Performing the substitution, the Erlang C version of the $\mathbf{M}$ operator reads

$$\underset{N}{\mathbf{M}}\ P_{path} \equiv C(N,NP_{path})$$

[Friesenborg 1985] used the Erlang C formula to predict the reconnect failure probability in the IBM 3880 controller model.

The M/M/N/N loss system provides probably a better approximation for the reconnect failure probability, since a customer that arrives during a busy period in this system is turned away, just like a failed reconnection in the disk system. The probability that all servers are busy is written as

$$B(N,u) = \cfrac{u^N/N!}{1+u+u^2/2!+\cdots+u^N/N!}$$

B(N,u) is called the Erlang's B formula. This result is valid for any service time distribution. Contrary to the Erlang C system, the traffic intensity u cannot be directly computed from the utilization ρ. Instead, the average server utilization ρ for this system is a function of u:

$$\rho = \frac{\lambda_a}{N\mu} = \frac{\lambda(1-B(N,u))}{N\mu} = \frac{u(1-B(N,u))}{N}$$

with λ_a the rate of successful arrivals to the system. Rewriting the equation above as

$$u = \frac{N\rho}{1-B(N,u)}$$

shows how to obtain the u once the number of servers N and the average server utilization ρ are known, as is the case for our problem. This equation is easily solved by iteration. The Erlang B version of our multipath operator now reads

$$\underset{N}{\mathrm{M}}\, P_{path} \equiv B(N,u)$$

with u the solution of

$$u = \frac{NP_{path}}{1-B(N,u)}$$

The loss system approximation is used, in a different setting, by [Brandwajn 1986].

The Product, Erlang B and Erlang C versions of the multipathing operator will all be used with our model, to evaluate their accuracy.

6. Blocking Probabilities

In the previous sections the utilizations for the various path components were defined in terms of the disk workload parameters. Also, we have defined the multipathing operator $\mathbf{M}$. In this section, conditional path busy probabilities are defined, and used with the $\mathbf{M}$ operator to compute blocking probabilities.

A reconnect request from a device d fails when none of the internal paths is available.

$$P_{miss}[d,p] = \underset{N_i[d]}{\mathrm{M}}\, P_{miss,i}[i,p\,|\,d]$$

In the equation above, $P_{miss,i}[i,p\,|\,d]$ denotes the conditional probability that a reconnection request from device d for system p at internal path i will fail, when it is known that the device is ready to transmit (i.e., not busy). Since the internal path load is assumed to be balanced, it is sufficient to compute the blocking probability for one of the paths.

The failure may be caused by internal path busy, but also by a storage director or channel busy condition that blocks the internal path. The formula can be refined to distinguish between these busy conditions, as

$$P_{miss}[d,p] = \underset{N_i[d]}{\mathrm{M}}\left\{ P_i[i\,|\,d] + (1-P_i[i\,|\,d])\underset{N_s[i]}{\mathrm{M}}\, P_{miss,s}[s,p\,|\,i] \right\}$$

In the improved formula, $P_i[i\,|\,d]$ denotes the conditional internal path busy probability, if the device d is known to be free. The storage director blocking probability $P_{miss,s}[s,p\,|\,i]$ is added to the path blocking probability, when the internal path is known to be free. $P_i[i\,|\,d]$ is defined as

$$P_i[i\,|\,d] = \frac{\rho_i[i] - \rho_d[d]/N_i[d]}{1 - \rho_d[d]/N_i[d]}$$

where $\rho_{[d]}/N_i[d]$ denotes the path busy probability as caused by disk d. This formula states that a disk does not see its own path load when it tries to reconnect to an internal path.

224

In the same way as for the internal path blocking, the storage director blocking probability $P_{miss,s}[s,p \mid i]$ can be evaluated. The complete reconnection failure probability can be written as

$$P_{miss}[d,p] = \underset{N_i[d]}{\mathbf{M}} \left\{ P_i[i \mid d] + (1 - P_i[i \mid d]) \underset{N_s[i]}{\mathbf{M}} \left\{ P_s[s \mid i] + (1 - P_s[s \mid i]) P_c[c,p \mid s] \right\} \right\}$$

In this equation, the conditional probability that an internal path cannot reconnect to a storage controller, written as $P_s[s \mid i]$, accounts for the fact that an internal path does not see its own load.

$$P_s[s \mid i] = \frac{\rho_s[s] - \rho_i[i]/N_s[i]}{1 - \rho_i[i]/N_s[i]}$$

Since the channel sits at the end of the controller chain, its conditional busy probability $P_c[c,p \mid s]$ need not be decomposed. Furthermore, since the controller cleanup overhead does not load the channel, it uses the utilization figures without the storage director cleanup overhead.

$$P_c[c,p \mid s] = \frac{\rho_c[c,p] - \rho_s^c[s \mid p]}{1 - \rho_s^c[s \mid p]}$$

with p the system to which channel c is connected. Note that the channel will never block a transfer if only one storage director is connected to it.

[Lazowska 1984] uses a quite different method to compute the conditional probabilities. A major problem with the approach is that the **added** path busy probabilities in his model may exceed one. Also, it seems that shared channels (more than one storage director on a channel) are not modelled properly, since all conditional probabilities only use the information that the device is free.

7. RPS Model validation and discussion

In this section simulation and model results are presented for the blocking probabilities at the device level, as a function of the channel load in the 6 different configurations described in section 2. The workload parameters used were

S_{seek}	0.0050	ms
$S_{latency}$	0.0083	ms (half a rotation)
$S_{connect}$	0.0050	ms
$S_{cleanup}$	0.0000	ms (neglect overhead)

A balanced load was assumed, and the disk arrival rate was chosen such that the channel utilization specified was reached. For each of the systems A – F defined in section 2, simulations were done with channel loads from 10% and up to determine the average reconnect miss probability. The model discussed above was applied to each situation, using the three probability operators defined above. No attempt was made to differentiate between the probability for the first and subsequent reconnect misses; the miss probabilities reported are the averages over all reconnection attempts. The results are shown graphically in Figure 4.

For all systems with 1 or 2 channels paths (configuration A-E) both the Erlang B and Erlang C approximations yield accurate results. The Erlang B approximation yields the most accurate results for low channel utilizations, while the Erlang C approximation is more accurate for high channel utilizations. The Erlang B approximation tends to underestimate the miss probability, in particular at high controller utilizations.

The Erlang B approximation shows the best results by far for the system with 4 channel paths. The property that arriving customers are turned away when the system is busy, is apparently important in this situation.

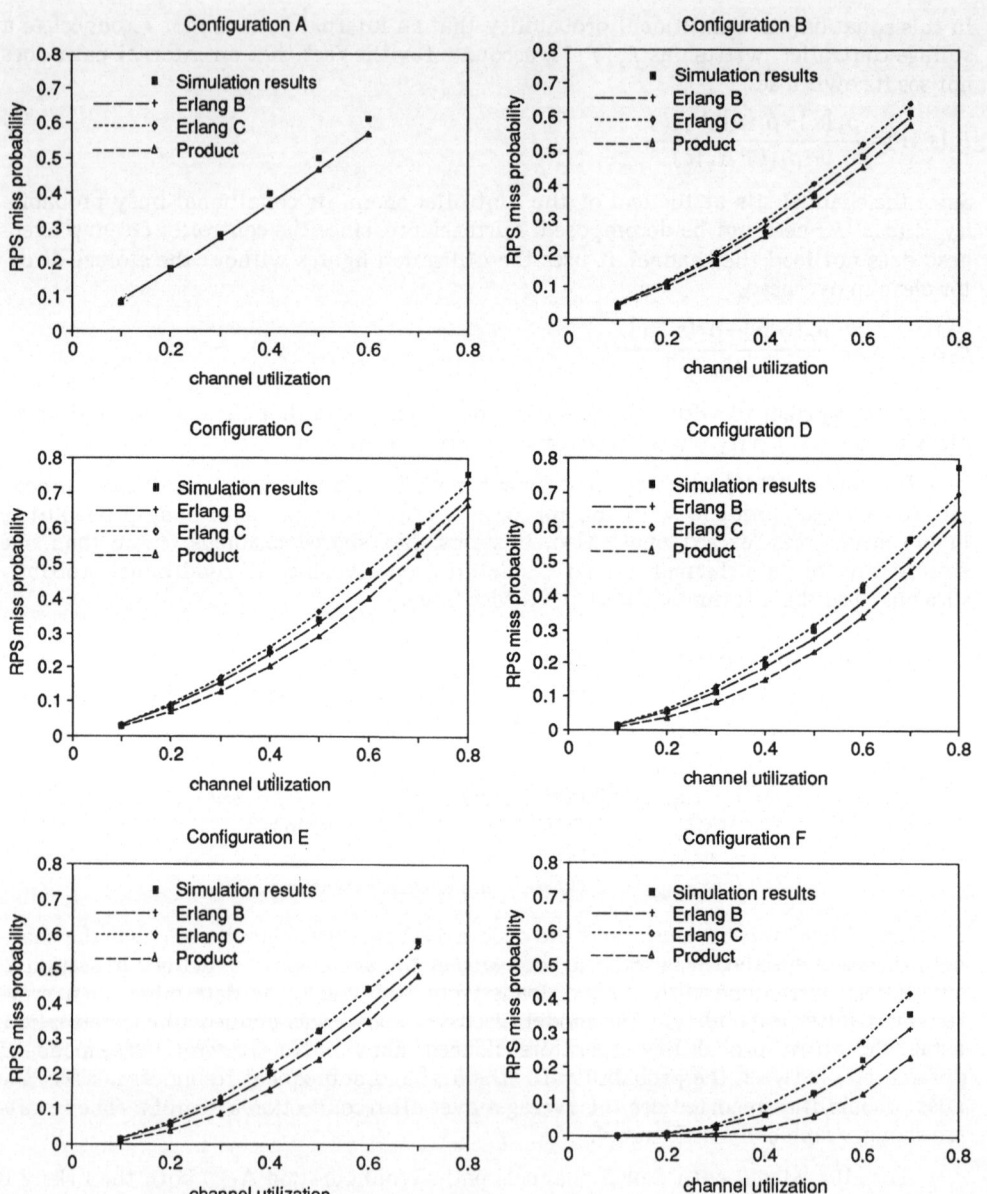

Figure 4. Simulation and numerical results for the RPS miss probability for the configurations A to F.

The Product approximation yields the largest errors, in particular for the configurations D, E and F, corresponding with the disk drives with the device level select feature (dual port).

Overall, the Erlang B (loss system) approximation seems the most useful for our model, since it handles a wide range of configurations with sufficient accuracy. This confirms the remarks made on theoretical basis in the section on the multipathing operators.

It is interesting to compare the results for the configurations A, D and F with the results from the model in [Brandwajn 1983]. In that paper, a *closed* system model is used for the blocking points, where the arrival rate is chosen such that the system throughput equals the arrival rate. Our model uses an open model with a multipathing operator derived by analogy from a loss system model. Table 1 below shows the simulation results, the results based on Brandwajn's closed model and results for our open model with the Erlang B approximation.

TABLE 1. Comparison of simulation results, with the results from Brandwajn's closed model and our open Erlang B model.

Configuration	Channel Util	Simu-lation	Closed model	error	Open model	error
A	10%	0.083	0.089	7%	0.089	7%
A	20%	0.182	0.179	-1%	0.179	-2%
A	30%	0.282	0.273	-3%	0.273	-3%
A	40%	0.400	0.368	-8%	0.368	-8%
A	50%	0.500	0.467	-7%	0.467	-7%
A	60%	0.612	0.568	-7%	0.568	-7%
D	10%	0.015	0.014	-5%	0.015	-
D	20%	0.054	0.052	-4%	0.054	-
D	30%	0.112	0.108	-4%	0.112	-
D	40%	0.197	0.181	-8%	0.187	-5%
D	50%	0.302	0.270	-11%	0.277	-8%
D	60%	0.418	0.375	-10%	0.382	-9%
D	70%	0.566	0.497	-12%	0.504	-11%
D	80%	0.775	0.639	-17%	0.644	-17%
F	10%	0.001	0.001	-	0.001	-
F	20%	0.007	0.006	-9%	0.007	-
F	30%	0.025	0.024	-4%	0.027	8%
F	40%	0.063	0.058	-8%	0.063	-
F	50%	0.127	0.113	-11%	0.121	-5%
F	60%	0.224	0.194	-13%	0.203	-9%
F	70%	0.359	0.306	-14%	0.316	-12%

The results for both models are almost the same for all three configurations, over the entire load range. Our open model is somewhat more accurate, in particular at high utilizations. The table illustrates that our approach with the multi-pathing operator yields results that are at least as accurate as for a closed loss system model.

Simulation results for systems with a non-balanced load indicate that the model is accurate for these situations as well. This was to be expected, since neither the multipathing operator nor the conditional probabilities depend on balanced load assumptions. In part, the accuracy of the method for a large range of configurations and system loadings will be a result of the loss system's insensitivity to the service time distributions: the Erlang B formula is valid for a general service discipline.

Table 2 below shows simulation and model results for a type D system with non-balanced load. In this particular example, the arrival rate for disks 1..4 is 2 times the arrival rate for the disks 5..8, and 4 times the arrival rate for the disks 9..16.

TABLE 2. Simulation and Model Results for Type D System with non-balanced load.

Channel Util	disk no	Simulation results	Erlang B results	error	Erlang C results	error	Product results	error
10%	1-4	0.012	0.013	16.4%	0.014	24.1%	0.008	-31.9%
	5-8	0.015	0.015	4.8%	0.016	12.4%	0.009	-38.6%
	9-16	0.015	0.016	8.1%	0.017	16.2%	0.009	-36.5%
20%	1-4	0.046	0.049	7.0%	0.055	18.7%	0.032	-30.0%
	5-8	0.052	0.054	4.8%	0.061	16.8%	0.036	-30.4%
	9-16	0.053	0.057	8.4%	0.064	20.9%	0.038	-27.8%
30%	1-4	0.096	0.103	7.2%	0.117	21.7%	0.074	-22.6%
	5-8	0.109	0.113	3.7%	0.128	17.4%	0.082	-24.6%
	9-16	0.120	0.117	-2.5%	0.133	10.8%	0.086	-28.3%
40%	1-4	0.178	0.174	-2.2%	0.198	11.2%	0.136	-23.6%
	5-8	0.196	0.187	-4.6%	0.214	9.2%	0.148	-24.5%
	9-16	0.206	0.194	-5.8%	0.221	7.3%	0.154	-25.2%
50%	1-4	0.266	0.260	-2.3%	0.297	11.7%	0.212	-20.3%
	5-8	0.291	0.277	-4.8%	0.316	8.6%	0.234	-19.6%
	9-16	0.306	0.285	-6.9%	0.325	6.2%	0.242	-20.9%
60%	1-4	0.383	0.364	-5.0%	0.411	7.3%	0.322	-15.9%
	5-8	0.414	0.382	-7.7%	0.431	4.1%	0.342	-17.4%
	9-16	0.428	0.391	-8.6%	0.440	2.8%	0.351	-18.0%

8. Pending Delay Model

A pending delay occurs when no path is available to a disk drive the moment a new I/O request must be started, because transfers for other disks are in progress. The pending period starts when the start command is issued to the channel subsystem (XA definition), and it ends when the disk accepts the command. A pending delay can occur only if the drive is free, since the operating system will not attempt to start an I/O request to a disk which is busy for that system, instead it will queue the request. In the latter case, the operating system will issue the request as soon as the device becomes available. Upon completion of the previous request, the device *and* the path become available. If the operating system reacts fast enough, the queued request will not experience a pending delay since a path is available ready for use.

On the assumption that the operating system reacts immediately as a path becomes available, the probability for a pending delay to occur is proportional with the all path busy probability and the probability that the device is free. The all path busy probability has been computed before: it is the $P_{miss}[d,p]$, as defined above for disk d at system p.

Once it is known that a pending delay occurs, the average wait time depends on the remaining service time for a transfer which is in progress, if there is just one path. If there are more paths, the I/O request can be started as soon as one path is available.

Assuming exponential service times, the remaining service time equals the average service time [Kleinrock 1975]. In our system, the service time corresponds to the path connect time. With multiple paths and exponential service time for each path, the remaining connect time can be divided by the number of paths, since the paths are parallel servers with exponential service times. In the equations below, $s_{connect}$ is used to denote the average path connect period for the path studied.

If each internal path has only one storage director connection ($N_s[i]=1$) the pending time can be estimated with

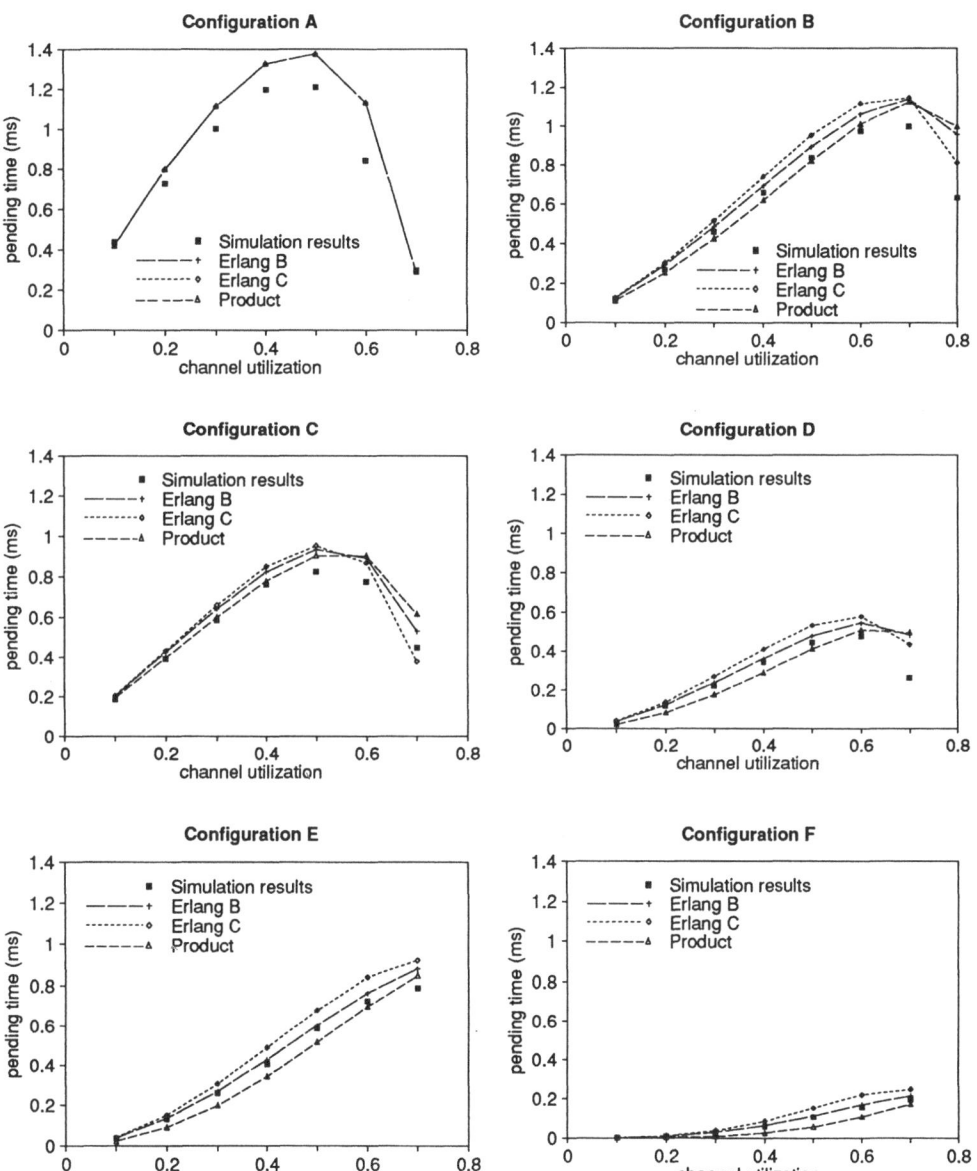

Figure 5. Simulation and numerical results for the Pending Delay for the configurations A to F.

$$S_{pending}[d,p] = (1-\rho_{disk}[d])P_{miss}[d,p]\frac{S_{connect}}{N_i[d]}$$

In a more general setting, both $N_s[i]$ and $N_i[d]$ can be greater than 1. The factor $P_{miss}[d,p]$ still represents the probability that a delay occurs, but the remaining service time will depend on the number of controllers concurrently active. If blocking occurs because of an internal path busy condition, the number of transfers active is $N_i[d]$. If blocking occurs because of a storage director busy condition, the number of transfers active is $N_i[d]N_s[i]$. A general expression for the pending time is thus

$$S_{pending}[d] = (1-\rho_{disk}[d])P_{miss}[d,p](\frac{P_i[i\mid d]}{P_d^{one\ path}[d]} + \frac{P_d^{one\ path}-P_i[i\mid d]}{P_d^{one\ path}[d]N_s[i]})\frac{S_{connect}[d]}{N_i[d]}$$

with

$$P_d^{one\ path} = P_i[i\mid d] + (1-P_i[i\mid d])\underset{N_s[i]}{M}\left\{P_s[s\mid i] + (1-P_s[s\mid i])P_c[c,p\mid s]\right\}$$

the probability that a single path is busy.

9. Pending Delay Model Validation and Discussion

Using the same configurations, and the same set of input parameters, simulations and numerical results were obtained for the average pending delay. The results are shown graphically in Figure 5.

Like for the RPS miss probability, the average pending delay model is most accurately approximated with the model using the Erlang B approximation for the multipathing operator. The errors are usually less than 15% for this model, while they are significantly larger for both the Erlang C and product approximations. Large errors occur for all models at high device loads, since a small error in the RPS miss probability causes a large variation in the device utilization (the factor $1-\rho_{disk}$). Nevertheless, the figures show that the model follows the shape of the pending time curve accurately for all configurations.

10. Discussion and Conclusions

A model for the disk service time of the IBM System/370 I/O subsystem has been presented. The model handles most of the current I/O configurations using the 3380 type disk drives, with dynamic reconnect.

Multipathing is modelled using a *multipathing operator*, which defines the probability that all available paths are busy. The multipathing operator based on the Erlang B formula was found to be the most accurate one. A set of conditional blocking probabilities is defined to account for internal path, storage director and channel contention.

The method presented yields accurate results for complex I/O subsystems, using an easy to understand method. The definition of the multipath operator allows us to combine accuracy of closed models with the easy of use of an open throughput driven model in an numerically efficient method.

As any open (throughput driven) model, this model can be used in closed models using an iterative scheme, with an approach as suggested in [Lazowska 1984].

Acknowledgements

This research is part of my Ph.D. study at the Delft University of Technology. I would like to thank my supervisor prof.ir. G.L. Reijns, Guus Bonnes and Hans Schoone for the helpful discussions I have had with them regarding this project.

References

[Allen 1978] A.O. Allen, **Probability, Statistics and Queueing Theory**, Academic Press, New York 1978.

230

[Bard 1980] Y. Bard, **A Model of Shared DASD and Multipathing**, Communications of the ACM, Vol 23, 1980, pp 564-572.

[Brandwajn 1981] A. Brandwajn, **Models of DASD Subsystems: Basic Model of Reconnection** Performance Evaluation, Vol 1, November 1983, pp 263-281.

[Brandwajn 1983] A. Brandwajn, **Models of DASD Subsystems with Multiple Access Paths: A Throughput Driven Approach**, IEEE Transactions on Computers, vol C-32, May 1983, pp 451-463.

[Brandwajn 1986] A. Brandwajn, **Modeling DASD and disk caches**, Proceedings CMG'86 Conference, December 1987, pp 206-216.

[Friesenborg 1985] S. Friesenborg and R. Wicks, **DASD Expectations: The 3380, 3880-23 and MVS/XA**, IBM Technical bulleting GG22-9363-2, Washington Systems Center, 1985.

[Houtekamer 1986] G.E. Houtekamer, **Measuring I/O workload characteristics in IBM/MVS systems**, Proceedings CMG'86 Conference, December 1987, pp 307-315.

[Houtekamer 1988] G.E. Houtekamer, **CCWANAL Release 1.5.6 User Manual**, Consul Risk Management B.V., 1988.

[Hunter 1982] D. Hunter, **Modelling Real DASD Configurations**, in Applied Probability-Computer Science, R.L. Disney and J.O.Ott (eds), Birkhauser, Boston 1982.

[IBM 1981] **OS/VS2 MVS System Programming Library: Service Aids**, IBM publication GC28-0674, 1981.

[IBM 1983a] **IBM System/370 Extended Architecture, Principles of Operation**, IBM publication SA22-7085, March 1983.

[IBM 1983b] **IBM 3880 Storage Control Models 1, 2, 3, and 4, Reference Manual**, IBM publication GA26-1661, April 1983.

[IBM 1985a] **Resource Measurement Facility (RMF), Version 3, General Information Manual**, IBM publication GC28-0922, 1985.

[IBM 1985b] **IBM 3380 Direct Access Storage Models AD4, BD4, AE4, and BE4, General Information** IBM publication GA26-4193, 1985.

[IBM 1987] **Overview: New dimensions in IBM storage subsystems**, IBM Product Information, ZA87-0216, ZG87-0225 and ZG87-0226, September 1987.

[Kleinrock 1975] L. Kleinrock, **Queueing Systems, Volume 1: Theory**, Wiley, New York 1975.

[Lazowska 1984] E.D. Lazowska et al, **Quantitative System Performance**, Prentice Hall, Englewood Cliffs NJ, 1984.

A UNIFIED APPROACH TO THE PERFORMANCE
EVALUATION OF MULTIPROCESSORS

E. Sanvicente, M.A. Fiol and J.L. Melús

Dep. de Matemàtica Aplicada i Telemàtica
Universitat Politècnica de Catalunya
08034 Barcelona, Spain

ABSTRACT

This paper introduces a unified approach to approximately compute the bandwidth of tightly coupled multiprocessors, working either synchronously or asynchronously. Several types of interconnection networks are considered, namely: crossbar, multiple-bus and multiple-bus with partial-busses. The analysis is carried out for both constant and exponential memory service times. Simulation runs are also included to validate the approximation used in the model. Although the analysis is asymptotic, the computations turn out to be quite accurate for moderate, or even small, system sizes.

I. INTRODUCTION

Analytic models and simulation are necessary to assess the performance of multiprocessor systems before the actual machine is built. These models can not include all the details of the real system, but rather concentrate on the most relevant features that have a bearing on the contention for shared resources (memory modules and communication paths). To that end, many articles have been appearing in the literature. Bhandarkar [1], for instance, discusses discrete Markov chain models to numerically study the extent of interference in multiprocessors with a crossbar switch. Also for the crossbar switch under synchronous operation, an asymptotic model using generating functions is derived in [2] when each processor issues a memory request immediately after memory service completion. This formula is generalized in [3] for the case of internal processing using an expression for the average number of processors referencing a given memory module. As shown in this paper, the same technique, properly modified, can also be used to obtain the bandwidth in the asynchronous case.

When the number of processors and memory modules is large, the crossbar organization is too expensive, and this led researchers to propose and study other kinds of interconnection networks with a better

Work supported in part by the Spanish Research Council (Comision Interministerial de Ciencia y Tecnologia, CICYT) under projects 1180/84, 0261/86 and 0173/86.

cost/performance ratio like, for instance, the multiple-bus and multiple-bus with partial-busses. The synchronous multiple-bus network was analyzed in [3], whereas [4] and [5] present, respectively, exact and approximate models to evaluate the asynchronous operation of such organization. In this paper, we also unify the evaluation for both operation modes, using a simple model that runs fast and produces accurate answers.

The multiple-bus with partial-busses network was introduced in [6] as a means of further reducing the system cost. The performance analysis of such network was also carried out in [6] through simulation. To evaluate this organization we present here formulas that are based on the unified model obtained in the paper for the multiple-bus system.

In Section II we state the system hypotheses, and present our unified approach to the performance evaluation of those three networks. Numerical results are collected and compared in Section III. Finally, some conclusions are drawn in Section IV.

II. AN ASYMPTOTIC ANALYTIC MODEL

Several performance indexes could be considered to evaluate the system, and in this paper we have chosen *bandwidth* or average number of busy memory modules, *B.*

The system we analyze consists of n processors and m memory banks connected by an interconnection network of the crossbar, multiple-bus or multiple-bus with partial-busses type. See Fig. 1. More details about these organizations can be found in [1-6].

The memory service time is either constant, taken as the time unit, or exponentially distributed with parameter μ. As usual, arbitration times and propagation delays are supposed to be negligible. Once a service completion occurs, the processor remains thinking (active) for an integer number of time units geometrically distributed with mean q/p, $q=1-p$, (*synchronous* operation), or for an exponential random variable with parameter λ (*asynchronous* operation).

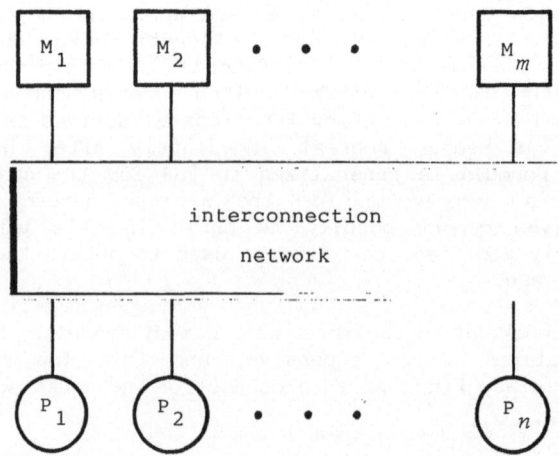

Fig. 1. Multiprocessor system organization.

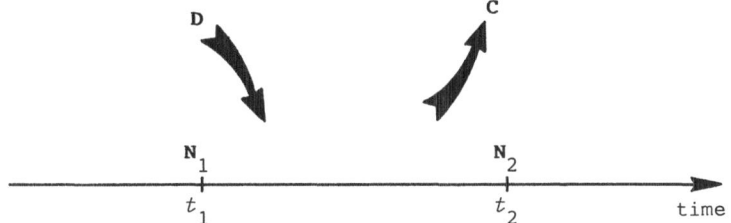

Fig. 2. Demands and completions during a time interval.

All memory modules are equally referenced by all the processors, and modules and communication paths are granted randomly among contending requests.

We now proceed with our unified analysis of these switches.

A) Crossbar Organization

Let N_1 and N_2 be the number (random variable) of processors referencing a given memory module at times t_1 and t_2 respectively. See Fig. 2. If we call D and C the number of demands and completions during the time interval $t_2 - t_1$, we have

$$N_2 = N_1 + D - C. \tag{1}$$

Times t_1 and t_2 are chosen so that C is at most 1.

Taking expectations in (1), and assuming the system in steadystate, we can write

$$E(D) = E(C). \tag{2}$$

Squaring (1), and taking expectations again, we have

$$E(N_2^2) = E(N_1^2) + E(D^2) + E(C^2) + 2E(N_1 D) - 2E(N_1 C) - 2E(DC). \tag{3}$$

Since C is either 0 or 1, we can write

$$E(C^2) = E(C). \tag{4}$$

Asymptotically, we can suppose that N_1 and D (and D and C) are independent. This yields

$$E(N_1 D) = E(N_1)E(D), \tag{5}$$
$$E(DC) = E(D)E(C). \tag{6}$$

On the other hand,

$$E(N_1 C) = \sum_{i=1}^{n} i P(N_1 C = i) =$$

235

$$= \sum_{i=1}^{n} i P(\mathbf{N}_1 = i) P(C = 1 | \mathbf{N}_1 = i) =$$

$$= P_c E(\mathbf{N}_1) \tag{7}$$

where $P_c = P(C = 1 | \mathbf{N}_1 = i)$ is the probability of service completion at t_2 when the memory is busy at t_1. Therefore, we also have

$$E(C) = P(\text{busy memory}) P_c = \frac{B}{m} P_c \ , \tag{8}$$

see [3].

In steady state, using equalities (2), (4), (5), (6) and (7), condition (3) becomes:

$$0 = E(\mathbf{D}^2) + E(\mathbf{D}) + 2E(\mathbf{N})E(\mathbf{D}) - 2E(\mathbf{N})P_c - 2[E(\mathbf{D})]^2$$

where $E(\mathbf{N}) = E(\mathbf{N}_1) = E(\mathbf{N}_2)$. Therefore

$$E(\mathbf{N}) = \frac{V(\mathbf{D}) + E(\mathbf{D})[1 - E(\mathbf{D})]}{2[P_c - E(\mathbf{D})]} \tag{9}$$

where $V(\mathbf{D})$ stands for the variance of $\mathbf{D}$.

Alternatively, since all the memory modules are statistically equivalent, $E(\mathbf{N})$ can be computed as follows:

$$E(\mathbf{N}) = \frac{n - A}{m} \tag{10}$$

where A is the so-called *processing power*, or average number of active processors.

Equating the quantities (9) and (10) we have the basic expression to evaluate the crossbar network. The details follow.

A1) Synchronous case

Take as t_1 any positive integer, and $t_2 = t_1 + 1$. Then,

$$P_c = 1. \tag{11}$$

Now, using (2) and (11), (8) becomes

$$E(\mathbf{D}) = \frac{B}{m} \ . \tag{12}$$

To compute $V(\mathbf{D})$, we will approximate the probability $P(\mathbf{D} = i)$ by the binomial distribution

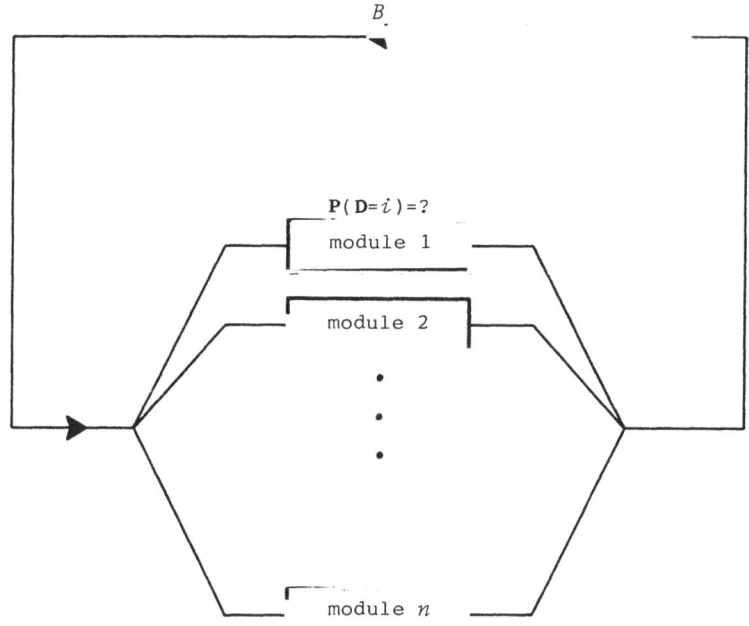

Fig. 3. Distribution of demands among the different memory modules.

$$P(D=i) = \binom{[B]}{i}(\frac{1}{m})^i(1 - \frac{1}{m})^{[B]-i}. \tag{13}$$

where $[B]$ is the closest integer to B.

The idea behind (13) is that, out of the n processors, in each cycle there are only B demands (on the average) uniformly distributed among the m modules. See Fig. 3.

The mean of D is

$$E(D) = \frac{[B]}{m} \simeq \frac{B}{m} , \tag{14}$$

as it should. The variance is

$$V(D) = [B]\frac{1}{m}(1-\frac{1}{m}) \simeq \frac{B(m-1)}{m^2} . \tag{15}$$

Entering (11), (14) and (15) in (9), we get

$$E(N) = \frac{B}{2m} + \frac{(m-1)B}{2m(m-B)} . \tag{16}$$

To compute A, we use the equilibrium condition

$$(A + B)p = B,$$

which yields

$$A = \frac{q}{p} B. \tag{17}$$

Substituting this value in (10), and equating the resulting expression to (16), we can write

$$\frac{n - \frac{q}{p} B}{m} = \frac{B}{2m} + \frac{(m-1)B}{2m(m-B)} .$$

Solving for B, we finally have

$$B = \frac{\frac{m}{p} + n - \frac{1}{2} - \sqrt{(\frac{m}{p} + n - \frac{1}{2})^2 - (\frac{2}{p} - 1)2mn}}{\frac{2}{p} - 1} \tag{18}$$

which generalizes a result obtained in [2] for $p=1$ using generating functions.

If instead of computing $P(D=i)$ according to (13) we had used the Poisson distribution

$$P(D=i) = e^{-\frac{B}{m}} \frac{(B/m)^i}{i!} , \tag{19}$$

we would have obtained

$$B = \frac{\frac{m}{p} + n - \sqrt{(\frac{m}{p} + n)^2 - (\frac{2}{p} - 1)2mn}}{\frac{2}{p} - 1} \tag{20}$$

which is the same as (18) with the 1/2 terms discarded.

A2) Asynchronous case

Take as t_1 any instant in time, and $t_2 = t_1 + \Delta t$ where Δt is an infinitesimal increment. In view of the exponential service time assumption stated before, we have

$$P_c = \mu \Delta t. \tag{21}$$

From (2) and (21), (8) can be written as

$$E(D) = \frac{B}{m} \mu \Delta t. \tag{22}$$

To compute $V(D)$ we will assume that D follows a Bernoulli distribution. Then,

$$P(D=1) = \frac{B}{m} \mu \Delta t,$$

$$P(D=0) = 1 - \frac{B}{m} \mu \Delta t,$$

and therefore

$$V(\mathbf{D}) = \frac{B}{m}\mu\Delta t(1 - \frac{B}{m}\mu\Delta t) = \frac{B}{m}\mu\Delta t. \tag{23}$$

Entering (21), (22) and (23) into (9) we have

$$E(\mathbf{N}) = \frac{B}{m-B}. \tag{24}$$

The balance equation to compute A is now the following:

$$A\lambda = B\mu,$$

or

$$A = \frac{B}{\rho}. \tag{25}$$

where $\rho=\lambda/\mu$ is called the *load factor*.

Equating (24) to the expression obtained substituting (25) in (10), we get

$$\frac{n - \dfrac{B}{\rho}}{m} = \frac{B}{m - B}. \tag{26}$$

Solving for B, we finally have

$$B = \frac{\dfrac{1+\rho}{\rho}m + n - \sqrt{(\dfrac{1+\rho}{\rho}m + n)^2 - \dfrac{4mn}{\rho}}}{\dfrac{2}{\rho}}. \tag{27}$$

The case of no internal processing can be obtained taking limits in (27) (or, more easily, in (26)) when $\rho \rightarrow \infty$. The result is

$$B = \frac{mn}{m+n},$$

which asymptotically coincides with the following exact formula reported in [7]

$$B = \frac{mn}{m+n-1}.$$

If formula (27) were not available, one could approximately compute B using (18) or (20) with

$$p = \frac{\rho}{1+\rho}. \tag{28}$$

See Fig. 4. Expression (20), for instance, yields

$$B = \frac{\dfrac{1+\rho}{\rho}m + n - \sqrt{(\dfrac{1+\rho}{\rho}m + n)^2 - (\dfrac{2}{\rho} + 1)2mn}}{\dfrac{2}{\rho} + 1}. \tag{29}$$

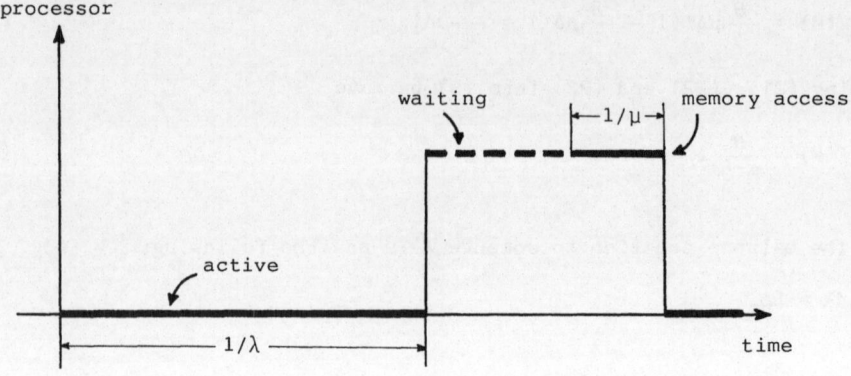

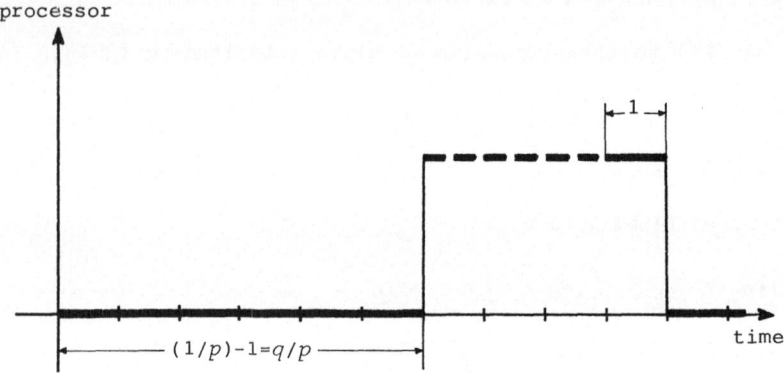

Fig. 4. Relationship between the load factor
and the demand probability.

which is almost the same as (27) except for the extra 1 in the two terms
$\dfrac{2}{\rho} + 1$.

B) Multiple-bus organization

The bandwidth of the multiple-bus interconnection network, B_{MB}, can
be computed as

$$B_{MB} = \sum_{i=1}^{b} i\beta(i) , \tag{30}$$

where b is the number of busses, and $\beta(i)$ is the probability that i busses
are busy. Denoting by $r(i)$ the probability that i different memory modules
are requested by the processors, we have

$$
\beta(i) = \begin{cases} r(i), & i<b \ ; \\[10pt] \displaystyle\sum_{j=b}^{m} r(j), & i=b \ . \end{cases} \qquad (31)
$$

The average number of <u>different memory modules referenced</u> by the processors can be approximated by B_c, where B_c is given by (18) or (27) depending upon the case. Assuming that the distribution of this random variable is binomial and $m \leq n$, we write

$$
r(i) = \binom{m}{i} \left[\frac{B_c}{m} \right]^i \left[1 - \frac{B_c}{m} \right]^{m-1} , \qquad (32)
$$

Using (31) and (32), we can now compute bandwidth according to (30).

C) Multiple-bus with partial-busses

This network is similar to the multiple-bus network. The difference is that, for this organization, each of the b busses is connected to all n processors but only to a subset of m/g memory modules. See [6] for more details. The load offered to each subset of memories by every processor is now p/g or ρ/g, depending upon the mode of operation. Therefore, we can write

$$
B_{PB} = g B_{MB}(m/g, \ n, \ b/g, \ p/g) \qquad (33)
$$

for the synchronous case, and

$$
B_{PB} = g B_{MB}(m/g, \ n, \ b/g, \ \rho/g) \qquad (34)
$$

for the asynchronous case, where $B_{MB}(m/g, \ n, \ b/g, \ \rho/g)$ is the bandwidth of a multiple-bus network with m/g memory modules, n processors, b/g busses and load factor ρ/g; and similarly for the formula (33). Such a formula was suggested previously in [8].

III. NUMERICAL RESULTS

In this section we comment upon the results obtained using the model introduced in Section II.

Figs. 5 and 6 show, for the synchronous and asynchronous case respectively, the crossbar bandwidth versus the number of processors. The number of memory modules is also equal to n, $p=0.5$ and $\rho=1$. We have also included simulation values. Observe that the agreement between model and simulation is so good that the two curves can not be told apart. Fig. 7 illustrates the discrepancies between the two models, as we vary p and ρ ($\rho=p/q$), for $m=n=32$. As can be seen, the differences are quite small, but increase as p approaches 1 (see (29)).

Similar results for the multiple-bus organization, with $b=8$, are plotted in Figs. 8, 9 and 10. Notice the degradation with respect to the crossbar. Finally, Figs. 11, 12 and 13 correspond to the multiple-bus with partial-busses with $g=2$. Again, note the extra degradation between this organization and the multiple-bus interconnection network.

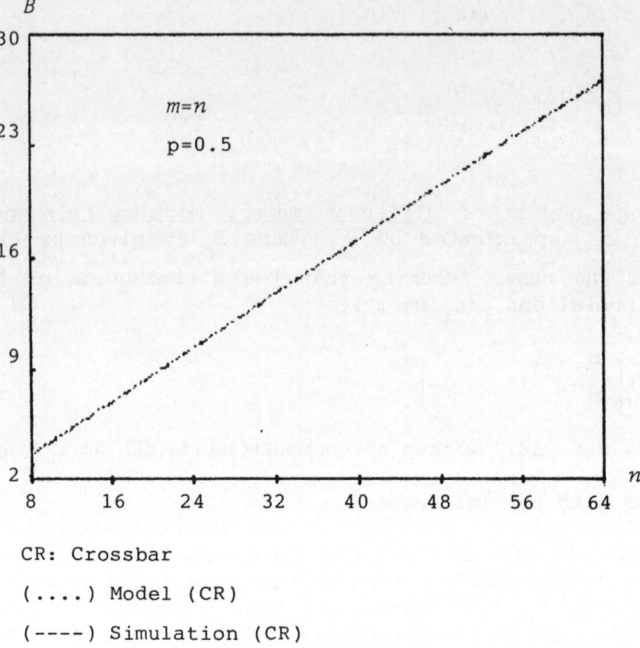

CR: Crossbar

(....) Model (CR)

(----) Simulation (CR)

Fig. 5. Bandwidth for the synchronous crossbar network.

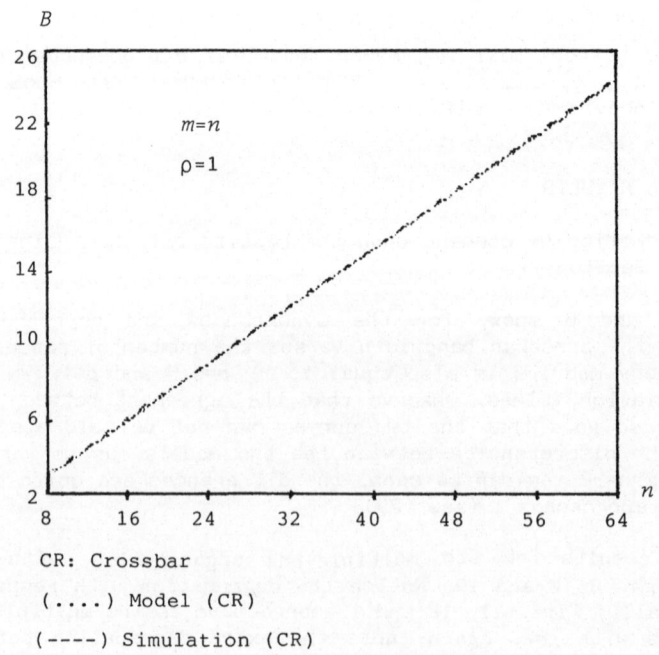

CR: Crossbar

(....) Model (CR)

(----) Simulation (CR)

Fig. 6. Bandwidth for the asynchronous crossbar network

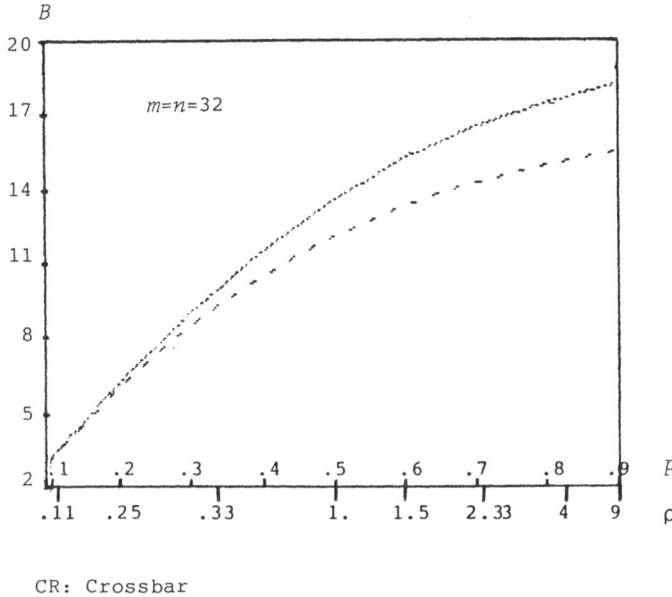

CR: Crossbar

(....) Synchronous model (CR)

(----) Asynchronous model (CR)

Fig. 7. Comparison between synchronous and asynchronous
crossbar models.

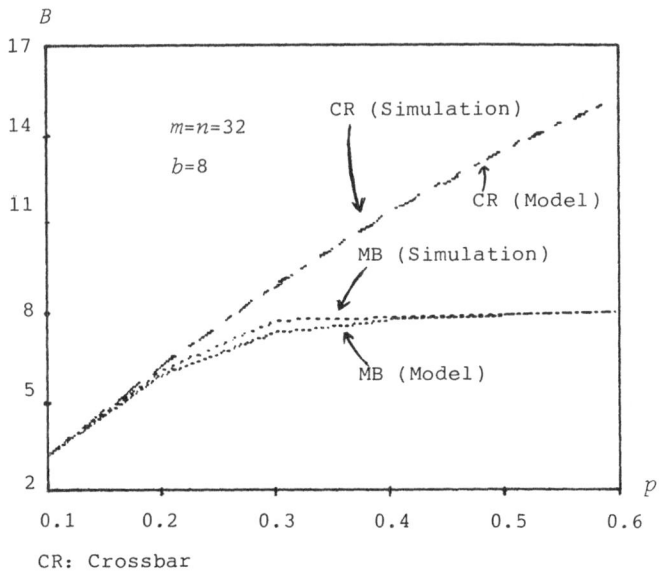

CR: Crossbar

MB: Multiple-Bus

Fig. 8. Crossbar versus multiple-bus:
synchronous case.

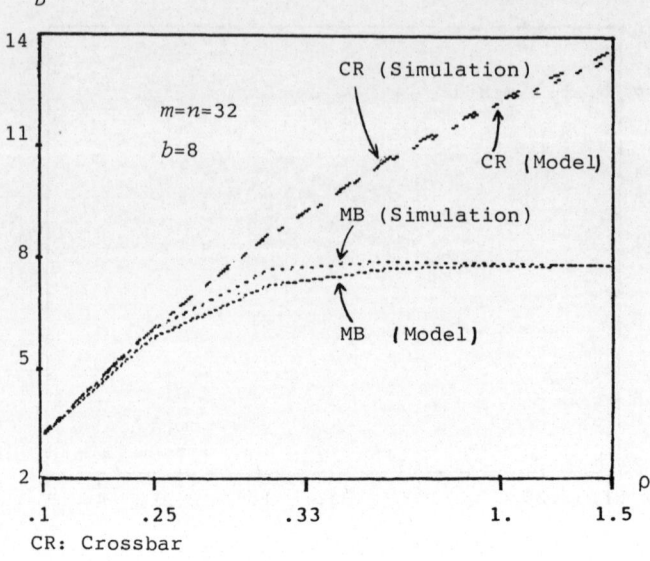

CR: Crossbar

MB: Multiple-Bus

Fig. 9. Crossbar versus multiple-bus:
asynchronous case.

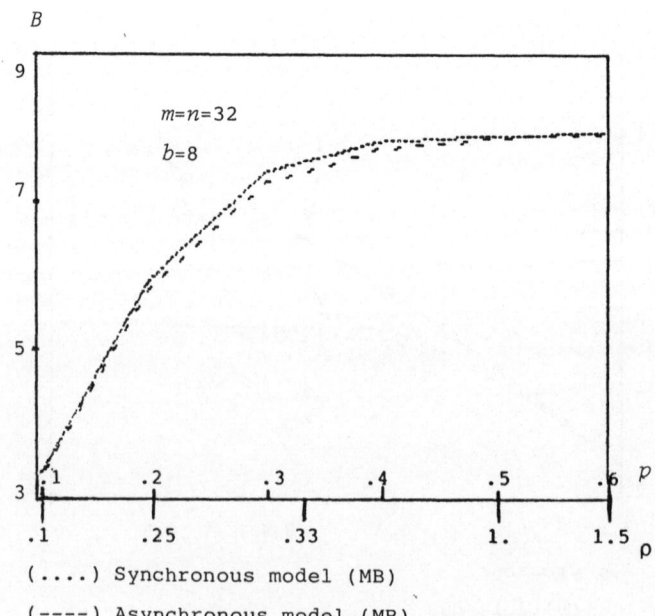

(....) Synchronous model (MB)

(----) Asynchronous model (MB)

Fig. 10. Comparison between synchronous and
asynchronous multiple-bus models.

244

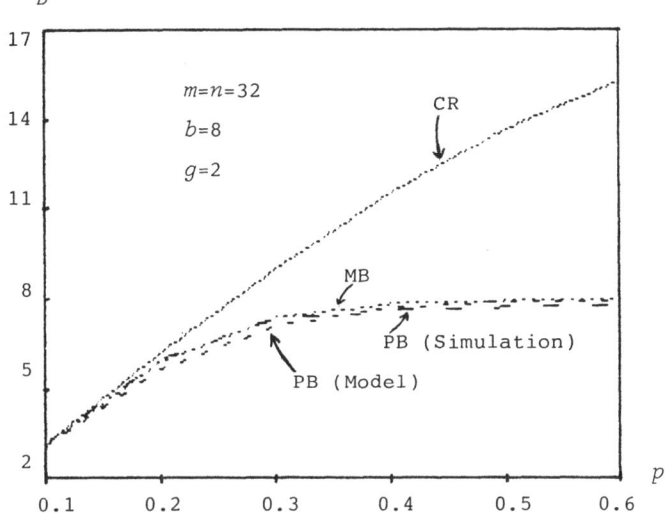

CR: Crossbar

MB: Multiple-Bus

PB: Multiple-Bus with partial busses

Fig. 11. Crossbar versus multiple-bus and multiple-bus
with partial-busses: synchronous case.

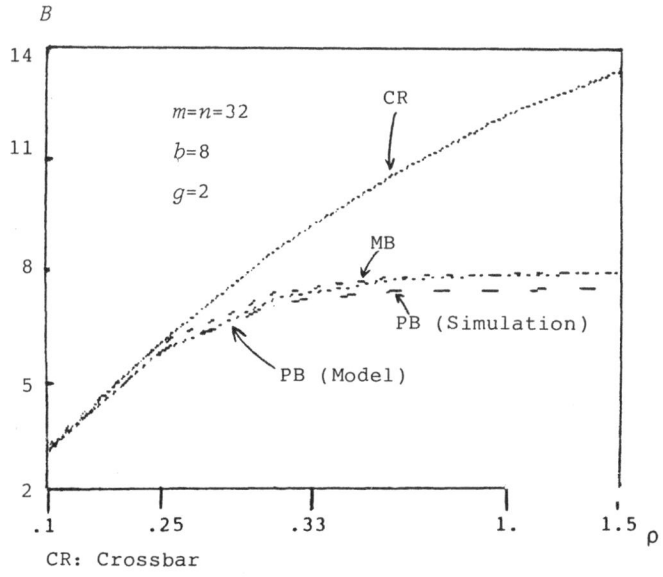

CR: Crossbar

MB: Multiple-Bus

PB: Multiple-Bus with partial busses

Fig. 12. Crossbar versus multiple-bus and multiple-bus
with partial-busses: asynchronous case.

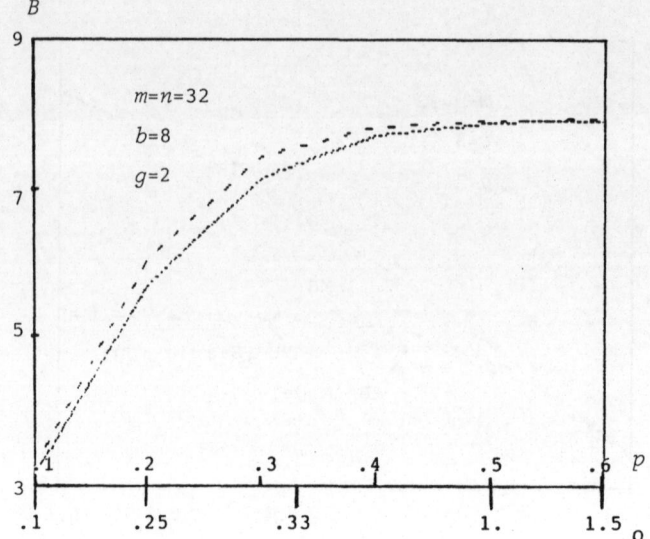

PB: Multiple-bus with partial busses

(----) Synchronous Model (PB)

(....) Asynchronous Model (PB)

Fig. 13. Comparison between synchronous and asynchronous
multiple-bus with partial-busses models.

IV. CONCLUSIONS

We have presented in this paper a unified method to evaluate the
performance of multiprocessor systems. The model is asymptotic and, using
only basic steady state equations, yields closed form expressions for the
evaluation of the crossbar network. Although not in closed form, the
computations for the multiple-bus and the multiple-bus with partial-busses
are also straightforward. In spite of the asymptotic approach, the
agreement between model and simulation is quite good for moderate system
sizes. Therefore, we conclude that our model is a valid approximation, and
that it should be used, rather than recurring to simulation, when quick
answers about the system behaviour are needed.

REFERENCES

[1] D.P. Bhandarkar, "Analysis of memory interference in
    multiprocessors", *IEEE Trans. Comput.*, vol. C-24, pp. 897- 908,
    Sep. 1975.
[2] F. Baskett and A.J. Smith, "Interference in multiprocessor computer
    systems with interleaved memory", *Comm. of the ACM*, vol. 19, pp.
    327-334, Jun. 1976.
[3] M. Valero, J.M. Llaberia, J. Labarta, E. Sanvicente and T.
    Lang, "A performance evaluation of the multiple bus network for
    multiprocessor systems", *Proc. 1983 ACM Sigmetrics Conf.*,
    Minneapolis, USA, pp. 200-206, Aug. 1983.

[4] K.B. Irani and I.H. Önyüksel, "A closed-form solution for the performance analysis of multiple-bus multiprocessor systems", *IEEE Trans. Comput.*, vol. C-33, pp. 1004-1012, Nov. 1984.

[5] M.A. Marsan and M. Gerla, "Markov models for multiple bus multiprocessor systems", *IEEE Trans. Comput.*, vol. C-31, pp. 239-248, Mar. 1982.

[6] T. Lang, M. Valero and I. Alegre, "Bandwidth of crossbar and multiple-bus connections for multiprocessors", *IEEE Trans. Comput.*, vol. C-31, pp. 1227-1234, Dec. 1982.

[7] D.P. Bhandarkar, "Markov chain models for analyzing memory interference in multiprocessor computer systems", *Proc. I Ann. Symp. Comp. Architecture*, pp. 1-6, Dec. 1973.

[8] Y.-C. Liu and C.-J. Jou, Effective memory bandwidth and processor blocking probability in multiple-bus systems, *IEEE Trans. Comput.*, vol. C-36, pp. 761-764, Jun. 1987.

A HARDWARE INSTRUMENTATION APPROACH FOR PERFORMANCE MEASUREMENT OF A SHARED-MEMORY MULTIPROCESSOR

George Nacht and Alan Mink

National Computer and Telecommunications Laboratory
National Institute of Standards and Technology
(formerly National Bureau of Standards)
Gaithersburg, MD 20899   USA

INTRODUCTION

Performance measurement requires a mechanism (tool) to obtain performance information (raw samples). The performance information can be placed into two orthogonal categories: (1) trace measurement, and (2) resource utilization. Trace measurement is concerned with the activities of the application or system processes, and provides information such as program execution time, execution path, response time, etc. Resource utilization is concerned with the detailed operation of the hardware, and provides information such as cache hit ratios, access delays, duty cycles, etc. Roberts [ROB86] provides a more complete discussion on performance information to be measured.

Ferrari [FER78] has classified measurement tools as either hardware, software/firmware, or hybrid. Measurement tools in all three of these categories can be used to obtain trace information but hardware measurement tools are required to obtain resource utilization information because of two major factors: (1) the high signal speeds involved and (2) the fact that these signals are not visible to software measurement tools. Software and hybrid tools are intrusive in that some additional code is executed either in the measured program or in the operating system. This affects the timing characteristics of the measured program. Hardware tools are non-intrusive, as they do not change the operating characteristics of the program.

A common feature of these measurement tools is the triggering facility. A trigger is the mechanism which causes a measurement sample to be taken. Hardware measurement tools constantly monitor the signal lines to which they are attached and cause a trigger when specific, predetermined signal patterns occur. Software and hybrid tools use either interrupts or embedded code to cause a trigger. One example of a software trigger is where each interrupt that occurs causes a measurement sample to be

---

This work was partially sponsored by the Defense Advanced Research Projects Agency.

taken which consists of the current program location. These samples are used to generate a program execution profile. Another example is the more standard software approach where the execution time of a known segment of code is desired. Two events, the beginning and the end points of the code segment to be measured, would be marked by the addition of extra code. This extra code requests from the operating system a timestamp which it stores along with information which identifies that event in the code. The time difference between the first and second events is the execution time of that code segment. In the first example the trigger is the interrupt which was caused by a device external to the measured program. In the second example the trigger is the additional code in the measured program, and is a function of the location of that code. Carpenter [CAR87] provides a more complete discussion on the entire range of multiprocessor measurement techniques and their associated trigger mechanisms.

The above measurement techniques are applicable to both uniprocessor and multiprocessor systems. For multiprocessor systems, the process of measurement is more complex due to the additional processors and the cooperating processes they are executing. Measurement tools which cause perturbations, or artifacts, in the timing characteristics of these cooperating processes can alter their execution and thus their performance. For this reason, hardware measurement tools which cause no perturbation or hybrid measurement tools which cause minimal perturbation are deemed the most desirable tools for multiprocessor systems. The threshold of perturbation that any given program can tolerate without significantly altering its execution is program dependent. In general, the larger the granularity [KRU87] of each of the cooperating processes and the less frequently communication/synchronization occurs between them, the higher the perturbation tolerance. For example, take the case of a program consisting of two parallel cooperating processes which periodically communicate/synchronize, and a measurement goal of determining this period using a measurement tool that requires 100 µsec of CPU time to acquire a sample. If this is a small grain program with an average communication/synchronization every 100 µsec, then this tool will significantly perturb the program execution, on the average 100%. On the other hand, a similar but larger grain program with an average communication/synchronization every 100,000 µsec, will only have a slight perturbation, on the average 0.1%.

Our model of the use of multiprocessors is one in which a single application program is broken into a number of cooperating processes. These processes are then distributed among the available processors to reduce the execution time. The performance concerns are focused not only on the application program, but also on the multiprocessor architecture and the implementation of that architecture. There is generally a performance hierarchy that starts at the application level. As performance is characterized at that level, there is a desire to delve into the underlying causes of the measured performance. Thus performance is measured from the application, through the operating system, down to the hardware operation. Because of this performance hierarchy, a measurement tool that is capable of acquiring performance information on both trace measurement and resource utilization is necessary.

Although hardware tools were popular in the 60's and early 70's [AGA75, FED75, NOE74, NUT75], commercial versions are almost extinct for uniprocessors [ABL85] and do not exist for multiprocessors. Some degree of uniprocessor performance measurement can be accomplished with hardware instruments such as logic analyzers and in-circuit emulators, but their ability to provide useful trace measurement information is limited and they are not currently applicable to multiprocessors.

A number of hybrid measurement tools have been designed recently, some of which are applicable to multiprocessor architectures. Hughes [HUG80] has developed a hybrid measurement tool for a uniprocessor. A similar hybrid measurement approach was used for the experimental EGPA pyramid multiprocessor [FRO83, HER82] through the integration of their hardware (ZAHLMONITOR III) and software monitors. In an attempt to measure the performance of a real-time system with but a single processor, Schrott [SCH83] has used a hybrid approach to measurement. A hybrid measurement tool developed for the CONCERT multiprocessor system [AND82] is described by Mitchell [MIT86]. We have developed a hybrid measurement tool [MIN86, MIN87] for a tightly coupled, shared memory multiprocessor which captures timestamped trace measurement data.

Our present focus is on multiple-instruction-stream, multiple-data-stream (MIMD), tightly coupled, shared memory multiprocessor systems. Based on our hybrid measurement experience and the fact that both non-intrusive trace measurements and resource utilization measurements are needed, a hardware measurement tool that is capable of accomplishing these measurements has been designed. This paper describes a design and implementation of a hardware performance measurement tool for commercial MIMD, tightly coupled shared memory multiprocessors, which is based on extensions to existing uniprocessor techniques. Although designed independently this measurement tool is similar in concept to one designed by Gregoretti [GRE86], but differs significantly in its implementation. As a result of developing this tool, we have realized that some technology trends limit its applicability and thus the ability to obtain a number of performance metrics.

HARDWARE APPROACH

Events are defined by the state (value) of certain signals. These states are called *patterns* and are user defined prior to an experiment. Dedicated hardware searches for these *patterns*, and cause samples to be taken when they occur. As these are signal states, they may be used to define not only trace information (e.g., program location), but also resource utilization (i.e., machine hardware activities).

Overview

The REsource Measurement System, REMS, consists of a number of Sample Units (SU) connected to an analysis computer via a bus, see Figure 1. An SU is the logic that captures, processes, and stores measurement samples. There is one SU for each CPU in the multiprocessor under test. Each SU connects directly to the hardware signals of a processor under test via a set of wires called probes. An SU consists of three major modules, a Pattern Matcher, a Preprocessor and a Sample Memory.

The Pattern Matcher is the logic that constantly monitors the hardware signals of the processor and compares those signal patterns against a set of stored signal patterns. When a match occurs, a trigger is generated that causes a measurement sample to be taken. The data output from the Pattern Matcher is the pattern that was matched. In general the Pattern Matcher module is concerned with obtaining trace measurement performance information acquired from the CPU bus.

The Preprocessor performs a data reduction on resource utilization events to decrease the number of samples required and/or the number of bits in a sample. There are different types of Preprocessors, but their common function is to maintain cumulative counts of the occurrence of specific hardware events. The Preprocessor, therefore, relieves the measurement system from the burden of monitoring and triggering on these frequent events and filling the sample memory with all of their occurrences, which would be reduced to cumulative counts during postprocessing. The data output of the Preprocessor is the current count values. *The Preprocessor and the Pattern Matcher of any single SU do not have to be attached to signals from the same processor.* In general the Pattern Matcher module is concerned with obtaining trace measurement performance information, while the Preprocessor is concerned with obtaining resource utilization performance information.

The Sample Memory is a large local memory which stores every measurement sample. A sample from a single SU consists of the combined data output of the Pattern Matcher and the Preprocessor. When a trigger is generated at any of the SUs, all of the SUs take a measurement sample. In this way the global activities of each of the processors under test may be correlated when any of them reach a critical point in the test program.

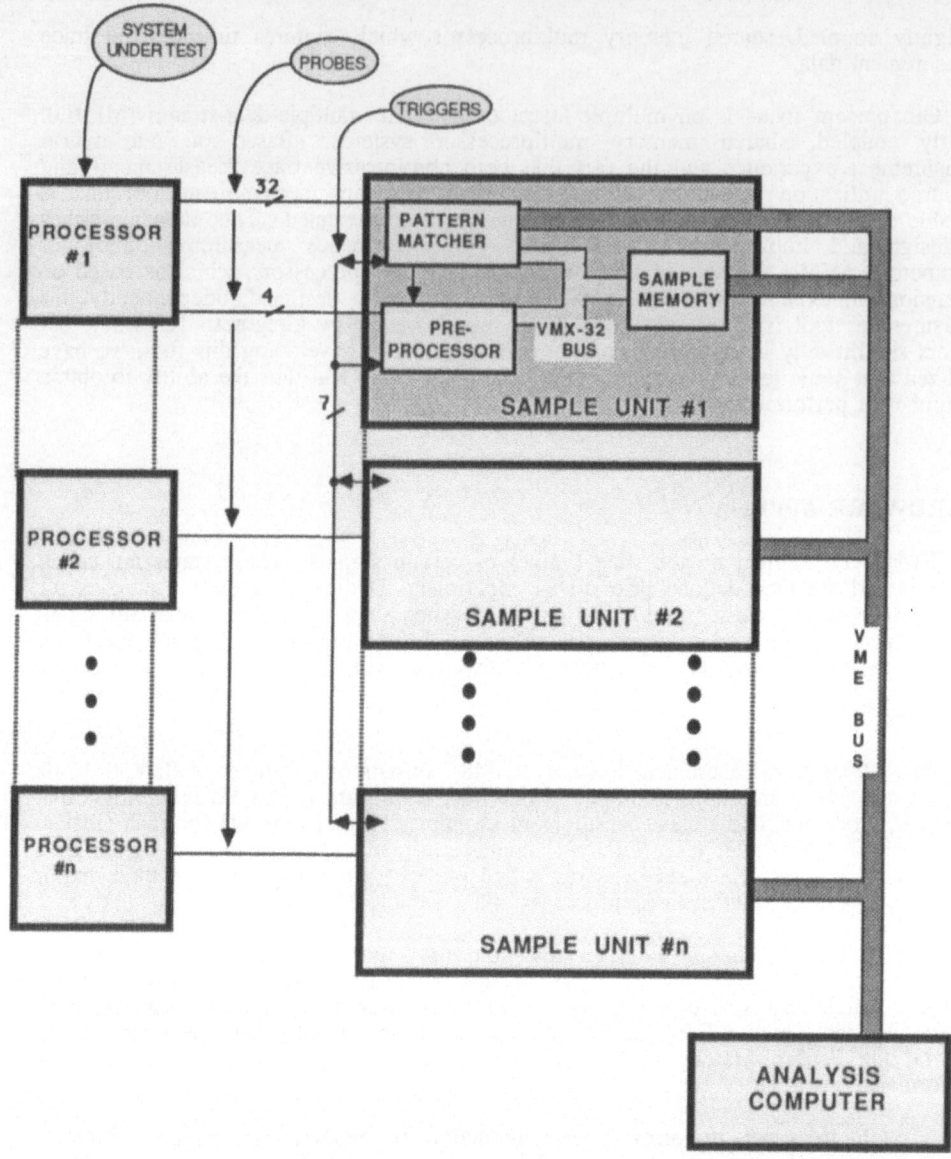

**Fig. 1. Resource Measurement System, REMS, for an 'n' CPU
Testbed System.**

Probes

Each SU is connected to the hardware signals of a processor via a set of probes. The probes have a two-fold purpose: they reduce electrical loading on the signals to which they are attached and they contain combinatorial logic with which a sample clock and state information are extracted from various timing signals. The sample clock is used to strobe a signal pattern (Trigger Data) into and through the Pattern Matcher.

The most likely hardware signals of interest to the Pattern Matching module are the CPU bus signals along with the necessary control and timing signals. The current format of this 32 bit Trigger Data is 24 bits for bus information, 4 bits for bus qualifier, and 4 bits for user selected signals. In the multiprocessor we currently use as a testbed, the 24 bits of bus information can be any one of three types: virtual address, physical address, or data. All three types of information are multiplexed onto the same signal lines, therefore, the information on the bus is timing (state) dependent. Combinatorial logic on the probes constantly monitors and interprets the bus timing and control signals and generates 4 bits of bus qualifier data. Two bits are encoded to indicate the type of bus information and the remaining two bits indicate current and previous processor mode (user/supervisor). The use of the latter two bits allows samples to be taken on the transitions into and out of the operating system. Each time the information on the bus changes, the probes generate a new 4 bit bus qualifier and cause a sample clock to capture the new Trigger Data.

Each time the information on the bus changes, the probes generate a new 4 bit bus qualifier and cause a sample clock to capture the new Trigger Data. As the bus qualifier is part of the pattern to be matched (Trigger Data), any combination of bus information types can be acquired during a single experiment.

Pattern Matcher

The probes provide a sample clock and the Trigger Data to the Pattern Matcher. The Pattern Matcher latches the Trigger Data and compares it against a set of stored signal patterns. If a match occurs, a global trigger is generated that causes every SU to take a measurement sample which provides a global view of activities. The output of the Pattern Matcher, which is used as part of the measurement sample, is the Trigger Data which caused the match.

Two design issues of the Pattern Matcher were its operational speed (100 nsec per pattern) and the ability to match an arbitrary set of 32-bit patterns which may be changed for each experiment. Either combinatorial logic or memory could be used to construct a matcher. Combinatorial logic was ruled out since it could only operate on patterns fixed at design time. Of the memory approaches, associative memory was ruled out since it is not commercially available in a size useful for this application and a custom designed one would be too expensive. Gregoretti [GRE86] used a custom designed associative memory in the implementation of his OBSERVER module (functionally similar to our SU), but was limited to only 16 patterns of 16 bits per pattern. Both Gregoretti's approach and our approach allow arbitrary don't cares to exist in the patterns. A direct memory lookup technique utilizing a random access memory (RAM) could be used where the trigger pattern is the RAM address and the contents of each memory location is a true/false indicator; true if the pattern corresponding to the RAM address is in the required Trigger Data pattern set, false otherwise.

An apparent problem with the above RAM approach is that the Trigger Data is 32 bits wide, requiring a memory of 2**32 (over 4 billion) locations. But the trigger pattern set occupies a sparsely populated state space. The trigger pattern set is very small (hundreds) compared to the universal set (billions) of potential patterns. Therefore the trigger pattern set can be recoded into a smaller state space and the above direct memory lookup technique can be used employing a smaller, thus more feasible, RAM.

A mapping is needed between the original trigger pattern set and the recoded pattern set. This can be accomplished in parallel on disjoint pieces of the trigger pattern using a direct memory lookup. This is similar to the decomposition of a single-stage combinatorial logic sum-of-products expression into a multi-stage sum-of-products expression.

Figure 2 shows a block diagram of the Pattern Matcher memory which contains two Trigger Data latches and three levels of RAM, one level for each sum-of-products stage. The first two levels of RAM handle the mapping into the recoded, reduced state space. The third level does the pattern match on this reduced state space. The 32-bit Trigger Data are latched at the input of the Pattern Matcher. This data is then divided into three disjoint segments, each of which is used as the address to one of three 2K x 8 RAMS at LEVEL 1. Only 22 bits in the output from LEVEL 1 contain recoded information.

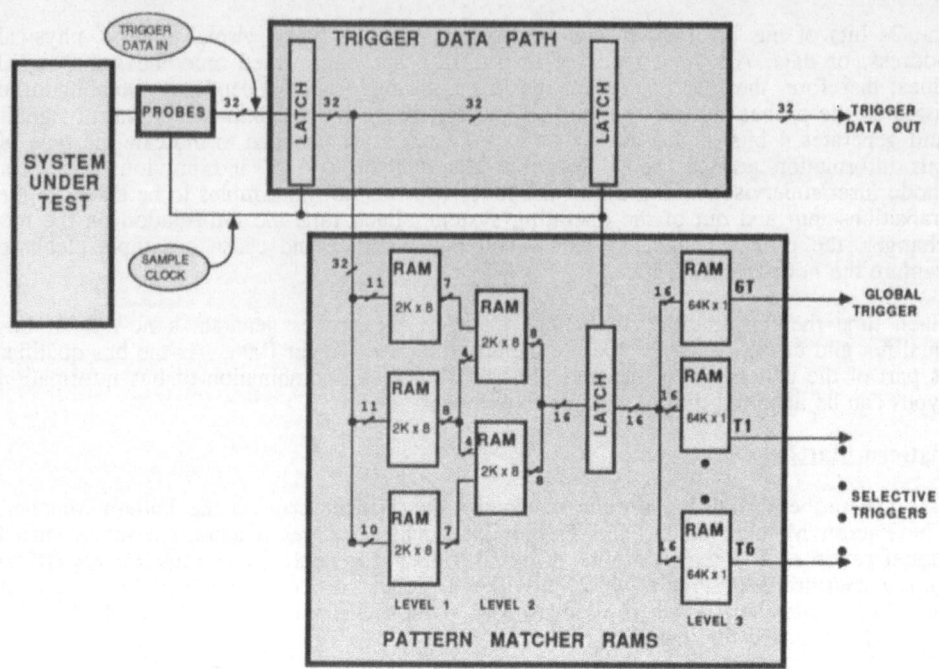

Fig. 2. Block Diagram of the Pattern Matcher Memory Which Effects an Associative Match.

They are then divided into two disjoint segments, each of which is used as the address input to one of two 2K x 8 RAMs at LEVEL 2. The 16 bit output from the LEVEL 2 RAMs is used as a common address input to seven 64K x 1 RAMs at LEVEL 3. The output from one of the LEVEL 3 RAMs is the "Global Trigger", which causes all the SUs to take and store a measurement sample. The output of the other LEVEL 3 RAMs represent "Selective Triggers" which are control signals for the Preprocessors.

The Pattern Matcher must acquire samples at a 100 nsec data rate. Since the Pattern Matcher is implemented using 45 nsec RAMs, the data needs to be buffered between LEVEL 2 and LEVEL 3 RAMs. When a Global Trigger is generated at the output of LEVEL 3, the data which caused that trigger must be available as output data. Therefore a similar buffer is used in the Trigger Data Path. The addition of a buffer between LEVEL 1 and LEVEL 2 RAMs and another buffer in the Trigger Data Path would provide a data rate of 50 nsec.

Pattern generation. Each of the SUs is assigned a 256K byte (64K long word) address block within the VME address space of the analysis computer. The analysis computer loads a new pattern set into a Pattern Matcher by doing memory writes to the assigned address block of that Pattern Matcher.

The pattern set represents events on which measurement samples are to be taken. Each bit position of a pattern may be *true, false* or *don't care*. Although a pattern may represent a virtual or a physical address, or data, along with other signals of interest, for the sake of simplicity the following discussion will assume that it represents a virtual address. A programmer will select a set of *events* within a program of interest. An *event* is normally the beginning or the end point of a section of code which is to be measured and is specified by its virtual address. The virtual address may be obtained from the compiler or linking loader outputs. A 24 bit virtual address is converted to a 32 bit pattern by the addition of the proper 4 bit bus qualifier and (currently) zeros for the remaining 4 bits. The resultant pattern set is reduced and recoded to generate the contents for the RAMs of the Pattern Matcher. A program, outlined below, does the recoding of the 32 bit pattern set and downloads the codes into the RAMs of the Pattern Matcher. The user is required to select the desired *events*, determine the virtual addresses, transform them into patterns and use these patterns as the input to the program.

The procedure used in the download program requires that any state space overlaps between patterns be eliminated, although subsets are acceptable. Patterns will overlap only when *don't cares* occur. A pattern that overlaps another pattern is decomposed into a subset pattern and one or more disjoint patterns by eliminated the offending *don't cares*, thus expanding the pattern set. The expanded pattern set is then divided into three disjoint sets corresponding to the three LEVEL 1 RAMs. Each 11 bit element of a set need not be unique but all lie within the range of 0 to 2047. The recoding procedure assigns to each unique 11 bit value a new unique 7 bit value in the range of 1 to 127. Many of the unpopulated states of the original set are mapped into a new unique value of *zero*. The original value is the address for the LEVEL 1 RAMs while the new, recoded value is the contents at that address. The recoded value for each original pattern is the concatenation of the corresponding values from all three sets, that is, the combined output of all three LEVEL 1 RAMs. The original 32 bit pattern has now been recoded and reduced to 22 bits.

The recoded pattern from the LEVEL 1 RAMs is again recoded in a similar fashion through the LEVEL 2 RAMs and reduced to 16 bits. This 16 bit representation of the original 32 bit pattern set is then used in a single-RAM, look-up technique pattern search. A value of *one* is assigned to each location in the 64K x 1 RAM which corresponds to a recoded trigger event pattern. The value of *zero* is assigned to all other addresses. When the recoding procedure is completed, the values are downloaded into the RAMs of the Pattern Matcher by writing into their memory mapped locations.

Preprocessor

The predominant function of a Preprocessor is to acquire resource utilization performance information. One fundamental type of measurement for resource utilization is accumulated counts. The main items being counted, which may occur at a rapid rate, are event occurrences and time. Some examples of typical resource utilization performance metrics that require such measurement counts are cache hit ratios, access latencies, duty cycles and elapsed time.

Although the pattern matcher could be programmed to detect and trigger on each occurrence of these events, the large quantity of data would rapidly flood the sample memory. Thus, the Preprocessors, by accumulating these counts rather than reporting each individual occurrence, relieves the Pattern Matcher from taking these samples and filling the Sample Memory with large volumes of unprocessed data.

We currently have two classes of Preprocessors. One type accumulates a single independent count whose value must be maintained and reported in full precision. An example of this type of Preprocessor is a timestamp generator, which accumulates counts of time ticks in 32 bit precision and reports the current full 32 bit value each time a trigger occurs. The current clock rate is 4 MHz, one tick every 250 nsec.

The other type of Preprocessor is used to count pairs of related events whose values must be maintained in full precision, but need not be reported in full precision. An example of this type of Preprocessor is a ratio counter, which accumulates a pair of counts to measure cache hit ratios. In this example, one of the counters accumulates memory accesses, while the other accumulates cache hits. Both counters accumulate 32-bit-precision counts. Only a single value, the ratio, is of interest and its accuracy does not require the full 32 bit precision. Since division is a very time consuming operation, the decision was made to report both numbers rather than the ratio of the two. The division is done during postprocessing by the analysis programs. The ratio is reported as two floating point numbers with separate, truncated mantissas and a common exponent. The total number of bits required to represent this pair is dependent on the accuracy required of the ratio. We expect a 3% error to be acceptable. This requires a total of 16 bits (6 bit numerator, 5 bit denominator, and 5 bit exponent) reported for a pair each time a trigger occurs, thereby allowing two independent counter pairs for each 32 bit Preprocessor sample output.

There are four types of measurements which the ratio counter Preprocessor can perform: duty cycle, average duration, ratio of events and cumulative count. For the purposes of this discussion, time is the cumulative count of some regularly occurring signal, such as a CPU clock or bus cycle clock. Duty cycle is the time a signal is active divided by the total time. Duty cycle, for example, may be used to measure bus utilization which is the number of bus cycles the bus is busy, divided by the total number of bus cycles. Average duration, such as average bus access latency, is the number of occurrences of an event, divided by the cumulative time that event is active. Ratio of events is the quotient formed by a subset of events of type A divided by the entire set of events of type A. For example, hit ratio is the number of access hits, divided by the number of accesses. Cumulative count is the total number of times an event has occurred.

The measurements taken with the Preprocessors are of more interest if taken during specific periods of an experiment rather than over the entire duration of the experiment. In order to correlate resource utilization with segments of the test program, The Pattern Matchers generate Selective Triggers which are connected to individual Preprocessors through switches that are set prior to each experiment. Like the Global Trigger from each SU that are "wire ORed" together, the corresponding Selective Triggers from each SU are similarly "wire ORed". Thus a Global Trigger occurring at any SU will cause a measurement sample to be taken at every SU. Similarly, a Selective Trigger occurring at any SU will cause the counters of all of the Preprocessors attached to that Selective Trigger to be reset immediately after a measurement sample, if any, is taken. Each of the above measurements can be taken over a specific segment of the test program if a Selective Trigger is generated to reset the counters of the Preprocessor at the beginning of the segment. The next section discusses the design of the ratio counter Preprocessor since, unlike the timestamp generator, it is a non-standard concept.

Ratio counters. Two major design constraints of the ratio counter Preprocessor are operational speed and the size of the output sample. The ratio counters have to be able to accumulate counts of 10 MHz signals, that is, 100 nsec per event. There are 32 bits allocated for the output sample. In order to accumulate counts over a reasonable experimental duration, counters of 32 bits in length are required. No practical techniques were found to keep running ratios, that is, perform the division each time a new count occurred. An alternative approach is to accumulate the two counts and then perform the division only when a sample is requested. This is possible but, due to the complexity, it is much too expensive in both cost and real estate. A remaining choice is to sample and store both 32 bit counts of the ratio and perform the division in the analysis computer post experiment. But this requires a 64 bit sample.

A pair of self normalizing counters was designed which accumulate two counts of 32 bits each. The output is the two related values represented as two truncated mantissas with a common exponent. A normalizing counter pair consists of three registers and a sliding incrementer, see Figure 3. The three registers are the 32 bit denominator register, the 32 bit numerator register, and the 5 bit scale factor register which contains the common exponent value. The numerator and denominator registers do not use a standard structure in which the least significant bit is fixed in the right-most bit position of the register and the most significant bit moves from right to left when a high order carry occurs. Instead, the denominator register uses a structure which keeps the most significant bit in the leftmost position of the register and the least significant bit moves from left to right by a right shift when a high order carry occurs. The numerator is always right shifted along with the denominator and, therefore, they may share a common exponent. A sliding incrementer is necessary to support this register structure, since the position of the least significant bit is no longer fixed but moves one bit position to the right each time a high order carry occurs. Thus, on each high order carry out of the denominator register, the denominator register, the numerator register, and the sliding incrementer are all right shifted and the scale factor (exponent) register

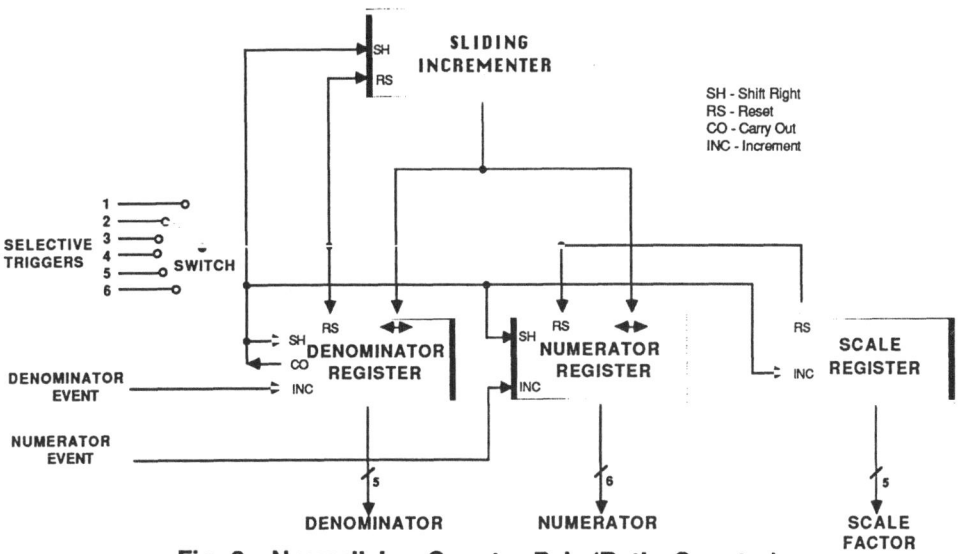

Fig. 3. Normalizing Counter Pair (Ratio Counter).

is incremented. As a result of this design the ratio counter output is always directly available without the need of additional manipulation. The exponent is in the scale factor register and the mantissas are always in the 6 most significant bit positions of the numerator and denominator registers.

This technique allows the original 64 bits (the pair of numbers) to be represented in a total of 17 bits (6 denominator bits, 6 numerator bits, and 5 exponent bits). This is further reduced to 16 bits by not outputting the most significant bit of the denominator, since it is always set (when the exponent is non-zero). A ratio counter Preprocessor output sample therefore consists of 16 bits, and, due to this condensation, two independent sets of ratio counters may be placed in a single Preprocessor, for a total of 32 output bits. The worst case measurement error is 1/D, where D is the truncated denominator count. For this case the minimum value of D is 32 which yields a maximum error of 3.125%. Higher precision ratios may be acquired by using higher precision mantissas. This limits the output of the Preprocessor to a single ratio pair in the 32 bit sample. For example, 14 bit precision in the mantissas requires 32 bits (14 bit numerator, 13 bit denominator and 5 bit exponent) and yields a maximum error of 0.013% of full scale.

<u>Sample Memory</u>

Each 64 bit SU measurement sample, which consists of the output from the Pattern Matcher and the Preprocessor, is stored in a 2M byte, dual ported Sample Memory. One port is used for inputting samples and the other port is connected to the analysis computer which extracts the samples for data reduction, storage, and analysis. Samples are taken at a maximum rate of 10 MHz. Since the Sample Memory is not fast enough to accept data at this rate, a FIFO is used to buffer the measurement samples. The global trigger causes a measurement sample to be immediately shifted into the FIFO. The measurement sample is shifted from the FIFO into the Sample Memory when the Sample Memory is available. The Sample Memory word is only 32 bits wide. Therefore the two 32 bit words of the sample (32 bits each from the Pattern Matcher and the Preprocessor) are written sequentially into the Sample Memory under control of a state sequencer, see Figure 4.

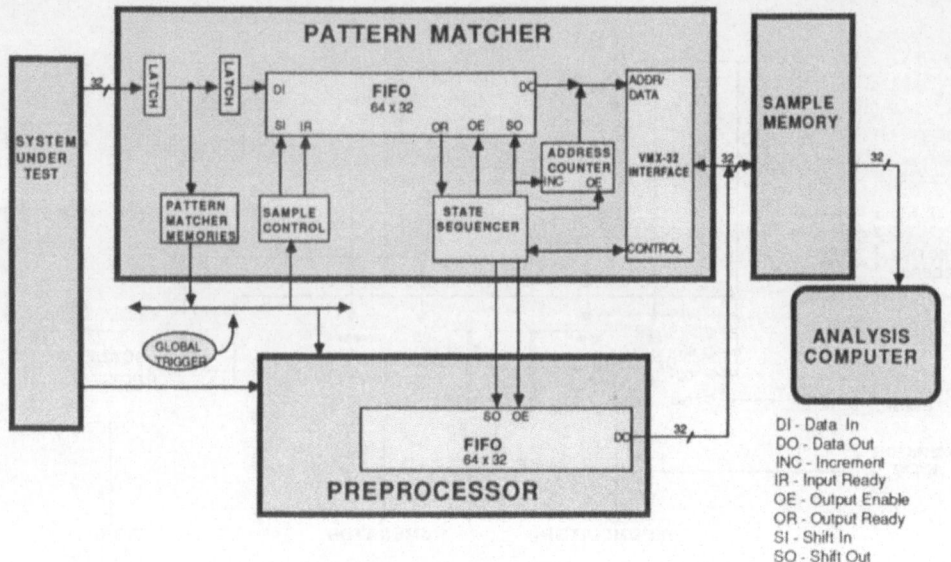

Fig. 4. Data Path of a Measurement Sample.

The Sample Memory is dual ported, thus allowing simultaneous connection and interleaved access to both the SU and the analysis computer. As can be seen in Figure 1, there is a separate VMX-32 bus segment for each SU, but only one VME bus connecting all of the Sample Memories and the SUs to the analysis computer. The VME bus is the path by which the pattern sets are downloaded from the analysis computer to the Pattern Matcher and the path by which the analysis computer reads both the measurement samples from the Sample Memory and the sample memory address counter, which indicates the number of samples taken.

A complete measurement sample, for our six processor testbed, is 384 bits wide, see Figure 5, which consists of 64 bits from each of the SUs. Each of the SUs' samples consists of 32 bits of Trigger Data and 32 bits of Preprocessor data which are stored in successive addresses in the sample memory. Note that the 32 bits of Preprocessor data from SU #6 is the timestamp for a complete measurement sample.

LIMITATIONS

In general a hardware measurement approach for shared memory multiprocessors is attractive because it is non-intrusive and can provide more detailed measurement information than either software or hybrid approaches, albeit at a relatively high cost. However, a hardware measurement tool like the REMS may have limited applicability because of three classes of problems: signal accessibility, processor architecture, and physical size of the measurement tool. Architectural problems deal with the way the software handles multiple processes and the way the hardware internally handles the data and instruction streams. Accessibility problems have to do with the way the measurement tool is integrated into or attached to the processor to be tested. Most of these problems have solutions but many must be resolved during the design phase of both the processor and the VLSI integrated circuits.

Accessibility Problems

All hardware measurement tools must connect to various signals of the system under test. For any useful tool this is really two requirements. The first requirement is to have access to the signals to be measured. Without these signals, measurement is not possible. The second is to have some means of connecting to these signals.

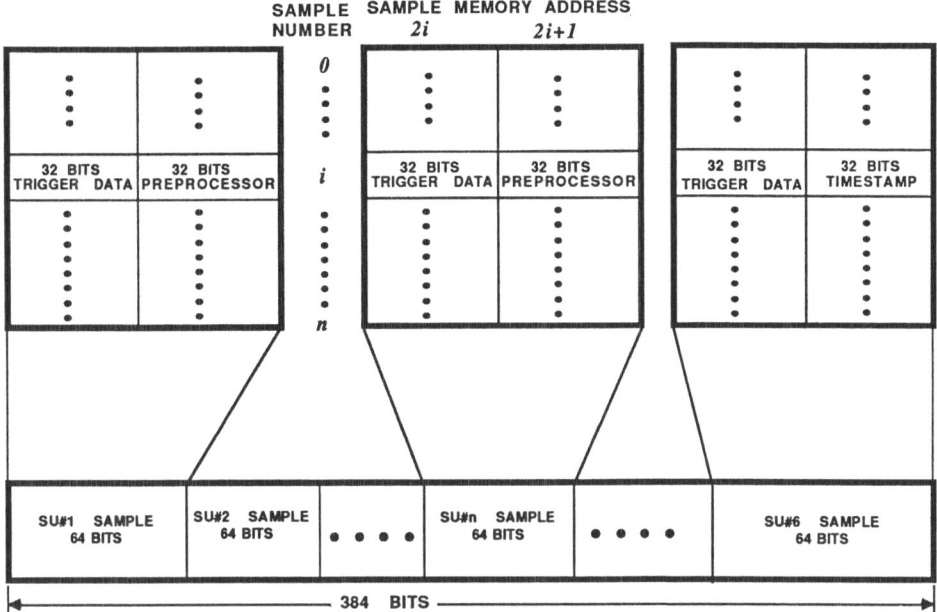

Fig. 5. Measurement Sample Format for a Six CPU Testbed.

Signal access. Among other things, hardware measurement tools need access to the virtual address signals in order to capture trace measurement information. Since all program locations referred to by the compiler, link editor, and debugger use the virtual address, physical addresses are, in general, too difficult to relate back to the program under test. Also, the physical address of a program is not known prior to run time and in many environments is dynamic and may change a number of times during execution. Some of the newer VLSI microprocessor chips have the memory management unit and/or both data and instruction caches designed into the chip. Some examples of this trend include National Semiconductor's 32532, Motorola's 68030 and Intel's 80386. This means that neither the virtual address nor the cache "hit" and "miss" signals may be available for triggering or counting purposes. Even worse, a number of accesses (instructions and data) may occur that are satisfied by the on-board caches and will never be observed by the hardware measurement tool.

The best solution to this problem is for the Integrated Circuit (IC) designers and manufacturers to design-in the *hooks*, so that, as an option, these signals could be available for measurement purposes. The ICs could be designed with extra leads to which the measurement tool could connect. These leads would provide the virtual address and necessary timing signals. This is probably not economically feasible even as an optional special purpose IC offered at additional cost to those interested in performance measurement.

An alternative solution, which reduces the need for cooperation by the manufacturers and IC designers, is to augment the strictly hardware approach of the REMS tool with some of the hybrid concepts used in the TRAMS [MIN86, MIN87] measurement tool, Gregoretti [GRE86] discussed a similar approach. Specifically, use some embedded code to trigger the REMS, thereby eliminating the need to access the virtual address. The cost, of course, would be some perturbation to the program under test. This is only a partial solution, since resource utilization signals such as cache access, cache "hit", etc. would still be inaccessible.

Signal connections. For any useful tool, other than a laboratory version, a convenient means to connect to the signals is necessary, such as a plug or connector. Without such a connector, measurement is limited to highly knowledgeable and skilled individuals who have access to the internal design of the machine which might involve proprietary information. All of the processors signal lines are available at a connector on each CPU board of our current testbed multiprocessor. The REMS probes are designed with a matching plug which makes the physical and electrical connectivity a relatively simple matter. Only a few other signal lines are required, to which "flying" leads are attached.

This connector is not available on other manufacturers' CPU boards and on newer versions of the current testbed. Without this connector two choices remain: use *flying leads* for connection to each signal line or use a daughter board. The use of *flying leads* requires very detailed knowledge of the board design. The daughter board, on the other hand, connects into the socket on the CPU board where the processor is normally inserted. This daughter board has a socket for the processor so that normal CPU operation can be maintained and, in addition, would bring out the required signal lines of the processor. In both cases significant spacing is required between adjacent CPU boards. This may not be available and a CPU board may have to be put on an extender board. This has the negative effect of lengthening the signal propagation path causing delays in some signals and may change some critical timing, thereby introducing perturbations and possibly errors.

Manufacturers could lay out their CPU boards with measurement in mind and make a measurement connection available on the board. This could be in the form of a socket or possibly an edge board connector. This may not be feasible for two reasons, electrical and financial. The addition of an extra connector along with the additional signal path length may introduce unacceptable propagation delays and reflections (even if terminators are used). In addition, this may not be economically feasible since it would increase the cost of each board. Possibly an optional special purpose board may be offered at additional cost to those interested in performance measurement, although the anticipated limited production run of these special boards may still prove uneconomical. Certainly without a reasonable user base demonstrating demand, no manufacturer would even consider such a product.

Architectural Problems

Architectural problems have to do with the way the architecture functions. Solutions to these problems, when possible, require significant design modifications by both the manufacturer and IC designers. Due to current VLSI circuit technology, it is virtually impossible to provide access to every logic signal of a computer. It would be completely impractical for any manufacturer or IC designer to even consider making this access available. So there will be operations internal to CPU ICs that affect the accuracy of measurement and yet will never be observable. In other cases the operation is observable, but it is impossible under normal performance circumstances to distinguish between a number of possible source processes, resulting in inaccuracy of measurement.

Internal operations. Similar to the signal access problem in which signals internal to an IC are not available, hidden internal operations can erroneously indicate the occurrence of an event. Look-ahead and pipelining are used on the instruction stream in order to keep the instruction queue full. Instruction prefetch is used to implement this look-ahead. In some cases, data prefetch is used for similar reasons. This could cause inaccurate measurement in two ways. First, by detecting the address of an instruction or of data during prefetch, the time that will be sampled and recorded will be the time of the prefetch and not the time the event actually occurs. In most cases the time skew will not be significant, although when very fine grain measurements are attempted these few cycles may be significant. Second, since prefetch is only a statistical anticipation of potential use and not an assured use, there is always the possibility that, although fetched, the instruction or data will not be used. But the measurement tool will erroneously log the fetch operation as if the event had occurred. The error introduced by this false trigger is much more serious than the introduction of a slight time skew as in the first error type.

There is no feasible internal redesign that will alleviate this problem. Additional complexity can be added to the measurement tool to monitor for sequences, but this is at best a half solution. An alternative would be to modify REMS into a hybrid tool and allow software triggering similar to that used by the hybrid TRAMS [MIN86, MIN87] measurement tool.

Process distinction. When acquiring trace measurement information, virtual addresses are the predominant signals on which to trigger. When there are multiple processes executing it is impossible to determine which process accessed the virtual address that caused the trigger. This is bad enough if the only processes executing on the machine are part of the program under test, but will give totally erroneous results if there are other processes executing that are unrelated to the program under test.

A possible solution involves modification to the REMS measurement tool and to the scheduler within the operating system. A system call to the operating system would be inserted into each process to be measured which would be a signal to the scheduler. Then, each time a process to be measured is scheduled for execution, either the scheduler controls a dedicated signal line which would cause REMS to turn on and off all pertinent circuits, or the scheduler would write the process number of the process to be measured (else zero) to a dedicated memory location. The latter is similar to the approaches used in the EGPA [FRO83, HER82] experimental pyramid multiprocessor and by Hughes [HUG80] in the Diamond analyzer. Both of these approaches would require modifications to the Pattern Matcher and the Preprocessor so they would become inactive when the scheduler output is zero. Again, both these solution cause REMS to become a hybrid measurement tool, since some program perturbation occurs due to the embedded code in the operating system.

Physical Size Limitations

As the number of CPUs under test increases, the number of SUs also increases thereby expanding the physical size of REMS and the enclosure necessary to house it. The current SU implementation consists of three circuit boards, each plugging into a VME slot in a card cage. A single card cage can house six SUs of the current implementation. An increase of one order of magnitude in the current multiprocessor size, from 6 processors to 60, would require 10 card cages to house the REMS.

The size of an SU can possibly be condensed to a single circuit board using VLSI. If this were the case then manufacturers would only have to offer their machines with a double sized enclosure. That is one having twice as many slots as processors so that a measurement board could be located next to each processor. But this does not alleviate the problem of connection between the measurement system and the CPU board under test.

CONCLUSIONS

The design of the Resource Measurement System (REMS) prototype has been presented as an example of a non-intrusive hardware instrumentation approach for a shared-memory multiprocessor architecture. It is able to obtain both trace measurement and resource utilization measurements. It follows the design precepts of Franta [FRA82] in that it does not interfere with the executing program and provides a global view of program activities. Of interest in the hardware design is the Pattern Matcher, which is able to simultaneously search through hundreds of patterns. In contrast, logic analyzers can only search for a single pattern at a time, and other hardware/hybrid experimental monitors [FRO83,GRE86,HER82,KLA86] can only simultaneously search for sixteen or less. We have not planned an entire measurement environment as discussed by Segall [SEG83], although we have plans to expand the user/language interface tools as discussed by Burkhart [BUR84]. Our focus would initially be to integrate and expand the existing REMS pattern assembler program with the compiler, linker, and debugging facilities of our testbed multiprocessor, in a effort to provide user measurement facilities as part of the normal compilation and execution environment.

In addition, some of the limitations of using measurement tools like REMS on these architectures have been described, as have some potential solutions to overcome these limitations. These limitations may explain why hardware monitors for commercial (vs. experimental) computers are becoming extinct.

With the current high interest in multiprocessors, performance information has become a major concern to many users. The focus of the measurements is to ultimately increase performance. It may be argued that the resource utilization information is useless or irrelevant to users of commercial multiprocessors since they can't change the embedded hardware and it's the cost effectiveness of this VLSI embedded hardware that counts. We feel that this class of user needs tools to evaluate their algorithms on various architectures. They will select the "best" architecture for their algorithms and in addition will further tune those algorithms for that architecture. These evaluations require more than just "macro" trace measurement information, such as execution time, but in addition require "micro" measurement to determine the underlying execution characteristics which includes resource utilization information.

In general, the most realistic solutions to these limitations result in converting REMS into a hybrid tool by implementing a software triggering mechanism in addition to the existing hardware pattern matching. For our testbed multiprocessor we were able to avoid many of these limitations because: (1) signal accessibility was provided by the manufacturer through an extra CPU socket on the processor board through which signals of interest were visible; (2) architectural problems were avoided since the cache and the MMU are both external to the CPU chip; (3) process distinction was overcome by locking processes to CPUs in a controlled environment. Size (cost) limitations may become a problem in the future, as we consider expanding our testbed multiprocessor from 6 CPUs to 16 CPUs. We are currently pondering our alternatives. If manufacturers would give more consideration to performance measurement tools in their product designs, even as an extra cost option, many of these limitations would be alleviated.

We feel the REMS configuration as presented in this paper is too expensive a tool for a shared-memory multiprocessor environment, especially when the limitations discussed are considered. For a hardware measurement tool, a more feasible and cost effective configuration might be a single Pattern Matcher with a timestamp preprocessor on the system bus along with a number of ratio-counter preprocessors. We feel that the Pattern Matcher and the ratio-counter preprocessor are interesting and useful items by themselves. The Pattern Matcher effects an associative match on a relatively large number of patterns, where each pattern contains the equivalent of a separate don't care mask. This could provide an alternative to associative memory which, for a size large enough for many applications, is not commercially available and is expensive to build. The ratio-counter preprocessor provides a means of condensing 64 bits of counter data into 16 bits or 32 bits depending on the accuracy of the desired result. This can be important in VLSI situations where pins are a limitation and also in data storage situations where volume is a limitation.

ACKNOWLEDGEMENT

The Authors wish to thank R. J. Carpenter for his extensive editorial comments in the preparation of this paper and for raising some of the issues discussed herein.

REFERENCES

[ABL85] Ableidinger, B., Agarwal, N. and Nobles, C., *Real-time analyzer furnishes high-level look at software operation*, Electronic Design, Sept. 19, 1985, pp 117-131.

[AGA75] Agajanian, A., *A Bibliography on System Performance Evaluation*, IEEE Computer, Vol. 8, No. 11, Nov. 1975, pp 63-74.

[AND82] Anderson, T., *The Design of a Multiprocessor Development System*, Masters Thesis, MIT, Dept of Electrical Engineering and Computer Science, Sept. 1982.

[BUR84] Burkhart, H. and Millen, R., *High-Level Language Monitoring: Design Concepts and Case Study*, in Advances in Microprocessing and Microprogramming, Myhrhaug, B. and Wilson, D. (eds.), Elsevier Science Publishers B.V. (North Holland), 1984, pp 177-185.

[CAR87] Carpenter, R., *Performance Measurement Instrumentation for Multiprocessor Computers*, NBSIR 87-3627, National Bureau of Standards, Gaithersburg, MD, Aug. 1987.

[FRA82] Franta, W., Berg, H. and Wood, W. , *Issues and Approaches to Distributed Testbed Instrumentation*, IEEE Computer, Vol. 15, No. 10, Oct. 1982, pp 71-81.

[FED75] FEDSIM, *Hardware Monitor Specifications Comparison: Tesdata Systems Corp. and Comress, Div. of Comten, Inc.* Federal Computer Performance Evaluation and Simulation Center, 6118 Franconia Rd., Alexandria, Va. 22310, USA, Report No. R-75-1, Jan. 1975.

[FER78] Ferrari, D., *Computer System Performance Evaluation*, Prentice-Hall, Inc., Englewood Cliffs, N.J., 1978.

[FRO83] Fromm, H., et. al., *Experiences with Performance Measurement and Modeling of a Processor Array*, IEEE Trans. on Computers, Vol. C-32, No. 1, Jan 83, pp 15-31.

[GRE86] Gregoretti, F., Maddaleno, F. and Zamboni, M., *Monitoring Tools For Multiprocessors*, Euromicro Journal: Microprocessing and Microprogramming, Vol. 18, No. 1-5, Dec.86, pp 409-416.

[HER82] Hercksen, U., Klar, R., Kleinoder, W., and Kneibl, K., *Measuring Simultaneous Events in a Multiprocessor System*, Proc. of 1982 ACM SIGMETRICS Conf. on Measurement and Modelling of Computer Systems, Aug. 1982, Seattle, Wash., pp 77-87.

[HUG80] Hughes, J., *Diamond: A Digital Analyzer And Monitoring Device*, Perf. Evaluation Review, Vol. 9, No. 2, 7th Intern'l Symp. on Computer Performance Modelling, Measurement, and Evaluation, Toronto, Ontario, Canada, May 1980, pp 27-34.

[KLA86] Klar, R. and Luttenberger, N., *VLSI-based Monitoring of the Inter-process-Communication in Multi-Microcomputer Systems with Shared Memory*, EUROMICRO Journal: Microprocessing and Microprogramming, Vol 18, No. 1-5, pp 195-204, 1986.

[KRU87] Kruskal, C. and Smith, C., *On the Notion of Granularity*, NBSIR 87-3605, National Bureau of Standards, Gaithersburg, MD, July 1987.

[MIN86] Mink, A., Roberts, J., Draper, J. and Carpenter, R., *Simple Multi-Processor Performance Measurement Techniques and Examples of Their Use*, NBSIR 86-3416, National Bureau of Standards, Gaithersburg, MD, July 1986.

[MIN87] Mink, A., Draper, J., Roberts, J. and Carpenter, R., *Hardware Assisted Multiprocessor Performance Measurements*, to appear in Proc. of Performance 87, Brussels, Belgium, Dec. 1987.

[MIT86]   Mitchell, S., *SySM Functional Requirements Description*, Harris Corp., P.O. Box 98000, Melbourne, Fl. 32902, Feb. 1986.

[NOE74]   Noe, J., *Acquiring And Using A Hardware Monitor*, Datamation, Vol. 20, No. 4 (Apr. 1974) pp 89-95.

[NOE86]   Noelcke, G., *Debug System Targets Multiprocessor Design*, Computer Design, Nov 1, 1986, pp 105-114.

[NUT75]   Nutt, G., *Tutorial: Computer System Monitors*, IEEE Computer, Vol. 8, No. 11, Nov. 1975, pp 51-61.

[ROB86]   Roberts, J., *Performance Measurement Techniques for Multi-Processor Computers*, NBSIR 85-3296, National Bureau of Standards, Gaithersburg, MD, Feb 1986.

[SCH83]   Schrott, G. and Tempelmeier, T., *Monitoring of Real Time Systems By a Separate processor*, Proc. of the 12th Intern'l Federation of Automatic Controls/IFIP Workshop: Real Time Programming 1983, Hatfield, UK, Mar. 1983, pp 69-79.

[SEG83]   Segall, Z., Singh, A., Snodgrass, R., Jones, A., and Siewiorek, D., *An Integrated Instrumentation Environment for Multiprocessors*, IEEE Trans. on Computers, Vol. C-32, No. 1, Jan 83, pp 4-14.

ARTIFICIAL INTELLIGENCE MODELLING OF COMPLEX SYSTEMS

Patrice Poyet and Pierre Haren

ILOG S.A.
2, av Galliéni, B.P. 85
94253 Gentilly Cédex

ABSTRACT

In this paper, we present an Artificial Intelligence (AI) perspective on the potential benefits to be drawn from the integration of knowledge-based simulation and computer systems modelling. A growing interest in the use of AI techniques in the modelling and simulation fields is discernible in both scientific communities. As AI and simulation both strongly rely on models, and as a large degree of similarity exists between the two fields at the knowledge structuring requirements level, a merging of the separate know-how is desirable. In this paper, we compare simulation with knowledge-based simulation, we describe examples of an AI approach to the simulation of complex systems, and present the related environments. We conclude with an appraisal of the possible impact of knowledge-based simulation techniques on computer networks simulation.

1. INTRODUCTION

When asked to present a paper for this conference, we were quite conscious of the challenge that faced us: we are not computer systems specialists, and we quickly discovered that the amount of reading that had to be done in order to simply master the proper vocabulary of that domain was prohibitive.

That is the reason why we chose to stick to our field, namely artificial intelligence applied to knowledge-based design and simulation of complex systems involving autonomous agents, and to the vocabulary attached to it. Therefore, this paper should be considered only as a somewhat naive analysis of the changes that AI tools and techniques could bring in the future to the design and simulation of complex computer networks and to the domain of computer performance evaluation.

Computer simulation has been a very active field, ever since 1955, when Selfridge decided to transpose simulation programs from analog computers to digital ones (Selfridge, 1955), using the new capabilities offered by programmable devices. During the same period, artificial intelligence attracted much attention as well, from journalists and scientists altogether.

The two fields evolved in separate directions until recently (Elzas *et al.*, 1986), mainly because high level languages were not mature enough, and as a consequence no complete and powerful dedicated AI tool for discrete event simulation was available.

Indeed, until recent progresses (i.e. both in hardware and software), AI methodologies were not able to offer the complex environments needed for multifacetted simulation and variable structure modelling which represent the current requirements for state-of-the-art simulations (Zeigler, 1986).

A comprehensive taxonomy of feasable synergies between artificial intelligence and simulation can be found in (Oren, 1984). This author supported the view that the models elaborated through years of research by the AI community could bring important benefits to simulation and modelling of complex systems. This should not be considered as surprising, as the main concern of simulation, generally speaking, has been to create and define models that could give a compact representation of real world entities, thus generating simulated behaviors comparable in some ways to real systems and displaying some of their key characteristics.

However simulation is a large domain and little work has been done in the specific area of computer modelling using AI techniques. We believe this is due to the fact that the majority of AI research funding was focussed on military developments such as intelligent diagnosis and classification, automated assistance (pilot's associate program), VLSI design and wargames. In the mean time, computer systems simulation continued to rely mainly on its traditional (and complex) practice. In this we include very general tools such as Simula (Dahl *et al.*, 1966), Simscript (Dimsdale *et al.*, 1964), GASP (Pritsker, 1974) and Slam (Pritsker *et al.*, 1979) or more dedicated ones as the Extended Computer Systems Simulator (ECSS) (FEDSIM, 1978), the Information Processing System Simulator (IPSS) (DeLutis, 1977) (Kosy, 1975) or even other in-house products.

Military support for hardware research and development has been available as well, but it concentrated on specialized add-on, dedicated chips, or symbolic processing architectures as the Compact Lisp Machine of T.I. (Amundsen *et al.*, 1986), or the french MAIA effort. Little was left for complex AI-based computer systems simulations, as the subject was supposed to be tackled by the computer manufacturers with conventional, well mastered and validated approaches.

This is the reason why AI languages and environments that were developed for the specific purpose of modelling complex systems, addressed other military problems such as the Strategic Warfare In the Ross Language (SWIRL) (Klahr *et al.*, 1986), the Mark system (Davis, 1986), many other research programs referenced by (Marsh, 1986), or in France the SESANE and SATAN simulators respectively concerned by the validation of weapon systems and by tactical submarine warfare (Poyet *et al.*, 1987a-b) (Poyet *et al.*, 1988a) (LLIA, 88).

The defense industry, backed by government research funding and immediate applications needs for the ambitious military programs of smart weapons, led the way in many areas such as natural language, logic, simulation and wargames, vision, pattern and voice recognition, and specialized computer architectures.

As AI researchers and developpers, we gained experience in some of the aforementionned domains (which did not include AI-based computer systems modelling), and we hope that there are enough similarities between the topics of this conference, and other aspects of AI complex simulation systems, for the analogy to be fruitful or at least provocative enough to foster some discussions...

2. SIMULATION COMPARED TO KNOWLEDGE-BASED SIMULATION

As we mentioned in § 1., both analog and digital computers have been used heavily to support simulation activities for some time now. As a consequence, specific languages have been developed to ease the modeller's work and to increase the overall complexity that could be reached by simulation systems.

We shall recall in §2.1 the motivation for simulation experiments, then give in §2.2 an overview of the current simulation systems in order to emphasize later on the differences that exist with AI approaches. This survey will be focussed on discrete event simulation techniques even if the tools described in § 2.3. present some forms of continuous processing.

2.1. Simulation - What for ?

Simulation is the process of designing a model of an arbitrarily complex real entity or phenomenon, and conducting experiments with this model for the purpose, either of understanding the behavior of the entity itself, or of evaluating various strategies for the operation of the system. Close definitions may be found in (Shannon, 1975) and in (Elzas et al., 1986).

This general definition hides the tremendous conceptual diversity of simulation systems which can be built. We gave in (Poyet et al., 1988) a taxonomy of the AI simulation systems based on an "intelligent and autonomous behavior" scale.

Another partition of the simulation systems can be done in the context of computer performance evaluation, depending on whether the objective of the study led through simulation is to characterize the steady state of any sort of queueing system, or if the concern is to simulate intelligent behaviors of individual components.

We discuss in sections § 3. and § 4. how the second objective could lead to a new appraisal of the autonomy level that should be conferred to the different sorts of components involved in computer-architectures or computer-networks.

For now, we will sketch the potential applications of AI techniques on simulation problems concerned with any one of the two objectives.

The purpose of developments on the first type of systems could be to include some "intelligent features" to existing environments devoted to queueing networks or systems modelling. This could lead to the birth of hybrid environments offering AI knowledge representation as a support to the modelling of servers, customers, queues, solvers and related components, and at least rule-based reasoning which would allow high level functionalities such as automated checking of the integrity and validity of the current design, or "intelligent" selection of the solvers. These aspects and other related possibilities will be considered in section § 2.3.

The second type of developments are concerned by a family of systems that we are more familiar with. These systems involve numerous entities whose behavior is determined by complex sets of rules dynamically allocated either by a pre-programmed task scheduler (Poyet, 1987c) or by a temporal supervisor which is acting as a discrete event simulator engine (De La Cruz, 1988). In this case, we are not any more concerned by the steady state of the system, if there is any, but by an assessment of the overall integrity of the model, and the validation of the individual behavior of each component when confronted to a realistic representation of its external environment. Applications may concern multi-processing environments, complex networks with enhanced failure-recovering capabilities, fault diagnosis, and so on.

Before considering an AI approach to computer simulation, we will present the different stages followed by a modeller, and comment on some of the present tools, with more atttention to the Queueing Network Analysis Package (QNAP2) which includes advanced functions presenting some similarities with AI concepts (Merle *et al.*, 1978), (Potier, 1984), (Potier *et al.*, 1985a-b), (Veran *et al.*, 1984), (SIMULOG, 1988).

In the modelling and simulation context, knowledge has to be extracted from a rich set of competing fields, by a multidisciplinary team of persons leading to the multifacetted concept (Zeigler, 1984). Thus, several layers of knowledge have to be collected and conflicts can arise from this heterogeneity. When faced to this too common situation, the modeller usually has to give an appraisal of one or more of the following factors:

- *Cost*:
    When a large set of design alternatives exist, a prototype may be too costly to build to reflect the overall possibilities; or the configuration studied can require daunting means as for the study of tactical situations with cooperative agents.

- *Technology*:
    When current technology cannot be used to manufacture the projected system, a model can give some indications on the behavior of future designs incorporating next generation components.

- *Applicability*:
    This is perhaps the most interesting point, as it requires reasoning capabilities from the simulation system or from a meta-system, in order to determine the appropriateness of actions or of selections embedded within sub-components of the model or of the model itself. Often simulation is performed when a formal description of the problem cannot be obtained, and the model will allow the user to understand the level of design or behavioral brittleness of the real system. This validation problem will be pointed out in section 2.4.4.

Moreover some simulation studies are carried out for obvious reasons which may concern the following factors:

- *Morality*:
    Many experiments can only be executed with models: pilot crash-landing procedures, weapon capabilities and efficiencies, war games, and son on.

- *Risk*:
    Some experiments are highly risky, as structure-stress designs.

Effective simulation is obtained by the combination of an accurate modelling phase, followed by valid testing procedures. In most systems, the observability of the model offered by the software environment allows the verification of the structural similarities between the model and reality. As previously mentioned, the gathering of statistics and many other specialized tasks such as confidence interval estimation should also be carried out thanks to the functionalities of a powerful simulation-shell and these specific requirements have led to the analysis, the definition and the implementation of dedicated simulation systems which allow efficient modelling (Potier, 1985a), (Veran *et al.*, 1984) (SIMULOG, 1988).

Nevertheless, most simulations are no trivial exercices as they are time and resource-consuming, labor-intensive and expensive. The potential gains are found in the ability of the simulator to affect decisions of some larger magnitude order in a positive way. In this context it is easy to understand that powerful tools improving the productivity of engineers, have always been considered as worthwhile and represent an economic stake and a technical challenge.

2.2. Current tools

Any kind of computer language can be used to program simulation systems, even procedural and general purpose languages such as FORTRAN, COBOL, and PL/1. These are effectively used, even if they were not specifically designed for simulation, and if they have no particular facility to reproduce systems changing over time, as it is generally required for dynamic models. Their knowledge representation capabilities are intrinsically low, as complex structures built up with nested group of pointers are rarely possible, and recursive constructions not always allowed.

The models written with these general purpose languages lack flexibility, and do not accurately reflect the modelized concepts. Therefore they should be considered as "black-boxes" that can represent numerical components of higher level systems. Their scope of application should be limited, according to the AI view presented here, to restricted sub-parts of an overall complex system, where well delineated tasks have to be performed by efficient existing "library" modules usually devoted to number-crunching.

Because these general purpose languages are unable to manage simulation-specific concepts, super-sets have been built on the top of them to provide more friendly environments for simulation purposes. They belong either to the continuous or to the discrete simulation languages classes.

Continuous simulation systems are used when functional definitions of the simulated processes are available with time as a key parameter. This class of processes is normally described by a series of difference equations or differential equations and the reliability of the model relies upon the veracity of each equation, and the assumptions on which it holds. This area will be considered as intrinsically numeric and is therefore well supported by conventional techniques.

On the other hand, discrete simulation languages have led to huge developments in order to provide the modeller with features such as time clocks, event queues, data models and structures with extended data types, analytical solvers, statistic packages, dynamic transactions, synchronization mechanisms, validation procedures, etc. They offer some flexibility at the knowledge representation level, including the definition of static entities in an object-oriented manner, and description of their associated "daemons" that should be triggered automatically by the shell when necessary. The modeller can therefore concentrate on the definition of the simulation instead of spending tedious efforts for the resolution of inappropriate problems due to some alien language. These features border those found in AI environments (§ 2.3 and § 2.4.).

Following (Rose, 1980) and (Overstreet *et al.*, 1986), four major types of discrete event simulation languages can be found:

- Event-oriented languages rely on the definition of a set of events' types and of the actions that should be triggered when the corresponding event occurs. Events to be scheduled can be managed and updated using ad-hoc policies. This event world view is very straightforward and enables powerful implementations which can deal with arbitrarily complex systems and lead to easy AI modelling.

   The knowledge-based temporal supervisor (K.B.T.S.) described in (De La Cruz, 1988) is event-based and built in with the SMECI shell (SMECI, 1988). The SESANE simulator will be described in this paper as an AI example of this class of systems (§ 2.4.3.).

- Activity-oriented languages require the programmer to identify all the different sets of parameter conditions to which the model must respond. The background task of the shell is to determine which activity is to occur depending on the current state of the simulation, then to update this state, including time conditions. We can assert that the normal behavior of the AI SMECI environment (§ 2.4.1.) is activity-oriented as the shell determines, dynamically or not, depending on the strategies used (Poyet, 1987c), which set of rules is to be pushed on the task-stack in order to be declared current. For each activity (i.e. task or set of rules) to be executed, the shell fires the proper rule (§2.4.1.), updates the state, and generates the transition necessary to restore the former state, if needed for later backtracking. The SATAN simulator is an operational illustration of these concepts and will be briefly overviewed in section 2.4.4..

- Process-oriented languages use object-based world views, and require the programmer to identify all the sequences of actions named processes, which can be attached to active objects. Processing units are attached to the proper objects, if some of their triggering conditions involve the related objects. The K.B.T.S. is also representative of this kind of system, as the rule-bases which are triggered by an event processing are selected according to the class, in the AI sense, of the object associated to the triggering event (§ 2.4.3.).

- Transaction-flow-oriented languages use the block structure of flowcharts designed to describe a simulation, and to match it with a model. Blocks are substituted by stations, and paths between the stations are defined so as to account for the observed flows. Activities lie at each station, and concurrent paths can be defined and weighted thanks to adequate probabilities reflecting the related occurrences. The QNAP2 system can be viewed as such a kind of system, even though it includes many other features.

   Event-oriented, activity-oriented and transaction-flow oriented approches will be considered from a AI point of view in section 2.4.2.; examples of such kind of AI systems will be shortly given in the weapon-efficiency and submarine warfare domains, as well as in manufacturing. Possible applications to the computer modelling field will then be discussed.

   We will now provide a short overview of conventional transaction-oriented tools as GPSS or QNAP2, as an introduction to the potential improvements AI could bring in the field of queueing-systems modelling, where the steady state or the transient states of the studied configuration are key factors.

   The QNAP2 system is a very powerful tool dedicated to the modelling of queueing-systems (Potier, 1984), especially suitable for the representation of computer systems as a network of queues and servers for the analysis of which a set of solvers is provided. This shell can be also used for other classes of discrete-flow systems.

This conventional tool (written in Fortran 77), already offers many AI-like features among which should be mentionned the following:

- an object-oriented language to describe the entities manipulated through the analysis process thanks to the command language level. This object-oriented data definition level is quite powerful: instances can be created at run-time (i.e. thanks to the "new" statement of the algorithmic language); inheritance within the classes (properties and attributes) and a form of dynamic binding, limited at the class level, are also handled by the system (for example, transactions of a given class are processed according to a behavior specific to this class). All these characteristics are very useful to perform the construction of complex models;

- predefined behaviors can be attached to the objects thanks to standard policies as scheduling, queueing disciplines, predefined routing mechanism, default solvers, default confidence interval methods, etc., all which can be viewed as a kind of logic for default reasoning, a common feature of AI incompletely specified worlds (Reiter, 1980);

- the algorithmic language level is Pascal-like, but has been extended to cope with data types such as lists, or logical selections, and offers procedural attachments to the objects in order to describe some of their properties or behaviors when processed by the simulation;

- the system offers a hierarchical modelling structure. This approach is very often taken for AI systems, and leads to represent the sub-systems as very high level abstractions;

- finally a kind of similarity could be advanced between the states of a markov-chain representing the system in changing configurations, and the views, precisely named states, of AI tools as the SMECI workbench, for example, which memorize the transient states of the modelled system between rules firing...

All these characteristics are similar to the current AI paradigms. One could envision AI extensions of the previous conventional tools, or even research developments so as to specify and develop new dedicated AI tools for computer systems modelling. The solvers could become numerical modules as mentioned in section 2.1. and be merged into the new environments as processing facilities. Section 2.3. will partially explore these exciting perspectives.

2.3. Potential AI Improvements to conventional environments

As we suggested in section 2.2., complete and powerful conventional discrete-flow modelling tools have a lot of in common with AI concepts. From this point on, we shall emphasize the possible improvements that could be proposed in order to confer more autonomy and more intelligent support to the modelling process.

The whole knowledge representation framework could rely more heavily on AI techniques, using frames or extended object-oriented facilities (Hullot, 1985) (Booch, 1986) (Cox, 1986).

For example, the powerful facilities for data encapsulation offered by the QNAP2 system (§ 2.2.) could be enhanced by a more radical object-oriented approach.

A comprehensive definition of object-orientedness is provided in (Meyer, 1988). It includes: object-based modular structures which lead to modularize any system on the basis of its data structures, data abstraction which lead to define classes on the basis of abstract data types (Liskov *et al.*, 1974), automatic memory management policies as garbage collection, hierarchically organized classes of entities to provide powerful knowledge representation schemes, polymorphism and dynamic binding (see § 2.4.1.), and complex inheritance mechanisms. It is worthwhile noticing that object-oriented languages are often built on top of LISP and that they are used in turn to develop powerful A.I. tools; we could mention Flavors for Zetalisp, CEYX for Le-Lisp, Micro-CLOS for the emerging ISO-LISP.

Thus, servers, queues, customers, resources, semaphores, can be instances of sophisticated predefined classes offering complex inheritance mechanisms embedded within hierarchically organized trees of sub-classes.

The subclasses display varying properties from the root to the leaves of the hierarchy tree, and are more specialized and constrained from the top of the structure to the bottom. Acceptable slot values are more restricted for the specialized instances, so as the associated methods (i.e. computing means) should lead to more specific behaviors.

Inference rules should be devoted to the reasoning funtions:

- checking the validity of the constructs passed on to the solvers;

- testing the applicability terms of the services during the simulation process and the synchronization or preemption conditions;

- allocation of dynamic routing policies corresponding to the customers' characteristics;

- interpretation of the patterns embedded within the packets to allow dynamic services capabilities;

- analysis of the error reports from the solvers so as to give the user a high level failure diagnosis and to appropriately select another reso-lution-package according to its pre-conditions (this is currently achieved by an algorithmic dispatching mechanism);

- cross-checking of the results with fuzzy matching between results, to characterize individual results in an "intelligent way" so as to account for their accuracy, stability, etc.,

- automatic triggering of confidence intervals computation...

High level reasoning capabilities could also be provided to describe in a user oriented manner the steady state and the transient states, if there are any, of the system.

Powerful object-oriented interface-builders, such as the AIDA tool (AIDA, 1988) can be used to generate portable customized interaction panels to control the computer modelling expert system, in order to define in a transaction-oriented manner the computer configuration, to tailor specific classes or instances to particular needs, to manually activate the solvers, to trigger services so as to check their conformity to the specifications, to visualize the transit flow, to display the steady state or transient states, etc.

In fact, the powerful knowledge representation capabilities of AI environments and the flexibility of image languages as interface-builders, could progressively replace corresponding parts of current computer modelling tools, keeping a bridge over the numerical solvers which would be rule-activated. Even if the topic here addressed was more especially concerned with complex models (i.e. extended queueing network models) for which discrete event simulation is generally the only applicable resolution method (Potier, 1988), rule-based activation of solvers for simple service specifications (i.e. simple delays) should be moreover considered as giving valuable insights to the resolution process, thus preparing interesting computer-aided education capabilities.

After this general overview of the benefits to be obtained from an AI approach to computer modelling, we will turn our attention to more detailed examples of existing AI tools and results.

2.4. AI context for simulation studies

Artificial intelligence has long searched for methods to implement models of smart independent agents in computer software (Minsky, 1975), (Minsky, 1979). Computer networks designers also rely on this analogy, and the Ethernet protocol can be viewed as a good example of the results of such an analogy. However, the difference we perceive between these efforts and AI techniques lies in the degree of autonomy that is left to the agents.

AI techniques try to model subtle behaviors arising from the interaction between complex elementary chunks of knowledge and a changing world, which includes other independent agents. The overall behavior of any system built with a large (>= 10) number of these agents is quite difficult to predict, because of the very large amount of state variables in the model. The simulation systems we worked on (§ 2.4.2.) correspond to this description and their objectives are focussed towards component behavior validation.

Some of the advantages of AI tools are linked to the embedded software engineering techniques. Among these we emphasize the following:

- An expert system approach forces a very high level description of the components of a system. An explicit formalization of the abstract data types (Liskov et al., 1974) (Liskov et al., 1986) viewed as sets of classes is necessary. Processing capabilities accounting for the objects' behavior are locally packaged, either as methods or as tasks (i.e. sets of rules or rule-bases). Inference engine strategies embody very high level reasoning functions. Therefore, the methodical decomposition imposed by the structuring requirements of AI shells allows the developpers to master more easily the complex interactions that exist between the various components, and facilitates software maintenance.

- This structuration of the descriptions offer large evolution possibilities, and facilitates local modifications of any kind of application-dependant knowledge. This is a very desirable property as for multifacetted systems, knowledge belongs to diverse fields and endures frequent updates.

- This also leads to a high degree of adaptability at the conception and utilization level, and allows easy set up of a simulation and multiple use of blocks of knowledge.

- Finally, built-in features of AI shells can be very helpful, as the explanation expert system of the SMECI shell (Dieng et al., 1987). Sophisticated trace functions, and debugging aids contribute to the modeller's productivity.

We will now present a quick overview of the present state-of-the-art in knowledge-based simulation, and then describe in greater details examples of complex simulation systems developed for the french Navy and the Renault car manufacturer.

2.4.1. What can AI environments bring ?. Many AI environments can be bought or found in research laboratories. Each of them offers different knowledge representation capabilities and inference policies, depending on the target-hardware, and projected customers. We present here a brief description of the SMECI shell, which started as a research project at INRIA Sophia Antipolis in 1984, as a way to provide multi-expert environments derived from the blackboard model (Hayes-Roth, 1984) (Nii, 1986a-b). The project is still alive and active and a kernel of the research developments has been extracted and is commercially available as a powerful modelling tool.

A short description of SMECI is justified here, as the event-oriented, activity-oriented and transaction-oriented systems detailed in the following sections rely on this expert system toolkit. To understand the structure of these simulators, the reader needs some insights on the knowledge representation paradigms of the SMECI shell.

Presenting SMECI in a few lines is no little challenge. Therefore, we shall focus this description on the main features, as an introduction to the simulation systems described later.

SMECI was initially created for multi-expert CAD purposes (Haren et al. 1985b), and it quickly appeared to be also a suitable environment for knowledge based simulation. It offers strong knowledge-decomposition capabilities to represent elementary parts of complex configurations, multiple viewpoints facilities to account for the competing possibilities in a CAD design process, powerful rule-based and method-based deductive facilities to deal with complex reasoning, a blackboard working memory, reflexive control features that offer virtually unlimited inference strategies, highly portable graphic capabilities due to the Le-Lisp virtual bitmap layer, and easy connections to procedural languages such as C and Fortran.

The simulation systems overviewed in sections 2.4.3., 2.4.4. and 2.4.5. take advantage of all of these features.

The main characteristic of SMECI resides in its reflexivity, which means that the system concepts manipulated inside the shell are implemented with the same basic bricks as those offered at the user (i.e. here the modeller) level.

This is a fundamental option which implies larger flexibility, and allowed us to implement very different systems, ranging from CAD to simulation, and even to replicate some well known AI systems such as BB1 (Corby, 1987). For example, this allows the user to filter system objects with rules, and modify them. Of special interest are the frames representing the tasks-stack, the strategies used by the inference engine, the expert system object itself...

The event-oriented simulator presented in section 2.4.3. relies on this reflexive feature, since the event processing functions accomplished by the temporal supervisor are based on the management of SMECI system objects at the user level.

The modeller can create as SMECI knowledge bases many different sorts of dedicated systems for which AIDA-built smart interfaces hide the implementation level.

More precisely, SMECI's basic inference strategy is limited to the firing of rules packaged within frames named tasks so as to explore a search tree (named states-tree) which records incrementally the modifications endured by the working memory along the resolution process. Each task at the conceptual level embodies an activity, and is represented by a complex object describing the way in which the inference mechanism should use the related rules. This task frame contains in an object-oriented way numerous data stored in the following slots:

- *list-of-rules*: a list of the rules that contribute to achieve the activity, which is scanned at runtime by the inference engine so as to determine the conflict set (i.e. the rules that can be matched by current working memory objects);

- *nbr-unification?*: a local switch that determines locally for each task how rules can be used. From the current working memory, new state(s) is (are) being generated thanks to the activation of the rules. These state creations may be limited to the first firable rule, or restricted with respect to the first set of objects stored in the working memory that matches the first firable rule so as to limit the branching factor of the state-tree;

- *order?*: a local switch that controls the order used by the inference engine to fire the rules; among the firable rules of the conflict set, the engine can make several restrictions: it can use a rule once and only once for that task, or fire it whenever possible then never activate it again, etc.

- *branch?*: a local switch that masters, at the rule level, the creation of the competing world views; for a firable rule on multiple sets of matching objects, the engine can, for example, either produce all the working memory modifications within the same state or generate for each set a concurrent world view. This is a very attractive feature as it allows control of the generation of multiple viewpoints at the task level;

- *stopped?*: and last but not least, a slot used by the problem solver to determine the next task to be considered when the current one gets stuck. Some prededefined system tasks are offered to the developper.

It is worth noticing that each rule can override the control defined at the task level, and that all the aforementioned selections are restricted to the task for which they hold.

We mentioned earlier that at runtime all the tasks involved in the problem-solving process are stored within a stack. In fact, all the tasks have been structured previously in a logical way (i.e. a tree) by the modeller at conception-time, and for each, sons have been identified and fastened to it in a static way.

Sons (which represent sub-activities), are supposed to give valuable help to the resolution process when it is stopped for any reason in a task. In that case, the sons of the implicated task can be pushed on the stack and the rules examined by the inference engine would then belong to the top-most sub-activity. When the reasoning is stopped again in this sub-activity the system will either push in a recursive way the sub-activities of the sub-activity (exploring the tasks tree) or pop from the top of the stack the current task if the job that had to be achieved is done, according of the value stored in the *stopped?* slot, that reflects the way in which the control was specified by the modeller.

All the combinations for the slots' values are valid and lead to different states-trees, i.e. different explorations of the search-space, and generate different concurrent world viewpoints (Poyet, 1987c). The task structure is pointed to by a very high level object, the context, which is indeed a system-frame devoted to the control of the overall expert system and enables the inference engine to retrieve the correct tasks.

This would be a somewhat simple framework, if the rules themselves could not modify dynamically at runtime the scheduling of the tasks-stack according to the reflexive scheme presented above, when necessary.

One can easily imagine why an activity-oriented simulation system is quite naturally handled by the SMECI shell, but we will also demonstrate that the features we described facilitate the construction of event-oriented or transaction-oriented systems.

The working memory is used to determine the sets of objects matching the premisses of the rules pointed to by the current task. Thus, according to the prevailing strategy of the inference engine (i.e. another very high level system-frame), to the current task, to the firable rules, and to the sets of matching-objects, the transitions leading from the current state (i.e. the working memory) to its sons (i.e. concurrent world views) will be generated and stored so as to enable backtracking if needed. For each new competing view, the related overall set of objects (i.e. the working memory) is in a different state and the objects' slots values affected by the rule that generated the transition have changed.

Moreover, at each inference-cycle, competing world views are compared through an evaluation fonction to determine the most promising state from which the reasoning should be resumed. This can require backtracking, as any locally attractive direction can lead further to a deadlock.

Objects are stored in a blackboard-like manner in working memory and represent the current node of the state-tree. Each node is connected through transitions to its father and to its sons (for state management purposes).

The classes from which objects are instances of are static descriptions that model the various components of the modelled system. They are structured in a tree-like fashion and they exhibit inheritance facilities. Tied-up to the classes are methods that enable computing facilities according to a dynamic binding scheme (Meyer, 1988).

We hope that the basic concepts have been introduced, so we will now focus on AI-based discrete event simulation.

2.4.2. AI Expert discrete event simulation systems. The different reasoning facilities described in section 2.2., i.e. event-scheduling, activity-scanning, process-interaction and transaction-based, can be programmed in AI environments. As far as discrete event simulation is concerned, high-end commercial AI tools appear to be powerful enough, and can lead to straightforward modelling with the major advantages described in §2.4. As pointed out in section 2.3., dedicated tools for discrete-flow systems and especially for computer pérformance modelling, including complex solvers, could be linked to the AI system. This encouraging perspective should therefore lead to short term research work, and we are aware of progress in this direction.

We will focus more precisely on AI discrete event modelling, and give as an example some insights on three specific simulators: first, an event-based system devoted to the evaluation of weapon efficiency and to the validation of a target-assignment process is presented in § 2.4.3. (Poyet *et al.*, 1988a), then an activity-oriented model of a complex submarine wargame is described in §2.4.4. (Poyet *et al.*, 1988a) (Poyet *et al.*, 1987a-b), and finally a discrete-flow manufacturing simulation, which is the closest example to the topic of this conference we dispose of, is overviewed in section 2.4.5..

2.4.3. Event-oriented simulations: the SESANE simulator. The SESANE simulator is conceived for the off-line test of real-time modules devoted to the preliminary target-assignment phase of weapon-systems.

As such its architecture includes several complex sub-systems, some of which being replicates of operational codes that have moreover to work together with very different time scales. This is the reason why an event-oriented approach was chosen, and that a temporal supervisor was built inside the SMECI shell in order to accurately manage the successive events which occur during the simulation process (De La Cruz, 1988). A somewhat simplistic description follows.

The temporal supervisor was written with documented functions of SMECI, and did not require any specific enhancements of the shell. The supervisor is represented by a regular task (with § 2.4.1. meaning) that manages the flow of events, sorts them according to their future activation-timestamps, and focusses reasoning on the object associated to each event (that is the one responsible for the event generation) with a proper rule-base which is retrieved according to the "associated object" class.
When all the sorted events are successfully processed, specialized system rules pop the top of the task-stack, in order to trigger again the supervisor rule-base that was kept inactive at the bottom of the task-stack. Then a new cycle begins...

When the processing of one event aborts because no rule of the selected task can handle it, the inference recovering processes becomes more complex. The supervisor scans the class-tree and recursively selects the rule-base which is connected to higher level classes of the event's associated-object, until the top of the class structure is reached. In this very rare case, if the event is still unmanaged, an error condition is raised and reported to the user.

Following this framework, the more specific rules and methods are tried first, and more generic knowledge is used only in case of failure. Linked to the root of each object's class, resides general purpose knowledge.
It should be noted that the length of the time period between two successive events is unrestricted, and the supervisor is able to cope with systems working with very different time scales such as the refreshing of radar data (tenths of a second), aircraft guidance (about each second), or tactical and strategic decisions (minutes or hours).

Moreover some continuous features are provided by methods and enable to assess at any given time, when interrogated by message-passing procedures, key properties or characteristics of the simulation process as for example, the location of an extremely fast missile. The supervisor described has been sucessfully tested on actual data.

2.4.4. Activity-oriented simulations: the SATAN simulator. The SATAN simulator, a marine battlefield management system written in SMECI, can be described as an activity-oriented environment. The aim is to define tactical behaviors for the agents involved in a submarine warfare scenario and to check the quality of selected actions against statistical data or techniques.

As the system is oriented towards the validation of independant agents' behaviors, it is activity-oriented so as to qualify the relevance of blocks of knowledge. Each activity is described as a chunk of knowledge involving different classes, sub-classes and their related instances, rulebase(s) and task(s) devoted to the management of the objects concerned by this activity, sets of methods accounting for the objects' responses when solicited by message exchanges, Le-Lisp packages to implement custom functionalities, Fortran or C-based computing modules, etc...

These activities are scheduled according to a well-defined framework described in (Poyet, 1987c), that can be dynamically updated by task rules (Engelmore *et al.*, 1979) which modify the tasks-stack, and therefore the schedule of future activities (refer to § 2.4.1.).

We present here a toy example of such a task structure reflecting the previously mentioned activity-oriented programming; each task in italics is located within the hierarchy according to the indentation used in Table 1., *Ship_motion* being the lowest leave of this small three level tree and *Starting_point* the topmost (Fig. 1.).

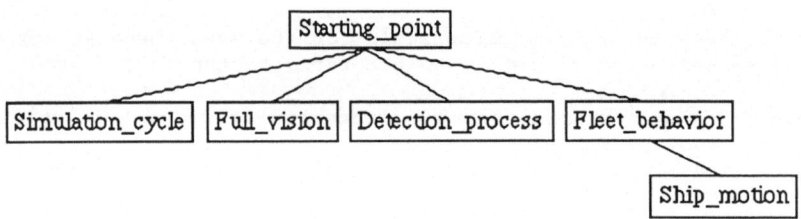

Figure 1. The tasks tree for the activity-oriented example (wargame).

We recall that for each task (a system-frame described §2.4.1.), the slot *stopped?* indicates to the inference engine which other task should be activated if the reasoning process is stopped in this context (i.e. no rule can be applied in the current task), the slot *nbr-unification?* reflects the number of times a rule should be fired, the slot *branch?* chooses to generate the transitions between the states that record the incremental modification made to the simulation (through rule firing) sequentially or in a parallel manner, and finally the slot *order?* signals in which order the rules of the task should be triggered.

Table 1. The framework of the activity-oriented example.

task-name	*stopped?*	*nbr-unification?*	*branch?*	*order?*
Starting_point	push-on-stack	first-rule-fired	parallel	strict
Simulation_cycle	pop-stack	first-rule-fired	sequence	strict
Full_vision	pop-stack	first-rule-fired	sequence	strict
Detection_process	pop-stack	first-rule-fired	sequence	strict
Fleet_behavior	push-then-pop	first-rule-fired	sequence	strict
Ships_motion	pop-stack	first-rule-fired	sequence	strict

For this simplified example, the only interesting slot is _stopped?_ which controls the way in which the activity will be scheduled by the inference engine. Very simple flags have been chosen for the other slots (Table 1.), and the incremental alterations of the model will be recorded sequentially (i.e. no alternative will be explored in the search-tree by the expert system).

So what's going to happen in this activity-oriented framework ? At the begining of the simulation, the reasoning is already stopped as no rule is available for the _starting_point_ task (of course we did it on purpose...); so the inference engine looks at the _stopped?_ slot and "push-on-stack" (Table 1.) the sons of the current task (i.e. the whole sub-tree). Then all the sub-tasks will successively pop the task-stack, with the exception of _fleet_behavior_ that will push its son when the reasoning will stop there. Finally, the system will come back in the _starting_point_ state, where a new cycle begins (Fig. 2.).

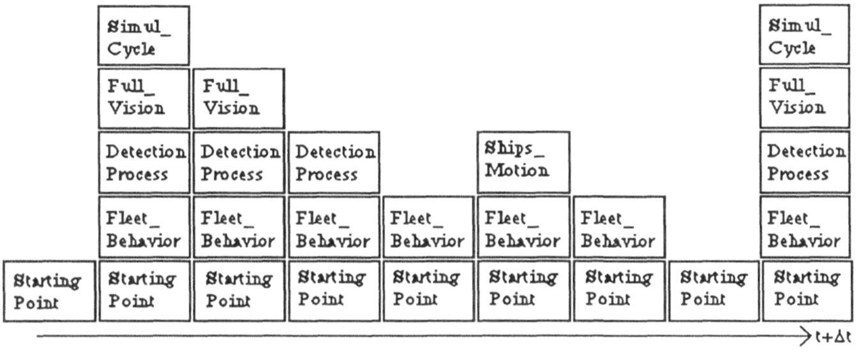

Simul_ Cycle								Simul_ Cycle
Full_ Vision	Full_ Vision							Full_ Vision
Detection Process	Detection Process	Detection Process		Ships_ Motion				Detection Process
Fleet_ Behavior	Fleet_ Behavior	Fleet_ Behavior	Fleet_ Behavior	Fleet_ Behavior	Fleet_ Behavior			Fleet_ Behavior
Starting Point	Starting Point	Starting Point	Starting Point	Starting Point	Starting Point	Starting Point	Starting Point	Starting Point

$\longrightarrow t + \Delta t$

Figure 2. The evolution of the simplified task-stack example (activity-oriented).

As you can imagine this kind of simulation never ends, and appropriate rules should test for a termination condition (no more threats for the reference-ship in the wargame example could be a reasonable test).

The actual system is much more complex, because in this case each task is a sophisticated compound frame pointing to the related rules, to the proper parameters used for the inference engine, and can develop competing worlds in the simulation process (refer to the parallel flag of § 2.4.1.), leading the way to non-deterministic behaviors. Moreover the triggering of the activities is not as static as described above, and rules can themselves alter the task-stack in order to react to any kind of event (i.e. the whole event-oriented system described in section 2.4.3. relies on this ability).

Nevertheless, the control structure of SATAN is made of the same building-bricks as those of the toy-example, and is devoted to an activity scheduling which only ends when one of the termination conditions is satisfied.

What should be emphasized here, is that the objective of this kind of simulation is of a higher level than what we have discussed so far. Among the components involved by the system, many of them have a completely autonomous behavior, not such as the one conferred for any class of usual automaton, but have access to the decision level for the simulation purposes. These modules aim to be on a par with human specialists (i.e. captains) and have to take difficult decisions (i.e. piloting, resources

279

allocation) with respect to the fuzzy world-view they possess through sophisticated filters (i.e. processed signals coming from sensors, etc.).

What should be kept in mind here, in respect of computer modelling, is that, in this case, we deal with very autonomous agents influencing each other through their changing observable state variables. Indeed, each agent, according to its fuzzy world-view, has to decide of some actions which will subsequently modify the world-view of other agents.

For doing so, each agent uses various knowledge, among which heuristic rules and non-deterministic sequences of trials-errors, so as to determine the "best" action (in a non-optimal sense).

The bottleneck for this kind of system is of course validation, as a heuristic component is part of the model and accounts for its internal "intelligent activity"; following (de Kleer, 1986), "as most problem-solvers search", the system will behave in a non-deterministic manner, in order to explore different search-trees for which many sequences of trials and errors can be required.

The validation of a complete system presenting such a behavior is complex and can affect various levels. An isolated action can involve some local search-tree representing, for a war-game, a "game within the game" or look-ahead phases leading to choices difficult to justify because of the fuzzy perception of each agent. For a complete model which relies on fuzzy logic and includes some randomness, the validation should lead to an evaluation of a "statistical behavior" deemed to be satisfying, thanks to monte-carlo techniques.

Of course, as for most difficult problems of this kind, a step by step approach is followed and successive validations for simulations of increasing complexity are attempted. For each step traditional validation techniques are used. For this purpose, a very high level interface is developed so as to control more and more complex simulations involving more and more sub-tasks. The first steps are dependant of simple toggles that influence greatly simulation runs. The following incremental steps can be adopted, for example, for the easy-to-understand target-location problem:

- the observer possesses the accurate position of the targets;

- the system simulates approximate positions and kinematic-parameters in agreement with the observer's bearing-measurements;

- each observer tries to determinate its targets' position and kinematic according to target motion analysis techniques for simple noise distribution and fixed standard-deviation;

- same as above, but the noise on the bearing-measurements is characterized by a variable standard-deviation;

- same as above for different biased-distributions of external noises;

- etc ...

Of course, many other topics are relevant for such a simulation, and our approach has been to include within the simulation system some sorts of expert aids (Sargent, 1986) (Balci et al., 1984), accessible through very sophisticated control panels. The need for very high level interfaces appeared early, to give a flexible and accurate account of the parameters of the simulation: i.e. to proceed to incremental validation procedures, to offer a suitable control on the running process, and to give an understandable picture of the simulation.

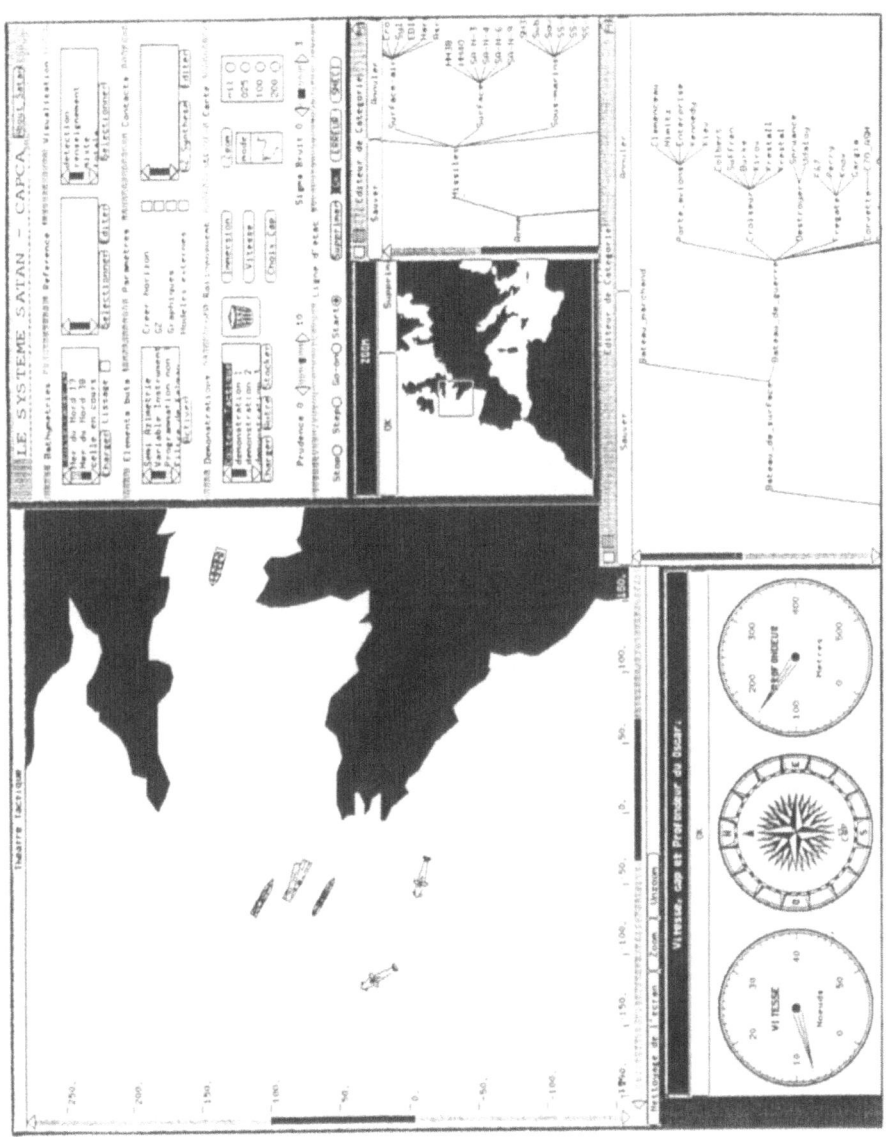

Figure 3. An overview of the submarine warfare simulator: SATAN.

Figure 3. is an illustration of the aforementioned concepts, and presents a hardcopy of the running process for the SATAN system, showing some of the very high level functions offered at the user level so as to control the simulation.

This interface is naturally object-based, and abstract entities have been modelled as SMECI frames (i.e. scale, map, coasts, polygons, points and other objects as the SATAN control panel), each of them being hierarchically-linked, and having a corresponding AIDA frame interpreted by the graphical manager as an instance of an image (Schneider, 1988). When a user's request, or a reasoning action, modifes the SMECI structures, daemons automatically updates the AIDA level, thus enabling the image manager to modify the view of the different elementary pictures which forms the current screen.

We hope this system gives a good insight on the ability of AI techniques to modelize activity-oriented systems, even if an extrapolation is needed with respect to computer systems modelling. The last simulator presented will try to bridge part of this gap, with a discrete-flow manufacturing example based on the same basic techniques (in the AI sense), but leading to a transaction-oriented world view.

2.4.5. Flow-oriented simulations: a manufacturing example. The STICS project, conducted in cooperation with Renault's Research Laboratories, is an example of a manufacturing problem. The "Régie Renault" after a survey of different general purpose simulation packages, used as a first approch the QNAP2 system (§ 2.2.) to cope among other objectives with production forecasts of flexible workshops, then developed in-house software able to handle in a more specific way their applications. The approach chosen for the STICS project is very similar to the one that could be used so as to develop an AI-based computer-modelling system.

Indeed, the workbench is described according to a transaction-oriented view, thanks to a very high level AIDA-interface that enables to configurate interactively the production line.

Machines (respectively servers), pieces to be produced (respectively customers), paths between the stations (respectively lines), are created thanks to graphical functions accessed through a pointing device.

Corresponding SMECI frames are automatically created taking into account the classes and sub-classes of the specified items, and linked together with respect to the configuration defined at the interactive level. The assembly is then rule-tested in order to check for the quality of the user data, and the corresponding memory-structures are produced so as to activate the in-house solvers mentioned above. When the input is not in solver-acceptable form, but that knowledge exists to rewrite the schema to make it acceptable, the rules also perform automatic data rewriting before the computation phase.

As in traditional computer-modelling, different solvers are used depending on the refinements of the model. The exact analysis of limited-size/limited-complexity configurations can be achieved thanks to a markovian solver, and for very sophisticated models, discrete event simulation can be used (of course this could be handled by AI techniques as well but the previously in-house solvers had to be reused).

Current design flaws are detected during the analysis, and the system can be used to modify the current configuration, and to iterate the process

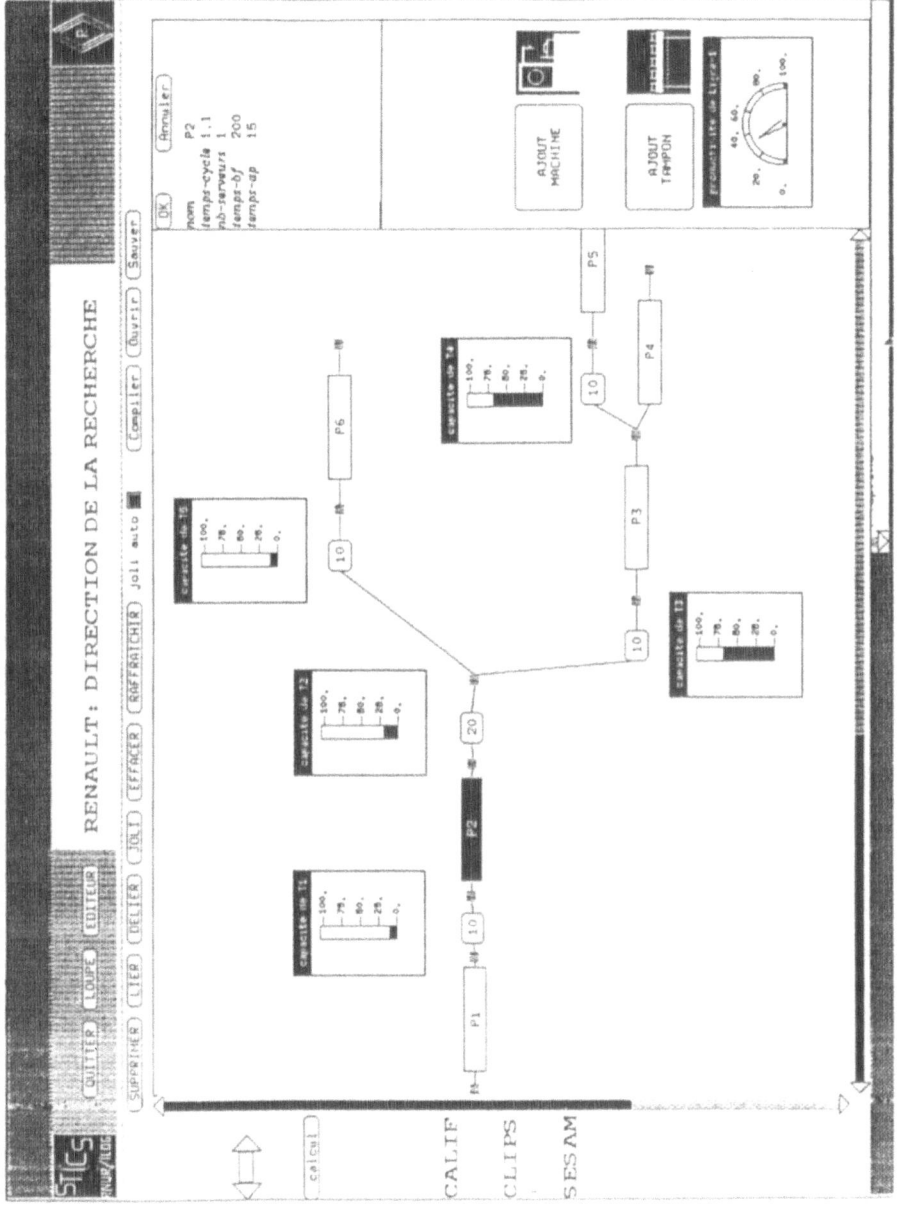

Figure 4. A manufacturing example of a discrete-flow system: the STICS project.

until a satisfying design is reached. Iteration cycle is very fast (less than a second for a graphic modification of a value, recomputation through the markovian solver and upgrade of the display).

Figure 4 gives an overview of the system and illustrates some of the concepts presented in section 2.4.4.

3. WHICH CHANGES WILL AI BRING TO COMPUTER NETWORKS

We believe that AI will bring a few changes to the design and simulation of complex discrete-flow systems, and of course sophisticated computer-networks modelling falls within this scope:

- first, the design of elementary components will rely more and more on AI techniques, that will in turn be incorporated into these components;

- consequently, these elementary components, whose behavior was modeled rather simply as on/off systems, will become more and more autonomous, and this will in turn modify the overall behavior (and model) of computer networks. A parallel can be drawn with the submarine warfare simulator described § 2.4.4. that involves very autonomous components simulating human decisions ;

- third, the design and operation of large computer networks will certainly benefit from AI simulation techniques such as the ones we described in the previous chapter in sections 2.3., 2.4.1. and 2.4.2.

For all these reasons, we are quite certain that in the future, the majority of the tools that will be used for computer networks design and performance prediction will mix AI techniques with the firmer mathematical theories that are developed and presented in this conference.

3.1. Elementary component behavior

By "elementary component", we mean a part of a computer network of the size and complexity of, for example, a modem. The point we shall make here is that the complexity of the behavior of such components in case of failure will dramatically increase due to the integration of AI techniques into such components.

Two years ago, we worked with researchers of IBM-LaGaude on an expert system for modem failure diagnosis (Eike *et al.*, 1986). The modems they designed were usually linked to mainframes where a complex maintenance program was activated in case of failure along the connexion links (Huon *et al.*, 1981).

This program was difficult to maintain partly because it was written in a procedural language and partly because of the length of the chain of transformations that was imposed on the knowledge of the expert modem designers before it became machine executable. In other words, so many people were involved in the creation process of this maintenance software that the propagation of any modification of the design of the modems to the maintenance software was extremely slow.

We were involved in a joint program during which we rewrote a large part of this maintenance software with expert system technology. This project was successful (we believe it became an internal IBM project), and brought forth a few interesting conclusions:

- in order to produce a good maintenance program, an equally good configurator was needed: to test the expert system maintenance program on numerous different configurations, an assistant configurator was needed, to correctly set the tens or hundreds of parameters that had to be known to correctly describe a network. During the validation phase, this correct description was locally altered to simulate different failure modes. Producing the configurator with AI techniques was neither new (McDermott, 1980), (McDermott, 1981), nor difficult. It showed however that even diagnosis tasks could require simulation techniques in order to build the associated maintenance program ;

- maintenance of such an expert system seemed much easier for the modem designers than maintenance of their former software ;

- failure of a component in a complex link involving several modems and telephone lines could foster a flurry of activities on the network during the fault detection phase. Facilitating the comprehension of the maintenance algorithm to the modem designers allowed them to think of more complex queries to refine the diagnostic, and these queries in turn required more information transmission...

In this project, the maintenance software was executing on a mainframe to which the faulty modem was linked. However, current microprocessors are powerful enough to run large AI programs. The japanese software manufacturer CSK already records educational AI programs on PROMs that eliminate the necessity of magnetic mass memory. It is therefore quite obvious that in the near future "elementary" components will be given some autonomy for failure recovery. One can even assume that normal operation will increasingly rely on "smart" local decisions.

As a consequence, the information transmission pattern of networks of such autonomous agents could behave quite differently than that of present systems. If each individual behavior is quickly adjusting to the multiple parameters describing its environment, and if the decision process is complex enough, it is not clear to us that any mathematical model of the behavior of large populations of these entities will have more predictive abilities than economics, for example !

As usual, fortunately, the same technology that improved the missile can also improve the anti-missile, and the AI-based modelling of complex systems, using the techniques presented in sections 2.3. and 2.4., can be considered as a possible way to help the design phase of such nets involving multiple interacting autonomous agents.

3.2. AI techniques for network management

We are aware of as yet unpublished work on the use of AI techniques for computer network management.

It is a large private project concerned with real-time management of a cluster of mainframes. The project used extensively the blackboard concept. This concept is particularly useful in the cases where a "democratic supervisor" is required: multiple "knowledge sources" continuously observe a common database of facts about the local world, and ask for the right to modify these facts when some conditions are met in the data base. The central controller chooses among the currently active knowlege sources and let the most interesting one modify the database.

This general scheme is quite adapted to constantly changing data, multiple semi-independant agents, with the presence of an "opportunistic scheduler". The latter will not distribute scarse ressources according to a master plan, but as the need arises, and to the most needed places.

The network supervisor we observed achieved a very good performance (about a hundred decisions per second) and appeared quite easy to maintain thanks to its modular architecture. We believe it is only the first of a large number of such AI network management tools.

4. IMPACT OF KB-SIMULATION ON COMPUTER-NETWORK SIMULATION

We believe that knowledge-based simulation can be used economically as a tool to model all sorts of discrete-flow systems involving resource contention problems (§ 2.4.5.), as for example, large computer networks during their design phase. In this context, an AI simulation program would bring the following benefits :

- a powerful support for knowledge structuring (§ 2.4.1.), offering the complete functions of an object-oriented language, with specific AI-based capabilities such as daemons to master side-effect requirements (i.e. as siblings synchronization for computer modelling for example), active values (especially useful for graphical side-effects) (Stefik et al., 1983), symetric links between objects (SMECI, 1988), automatic management of objects' dependencies, reflexivity to build powerful and specialized-models made of reusable bricks, etc. ;

- an easy access to data-bases describing a comprehensive behavior of individual components of the network ;

- very high level reasoning functions, obtained by powerful rule-based mechanisms (§ 2.3.) ;

- new validation techniques, relying on embedded incremental expert-assistants (§ 2.4.5) accessible through custom graphic interfaces (Fig. 3 and Fig. 4) ;

- hybrid, hierarchical and cost effective approaches, either event-oriented, activity-oriented or transaction-oriented, built on the top of the same reflexive tools, to offer different world-views of complex models for which discrete-event simulation is often the only possible resolution-method ;

- object-based interfaces to edit and modify networks in various ways (§2.4.5.), and powerful control panel to control the simulations.

Developers now have the choice between two approaches:

They can create "smart front-ends" to advanced traditional simulation softwares that would become easier to use thanks to, for example, automatic rule-based solver selection, or automatic hierar-chical decomposition to simulate parts of the designed networks.

They can also develop specific AI tools for computer modelling purposes taking advantage of the experience acquired in both domains. These two approaches can lead to comprehensive software which would include numerous exact or approximate solvers, handle different world views as discussed in sections 2.4.3, 2.4.4, 2.4.5., and offer high level functions for control, representation, education, validation, etc.

5. CONCLUSION

We hope we gave the (courageous) reader a feel for the reasons why AI could be increasingly involved in the design of complex systems. We sketched current achievements of knowledge-based simulation techniques (§2.3. and § 2.4.1.) and results (§ 2.4.2.). We projected these known trends to computer network design and simulation (§ 3.), and proposed a somewhat optimistic view of the benefits and pains for the field of computer modelling brought forth by new AI software engineering techniques.

It is mentionned in (Potier, 1988) that queueing network theory can solve 25 % of the problems submitted by the end-users with efficient and exact methods. We tried to show why AI techniques can contribute to the resolution of a fraction of the remaining 75 %. It is now simply a matter of hard work, substantial financial backing and stronger communication between the specialists of the two fields before these sketchy directions become operational programs...

Acknowledgments

Quotations from the papers listed in the bibliography have sometimes been freely made when compiling this paper and the help of their authors is gratefully acknowledged. The opinions expressed are however, those of the authors, and do not necessarily represent those of any other person who bear no responsibility for any remaining flaws. Valuable support for the writing, the illustration of this paper, and the development of the presented systems, was provided by the whole staff of ILOG S.A., and it is a pleasure to acknowledge the major contributions of Philippe De La Cruz for the SESANE system, of Manuel Montalban and Patrick Albert for the manufacturing simulator and the related illustrations, of graduate students from Ecole Supérieure de Physique de Marseille (ENSPM) among whom special thanks are due to Jean-Yves Schneider, Bruno Favennec, Jean Stéphane Villiers and to Louis Arrivet from ESIEA (Paris) for their contribution to the SATAN system. Work on the SESANE and SATAN systems was supported by the French Navy (CAPCA), and the manufacturing research system was financed by Renault's Direction de la Recherche.

REFERENCES

Note: *for all publications of historical importance, the oldest retrievable reference has been selected.*

AIDA, 1988. AIDA a Powerful LISP Portable Interface Builder, ILOG S.A., manuel de référence v 1.2.

Amundsen, M., Kastner B., Krueger, S., Manuel, G., Matthews, G., Prentice, R., Watson, M., 1986. Compact Lisp Machine, T.I. Engineering Journal, January-February 1986, Vol 3, n° 1, pp. 116-121.

Balci, O., Sargent, R. G., 1984. A bibliography on the credibility, assessment, and validation of simulation and mathematical models. Simuletter, Vol 15, n° 3, pp.15-27.

Boock, G., 1986. Object-Oriented Development, IEEE Trans. on Software Engineering, vol. SE-12, n°2, pp. 211-221.

Charniak, E., Riesbeck, C. K., Mc Dermott, D. V., 1980. Artificial Intelligence Programming. Lawrence Erlbaum Associates, Publishers, Hillsdale, New Jersey, 323 pp.

Clayton, B., 1985. The ART Programming Tutorial, Vol 1, 2, 3, respectively: 138 pp., 158 pp., 102 pp.

Corby, O., 1987. BB1 en SMECI, 6ème Congrès Reconnaissance des Formes et Intelligence Artificielle de l'Association Française de Cybernétique Economique et Technique, Dunod ed., pp. 581-586.

Cox, B. J., 1986. Object-Oriented Programming: An Evolutionary Approach, Addison-Wesley, Reading (Mass.).

Dahl, O. and Kristen Nygaard, 1966. SIMULA - An ALGOL-Based Simulation language, Communication of the ACM, Vol 9, n° 9, pp. 349-395.

Davis, P. K., 1986. Applying Artificial Intelligence Techniques to Strategic-Level Gaming and Simulation, in: (Elzas et al., 1986), pp. 315-338.

de Kleer, J., 1986. An Assumption based Truth Maintenance System. AI Journal 28, pp. 127-161.

De La Cruz, P., 1988. Intelligent Event Oriented Simulations, ILOG S.A., to be published

DeLutis, T. G., 1977. A Methodology for the Performance Evaluation of Information Processing Systems", Final Report to the National Science Foundation, OSIS, GN36662.

Dieng, R., Corby, O., Haren, P., 1987. Un Système Expert Explicateur, Cognitiva 87.

Dimsdale, B. and Markowitz, H. M., 1964. A description of the SIMSCRIPT language, IBM Systems Journal, Vol 3, n° 1, pp. 57-67.

Eike, J. K., Cayeux, E., 1986. DIANES Project, DESS-ISI Project Report, INRIA Sophia Antipolis, 30 pp.

Elzas, M. S., Ören, T. I., Zeigler, B. P., 1986. Modelling and Simulation Methodology in the Artificial Intelligence Era, in: Elzas, Ören, Zeigler (Eds), Elsevier Science Publishers, North-Holland, 423 pp.

Engelmore, R., Terry, A., 1979. Structure and Function of the CRYSALIS System. Proc. 6 th Int. Joint Conf. on Artificial Intelligence, pp. 250-256.

Haren, P., Neveu, B., Corby ,O., Montalban, M. , 1985a. "MEPAR: Un moteur d'inférences pour la conception en ingenierie". 5 ème Congrès Reconnaissance des Formes et Intelligence Artificielle de l'AFCET, Grenoble, 27-29 Novembre 1985, Dunod ed., pp 1273-1280.

Haren, P., Neveu, B., Giacometti, J.P., Montalban ,M., Corby, O., 1985b. "SMECI: Cooperating Expert Systems for Civil Engineering Design". SIGART Newsletter, April 1985, Number 92, pp 67-69.

Hayes-Roth B., 1984. BB1: An architecture for blackboard systems that control, explain and learn about their own behavior". HPP Report n° HPP-84-16, 22pp.

Hopper, G. M., 1952. The Education of a Computer. in: Proceedings Pittsburg Meeting of the ACM, May '52.

Hullot, J. M., 1985. CEYX - Version 15. Rapports de Recherche INRIA n° 44 et n° 45, pp. 19 et pp. 83.

Huon, S., Smith, R., 1981. Network Problem-Determination Aids in Microprocessor-Based Modems, IBM Journal of Research and Development, n°1, 25, 1981.

Klahr, P., Waterman, D. A., 1986. Expert Systems, Techniques, Tools, and Applications, Addison Wesley, 441 pp.

Kosy, D. W., 1975. The ECSS II Language for Simulating Computer Systems, R-1895-GSA, December, 1975, Rand Corporation, Santa Monica, CA.

Liskov, B. H., Zilles, S. N., 1974. Programming with Abstract Data Types, Computation Structures Group, Memo n° 99, MIT Project MAC, Cambridge (Mass.).

Liskov, B. H., Guttag, J., 1986. Abstraction and Specification in Program Development, MIT Press, Cambridge (Mass.), 1986.

LLIA 1988. *La Lettre de l'I. A.*, n° 40, Juillet-Août 1988, Chez qui ?: DCN de Toulon, pp. 4-5.

Marsh, A. K., 1986. Guide to Defense and Aerospace Expert Systems, High Technology, Pasha Publications, Arlington, VA, 136 pp.

McDermott, J., 1980. R1: a Rule-Based Configurer of Computer Systems, Carnegie Mellon University, Report cs-80-119, April 1980.

McDermott, J., 1981. R1's Formative Years, *AI Magazine*, Vol. 2., n° 2, summer 1981, pp. 21-29.

Merle, D., Potier, D., Veran, M., 1978. A Tool for Computer Performance Analysis. Proc. Int. Conf. on Performance of Computer Installations, North-Holland, pp. 195-213.

Meyer, B., 1988. Object-oriented Software Construction, Prentice Hall International Series in Computer Sciences, 534 pp.

Minsky, M., 1975. A framework for representing knowledge, *in*: P. Winston (Ed.), The Psychology of Computer Vision, McGraw-Hill, New York.

Minsky, M., 1979. K-lines: A theory of memory, MIT AI Lab., Memo 306.

Nii, P., 1986a. "Blackboard systems: the blackboard model of problem solving and the evolution of blackboard architectures". *AI magazine*, summer 1986, pp. 38-53.

Nii, P., 1986b. "Blackboard system, blackboard application system, blackboard systems from a knowledge engineering perspective". *AI magazine*, august 1986, pp. 82-106.

Ören, T. I., 1984. Model-Based Activities: A Paradigm Shift. *in*: Simulation and Model-Based Methodologies: An Integrative View. Ören, Zeigler, Elzas (Eds), Springer Verlag, Heidelberg, pp. 3-40.

Overstreet, C. M., Nance, R. E., 1986. World View Based Discrete Event Model Simplification. *in*: loc. cit. (Elzas *et al.*, 1986), pp. 165-179.

Potier, D., 1984. New User's Introduction to QNAP2, Rapport Technique INRIA n°40.

Potier, D., (Ed.), 1985a. Modelling Techniques and Tools for Performance Analysis, North-Holland.

Potier, D., Veran, M., 1985b. The Markovian Solver of QNAP2, Rapport Technique INRIA n° 49.

Potier, D., 1988. The Modelling Package QNAP2 and Application to Computer Networks Simulation, Thomson-CSF, LCR, Orsay - France, 31 pp.

Poyet, P., De La Cruz, P., 1987a. "Simulation Navale en Environnement Hostile". Actes de l'Ecole d'Automne d'Intelligence Artificielle. Institut d'Expertise et de Prospective de l'Ecole Normale Supérieure de la rue d'Ulm - Société Thomson, 10pp.

Poyet, P., Haren, P. , De la Cruz, P., 1987b. "Un système expert de simulation navale". 6ème Congrès Reconnaissance des Formes et Intelligence Artificielle de l'AFCET, Dunod ed, pp. 587-592.

Poyet, P., 1987c. "La structure de contrôle dans les systèmes experts de simulation". 6ème Congrès Reconnaissance des Formes et Intelligence Artificielle de l'AFCET, Dunod ed., pp. 723-738.

Poyet, P., De La Cruz P., 1988a. "Une Nouvelle Classe de Simulateurs Destinée aux Aides Tactiques et aux Systèmes d'Armes". Actes des Conférences Spécialisées (Science et Défense), Huitièmes Journées Internationales sur les Systèmes Experts et leurs Applications - Avignon 1988, pp89-99.

Poyet, P., Mennecier, P., 1988b. Des codes de calcul au service de l'informatique symbolique. To appear *in*: Comptes Rendus de l'Académie des Sciences de Paris.

Pritsker, A., 1974. The GASP IV Simulation Language, Wiley Interscience, New York, N.Y., 451 pp.

Pritsker, A. and Pegden, D., Introduction to Simulation and SLAM, Wiley and Sons, New York, N.Y., 588 pp.

Reiter, R., 1980. A Logic for Default Reasoning. *AI Journal* 13, (1980), pp. 81-132.

Rose, L. L., 1980. Computer Systems Simulation: An Overview, Final Report to United States Army Institute for Research in Management Information and Computer Sciences, January 1980, 50 pp.

Sargent, R. G., 1986. An exploration of possibilities for expert aids in model validation. in: loc. cit. (Elzas et al., 1986), pp. 279-297.

Schneider, J. Y., 1988. Modélisation d'une connaissance cartographique dans un système expert de simulation. Projet de fin d'études, Ecole Nationale Supérieure de Physique de Marseille, Juin 1988, 36pp.

Selfridge, R. G., 1955. Coding a General Purpose Digital Computer to Operate as a Differential Analyser. in: Proceedings '55 Western Joint Computer Conference, pp. 82-84.

Shannon, R. E., 1975. Systems Simulation, Prentice Hall, Englewood, N.J., 387pp.

Shannon R. E., Mayer R., Adelsberger H. H., 1985. "Expert systems and simulation". Simulation June 1985, pp 275-284.

SIMULOG, 1988. QNAP2, A Portable Environment for Queueing System Modelling, Documentation de Référence tirée de (Veran et al., 1984), 38 pp.

SMECI, 1988. Le manuel de l'utilisateur SMECI V 1.3. ILOG S.A.

Stefik M., Bobrow D. G., Mittal S., Conway L., 1983. "Knowledge programming in LOOPS". The AI Magazine (Fall 1983) pp. 3-13.

Stefik M. J., Bobrow D. G., Kahn K. M. , 1986. "Integrating Access Oriented Programming into a Multiparadigm Environment". IEEE Software, January 1986, pp 10-18.

Swan Arons (de) H. , 1983. "Expert Systems in the Simulation Domain". Mathematics and Computers in Simulation XXV (1983), North-Holland Publishing Company, pp 10-16

Veran, M., Potier D., 1984. QNAP2: A Portable Environment for Queueing Networks Modelling. in: Colloque International sur la Modélisation et les Outils d'Analyse de Performance, May 16-18, Paris.

Zeigler, B. P., 1984. Multifacetted Modelling and Discrete Event Simulation. Academic Press, London, 372 pp.

Zeigler, B. P., 1986. Toward a simulation methodology for variable structure modelling. in: loc. cit. (Elzas et al., 1986), pp. 195-210.

PEPS: A PACKAGE FOR SOLVING COMPLEX MARKOV MODELS OF PARALLEL SYSTEMS

Brigitte Plateau *, Jean-Michel Fourneau * and ***, Kuei-Hsiang Lee **

* ISEM, Université de Paris XI, Orsay 91405, France
** Comp. Sci. Dept., Univ. of Maryland, College Park, MD 20842, USA
*** LRI, Université de Paris XI, Orsay 91405, France

The purpose of this paper is to present the ideas and the algorithms that sustain the modeling methodology of the Package for the Evaluation of Parallel Systems (PEPS). This methodology is based on Markovian assumptions and is efficient for very large systems. The state space explosion is handled by a decomposition technique using tensor algebra operators. The presentation is driven by an example.

1. Introduction

This work is motivated by the study of performance of parallel systems, which is of current increasing importance. Recently, there has been an abundant literature on this subject, addressing theoretical and computational issues as well as case studies. Concerning the methodologies, there exist well known techniques that have proved to be efficient to model parallel systems. Among them are Queing Networks models and Stochastic Petri Nets models.

Queuing Networks are very efficient to model resource contention among independent programs running on a computer system [4], [5]. Some analytical results are now available for single queues running parallel programs with fork-join structures [9], and subjected to sequencing constraints [1]. The strength of the queuing network formalism lies in its expressive power, which leads to compact models, and the efficiency of its known resolution methods. Sophisticated queuing packages are now available and usable by untrained users. But, on the whole, explicitly calculating a probability distribution of a queuing system under some synchronization constraint is rarely attainable. That is why recent work propose systematic methods to derive bounds for such systems [2].

Stochastic Petri Nets are another approach essentially suitable for the representation of synchronization constraints of parallel systems [8], [6], [15]. They have been successfully applied in many areas, and the specification tool "Petri Net" covers a wide range of systems. The major problem of Stochastic Petri Nets is that they do not generally lead to compact models. Plus, they do not provide any results to deal with the state space explosion of the underlying Markov chain, and so are computationally expensive. Petri Net Packages exist and differ one from another by the assumptions they use concerning the delays within the Petri Net.

This work has been supported by the French program C^3, Communication, Cooperation and Concurrency.

So, as with simpler, sequential systems, abstractly Markov models provide a reasonnable tools. But, unlike those systems, useful Markov models of parallel systems do not usually fall in the class of known efficiently solvable models. This paper presents a method to address this problem.

The approach we present here was originally applied to the performance evaluation of distributed algorithms [11]. In this formalism, the dynamic behavior of a process in the distributed algorithm is typically represented by one automaton. As a single automaton represents only the state of one process, additional information is used to express synchronization constraints among the processes. Labels on the transitions of each automaton concentrate information concerning the timing and probability of occurrence of events, and the synchronization between automata of the same network [12]. We showed that the dynamic behavior of these networks of automata can be represented by a multi-dimensional Markov chain, whose matrix description (the generator for a continuous time scale model, and the transition matrix for a discrete time scale model) has a structure that can be exploited to improve the computation efficiency. Constructs based on tensor algebra are used to express the structure of these matrices. This formulation is used to obtain a more efficient computation of the performance measures.

In this presentation we chose to have a different approach based on the following considerations. It has been shown that using tensor algebra, the generator matrix of a Jackson network has an compact formulation [7], and that many other useful Markovian queuing models have a convenient representation [10]. Additionlly, our experience in modeling distributed algorithms and protocols using stochastic automata networks has shown that the representation of the algorithm as a network of stochastic automatas is not always the most convenient. It can be easier instead to write down the Chapmann-Kolmogorov equations of the multi-dimensional Markov process modelling the algorithm. These are equivalent expressions of the same model, leading to the same matrix constructs. So, we do not assume any specific description of the model to analyze, and we try to introduce these tensor algebra constructs in an intuitive manner.

The Package for the Evaluation of Parallel Systems (PEPS) is a package whose editor allows one to describe various mathematical objects, that are used for these tensor constructs and for specifying the performance measures of interest. PEPS is essentially composed of three independent modules: the editor, the compiler and the solver. The goal of the editor is to build a compact description of the generator of a multi-dimensional, Markov chain. The compiler translate this description into a form which is executable by the solver. The solver is in charge of the numerical computation and does not need any human intervention.

The structure of the paper is as follows. Section 2 provides the basic tensor algebra definitions and show their usage with examples. Section 3 explains the basic results that are used to take advantage of the tensor constructs and that lead to a more efficient computation. Section 4 presents PEPS organization and the major functionalities.

2. Elements of tensor algebra and their extensions

This section states the definitions and gives a framework for using the tensor algebra constructs.

2.1. Basic definitions

Let $M(n)$ be the set of square matrices of size n with elements in R. The element of matrix A, $A \in M(n)$, on row i and column j is denoted $a_{i,j}$.

A matrix A in $M(np)$ can be decomposed into n^2 blocks of $M(p)$. An element of A can be located by the coordinates of its block, and its coordinates within this block. So,

$$A \in M(np) \quad A = (a_{\overline{i}\,\overline{j}})_{\overline{i},\overline{j} \in L(n,p)}$$

with $L(n,p) = \{\overline{i} \mid \overline{i} = (i_1, i_2) \ 1 \le i_1 \le n, \ 1 \le i_2 \le p\}$

The block coordinate of element $a_{\overline{ij}}$ is (i_1,j_1), and its situation within this block is (i_2,j_2). With a direct generalization procedure, elements of matrix $A \in M(p_1 p_2 \cdots p_c)$ are referenced as follows:

$$A = (a_{\overline{ij}})_{\overline{ij} \in L(p_1,\ldots,p_c)}$$

with $\quad L(p_1,\ldots,p_c) = \{ \overline{i} \mid \overline{i} = (i_1,\ldots,i_c) \text{ and } (\forall k \in [1,c]) \quad 1 \le i_k \le p_k \}$

With this indexing method, elements of A are ranked according to the lexicographical ordering in $L(p_1, \ldots, p_c)$.

Id_p is the identity matrix in $M(p)$.

Definition 1: *The tensor product and sum of matrix A in $M(n)$ and B in $M(p)$ are matrices C and D in $M(np)$ defined by:*

$$C = A \otimes B$$

with $\quad c_{\overline{ij}} = a_{i_1 j_1} b_{i_2 j_2} \quad$ and $\quad \overline{i} = (i_1,i_2) , \overline{j} = (j_1,j_2)$

$$\text{and} \quad D = A \oplus B = A \otimes Id_p + Id_n \otimes B$$

As an example consider,

$$A = \begin{bmatrix} a_{1,1} & a_{1,2} \\ a_{2,1} & a_{2,2} \end{bmatrix} \qquad B = \begin{bmatrix} b_{1,1} & b_{1,2} \\ b_{2,1} & b_{2,2} \end{bmatrix}$$

Then

$$A \otimes B = \begin{bmatrix} a_{1,1}b_{1,1} & a_{1,1}b_{1,2} & a_{1,2}b_{1,1} & a_{1,2}b_{1,2} \\ a_{1,1}b_{2,1} & a_{1,1}b_{2,2} & a_{1,2}b_{2,1} & a_{1,2}b_{2,2} \\ a_{2,1}b_{1,1} & a_{2,1}b_{1,2} & a_{2,2}b_{1,1} & a_{2,2}b_{1,2} \\ a_{2,1}b_{2,1} & a_{2,1}b_{2,2} & a_{2,2}b_{2,1} & a_{2,2}b_{2,2} \end{bmatrix}$$

and

$$A \oplus B = \begin{bmatrix} a_{1,1}+b_{1,1} & b_{1,2} & a_{1,2} & 0 \\ b_{2,1} & a_{1,1}+b_{2,2} & 0 & a_{1,2} \\ a_{2,1} & 0 & a_{2,2}+b_{1,1} & b_{1,2} \\ 0 & a_{2,1} & b_{2,1} & a_{2,2}+b_{2,2} \end{bmatrix}$$

Notice the embedded block structure of the result $A \otimes B$ and $A \oplus B$. It is clear from this last definition that operators $\otimes$ and $\oplus$ are not commutative.

Briefly, when the sums, ordinary matrix products and inverse are defined, the tensor operators have the following properties:

- Associativity: $(A \otimes B) \otimes C = A \otimes (B \otimes C)$ and $(A \oplus B) \oplus C = A \oplus (B \oplus C)$

  Associativity implies that $\overset{c}{\underset{m=1}{\otimes}} A_m$ is readily defined.

- Distributivity over the addition:
  $(A+B) \otimes (C+D) = A \otimes C + A \otimes D + B \otimes C + B \otimes D$

- Compatibility with the regular product: $(A \bullet B) \otimes (C \bullet D) = (A \otimes C) \bullet (B \otimes D)$

Compatibility with inversion: $(A \otimes B)^{-1} = A^{-1} \otimes B^{-1}$

Complementary information can be found in [3] concerning tensor algebra properties.

It can be easily shown that if X is a Markov chain (indexed by a discrete time scale) with transition matrix A, and Y is another Markov chain independent from chain X, with transition matrix B, the two-dimensional chain (X,Y) has transition matrix $A \otimes B$. Similarly, if X is a Markov chain indexed by a continuous time scale, with generator matrix A, and Y is another Markov chain independent of chain X, with generator matrix B, the two-dimensional chain (X,Y) has generator matrix $A \oplus B$.

In this paper, we restrict ourselves to the product operator. This is not a limitation as the sum, which we exclude, can be expressed in terms of products as stated in Definition 1.

2.2. Tensor algebra extensions

The classical tensor product has matrices arguments whose elements are real numbers. We generalize this operator for matrices with functional elements.

Let $F(p)$ be the set of real functions defined on the integer interval $[1,p]$, and $M[n+1,F(p)]$ the set of square matrices of size n with elements in $F(p)$.

Definition 2: *Given A in $M[n,F(p)]$ and B in $M[p,F(n)]$, the generalized tensor product of A and B is matrice C, $C \in M(np)$, defined by:*

$$C = A \otimes B$$

$$\text{with} \quad c(\overline{i,j}) = a_{i_1,j_1}(i_2) \cdot b_{i_2,j_2}(i_1) \quad \text{if} \quad \overline{i} = (i_1,i_2) \quad , \quad \overline{j} = (j_1,j_2)$$

For example, if $n = p = 2$

$$A \otimes B = \begin{bmatrix} a_{1,1}(1)b_{1,1}(1) & a_{1,1}(1)b_{1,2}(1) & a_{1,2}(1)b_{1,1}(1) & a_{1,2}(1)b_{1,2}(1) \\ a_{1,1}(2)b_{2,1}(1) & a_{1,1}(2)b_{2,2}(1) & a_{1,2}(2)b_{2,1}(1) & a_{1,2}(2)b_{2,2}(1) \\ a_{2,1}(1)b_{1,1}(2) & a_{2,1}(1)b_{1,2}(2) & a_{2,2}(1)b_{1,1}(2) & a_{2,2}(1)b_{1,2}(2) \\ a_{2,1}(2)b_{2,1}(2) & a_{2,1}(2)b_{2,2}(2) & a_{2,2}(2)b_{2,1}(2) & a_{2,2}(2)b_{2,2}(2) \end{bmatrix}$$

The ordinary tensor product is clearly a restriction of this generalized tensor product, when we identify a constant function with its value. So, from now on, we will use generalized operators with mixed arguments: matrices in $M(n)$ or $M[n,F(p)]$.

The generalized tensor sum of A in $M[n,F(p)]$ and B in $M[p,F(n)]$ is defined as: $A \oplus B = A \otimes Id_p + Id_n \otimes B$. The operators used in this last expression have mixed arguments.

We introduce the generalized tensor product with more than two arguments: for a sequence $\overline{p} = (p_1, \ldots, p_c)$ of integers, we denote $\overline{p_i}$ the sequence obtained from $\overline{p}$ where p_i has been removed. Given matrices $A^l = (a^l_{i,j})_{i,j \in [1,p_l]}$ in $M[p_l,F(\overline{p_l})]$, matrix $C = \overset{l=c}{\underset{l=1}{\otimes}} A^l$ is defined by:

$$c_{\overline{i,j}} = \prod_{l=1}^{l=c} a^l_{i_l,j_l}(\overline{i_l}) \quad \text{for} \quad \overline{i} = (i_1, \ldots, i_c) \in L(\overline{p}) \quad \text{and} \quad \overline{j} = (j_1, \ldots, j_c) \in L(\overline{p})$$

Among the algebraic properties that were true for the ordinary tensor product, only the compatibility with the addition still holds. The compatibility with the matrix product is generally wrong, and the inverse of a matrix in $M[n,F(p)]$ has no standard definition.

We already noticed the possible use of classical tensor algebra for multi-dimensional Markov chains with independent components. The generalized operations have the same use when the components are not independent. This will be introduce with the example in the next section.

3. A queuing model with synchronization constraints and failures

We present the basic model and two successive refinements. We consider an architecture with P processors running in parallel with a Processor Sharing (PS) discipline (Figure 1).

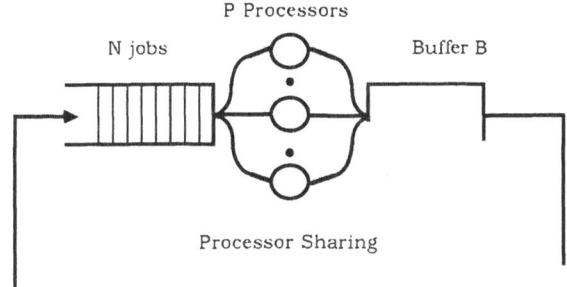

P Processors

N jobs

Buffer B

Processor Sharing

Figure 1. The closed multi-processor architecture

This is a closed system, and a set of N jobs are executed on this architecture, with $N > P$. These jobs perform fork-joins. A job can generate up to T tasks, which run in parallel or the multi-processor. Once terminated, a task wait in a buffer B for its siblings to complete. As soon as all siblings have completed, the job parent resumes its activity

3.1. Formulation of the basic model

We model this system by the current state of each job, denoted X_t^i for job i at instant t, $t \in R^+$: if the parent alone is processed, state variable $X_t^i = 0$. When k siblings are currently in execution, $X_t^i = k$. The behavior of state variable X_t^i is represented by the stochastic automaton of Figure 2.

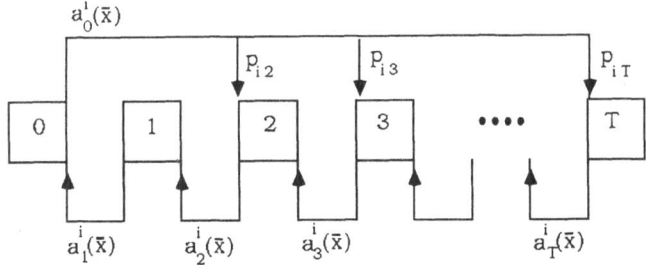

Figure 2. Behavior of job i represented by a stochastic automaton

The parameters of our model are the following:

- p_j^i, for $i \in [1,N]$ and $j \in [2,T]$, is the probability that job i generates j siblings. We notice that different jobs might have different probabilistic behaviors, and that we do not consider a fork with one child, so $p_1^i = 0$.

- c is the speed of each processor, and l^i the mean length of a task belonging to job i, so that a task has a duration which is exponentially distributed with parameter $\frac{c}{l^i}$, whenever it is the only one in execution.

Under the assumption of independence of all these random variables, process $\overline{X}_t = (X_t^i)_{i \in [1,n]}$ is a N-dimensional Markov chain. We denote $\overline{X}_t^i$ the vector obtained from $\overline{X}_t$ by removing component X_t^i.

With this representation, the total number of tasks (parents or siblings) in execution at instant t is:

$$N_t = \sum_{i=1}^{N} \left[\mathbf{1}\,(X_t^i=0) + X_t^i \right]$$

where $\mathbf{1}\,(X_t^i=0)$ is the characteristic function of event $\{X_t^i=0\}$.

Rate $a_{x_i}^i(\bar{x})$ is the rate at which a task is completed, when job i is in state x_i, and the global state is $\bar{x}$. It is defined by:

$$a_{x_i}^i(\bar{x}) = \frac{P\,c}{l^i \sum_{j=1}^{N} \left[\mathbf{1}\,(x_j=0) + x_j \right]}$$

We denote M^i the generator corresponding to the stochastic automaton of job i. Matrix M^i belongs to $M[T+1\,,\,F(\,(T+1)^{N-1}\,)\,]$, as its dimension is $T+1$, and its elements are functions with arguments in $[0\,,\,T] \times \cdots \times [0\,,\,T] = [0\,,\,T]^{N-1}$. For $T=4$, M_i is:

$$M^i(\bar{x}_i) = \begin{bmatrix} -a_0^i(\bar{x}) & 0 & a_0^i(\bar{x})p_2^i & a_0^i(\bar{x})p_3^i & a_0^i(\bar{x})p_4^i \\ a_1^i(\bar{x}) & -a_1^i(\bar{x}) & 0 & 0 & 0 \\ 0 & a_2^i(\bar{x}) & -a_2^i(\bar{x}) & 0 & 0 \\ 0 & 0 & a_3^i(\bar{x}) & -a_3^i(\bar{x}) & 0 \\ 0 & 0 & 0 & a_4^i(\bar{x}) & -a_4^i(\bar{x}) \end{bmatrix}$$

In matrix $M^i(\bar{x}_i)$, the functions $a_j^i(\bar{x})$, take $\bar{x}$ as arguments, but component x_i is defined by the location in the matrix.

Then, using the generalized tensor sum, the generator of Markov chain $\bar{X}_t$ is simply:

$$Q = \bigoplus_{i=1}^{N} M^i$$

The simplicity of that result should not hide that the size of the state space is $(T+1)^N$, and exponentially increasing . Plus, there is probably no close form solution to the system $\Pi\,Q=0$. Section 3 will show how to compute efficiently steady state probability vector Π.

Assume that we have computed Π. We denote E_Π the expectation related to steady state probability Π. To analyze the performance of the system pictured in Figure 1, we may want to compute, in steady state:

- The expected number of tasks in execution:

$$E_\Pi\,(\sum_{i=1}^{N} \left[\mathbf{1}\,(X^i=0) + X^i \right]\,)$$

- The expected number of tasks waiting in buffer B:

$$\sum_{i=1}^{N} \sum_{j=2}^{T} \frac{E_\Pi\left[p_j^i\,(j-X^i)\,\mathbf{1}\,(X^i \neq 0)\,\mathbf{1}\,(X^i \leq j) \right]}{E_\Pi\,(\,\mathbf{1}\,(X^i \leq j)\,)}$$

In the above expression, $(j-X^i)$ is the number job waiting in buffer B for job i, when the last fork has generated j children. This happens with probability p_j^i and under the condition $X^i \leq j$.

- The mean response time of job i can be evaluated as the inverse of the exit rate from state 1:

$$\left[P_\Pi\,(X^i = 1\,)\,E_\Pi\,(a_1^i(\bar{X})\,) \right]^{-1}$$

So, provided we know distribution Π, various performance measures can be computed as expectation of functions of the various parameters and components of vector $\overline{X}$. Similarly, moments of any order can be computed.

3.2. A multiprocessor with breakdowns

Now, the multiprocessor is subject to failures. No assumptions is made on the type of failure. All processors can stop at the same time, or the the multiprocessor can be gracefully degradable.

The state of the multiprocessor is described by an other automaton, which is pictured in Figure 3. The multiprocessor is in state j, $0{\leq}j{\leq}P$, when j processors are working, and $P{-}j$ are broken. Parameters $\beta_{i,j}$ are the rates of failure from state i to j, with $i{\geq}j$. Parameters $\alpha_{i,j}$ the rates of repair from state i to j, with $i{\leq}j$. All distributions are exponential and independent.

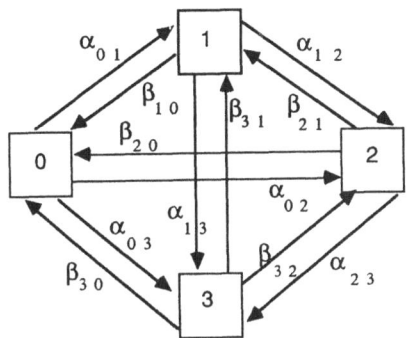

Figure 3. Behavior of the multiprocessor represented by a stochastic automaton (example with 3 processors)

We denote Y_t the random variable representing the state of this automaton at instant t. The generator of random variable Y_t is matrix M_Y in $M(P{+}1)$. If $P{=}3$, M_Y is equal to:

$$M_Y = \begin{bmatrix} \gamma_{0,0} & \alpha_{0,1} & \alpha_{0,2} & \alpha_{0,3} \\ \beta_{1,0} & \gamma_{1,1} & \alpha_{1,2} & \alpha_{1,3} \\ \beta_{2,0} & \beta_{2,1} & \gamma_{2,2} & \alpha_{2,3} \\ \beta_{3,0} & \beta_{3,1} & \beta_{3,2} & \gamma_{3,3} \end{bmatrix}$$

where coefficients $\gamma_{i,i}$ are such that the sum of the coefficients of a row is equal to zero.

The joint behavior of the multiprocessor with failure and the N jobs with fork-join is described by process $(\overline{X}_t,Y_t)$. Considering the assumptions, process $(\overline{X}_t,Y_t)$ is a Markov chain. In this chain, component Y_t is independent from components $\overline{X}_t$, but components $\overline{X}_t$ depend on the state of component Y_t. Precisely, as processors can fail, functions $a_{x_i}^i(\overline{x})$ need to be replaced by functions $a_{x_i}^i(\overline{x},y)$, which are equal to:

$$a_{x_i}^i(\overline{x},y) = \frac{y\,c}{i\sum_{j=1}^{N}\left[\mathbb{1}\,(x_j{=}0) + x_j\right]}$$

The generator of Markov chain $(\overline{X}_t,Y_t)$ is simply:

$$Q = \bigoplus_{i=1}^{N} M^i \oplus M_Y$$

The size of the state space is now $(T{+}1)^N(P{+}1)$. We notice that we have modeled a blocking situation: when all processors are failed, variable Y_t is equal to zero. Consequently, the rates $a_{x_i}^i(\overline{x},y)$ that govern job i behavior are also equal to zero. All jobs are blocked.

This non-trivial refinement show how, with very little effort, the model has been extended.

3.3. Jobs with checkpoints

Now, we assume that when all processors have failed, jobs have to repeat their activities from the last checkpoint. There is a checkpoint after each fork, before the parent resumes its activity. So, each time the multiprocessor fails entirely, all jobs jump to state 0.

We have here a new phenomenon: simultaneous jump among different automata for the same event, total breakdown of the multiprocessor. So, we introduce a new label (s) on the transitions involved in the same simultaneous jump. In models where different simultaneous jumps occur, symbol (s) is indexed to differentiate them.

The automaton representing the behavior of the multiprocessor is pictured on Figure 4. It is essentially the same as in Figure 3, except that we add a symbol (s) on the transitions to state 0.

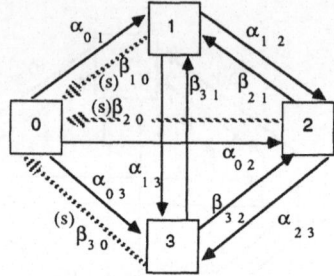

Figure 4. Behavior of the multiprocessor represented by a stochastic automaton with failures provoking roll-backs (example with 3 processors)

The automaton representing the behavior of job i is pictured on Figure 5. New transitions are added, which correspond to their roll-back.

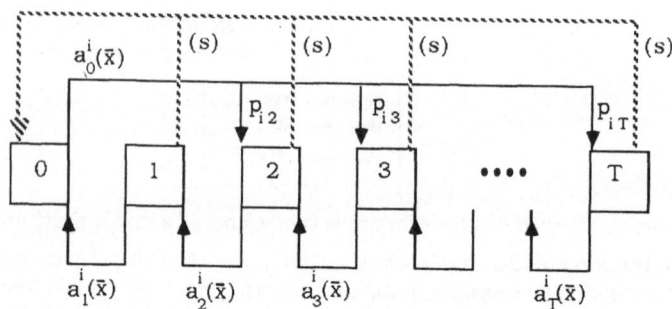

Figure 5. Behavior of job i with roll-back in case of complete failure of the processor

Again, in this case, process $(\bar{X}_t, Y_t)$ is a Markov chain. To express its generator, we have to consider separately the transitions that do not involve any simultaneous jump, and the transitions that involve simultaneous jumps.

We decompose generator M_Y defined in Section 3.2 in two matrices M_y' and M_Y'', such that $M_Y = M_Y' + M_Y''$. If $P=3$, we have:

$$M_Y' = \begin{bmatrix} \gamma_{0,0} & \alpha_{0,1} & \alpha_{0,2} & \alpha_{0,3} \\ 0 & \gamma_{1,1} & \alpha_{1,2} & \alpha_{1,3} \\ 0 & \beta_{2,1} & \gamma_{2,2} & \alpha_{2,3} \\ 0 & \beta_{3,1} & \beta_{3,2} & \gamma_{3,3} \end{bmatrix}$$

And,

$$M_Y'' = \begin{bmatrix} 0 & 0 & 0 & 0 \\ \beta_{1,0} & 0 & 0 & 0 \\ \beta_{2,0} & 0 & 0 & 0 \\ \beta_{3,0} & 0 & 0 & 0 \end{bmatrix}$$

Similarly, we replace the generator of component X_t^i by two matrices $M^{i'}$ and $M^{i''}$. We define $M^{i'} = M^i$, where M^i is as defined in Section 3.2. A new matrix has to be introduce for the new transitions labeled with (s). On automaton j there are no rates accompanying these labels. So, in the corresponding transition matrix, there are coefficients equal to one when the simultaneous jump takes place, and zero otherwise. So, if $T = 4$, we have

$$M^{i''} = \begin{bmatrix} 0 & 0 & 0 & 0 & 0 \\ 1 & 0 & 0 & 0 & 0 \\ 1 & 0 & 0 & 0 & 0 \\ 1 & 0 & 0 & 0 & 0 \\ 1 & 0 & 0 & 0 & 0 \end{bmatrix}$$

The generator of Markov chain $(\bar{X}_t, Y_t)$ is in this model:

$$Q = \overset{N}{\underset{i=1}{\oplus}} M^{i'} \oplus M_Y' + \overset{N}{\underset{i=1}{\otimes}} M^{i''} \otimes M_Y''$$

We notice the splitting in two parts: the tensor summation when no simultaneous jump occur, and the tensor product to express simultaneity. This last formula is less intuitive than the previous ones because of this splitting that requires a more detailed analysis.

In this case, the reachable state space is not the entire product space: the set of states $I = \{ Y = 0 \text{ and } \sum_{i=1}^{N} X^i \neq 0 \}$ is not reachable. When the multiprocessor is entirely down, all jobs have rolled back to their last checkpoint and are in state 0.

Through this example, we wanted to illustrate the expressive power of networks of stochastic automata. Each sequential activity is represented by one automaton. Then, various aspects of the architecture: sharing a common resource or failures of processors, and various aspects of program behavior: fork-joins and roll-backs, enforces the automata to depend on each other. The denomination network refers to these dependencies.

After abstraction, dependencies are of two types: the first type is called *stochastic dependency*, and covers the cases where the transition rates of one automaton depend on the current state of the rest of the Markov chain. The generalized tensor sum and products provide a convenient tool to introduce these dependencies in the generator. The second type is called *simultaneous-jump dependency*, and covers the case where more than one automaton proceed to a jump triggered by a common event. Here too, generalized tensor products are used to express the generator.

The constructs that were used in this example are very intuitive. This example is intended to help the reader to "learn by example". More formal derivations are presented in [12].

4. Numerical optimization

The previous section addressed the expressive power of our modeling technique. This section addresses the complexity aspect.

The analysis of a problem of dimension c, where component i has a state space of size p_i, leads to a matrix of the type:

$$Q = \overset{c}{\underset{i=1}{\oplus}} A_i + \sum_{j=1}^{K} \overset{c}{\underset{i=1}{\otimes}} B_{j,i}$$

with

$$\forall\ i\in[1,c]\ ,\quad A_i\in M(p_i)\quad\text{and}\quad B_{j,i}\in M(p_i)$$

Operator $\oplus$ arises only in problems on continuous time, and parameter K can be interpreted as a distance to pure parallelism: the more simultaneous-jump dependencies there are, the bigger K is.

4.1. The power method

Steady state probability vector Π is computed in PEPS using a power method [13]. PEPS interface requires that the user specifies the reachability space $R\subset L(p_1,\ldots,p_c)$, and initial probability vector Π^0 is chosen such that,

$$(\forall \overline{i}\notin R)\quad \Pi_{\overline{i}}^0=0$$

and is uniformly distributed on R. As R is the reachability space, generator Q has the following property:

$$(\forall \overline{i}\in R)\quad\text{and}\quad(\forall \overline{j}\notin R)\quad Q_{\overline{ij}}=0$$

Vector $\Pi^1=\Pi^0\,Q$ has its components equal to:

$$\Pi_{\overline{i}}^1=\sum_{\overline{j}\in L(p_1,\ldots,p_c)}\Pi_{\overline{j}}^0\,Q_{\overline{j}\overline{i}}=\sum_{\overline{j}\in R}\Pi_{\overline{j}}^0\,Q_{\overline{j}\overline{i}}$$

It is clear from this formula, that $\overline{i}\notin R$ implies $\Pi_{\overline{i}}^1=0$. So, Π^1 is also in reachability set R.

We assume that R is an irreducible class. For a problem on discrete time, PEPS computes the sequence:

$$\Pi^n=\Pi^{n-1}\,Q$$

On continuous time, let ω the maximum of the absolute value of the diagonal elements of matrix Q, and ε be a small positive number, the sequence is:

$$\Pi^n=\Pi^{n-1}+\frac{1}{\omega\,(1+\varepsilon)}\ \Pi^{n-1}\,Q$$

In both cases, the power method converges to the steady state probability vector on reachability set R. Getting any knowledge on the speed of convergence of this method would require extra knowledge on the eigenvalues of matrix Q. PEPS provides only two stopping rules: one is based on a number of iterations and is used as a maximum barrier, and the second one is a convergence precision criteria using the norm L_1: $\displaystyle\sum_{\overline{i}\in L(p_1,\ldots,p_n)}\mid\Pi_{\overline{i}}^n-\Pi_{\overline{i}}^{n-1}\mid.$

4.2. Optimization for ordinary tensor products

As we use a power method to compute steady state vector Π, the basic operation to optimize is multiplication $\Pi\,Q$, or more basically multiplication $\Pi\ \overset{c}{\underset{i=1}{\otimes}}\ A^i$ (Remember that a tensor sum is reducible to tensor products). These multiplications are performed by PEPS solver.

The naive solution would be to compute explicitly matrix Q, which is a square matrix of size $\displaystyle\prod_{i=1}^{c} p_i$, and perform the product $\Pi\,Q$, which requires a number of operations of the order of $\displaystyle(\prod_{i=1}^{c} p_i)^2$.

For ordinary tensor products, we propose a solution that does not requires the effective calculation of matrix Q, but works on the tensor formula. So, the storage cost of our method is negligible. Plus, we propose an algorithm to compute $\Pi\ \overset{c}{\underset{i=1}{\otimes}}\ A^i$, whose complexity is of order of $\displaystyle\left[\prod_{i=1}^{c} p_i\right]\left(\sum_{i=1}^{c} p_i\right)$

To present this algorithm, we first proceed to the underlying algebra, and then we present briefly the algorithm.

Remark 1: We consider a multi-dimensional chain $\bar{X} = (X_1,...,X_c)$, whose matrix is $\overset{c}{\underset{i=1}{\otimes}} A^i$. The steady state vector components are indexed on $L(p_1,...,p_c)$, and we denote $\Pi_{\bar{i}}$ the component on rank $\bar{i} = (i_1, . . . ,i_c)$.

Let σ be a permutation of $[1,c]$. By permuting the components of $\bar{X}$ by σ, we do not change the problem: chain $\bar{X}_\sigma = (X_{\sigma(1)},...,X_{\sigma(c)})$ has the matrix $\overset{c}{\underset{i=1}{\otimes}} A^{\sigma(i)}$. The new steady state vector Π_σ has components that are indexed on $L(p_{\sigma(1)},...,p_{\sigma(c)})$.

We denote P_σ the permutation matrix such that $\Pi_\sigma = \Pi\, P_\sigma$. Matrix P_σ performs a perfect shuffle on the components of vector Π. In this transformation, we have:

$$\overset{c}{\underset{i=1}{\otimes}} A^{\sigma(i)} = P_\sigma^T \left[\overset{c}{\underset{i=1}{\otimes}} A^i \right] P_\sigma$$

because the inverse of P_σ is also its transpose.

So, PEPS uses this flexibility, and consider the components of chain $\bar{X}$ in the order that is more convenient for the computation.

Remark 2: We want to compute the product $\overset{c}{\underset{i=1}{\otimes}} A^i$ in a more convenient way. We have the obvious equality:

$$A_i = Id_{p_i} \, \cdots \, Id_{p_i} \, A_i \, Id_{p_i} \, \cdots \, Id_{p_i}$$

with $i-1$ factors equal to Id_{p_i} on the left side of A_i, and $c-i$ factors equal to Id_{p_i} on the right side. Then, using the compatibility of the tensor product and the regular matrix product, we get:

$$\overset{c}{\underset{i=1}{\otimes}} A^i = \overset{c}{\underset{i=1}{\otimes}} Id_{p_i} \, \cdots \, Id_{p_i} \, A_i \, Id_{p_i} \, \cdots \, Id_{p_i} = \overset{c}{\underset{i=1}{\bullet}} Id_{p_1} \otimes \cdots \otimes Id_{p_{i-1}} \otimes A_i \otimes Id_{p_{i+1}} \otimes \cdots \otimes Id_{p_c}$$

We denote σ_i the circular permutation that puts component X_i in the last position, and $q_i = \overset{c}{\underset{k=1,k\neq i}{\prod}} p_k$. Using Remark 1, we get:

$$\overset{c}{\underset{i=1}{\otimes}} A^i = \overset{c}{\underset{i=1}{\bullet}} P_{\sigma_i}^T \, (Id_{q_i} \otimes A_i) \, P_{\sigma_i}$$

This last equality is the basis of our optimaization.

Remark 3: To perform the product $\Pi_{\sigma_i} \, (Id_{q_i} \otimes A_i)$, one can perform, q_i products of size p_i, as $Id_{q_i} \otimes A_i$ is a block diagonal matrix. The complexity of this operation is of the order of $p_i \overset{c}{\underset{k=1}{\prod}} p_k$.

Remark 4: The cost of performing the permutations in the product $\Pi \, P_{\sigma_i} \, (Id_{q_i} \otimes A_i)P_{\sigma_i}^T$ is of the order of $\overset{c}{\underset{k=1}{\prod}} p_k$. It can be done naively by re-computing addresses, or more cleverly by scanning vector Π using appropriate translations.

In conclusion, to perform the product $\Pi \overset{c}{\underset{i=1}{\otimes}} A_i$, where only ordinary tensor products occur, PEPS performs actually the product $\Pi \overset{c}{\underset{i=1}{\bullet}} P_{\sigma_i}^T (Id_{q_i} \otimes A_i) P_{\sigma_i}$. In this computation, many steps can be done in parallel, and the sequential complexity is of the order of $(\overset{c}{\underset{i=1}{\prod}} p_i) (\overset{c}{\underset{i=1}{\sum}} p_i)$.

4.3. Optimization for generalized tensor products

The optimization procedure for ordinary tensor products was based on the compatibility between tensor product and regular matrix product (Remark 2). As we already mentioned in Section 2, this property does not hold for generalized tensor products. So, the idea here is to

301

transform generalized tensor product into ordinary tensor products for the numerical solver. Then, we apply the computation method presented in Section 4.3 to the result of this transformation. The problem is that the transformation of generalized tensor products into ordinary tensor products might be very costly. The optimization here concerns this transformation, and is done in the compiler module of PEPS.

The basic algebraic identity we use is the following. Matrix $l_i(A)$ denotes the matrix obtained from A by keeping the i–th row, and letting all other components being equal to zero. Matrices A and $l_i(A)$ are of the same dimension. Given matrices $A^l=(a^l_{i,j})_{i,j\in[1,p_l]}$ in $M[p_l,F(\overline{p}_l)]$, we have

$$\overset{c}{\underset{k=1}{\otimes}}\ A^k = \sum_{\overline{i}\in L(p_1,\ldots,p_c)} \overset{c}{\underset{k=1}{\otimes}}\ l_{i_k}(A(\overline{i}_k))$$

This identity simply says that, to perform a tensor product (generalized or not) of c matrices, one can perform it row by row, for all the $\prod_{i=1}^{c} p_i$ combinations. In this "row by row" procedure, the functions imbedded in the matrices of the generalized tensor products can be instanced. So, on one side of the equality, we have generalized tensor products, and on the other side, ordinary tensor products, to which the previous optimization procedure can be applied. But, the size of the summation $\prod_{i=1}^{c} p_i$ involved is such that this transformation does not reduces the complexity, as compared to the naive multiplication.

So, the objective of the next remarks is to reduce the size of this summation. In order to avoid heavy notations, we will consider a multi-dimensional problem with four components, and work on examples. So we consider the term

$$S = \overset{4}{\underset{k=1}{\otimes}}\ A^k = \sum_{i_1=1}^{P_1} \sum_{i_2=1}^{P_2} \sum_{i_3=1}^{P_3} \sum_{i_4=1}^{P_4} \overset{4}{\underset{k=1}{\otimes}}\ l_{i_k}(A(\overline{i}_k))$$

Remark 5: In the above formula, we are in the most general case, where any component i depends on all the others. Assume that, for reasons of locality, we have the following functional dependencies: Matrix A^1 has arguments i_2 and i_3 only, and matrix A_3 has arguments i_2 only. Matrices A_2 and A_4 are constant. Using the distributivity of the tensor products over the addition, we can write:

$$S = \sum_{i_2=1}^{P_2} \sum_{i_3=1}^{P_3} \left[\sum_{i_1=1}^{P_1} l_{i_1}(A^1(i_2,i_3))\right] \otimes l_{i_2}(A^2) \otimes l_{i_3}(A^3(i_2)) \otimes \left[\sum_{i_4=1}^{P_4} l_{i_4}(A^4)\right]$$

And, by recomposition,

$$S = \sum_{i_2=1}^{P_2} \sum_{i_3=1}^{P_3} A^1(i_2,i_3) \otimes l_{i_2}(A^2) \otimes l_{i_3}(A^3(i_2)) \otimes A^4$$

In this case, the set of components (X_2,X_3) can be identify as a Dependency Set (DS), and the summation reduces to this set. The complexity of the product $\Pi\ S$ is of the order $(\prod_{DS} p_i)\ (\prod_{i=1}^{c} p_i)(\sum_{i=1}^{c} p_i)$.

PEPS compiler is capable of computing the dependency set of a term $\overset{c}{\underset{k=1}{\otimes}}\ A^k$, and to reduce the summation accordingly. We notice that if the dependency set is empty, it means that the tensor products do not have any functional arguments, and reduces to an ordinary tensor product.

Remark 6: In the case of Remark 5, component X_4 is not in the dependency set, and matrix A_4 is constant. In this case, one can operate a permutation σ to place the constant term in the first

302

position, and S becomes:

$$S = P_\sigma A_4 \otimes \left[\sum_{i_2=1}^{P_2} \sum_{i_3=1}^{P_3} A^1(i_2,i_3) \otimes l_{i_2}(A^2) \otimes l_{i_3}(A^3(i_2)) \right] \otimes P_\sigma^T$$

So, PEPS compiler detects constant terms that are not in the dependency set, and factorizes them. The complexity is reduced to the order of: $(\prod_{i=1}^{c} p_i) \left[\sum_{i \notin DS} p_i + (\prod_{DS} p_i)(\sum_{i \in DS} p_i) \right]$.

Remark 7: When tensor sum $\overset{4}{\underset{k=1}{\oplus}} A^k$ occurs in a continuous time model, PEPS analyzes it as

$$A^1 \otimes Id_{p_2} \otimes Id_{p_3} \otimes Id_{p_4} + Id_{p_1} \otimes A^2 \otimes Id_{p_3} \otimes Id_{p_4} + Id_{p_1} \otimes Id_{p_2} \otimes A^3 \otimes Id_{p_4} + Id_{p_1} \otimes Id_{p_2} \otimes Id_{p_3} \otimes A^4$$

Each of these terms is analyzed the same way, for example,

$$S = Id_{p_1} \otimes Id_{p_2} \otimes A^3 \otimes Id_{p_4} = \sum_{i_1=1}^{P_1} \sum_{i_2=1}^{P_2} \sum_{i_4=1}^{P_4} l_{i_1}(Id_{p_1}) \otimes l_{i_2}(Id_{p_2}) \otimes A^3(i_1,i_2,i_4) \otimes l_4(Id_{p_4})$$

which can be transformed in

$$S = P_{\sigma_3} (\sum_{i_1=1}^{P_1} \sum_{i_2=1}^{P_2} \sum_{i_4=1}^{P_4} l_{i_1}(Id_{p_1}) \otimes l_{i_2}(Id_{p_2}) \otimes l_4(Id_{p_4}) \otimes A^3(i_1,i_2,i_4)) P_{\sigma_3}^T$$

Applying the operator $l_{i_1}(Id_{p_1}) \otimes l_{i_2}(Id_{p_2}) \otimes l_4(Id_{p_4})$ is just selecting components $\Pi_{\overline{k}}$ of Π, such that $k_1=i_1$, $k_2=i_2$, and $k_4=i_4$. So, interpreting the first part of this operator as a selection reduces the complexity of the product ΠS to $p_3 \prod_{i=1}^{4} p_i$. The complexity of the entire tensor sum is of the order of $(\prod_{i=1}^{c} p_i) (\sum_{i=1}^{c} p_i)$.

In conclusion, optimization in PEPS occurs at two levels: in the solver, through the multiplication of a vector by a matrix, and in the compiler, through the transformation of generalized tensor operators to ordinary operators.

5. The program PEPS

As we mentioned it already, PEPS is divided into three modules: the editor, the compiler, and the solver. It is written in Pascal, and runs on Sun and Vax machines under UNIX system.

5.1. The editor

The editor is a text editor based on a hierarchy of menus, and is logically divided in three parts: The object editor, the model editor, and the verification module.

The object editor permits the manipulation of objects. These objects have symbolic names, and are of four basic types: constants, functions, relations and matrices. Functions, relations, matrices have arguments, which can be constant names, component names, functions and relations. Functions and relations are parsed according to the usual grammatical rules of Pascal. The manipulations provided by PEPS are creation, change, visualization and deletion of an object, and deletion of all the objects of a type.

The model editor permits the definition of the model type (discrete or continuous time), the model size, the component size (the p_i), the description matrix (called Q in the paper) and the performance measures. All these are also defined as objects, but with a unique instance per model. Building them requires to use the constant names, functions, relations and matrices defined in the object editor. The same manipulations are provided for these unique objects.

The verification module checks that all the names that are used have a definition. Functions, relations and matrices used in the description matrix and the performance measures must have a symbolic definition, and constant names must be related to a value. This module also verifies that functions and relations definition are not recursive and realize a pre-compilation of these objects. The full compilation must be delaied until the component values are instanced.

Editing a model with PEPS produces two files: *SYM* contains all the symbolic definitions, and *DATA* contains the numerical values for the constant. This permits to create multiple *DATA* files for the same structural model, and to vary the parameters.

5.2. The compiler

The compiler takes as input the files *SYM* and *DATA*. It translates the matrix descriptor, which is in a symbolic form in *SYM*, in a form usable by the solver, called Q'. For this,

- it replaces the constant names by their values,
- it applies the rules of Remarks 5, 6 and 7, in order to replace generalized tensor products by ordinary tensor products,
- it uses tags for matrices of a special type, such as identity, which will be used in the solver to simplify the computation.

At the end of this transformation, the complexity of product $\Pi Q'$ is given.

The compiler generates the initial vector of the power method in the reachability set. It operates a semantic verification on Q' : it verifies that that the sum of the coefficients on a row of Q' is zero or one, depending if it is a model on continuous or discrete time model. It verifies that $\Pi^1 = \Pi^0 Q'$ is also a probability vector on the reachability set R, with positive components that sum up to one.

The compiler produces a file *READY*, containing Q', and a file *ERROR*, containing the results of the semantic verification.

5.3. The solver

The solver executes the power methods, performs the stopping tests, and the products as defined in Section 4.2. At the end of the power method, the solver computes the performance measures defined in *SYM*.

6. Conclusion

In this paper, we wanted to show the field of application of our modeling technique: if the system we model is composed by parallel activities with synchronization points, then it is convenient and natural to represent it by a network of stochastic automata. This method is efficient to handle the state space explosion. Plus, the complexity of the computation of the steady state performance can be reduced, using an adequate representation for the transition matrix. On the opposite, if in the system we model with a multi-dimensional state variable, the interactions between components are very dense, the network of automata can be very complex, and the gain of numerical method can be small: this method might be not adapted.

In the future, we want to expand PEPS functionalities. First, we want to improve its interface by adding editing facilities for the various objects of the model. We will complement this text interface by a graphical interface, where the user will input directly stochastic automata.

From the theoretical point of view, we want to extend the types of models PEPS can solve. For the time being, PEPS solves ergodic problems on finite state space. We want to introduce problems with one infinite component, using Neuts method [10], and problems with absorbing states to study their transient behavior. This last extension has an obvious interest for reliability or real-time constraints in parallel systems.

The numerical method we apply in PEPS provides exact results. Even if very much care has been brought in PEPS to the complexity aspect, computation is still very expensive for very large problems. In our experimentations, we have considered problems with up to 15 000 states. We want to adapt PEPS to compute bounds for the performance of our systems, at a lower cost, using stochastic dominance methods [14].

BIBLIOGRAPHY

[1]   F. Baccelli, E. Gelenbe, B. Plateau: "An end to end approach to the resequencing problem", *Journal of ACM, Vol 31, No 3, July 1984.*

[2]   F. Baccelli, A. Makowski: "Simple computable bounds for the fork-join queues", *The John Hopkins Conference on Information Science, 1985, Baltimore.*

[3]   M. Davio: "Kronecker products and shuffle algebra", *IEEE Transactions on Computers, Vol C-30, No 2, Feb 81.*

[4]   L. Kleinrock: "Queuing systems, Vol I and II", *Wiley-Interscience, 1975.*

[5]   J.Y. Le Boudec: "A BCMP extension to multiserver stations with concurrent classes of customers", *Proceedings of Performance 86 and ACM Sigmetrics 86, May 1986, Raleigh.*

[6]   M.A. Marsan, G. Balbo, G. Conte: "A class of generalized stochastic Petri nets", *ACM Transactions on Computer Systems, Vol 2, pp 93-122, May 1984.*

[7]   W.A. Massey: "Open networks of queues: Their algebraic structure and estimating their transient behavior", *Advances in Applied Probability, Vol 16, No 1, March 1984.*

[8]   M. Molloy: "Performance analysis using stochastic Petri nets", *IEEE Transactions on Computers, Vol C-31, No 9, Sept. 1982.*

[9]   R. Nelson, D. Towsley, A.N. Tantawi: "Performance analysis of parallel processing systems", *Proceedings of ACM Sigmetrics 87, 1987, Calgary.*

[10]   M.F. Neuts: "Matrix geometric solutions in stochastic models, an algorithmic approach", *The John Hopkins University Press, 1981.*

[11]   B. Plateau: "On the stochastic structure of parallelism and synchronization models for distributed algorithms", *Proceedings of ACM Sigmetrics 85, Aug. 1985. Austin.*

[12]   B. Plateau: "A method for handling complex Markov models of distributed algorithms", *Technical report, TR-SRC 86-39, University of Maryland, USA.*

[13]   W. Stewart, E. Gelenbe, J. Labetoulle, M. Metivier, G. Pujolle: "Réseaux de files d'attente, modélisation et traitement numérique", *Ed. des hommes et techniques, Monographies informatiques de l'AFCET, Chap 4, 1981.*

[14]   D. Stoyan: "Comparison methods for queues and other stochastic models", *John Wiley and Sons, 1983.*

[15]   M. Vernon, M. Holliday: "Performance analysis of multiprocessor cache consistency protocols using generalized timed Petri nets", *Proc. of Performance 86 and ACM Sigmetrics 86, May 1986 Raleigh.*

PERFORMANCE OF CONCURRENT RENDEZVOUS SYSTEMS

WITH COMPLEX PIPELINE STRUCTURES

C.M. Woodside, J.E. Neilson, J.W. Miernik,
D.C. Petriu, and R. Constantin

Real-Time and Distributed Systems Group
Carleton University, Ottawa, Canada

Abstract

The term "complex pipeline" describes a set of tasks which process incoming data in a sequence, like a pipeline, but have various kinds of parallel execution steps coupled into the main stream of execution. Examples are, splitting off of parallel streams, and shared server tasks. Examples are found in processing to interpret radar data, and other real-time systems. Rendezvous systems like Ada have static tasks, static processor allocations and synchronous inter-task communications, which can cause potential performance problems. The growing importance of rendezvous-based environments, including Ada, requires that we be able to predict these problems. Models such as Petri nets, are often too expensive to solve; fast approximation techniques are needed. The approach of "stochastic rendezvous networks" is adapted here to deal with complex pipelines. This paper describes an algorithm and evaluates its accuracy; the algorithm is the major feature of the paper, including a "Conditional Mean Value Analysis" step. It includes processor queueing, which was not modelled in the earlier work. The method is several orders of magnitude faster than Petri net analysis even on small examples. The accuracy obtained is generally better than 10%.

1 Introduction

In concurrent software written for multi-tasking, multi-processing environments such as Ada [DOD83], V [CHER83], or XMS [GAMM84], we often find a sequence of tasks operating as a pipeline on a stream of data. For example, a radar tracking system might have tasks for filtering, detection, track correlation, track update, display and storage updating for the track. It may be a simple sequence of tasks as illustrated in Figure 1(a) or a more complex pattern which we will term a "complex task pipeline".

Pipelines are introduced in hardware to obtain extra throughput by overlapping successive operations on successive items of data, and task pipelines can have the same effect when they are executed on a succesion of processors. Performance calculations and optimizations for deterministic clocked hardware pipelines are surveyed by Kogge [KOGG81].

However the previous studies miss out some important features of task pipelines. First, intertask communications may affect performance, particularly in a rendezvous system where there is no intertask buffering of communications. Second, it is common for task architectures to have the more complex structures already mentioned, perhaps with branching paths or shared resources. Examples of resources shared between stages are, a shared file, or a buffer pool, and in a rendezvous system they are likely to be managed by a separate task called a *server task*. Pipeline tasks must queue for access to server tasks, and in an extreme case there may be several levels of servers involved.

This paper shall define a complex task pipeline to be:

- a sequence or tree of tasks, possibly with branches in the flow to create parallel segments,

- data dependent (ie. stochastic) access to server tasks providing shared services or managing shared resources.

The analysis here will cover the features in the first item, leaving server tasks to a later paper. The complex pipelines will be made up of software tasks statically allocated to processors and communicating via rendezvous, interpreted as a send-receive-process-reply sequence (see Section 2). There may be waiting for a rendezvous or for processor scheduling; this waiting is estimated in order to determine the pipeline throughput capacity. Response times are also obtained as a by-product of the analysis.

This paper extends the method introduced in [WOOD84] and [WOOD88], by explicitly modelling processor contention sets and deterministic communication sequences along the

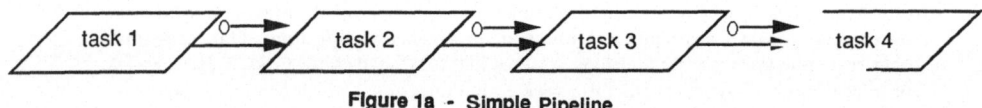

Figure 1a - Simple Pipeline

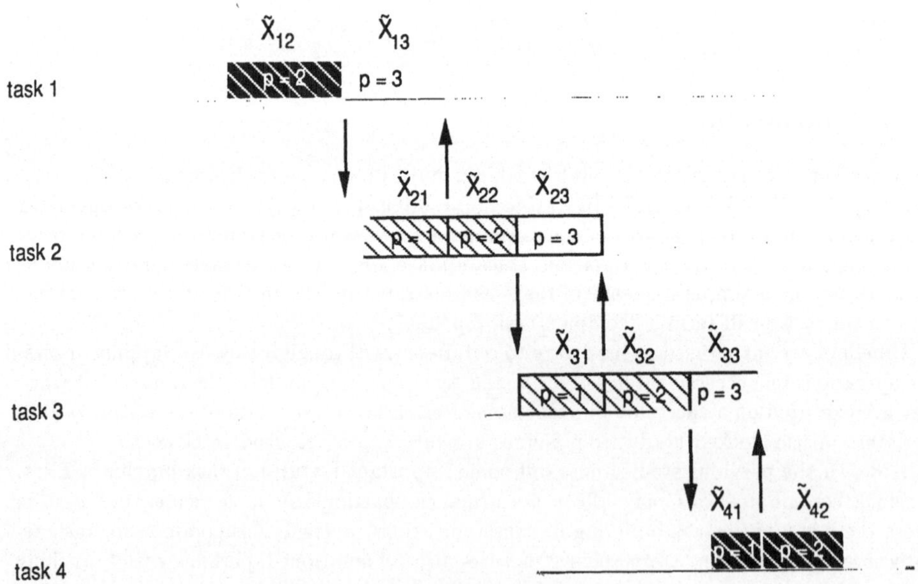

task 1 $\tilde{X}_{12}$ $\tilde{X}_{13}$
          $p=2$ $p=3$

task 2 $\tilde{X}_{21}$ $\tilde{X}_{22}$ $\tilde{X}_{23}$
          $p=1$ $p=2$ $p=3$

task 3 $\tilde{X}_{31}$ $\tilde{X}_{32}$ $\tilde{X}_{33}$
          $p=1$ $p=2$ $p=3$

task 4 $\tilde{X}_{41}$ $\tilde{X}_{42}$
          $p=1$ $p=2$

Figure 1b - Task Synchronization

pipeline. It also introduces a new method for analysis of queues in systems with arbitrary synchronization and static dependencies, called "Conditional Mean Value Analysis". The essence of the contribution of this paper is fast approximations for contention. With this method, systems of over 80 tasks have been modelled.

For tasks with rendezvous, timed Petri Nets have been used in [WOOD88], [SCHA88], and [KANT88]. In [WOOD88] the Generalized Stochastic Petri Net (GSPN) model of Ajmone Marsan, Balbo et al [AJMO84] was applied to a class of stochastic models of task behaviour called Stochastic Rendezvous Nets. Kant [KANT88] used a combination of timed Petri Nets and queues for a similar class of models. Other authors have used Petri nets to represent and analyze the flow of control between tasks in Ada programs. Schatz [SCHA88] proposed doing this, based directly on parsing of Ada code, followed by timed Petri Net modelling of performance. However he does not include modelling of processor dispatching delays.

In any case, it seems (see for instance [WOOD88] for a discussion) that Petri Net models are too large and computation-intensive for use on systems of practical scale, although hierarchical decomposition may overcome this obstacle. The present approach combines a degree of hierarchical decomposition with a delay approximation. It is a special case of approximation of Timed Petri Nets or other equivalent models by higher level constructs, with approximate delays for the subsystems. This is the purpose also of the Active Server Network family of algorithms described in [WOOD84] and applied to Stochastic Rendezvous Networks in [WOOD88]. The approach uses ideas from queueing network analysis, notably surrogate delays [JACO82] and approximate Mean Value Analysis [REIS79].

The Rendezvous Network Approach

The Rendezvous (abbreviated RNV hereafter) Network modelling approach identifies all the various waiting delays and approximates them by calculations adapted from approximate Mean Value Analysis [REIS79]. In the pipeline, each task waits for the following task to complete the RNV which passes on the data, plus there may be processor waiting and waiting for shared server tasks. In adapting the Mean Value calculation, conditions governing the state of the accepting task or processor are considered. The method reflects saturation of the pipeline back towards the beginning, and throughput is determined by how fast the source task can cycle.

The present research extends the previous work on stochastic sequences of rendezvous by examining deterministic sequences which occur along the pipeline, as well as processor contention. Shared server tasks are then a natural generalization which will be obtained by combining this and the earlier work. The goal of this paper is to show that the approach can be extended, and to evaluate its accuracy. The principal advantage of the method is speed which is several orders of magnitude faster than Petri net analysis even on small examples. The accuracy obtained is only modest, with errors generally under 10% but occasionally up to twice that.

Section 2 begins with a special model for simple pipelines, and Section 3 describes contention for processors by the pipeline tasks. Section 4 adds splits in the pipeline flow, to give the complete model. The approximations are compared to exact results found from GSPN analysis of the smaller examples and to simulation results for the others.

2   Simple Task Pipelines With Rendezvous

To introduce the approach to be taken for complex pipelines, first consider the more usual "simple task pipeline", illustrated in Figure 1(a) and described as follows:

- a sequence of N static tasks communicating in one direction by rendezvous, in pipeline style. The first task is a source, computing and generating data for the remainder of the pipeline, while the last task is a sink (after completing its computation).

- each task has a processor to itself (this will be relaxed shortly to allow tasks to be co-allocated), and there are no contention delays in communications. Communication delays can be included in the task execution times.

- each task executes in a cycle divided into three phases:

> *Phase 1 (synchronous):* (a) receive input data as a message, (b) check the data, (c) reply to sender, to acknowledge completion of the handshake;
>
> *Phase 2 (asynchronous execution):* execute the task function on the data, for this stage of the pipeline.
>
> *Phase 3 (transmit by RNV)* (a) send the data to next task in the pipeline, (b) wait for the reply, (c) make ready to receive the next input message (cycle back to phase 1)

- task 1, the source, omits phase 1 and task N, the sink, omits phase 3 in its cycle.

This pipeline always has input waiting and runs at its maximum rate. Poisson arrivals at a lower rate are a simple adaptation, described at the end. The following notation describes the sequence of activities in a single RNV and is illustrated in Figure 1(b):

> f = throughput or frequency of task cycling for all tasks in the pipeline;
>
> s_{ip} = mean execution time of task i in phase p;
>
> x_{ip} = mean duration of phase p of task i. For $p = 1, 2$, a phase consists purely of execution, and $x_{ip} = s_{ip}$.
>
> w_{ij} = mean delay to task i in a RNV with task j.
>
> y_{ijp} = the mean number of of messages sent to task j by task i in phase p. In this simplest version $y_{ij1} = y_{ij2} = 0$.
>
> y_{ij3} = 1 if task j succeeds task i in the pipeline, or 0 otherwise (i.e., $y_{i,i+1,3} = 1$).

The notation $\tilde{s}_{ip}$, $\tilde{x}_{ip}$, $\tilde{w}_{ij}$, etc. will be used for the random variable whose mean is s_{ip}, x_{ip}, w_{ij}.

Now we shall determine the delays experienced by a task in processing and in waiting at the RNVs. The only way a task can be made to wait is, if the successor task is still busy from the previous message. That is, the only reason task j can make task $j - 1$ wait is if task j is busy in its second or third phase. Define:

> E_{jp} = event that, at the moment task $j - 1$ sends to task j, the latter is busy in phase p, $p > 2$.
>
> E_j = the union of E_{j2} and E_{j3}; task $j - 1$ 'overtakes' task j.
>
> V_{jp} = the mean residual life of phase p of task j, called $MRL(\tilde{x}_{jp})$. In general, $MRL(\tilde{x}) = Exp\{\tilde{x}^2\}/2Exp\{\tilde{x}\}$ (see [KLEI75] Sec. 5.2 for a discussion of mean residual life). If $\tilde{x}$ is exponentially distributed, $MRL(\tilde{x}) = Exp\{\tilde{x}\}$.

Then for a simple pipeline the delays defined above are given by:

$$w_{j-1,j} = x_{j1} + Prob\{E_{j2}\}(V_{j2} + x_{j3}) + Prob\{E_{j3}\}V_{j3}, \quad j = 2, \ldots, N \qquad (1)$$

$$x_{j1} = s_{j1}, \quad x_{j2} = s_{j2}, \quad x_{j3} = w_{j,j+1}, \quad j = 1, \ldots, N \qquad (2)$$

with the exceptions that $x_{11} = x_{N3} = 0$. The MRL values are

$$V_{jp} = Exp\{(\tilde{x}_{jp})^2\}/2(x_{jp}), \quad j = 2, \ldots, N \qquad (3)$$

Two approximations will be used in (1), one for V_{jp} and one for $Prob\{E_{jp}\}$. The mean residual life value V is computed on the basis of an assumption that the request instant is random and independent of the state of task j. It is also assumed that $\tilde{w}$ is exponentially distributed, which means that (3) gives:

$$V_{j2} = Exp\{\tilde{s}_{j2}^2\}/2s_{j2}; \quad V_{j3} = w_{j,j+1} \quad j = 1,\dots,N \qquad (4)$$

For $j = N$, we use $V_{N3} = w_{N,N+1} = 0$. MRL values are not needed for phase 1.

The event E_{j2}, that task j is found to be busy in phase 2, is illustrated in Figure 2(a). The probability was found by analyzing the race between task j finishing this phase, and the generation of the next RNV request by task $j - 1$. Let $\tilde{t}_{j-1}$ denote the time from the end of the previous RNV to the instant of the next request from task $j - 1$; it has mean value $1/f - w_{j-1,j}$. Then:

$$Prob\{E_{jp}\} = Prob\{\tilde{t}_{j-1} < (\tilde{x}_{j2} + \dots + \tilde{x}_{jp})\}; \quad p = 2 \text{ or } 3$$

which depends on the distributions of $\tilde{t}_{j-1}$ and of $(\tilde{x}_{j2} + \dots + \tilde{x}_{jp})$. Figure 2(b) shows the random variables involved. An especially simple result is obtained if the distributions are

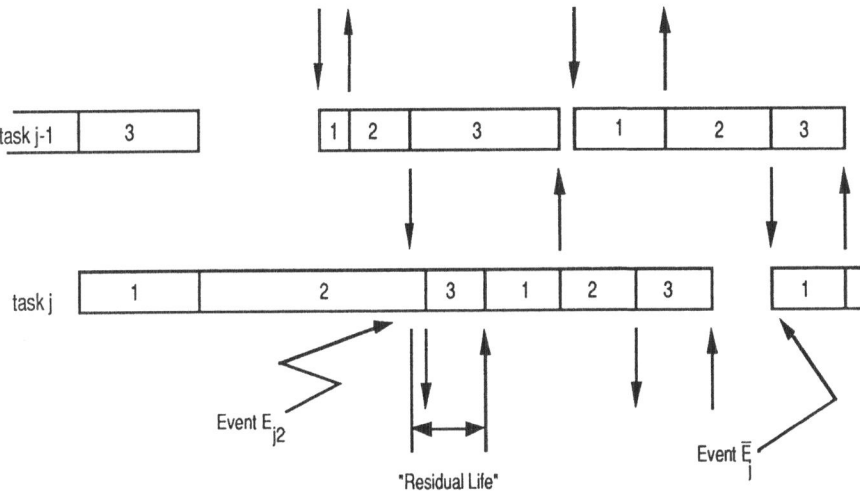

Figure 2a - Overtaking of Previous Computation

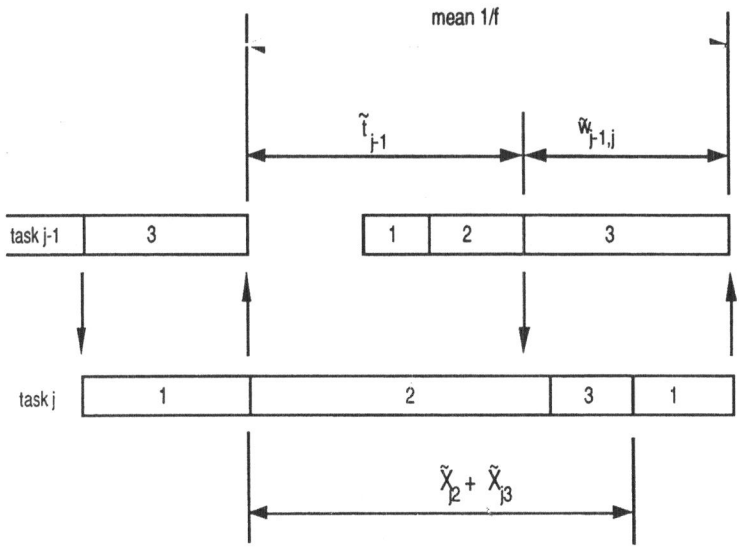

Figure 2b - Race

311

exponential, so for the sake of calculation this was assumed. With a little manipulation this gives the approximation:

$$Prob\{E_{j2}\} = (x_{j2})/(x_{j2} + (1/f) - w_{j-1,j}) \qquad (5a)$$

$$\begin{aligned} Prob\{E_{j3}\} &= (1 - Prob\{E_{j2}\})Prob\{E_{j3}|\bar{E}_{j2}\} \\ &= (1 - Prob\{E_{j2}\})x_{j3}/(x_{j3} + (1/f) - w_{j-1,j}) \end{aligned} \qquad (5b)$$

$$Prob\{E_j\} = Prob\{E_{j2}\} + Prob\{E_{j3}\} \qquad (5c)$$

Now (1)-(3) can be solved for the delay for each task in terms of the execution of the task which follows it. In order to solve for the throughput, the calculations for x and w are applied iteratively. At each iteration the overall throughput f is calculated from the time it takes the source task to cycle:

$$f = 1/(x_{12} + x_{13}) \qquad (6)$$

This throughput value is then used to find the other quantities for the next iteration, using the following algorithm. The starting value for f was taken as a bounding value found from a task saturation condition.

Algorithm 1, for Simple Pipelines

Step 1 – initialize $f = 1/max_i(s_{i1} + s_{i2})$; $x_{i1} = s_{i1}$, $x_{i2} = s_{i2}$, for $i = 1,.., N$; and V_N from (4).

Step 2 – for each value of j in the order $j = N-1, N-2, \ldots, 1$ determine $w_{j,j+1}$, x_{j3}, V_{j2} and V_{j3} using (1), (2), (4), (5).

Step 3 – set $f = 1/(x_{12} + x_{13})$. If within a preset percentage of the previous value, stop, else repeat from 2.

Examples and Accuracy

The algorithm was applied to the example of four tasks shown in Figure 1(a), and compared to an exact throughput analysis found by a Markov Chain analysis of a GSPN model [AJMO84]. For this purpose the distributions of execution times were taken to be exponential, although the algorithm is not limited to such cases. The parameter values and results are shown in the following table.

Table 1. Simple Pipeline Throughputs (No Processor Contention)

Four tasks as in Figure 1(a) with default parameters: $s_{i1} = 0.1sec$, $s_{i2} = 1.0$ sec, $y_{i,i+1,3} = 1$, all i.

Case	Parameters (differences from defaults)	Exact Throughput	Approximate Throughput
1	Default	0.474	0.461
2	$s_{12} = \frac{2}{3}$, $s_{22} = 2$	0.368	0.361
3	$s_{12} = \frac{1}{2}$, $s_{22} = \frac{2}{3}$ $s_{32} = 2.$	0.384	0.376
4	$s_{12} = 0.5$, $s_{22} = 0.8$ $s_{32} = 1.2$ $s_{42} = 1.5$	0.432	0.423
5	$s_{12} = 1.5$, $s_{22} = 1.2$ $s_{32} = 0.8$ $s_{42} = 0.5$	0.432	0.424
6	$s_{12} = 0.5$, $s_{22} = 1.5$, $s_{32} = 1.5$, $s_{42} = 0.5$	0.400	0.391

Case 1 is balanced, while cases 2 and 3 show various unbalanced patterns. Cases 4,5,6 have the same total workload as case 1 but redistributed systematically in increasing order (case 4), in decreasing order (case 5), and increasing first, then decreasing (case 6). The most balanced case, case 1, gives the largest error of about -2.7%, and all the approximate throughputs are less than the exact values. The nominal saturation rate can be found from the longest processing time s_{i2}, plus 0.1 sec. for communication in phase 1 (input) and another 0.1 in the RNV on output. This gives $1.2^{-1} = 0.833$ in case 1, $2.2^{-2} = 0.454$ in cases 2 and 3, and $1.7^{-1} = 0.588$ in cases 4, 5 and 6. The actual value is less than this because of random variations and the associated waiting caused by them and propagated by the rendezvous.

Notice that each task is busy only about half the time (execution time of 1.1 sec per cycle times rate of about 0.4 cycles per sec.). The rest of the time it is blocked, either waiting for input or waiting to pass on its output. This is a penalty of the rendezvous communications, which can be mitigated by introducing buffers between stages.

3 Processor Contention

The allocation of tasks to processors and the resulting queueing delays from the time a task is ready until it begins execution, are now considered. The notation $J(i)$ is used for the processor which executes task i. We suppose that when a task is ready to run it "makes a request" to its processor, is queued and served and "returns" at the end of processing. Processor contention only occurs when a task blocks and then resumes. This always occurs in phase 3 for passing on data, except in task N. It also occurs sometimes in phase 1 of tasks $2 - N$, when even the message from the previous task is not available. This condition "message from task $i - 1$ is not available when task i tries to receive it" has already been identified as the event E_i. The mean waiting for a single request depends on the loading of processor $J(i)$, described as the set K_i of tasks contending for the processor. We shall consider a certain degree of state dependence in K_i, for if task $i - 1$ is allocated to the same processor and if it is suspended attempting to RNV with task i, then it is removed from contention. Because these processor requests occur at the end of phase 3 of task i, this situation corresponds to the event E_i defined in the last Section, when task $i - 1$ is ready before task i is ready. Thus we denote the contention set as K_{iE}:

$$K_{iE} = \{k|J(k) = J(i); k \neq i; k \neq i - 1\} \tag{7}$$

and the corresponding mean wait for the processor is denoted W_{iE}. The opposite condition, in which task $i - 1$ is still running and in contention, has contention set $K_{i\bar{E}}$ and mean wait $W_{i\bar{E}}$, with:

$$K_{i\bar{E}} = \{k|J(k) = J(i); k \neq i\} \tag{8}$$

At a randomly chosen processor request instant the mean wait for the processor is the combination;

$$Processor\_waiting = Prob\{E_i\}W_{iE} + Prob\{\bar{E}_i\}W_{i\bar{E}} \tag{9}$$

Phase 3 always contains a processor request, for $i \leq N - 1$, so:

$$x_{i3} = w_{i,i+1} + Prob\{\bar{E}_i\}W_{i\bar{E}} + Prob\{E_i\}W_{iE}; \quad i = 1, \ldots, N - 1 \tag{10}$$

Phase 1 contains a processor request only in the event $\bar{E}_i$, for $i \geq 2$, and phase 2 never does, so

$$x_{i1} = s_{i1} + Prob\{\bar{E}_i\}W_{iE}; \quad i = 2, \ldots, N \tag{11}$$

$$x_{i2} = s_{i2}; \quad i = 1, \dots, N$$

and

$$x_{11} = x_{N3} = 0$$

as before.

Conditional Mean Value Analysis for Processor Delay

The equation (9) with the condition E_i will now be used in a "Conditional Mean Value Analysis" calculation for *Processor-waiting*. The general form for a "Conditional MVA" model with conditions $C_1, \dots, C_n$ (which depend in turn on various system state probabilities denoted $state - probs$) is:

$$waiting\ values = \sum_i \{waiting \mid C_i\} Prob\{C_i\} \quad (A)$$

$$state - probs \leftarrow waiting\ values \quad (B)$$

$$Prob\{C_i\} \leftarrow state - probs \quad (C)$$

and the solution approach used here is iterative.

The following development specifically for pipelines uses Eq. (5) for (B) and (C) together, and uses Eq. (9) together with the analysis to follow in the role of (A). Considering W_{iE} first, it is broken into two components, for the task-in-service and the queue:

$$W_{iE} = Pwait_{iE}(1) + Pwait_{iE}(2) \tag{12}$$

where

$Pwait_{iE}(1)$ = waiting due to the task in execution at processor $J(i)$ at the time task i is ready to run,

$Pwait_{iE}(2)$ = waiting due to tasks which are in the queue for processor $J(i)$ at the time task i is ready to run.

We will continue to assume a randomly chosen instant for making the request for execution, subject to some qualifications to be made below. Define:

$E_{iE,k}$ = the event that a request by task i finds task k being executed by processor $J(i)$, given the contention set K_{iE}. Its probability is

$$Prob\{E_{iE,k}\} = f(s_{k1} + s_{k2}) \text{ for all } k \in K_{iE} \text{ and zero otherwise}$$

$F_{iE,k}$ = the event that a request by task i finds task k waiting in the processor queue, given contention set K_{iE};

σ_k = mean residual life of the processor execution time of task k, $MRL(\tilde{s}_{k1} + \tilde{s}_{k2})$. From the definition of MRL,

$$\sigma_k = (Exp\{\tilde{s}_{k1}^2\} + Exp\{\tilde{s}_{k2}^2\} + 2s_{k1}s_{k2})/2(s_{k1} + s_{k2}) \tag{13}$$

Then the first component of processor waiting is:

$$Pwait_{iE}(1) = \sum_{k \in K_{iE}} Prob\{E_{iE,k}\}\sigma_k = f \sum_{k \in K_{iE}} (s_{k1} + s_{k2})\sigma_k \tag{14}$$

The second component $Pwait_{iE}(2)$ is the delay for tasks in the processor queue at the time of the request, and is given by:

$$Pwait_{iE}(2) = \sum_{k \in K_{iE}} \text{Prob}\{F_{iE,k}\}(s_{k1} + s_{k2}) \tag{15}$$

To find Prob $\{F_{iE,k}\}$, consider the queue for processor $J(i)$. At a randomly selected instant the probability that task k is in the queue (waiting, not executing) is given by Little's result and by (10) and (11) as

$$\text{Prob}\{task\ k\ in\ the\ queue\} = f \times (mean\ processor\ waiting\ by\ task\ k\ per\ cycle)$$

$$= f(W_{kE} + \text{Prob}\{\bar{E}_k\}W_{k\bar{E}}) \tag{16}$$

However this must be adjusted to account for the following subtle but important interaction: task k only waits when some other task is executing and on some occasions it is task i which it waits for. In the calculation of $Pwait_{iE}(2)$ we must exclude these occasions, since task i cannot be simultaneously both in execution and arriving to the processor queue. To adjust, we condition on the task in execution being some other task and not task i. The conditional probability is taken to be a ratio of partial processor utilizations by the tasks, and gives:

$$Prob\{F_{iE,k}\} = \text{Prob}\{task\ k\ in\ the\ queue\}\text{Prob}\{not\ task\ i\ in\ execution \mid task\ k\}$$

$$= f(W_{kE} + \text{Prob}\{\bar{E}_k\}W_{k\bar{E}})\frac{\sum_{l \in K_{iE}, l \neq k} u_l}{u_i + \sum_{l \in K_{iE}, l \neq k} u_l} \tag{17}$$

where $u_i = f(s_{i1} + s_{i2})$ is the partial utilization of processor $J(i)$ by task i. This adjustment is important because, if there are only two tasks allocated to processor $J(i)$, the right side is zero and $Pwait(2)$ is zero. When one task makes a request the other must be executing, or blocked and not ready; it cannot be queued.

This completes the determination of W_{iE} using (12) with (14) - (17). $W_{i\bar{E}}$ is found by the same process with $\bar{E}$ substituted for E in (12), (14), (15), and using (16) unchanged. Then Eq. (17) is replaced for case $\bar{E}$ by:

$$Prob\{F_{i\bar{E},k}\} = f(W_{kE} + \text{Prob}\{\bar{E}_k\}W_{k\bar{E}})\frac{\sum_{l \in K_{i\bar{E}}, l \neq k} u_l}{u_i + \sum_{l \in K_{i\bar{E}}, l \neq k} u_l} \tag{18}$$

Processor delay terms also enter the computation of the mean residual life V_{jp}. We will use the Appendix with $z_1 = w_{j,j+1}$ and $z_2 = W_{j,E}$ (since every waiting of task $j-1$ for task j involves event E_j) and the processor waiting will be assumed to be exponentially distributed. Then Eq. (4) is replaced with:

$$V_{j2} = MRL\{\tilde{s}_{j2}\}$$

$$V_{j3} = MRL(\tilde{w}_{j,j+1} + \tilde{w}_{j,E}) = \frac{w_{j,j+1}^2 + W_{jE}^2 + (w_{j,j+1} + W_{jE})^2}{2(w_{j,j+1} + W_{jE})},$$

$$j = 1, \ldots, N-1 \tag{19}$$

The computation of the throughput is similar to Section 2, with Eqs. (10), (11) in place of (2), and W and V computed as above. Note that, if a task has a processor to itself the W terms are zero and the analysis of Section 2 can be used for that task, ignoring the existence of the processor.

The algorithm for throughputs is similar to the algorithm in section 2, but with the processor delay calculations included in Step 2.

Examples and Accuracy

Examples were computed for the same four-task pipeline and for three different processor allocations, as shown in Figure 3(a),(b),(c). Cases 1–6 have the same task parameters as Cases 1–6 in Table 1, and these are repeated for the two other allocations, giving 18 cases in all. Table 1 can be considered a fourth allocation with one processor per task.

Cases 1, 4, 5 and 6 all have the same total execution time, equally balanced between the two processors but distributed differently among the tasks. The highest throughput is found in case 5, where the tasks are ordered by execution time s_{12}, longest task first; the worst is case 4, ordered the opposite way, and the balanced cases (cases 1 and 6) are between them. The approximation has the most error with the balanced case, as before.

When only one processor is used, all the corresponding cases (i.e. 7, 10, 11, 12) have the same throughput; the processor is the only constraint. With three processors (in cases 13-18) the middle one is more heavily loaded than the others and is the dominant influence on throughput.

Table 2. Simple Pipeline Throughputs with Processor Contention

Four tasks as in Figure 1(a) with default parameters: $s_{i1} = 0.1$, $s_{i2} = 1.0$, $y_{i,i+1,3} = 1$, all $i = 1,..4$. The processor allocation is given by a list $J(1)$, $J(2)$, $J(3)$, $J(4)$.

Case	Parameters (differences from defaults)	Processor Allocation	Exact Throughput	Approximate Throughput
1	Default	1,1,2,2	0.367	0.369
2	$s_{12} = \frac{2}{3}$, $s_{22} = 2$	1,1,2,2	0.302	0.282
3	$s_{12} = \frac{1}{2}$, $s_{22} = \frac{2}{3}$ $s_{32} = 2.$	1,1,2,2	0.304	0.332
4	$s_{12} = 0.5$, $s_{22} = 0.8$ $s_{32} = 1.2$ $s_{42} = 1.5$	1,1,2,2	0.328	0.331
5	$s_{12} = 1.5$, $s_{22} = 1.2$ $s_{32} = 0.8$ $s_{42} = 0.5$	1,1,2,2	0.389	0.339
6	$s_{12} = 0.5$, $s_{22} = 1.5$ $s_{32} = 1.5$ $s_{42} = 0.5$	1,1,2,2	0.347	0.343
7	Default	1,1,1,1	0.233	0.239
8	$s_{12} = \frac{2}{3}$, $s_{22} = 2$	1,1,1,1	0.201	0.200
9	$s_{12} = 0.5$, $s_{22} = 0.6667$ $s_{32} = 2.$	1,1,1,1	0.224	0.219
10	$s_{12} = 0.5$, $s_{22} = 0.8$ $s_{32} = 1.2$ $s_{42} = 1.5$	1,1,1,1	0.233	0.229
11	$s_{12} = 1.5$, $s_{22} = 1.2$ $s_{32} = 0.8$ $s_{42} = 0.5$	1,1,1,1	0.233	0.232
12	$s_{12} = 0.5$, $s_{22} = 1.5$ $s_{32} = 1.5$ $s_{42} = 0.5$	1,1,1,1	0.233	0.227
13	Default	1,2,2,3	0.398	0.393
14	$s_{12} = \frac{2}{3}$, $s_{22} = 2$	1,2,2,3	0.302	0.308
15	$s_{12} = 0.5$, $s_{22} = 0.6667$ $s_{32} = 2.$	1,2,2,3	0.332	0.304
16	$s_{12} = 0.5$, $s_{22} = 0.8$ $s_{32} = 1.2$ $s_{42} = 1.5$	1,2,2,3	0.384	0.378
17	$s_{12} = 1.5$, $s_{22} = 1.2$ $s_{32} = 0.8$ $s_{42} = 0.5$	1,2,2,3	0.368	0.374
18	$s_{12} = 0.5$, $s_{22} = 1.5$ $s_{32} = 1.5$ $s_{42} = 0.5$	1,2,2,3	0.309	0.308

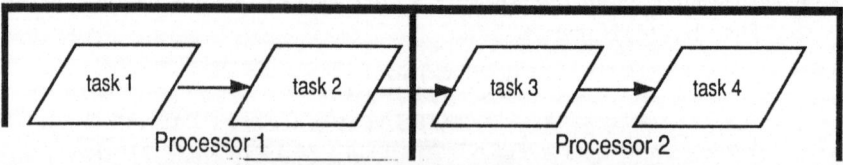

Figure 3a - 2 Processor System, Cases 1-6 in Table 2

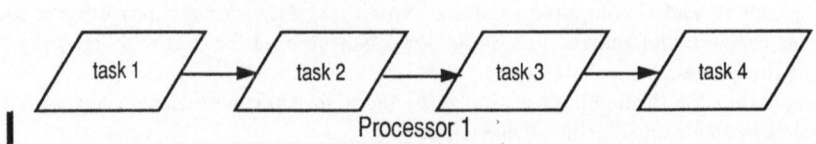

Figure 3b - 1 Processor System, Cases 7-12 in Table 2

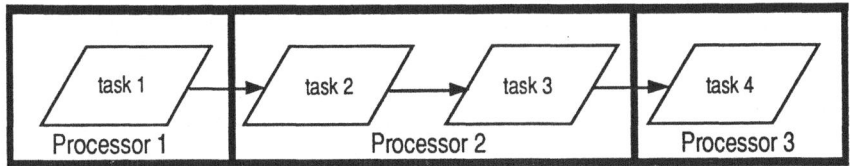

Figure 3c - 3 Processor System, Cases 13-18 in Table 2

Introducing the processor contention delays has increased the errors somewhat; they range from -8.5% in case 15 to +9.1% in case 3. The RMS percentage error is 3.6% and the mean is -0.6%.

4   Task Pipelines with Branching Flows

With flow branching there can be any number of parallel streams of pipeline tasks, as well as the features of the previous two sections.

Figure 4 shows an example. The joining of parallel flows is excluded from this study because it raises a distinct set of modelling problems which require special treatment, for instance in the split-join queue analysis of Flatto and Hahn [FLAT84].

The durations of phases 1 and 2 are the same as before, apart from differences in W described later. However the rest of the task is affected by splitting of the flow, for a task may now have several successors in the pipeline, and there will be a separate phase providing a RNV with each one (and a delay w) to pass on the data. Task j is a successor of task i if there is a phase p with $y_{ijp} = 1$, $p \in (3, P_i)$, where P_i is the number of successors of task i, plus 2. Without loss of generality the tasks are numbered so that data is passed only from lower-numbered tasks to higher-numbered tasks.

The phase durations are now:

$$x_{i1} = s_{i1} + (1 - Prob\{E_i\})W_{iE}, \quad x_{i2} = s_{i2}, \quad i \in (1, N) \tag{20}$$

$$x_{ip} = \sum_{j=i+1}^{N} y_{ijp}(w_{ij} + Processor\_waiting), \quad i \in (1, N), \ p \in (3, P_i) \tag{21}$$

$$w_{ij} = x_{j1} + \sum_{p=2}^{P_j} Prob\{E_{jp}\}(V_{jp} + \sum_{u=p+1}^{P_j} x_{ju}), \quad i, j \in (1, N) \tag{22}$$

$$Prob\{E_{jp}\} = (1 - Prob\{E_{j2}\}) \ldots (1 - Prob\{E_{j,p-1}\})x_{jp}/(x_{jp} + (1/f) - w_{ij}) \tag{23}$$

$$V_{jp} = MRL(\tilde{x}_{jp}) \tag{24}$$

There are two quantities in (20)-(24) which are affected by splitting of flows, *(Processor_waiting)* in x_{ip}, and V_{jp}; consider the former first. With more than one RNV, the probability π_{ip} of seeing contention set K_{iE} when task i is ready depends on the phase p in which the RNV takes place. As time goes on, the probability increases, as the sender task is progressively more likely to have finished. Thus in (21) the term *(Processor_waiting)* is given by the following (in place of (9)):

$$Processor\_waiting = (1 - \pi_{ip})W_{i\bar{E}} + \pi_{ip}W_{iE} \tag{25}$$

The value of π_{ip} is:

$$\pi_{ip} = Prob\{E_{i2}\} + \ldots + Prob\{E_{ip}\} \tag{26}$$

317

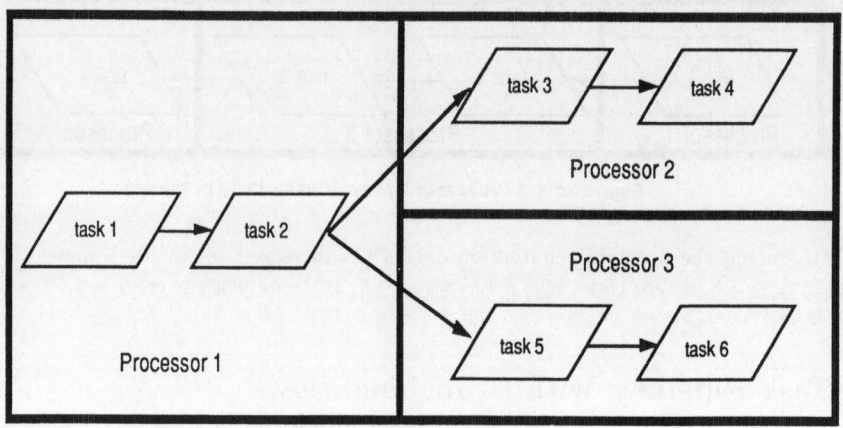

Figure 4a - Pipeline with Split

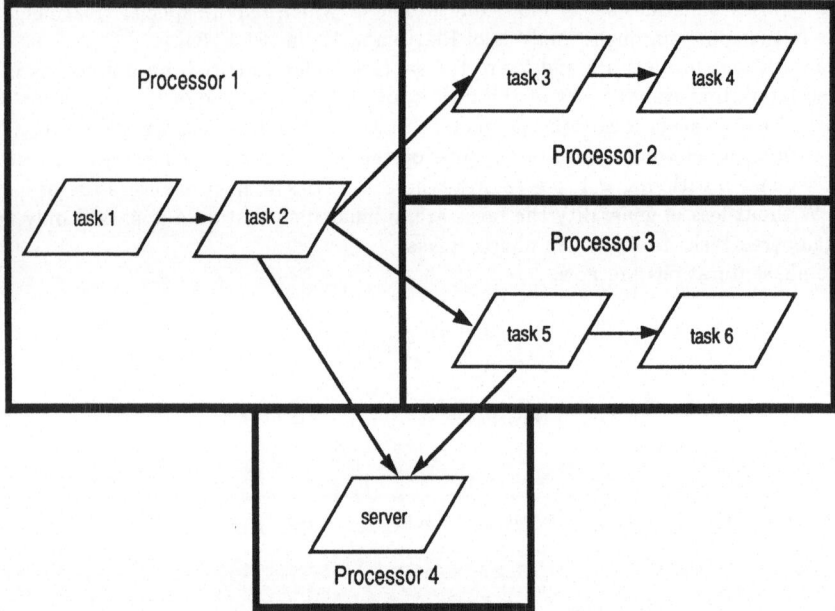

Figure 4b - Pipeline with Split and Server

V_{jp} is similar to (19), with task k being the successor task sent to by phase p when there are several successors at a split:

$$
\begin{aligned}
V_{j2} &= MRL\{\tilde{s}_{j2}\} \\
V_{jp} &= MRL\{\tilde{w}_{jk} + \tilde{W}_{jE}\}, \quad \text{for } p = 3, \ldots P_j \\
& \qquad\qquad j = 1, \ldots, N
\end{aligned}
\tag{27}
$$

The processor-waiting calculation is the same as in Section 3, except that the task which sends a message to task i (there is still only one) is not necessarily task $i - 1$. Thus the contention set definition (7) generalizes to:

$$
K_{iE} = \{k | J(k) = J(i); \ k \neq i; \ \sum_p y_{kip} = 0\}
\tag{28}
$$

318

The computation of *Pwait(1)* by (14) follows directly, and of *Pwait(2)* by (15) also, when (17) and (18) are modified appropriately. In both (17) and (18) the expression on the right side before the fraction generalizes to

$$\text{Prob}\{task\ k\ in\ the\ queue\} = f[(1 - \text{Prob}\{E_k\})W_{kE}$$

$$\sum_{p=3}^{P_k} \sum_j y_{kjp}((1 - \pi_{kp})W_{k\bar{E}} + \pi_{kp}W_{kE})] \tag{29}$$

This completely determines the W terms.

These component calculations are now assembled into the following algorithm.

Algorithm for Complex Pipeline Throughputs

Step 1: Initialize $f = 1/(max_i(s_{i1} + s_{i2}))$, V_{N4} from (4), and $x_{i1} = s_{i1}$, $x_{i2} = s_{i2}$, $x_{ip} = 0$, $(p = 3, P_i)$, for all $i \in (1, N)$.

Step 2: For each j in the order $j = N - 1, N - 2, ...1$ determine:

    (a) w_{jk} from (22), with (5), (27) for all $k \in (j + 1, N)$;

    (b) W_{jE} from (8), with (28), (12), (14), (15), and (17) as modified by (29);

    (c) $W_{j\bar{E}}$ from (8) with (22), equations symmetrical with (12), (14), (15) by interchanging E and $\bar{E}$, and (18) as modified by (29);

    (d) x_{jp} from (20), (21) with (22), (23), (24).

Step 3: set $f = 1/(x_{12} + x_{13})$. If within a preset percentage of the previous value, stop, else repeat from step 2.

Examples and Accuracy

An example system is shown in Figure 4(b), with six tasks and one branching point. Table 3 shows some results of using the full algorithm on this case.

The approximation shows a tendency to underestimate the throughput by around 6%, a larger error here than without the splitting of flow.

The mean error is -5.7% and the RMS error is 6.6%. The worst error occurred in case 16 with all tasks allocated to a single processor, which is odd. Cases with the execution bottleneck at the end of the pipeline, such as 4, 5, 10, 11, 15, 16, 21 showed a tendency to larger percentage errors; in these cases the effect of delay at the end is pushed back through the waiting calculations to the entry throughput, and errors have more opportunity to accumulate. But case 20 is similar, with a small error.

In an iterative algorithm convergence and computational complexity must be considered. Convergence was always obtained in a few steps, but a formal proof of convergence has not been found. It was necessary to modify the iteration update step to apply only a fraction (50% was used) of the calculated change in waiting values w_{ij} at each step. Time complexity is of the order of N^3, the same as in [WOOD88], and space complexity is also similar at N^2.

5   Conclusions

The various possible structures of contention for resources in a software pipeline using rendezvous communication have been studied in detail, including contention for processing resources and shared software resources. Approximations were found within a new framework for estimating queueing delays, called "rendezvous networks". Significant extensions to the rendezvous network approach were made in the process. The resulting analysis was extensively tested on examples and gives throughput accuracies from 1% to nearly 15%, but almost all under 10%.

Some direct generalizations can be described. Software pipelines often include shared server tasks with access from various points in the pipeline, as illustrated in Figure 4(b), but space limitations require that models for these cases be described elsewhere.

The mean delay for one path in a pipeline is easily calculated as the sum of phase durations:

$$Pipeline\ delay\ =\ x_{11} + \sum_{i=1}^{N}(x_{i2} + x_{i3})$$

The first phase of each task after the input is not included in the sum because it forms part of the preceding phase 3.

Table 3. Complex Pipeline Throughputs

Six tasks as in Figure 4(a) with default parameters: $s_{i1} = 0.1$, $s_{i2} = 1.0$, all $i = 1,..6$ and $y_{123} = y_{233} = y_{235} = y_{343} = y_{453} = 1$. The processor allocation is given by a list $J(1), J(2), J(3), J(4), J(5), J(6)$.

Case	Parameters (differences from defaults)	Processor Allocation	Exact Throughput	Approximate Throughput
1	Default	1,2,3,4,5,6	0.421	0.389
2	$s_{12} = 0.667$, $s_{22} = 2$	1,2,3,4,5,6	0.337	0.315
3	$s_{12} = 0.5$, $s_{22} = 0.667$ $s_{32} = 2$. $s_{52} = 2$.	1,2,3,4,5,6	0.310	0.292
4	$s_{62} = 2$.	1,2,3,4,5,6	0.353	0.336
5	$s_{12} = 0.3$, $s_{22} = 0.7$ $s_{42} = 1.3$ $s_{62} = 1.7$	1,2,3,4,5,6	0.392	0.371
6	$s_{12} = 1.7$, $s_{22} = 1.3$ $s_{42} = 0.7$ $s_{62} = 0.3$	1,2,3,4,5,6	0.354	0.343
7	Default	1,1,2,2,3,3	0.312	0.307
8	$s_{12} = 0.667$, $s_{22} = 2$	1,1,2,2,3,3	0.268	0.252
9	$s_{12} = 0.5$, $s_{22} = 0.667$ $s_{32} = 2$. $s_{52} = 2$.	1,1,2,2,3,3	0.247	0.258
10	$s_{62} = 2$.	1,1,2,2,3,3	0.258	0.248
11	$s_{12} = 0.3$, $s_{22} = 0.7$ $s_{42} = 1.3$ $s_{62} = 1.7$	1,1,2,2,3,3	0.291	0.273
12	$s_{12} = 1.7$, $s_{22} = 1.3$ $s_{42} = 0.7$ $s_{62} = 0.3$	1,1,2,2,3,3	0.281	0.271
13	Default	1,1,1,1,1,1	0.154	0.143
14	$s_{12} = 0.667$, $s_{22} = 2$	1,1,1,1,1,1	0.140	0.128
15	$s_{12} = 0.5$, $s_{22} = 0.667$ $s_{32} = 2$. $s_{52} = 2$.	1,1,1,1,1,1	0.130	0.113
16	$s_{62} = 2$.	1,1,1,1,1,1	0.133	0.119
17	Default	1,1,1,1,2,2	0.222	0.211
18	$s_{12} = 0.667$, $s_{22} = 2$	1,1,1,1,2,2	0.194	0.181
19	$s_{12} = 0.5$, $s_{22} = 0.667$ $s_{32} = 2$. $s_{52} = 2$.	1,1,1,1,2,2	0.196	0.183
20	$s_{62} = 2$.	1,1,1,1,2,2	0.203	0.195
21	$s_{12} = 0.3$, $s_{22} = 0.7$ $s_{42} = 1.3$ $s_{62} = 1.7$	1,1,1,1,2,2	0.236	0.216
22	$s_{12} = 1.7$, $s_{22} = 1.3$ $s_{42} = 0.7$ $s_{62} = 0.3$	1,1,1,1,2,2	0.197	0.185

For cases with Poisson arrivals at a fixed rate ("open" models) the throughput is known and it is delays that are of interest. One pass through the algorithm determines the phase durations and MRLs; then the input queue waiting time is found by considering only the first task as a server to the arrival stream. It is modelled as a special server, termed an M/G+G/1 server in [LENY88]. The result of Skinner [SKIN67] gives the mean input queue waiting time as:

$$Input\ wait\ =\ fExp(x_1^2)/2(1 - f\sum_{p} x_{1p})$$

where $Exp(x_1^2)$ is the mean square of the total service time of task 1, given by:

$$Exp(x_1^2) = (\sum_p x_{1p})^2 + Var(\sum_p \tilde{x}_{1p})$$

Because the phases are independent the variances add:

$$Exp\{x_1^2\} = (\sum_p x_{1p})^2 + \sum_p Var(\tilde{x}_{1p})$$

Total delay from arrival of a unit of input, to its completion, can be found by combining the input delay and the pipeline delay calculations.

6 References

[AJMO84] M. Ajmone Marsan, G. Balbo, and G. Conte, "A class of generalized stochastic Petri nets for the performance evaluation of multiprocessor systems", *ACM Trans. on Computer Systems*, v 2 n 2 May 1984.

[CHER83] D. R. Cheriton, W. Zwaenpol, "The distributed V-kernel and its performance for diskless workstations", *Proc. 9th Symp on Operating Systems Principles*, ACM Operating Systems Review v17 n 5, pp 129-140, Oct 1983.

[DOD83] U. S. Dept. of Defense, *Reference Manual for the Ada Programming Language*, MIL-STD-1815a, 1983.

[FLAT84] L. Flatto, S. Hahn, "Two parallel queues created by arrivals with two demands", *SIAM J. on Appl. Math.*, v 44, n 5, Oct. 1984.

[GAMM84] N. D. Gammage, L. M. Casey, "The software architecture of a distributed processing system", *Proc. 4th Int Conf. on Distributed Computing Systems*, IEEE Catalog 84CH2021-4, pp 414-431, May 1984.

[JACO82] P. A. Jacobson, E. D. Lazowska, "Analyzing Queueing Networks with Simultaneous Resource Possession", *Comm. ACM.*, v 25, no 2, Feb. 1982.

[KANT87] K. Kant, "Modelling Interprocess Communication in Distributed Programs", *Proc. Int. Wkshop on Petri Nets and Performance Models*, Madison, Wisc., Aug. 1987, IEEE Catalog 87TH0815-9, pp 75-83.

[KLEI75] L. Kleinrock, *Queueing Systems*, v 1, Wiley, 1975.

[KOGG81] P. M. Kogge, *The Architecture of Pipelined Computers*, Hemisphere, Washington, 1981.

[LENY88] L. M. Le Ny, C. M. Woodside, "Performance Modelling of Queues with Rendezvous Service", Report OCIEE-88-01, Dept of Systems and Computer Engineering, Carleton University, Ottawa, Canada, April 1988.

[REIS79] M. Reiser, "A queueing analysis of computer communication networks with window flow control", *IEEE Trans. on Communications*, v COM-27, pp 1199-1209, Aug. 1979.

[SCHA88] S. M. Schatz and W.K. Cheng, "A Petri Net framework for automated static analysis of Ada tasking behaviour", to appear in *J. Systems and Software*, 1988.

[SKIN67] C. Skinner, "A priority Queueing System with Server Walking Time", *Operations Research*, v 15 pp. 278-285, 1967.

[WOOD84] C. M. Woodside, E. Neron, E. D-S. Ho, B. Mondoux, "An "active server" model for the performance of parallel programs written using rendezvous", *Preprints of Int. Workshop on Modelling and Performance Evaluation of Parallel Systems*, pp 157-174, Grenoble, Dec. 1984. Also published in *J. Systems and Software*, v6 nos 1 and 2, pp 125-132, May 1986.

[WOOD88] C. M. Woodside, "Throughput Calculation for Basic Stochastic Rendezvous Networks"; to appear in *Performance Evaluation*, late 1988.

Appendix: Mean Residual Life

We consider the mean residual life V of a summation variable $\tilde{X}$ with mean X:

$$\tilde{X} = \tilde{s} + \sum_{i=1}^{M} \tilde{z}_i$$

where $\tilde{s}$ has a general distribution with mean s, $\tilde{z}_i$ has an exponential distribution with mean z_i, M is a constant and all the components of $\tilde{X}$ are independent of each other. It is well known (see e.g. [KLEI75]) that

$$V = Exp\{\tilde{X}^2\}/2Exp\{X\}$$
$$Exp\{z_i^2\} = 2z_i^2$$

Thus:

$$V = (Exp\{(\tilde{s} + \sum_{i}^{M} \tilde{z}_i)^2\})/2X = (Exp\{\tilde{s}^2\} + 2s\sum_{i} z_i + Exp\{(\sum_{i} z_i)^2\})/2X$$

$$= (Exp\{\tilde{s}^2\} + 2s\sum_{i} z_i + \sum_{i} z_i^2 + (\sum_{i} z_i)^2)/2X$$

If all the components are exponentially distributed we can set $s = 0$ in the above.

ON THE TRADEOFF BETWEEN

PARALLELISM AND COMMUNICATION

Andrzej Duda

IMAG
Laboratoire de Génie Informatique
BP 53 X
38041 Grenoble Cedex, France

ABSTRACT

The problem of the optimal partitioning of a computation into parallel tasks is studied. Tasks are created dynamically and there is a cost associated with the creation and with the transfer of parameters and results. In this case, increasing the number of tasks does not always decrease the execution time. We analyze quantitatively the tradeoff between parallelism and communication. Several processor interconnection structures are considered: the ring, the tree, the binary k-cube, the complete connection. The optimal number of tasks that maximizes the speedup and the quality is given.

INTRODUCTION

We consider the problem of the optimal partitioning of a computation into several independent tasks. Tasks may be executed in parallel. In this way, the execution time of the entire computation may be decreased. Theoretically, we may create as many of tasks as possible to minimize the execution time. The number of tasks will be limited by an indivisible unit of operation, e.g. instruction or procedure. However, if there is a cost associated with the creation of tasks and with the transfer of input data, increasing the number of tasks may not give the smallest execution time. Apparently, there is a tradeoff between the parallelism and the communication overhead. The optimal number of tasks depends on the problem size, on the structure of the communication subsystem, on the communication delays and on the execution times of tasks.

The problem of the optimal partitioning arises in parallel systems as well as in distributed systems. The two types of systems have different characteristics of the computational speed and the communication bandwidth, however, the granularity of tasks may be made so fine that the communication overhead becomes not negligible and should be taken into account during the decomposition of a computation. Especially, this is the case of networks of microprocessors such as the hypercube and distributed systems using high-speed local networks. The problem is much less important for shared memory multiprocessors, nevertheless, it does exist for growing number of processors [1, 3, 10]

The problem has been already studied in different contexts. Robinson analyzed the execution time of k-process algorithms for an asynchronous multiprocessor system [10]. He assumed that a central shared memory is used for communication and an optimal dynamic decomposition of an algorithm was analyzed. Reed [8] considered different interconnection structures of multimicrocomputer networks. Tasks are created dynamically and their execution times depend on the structure of the network and on the communication overhead. His simulation study shows the existence of a tradeoff between communication overhead and parallelism. Similar conclusions emerge from [9]. Lint and Agerwala discussed communication issues in the design of parallel algorithms [6]. They presented several examples emphasizing the influence of communication on the performance of parallel programs. The communication/computation tradeoff was compared to the idea of space-time tradeoffs in sequential programming. Axelrod [1] analyzed the performance of parallel algorithms having synchronization barriers. If there is a cost associated with the execution of the barriers, there is an optimal number of processors maximizing the speedup. Dubois and Briggs analyzed the performance of synchronized iterative algorithms executed on a loosely-coupled multiprocessor system [3]. They estimated the effect of the degree of decomposition of a given algorithm on the speedup. A method to determine an optimal grain size (i.e. task size) was proposed by Kruatrachue and Lewis [4]. They assumed the complete connection of processors and deterministic communication delays and task execution times.

The paper is organized as follows. First, Section 2 presents a model of the execution of parallel tasks on a multiprocessor system having different interconnection structures. Then, a deterministic model is analyzed in Section 3 to find the optimal number of tasks. Two optimization criteria are considered: the speedup and the quality. Another model assuming random task execution times is considered in Section 4. We present some numerical examples and comparisons. Finally, some conclusions are given.

MODEL OF A PARALLEL COMPUTATION

Consider the following model of a parallel computation. A given problem can be decomposed into n subproblems, each executed as a separate, independent task. We assume that tasks are created dynamically during the execution of the computation. They are executed on different processors reducing in this manner the execution time. The computation is terminated if all n tasks are finished. Theoretically, increasing the number of tasks decreases the execution time (remark that it is not possible to increase infinitely the number of tasks). Let τ denote the time needed to execute a given problem on one processor. It is a random variable with density function f_τ and mean T. The communication overhead related to the creation of one task and to the transfer of parameters and results will be denoted by μ. It is a random variable with density function f_μ and mean C. We assume that tasks do not communicate except for their creation and the transfer of results. Thus, the total communication overhead during a computation depends only on the structure of the communication subsystem.

We will consider the following interconnection structures: the ring, the tree, the binary k-cube (hypercube) and the complete connection. They are good representatives of many possible interconnections (for other interconnection structures see [7]). The optimization problem may be stated as follows: given an interconnection structure, execution time τ and communication overhead μ, find the optimal number of tasks. Optimal in the sense of maximizing a performance index. Note that the optimal number of tasks also determines the optimal granularity of tasks.

The results of the paper can be also used to analyze more complex structures of computation composed of phases of parallel execution of tasks with synchronization points between phases. In this case τ will denote the time needed to execute a phase on one processor and we will optimize the number of parallel tasks in one phase.

PERFORMANCE INDICES

In order to optimize the partitioning of a computation we will consider several performance indices. They are usually used to characterize parallel programs [5]. A basic measure is *total execution time* t_n, the time needed to execute n tasks on n processors. P_n will denote the sum of computations and communications during the execution of n tasks (for $n = 1$ we have $P_1 = t_1 = \tau$). If a stochastic model is considered, measures t_n and P_n will be expectations of random variables. The performance indices are defined as follows

speedup $\qquad S_n = \dfrac{t_1}{t_n}.$

efficiency $\qquad E_n = \dfrac{t_1}{nt_n}.$

redundancy $\qquad R_n = \dfrac{P_n}{P_1}.$

utilization $\qquad U_n = R_n E_n.$

quality $\qquad Q_n = \dfrac{S_n E_n}{R_n}.$

We will consider two models: A - deterministic execution times, B - random execution times. Random execution times permit to take into account synchronization delays between tasks.

DETERMINISTIC MODEL - A

We suppose that τ is constant and equal to T. The communication overhead is also constant: $\mu = C$. The execution time of n tasks on n processors will be expressed as

$$t_n = \frac{T + g(n)C}{n}, \tag{1}$$

where $g(n)$ represents the number of communications, each one of duration C. This function depends on a given interconnection structure. The total communication overhead is assumed to be equal to $g(n)C$. It results from the formulation of our problem: tasks are created dynamically and there is a constant overhead C related to the creation of a task. It is a realistic assumption for the ring, the tree and the complete connection, because each task is created on a different processor and there is no contention between requests for task creation. For the hypercube, it is an optimistic assumption valid only if $n \ll 2^k$. Relation (1) gives the smallest possible time needed to create and to execute an independent task. It corresponds to the allocation of computations to processors such as all tasks complete at the same time. t_n gives a lower bound for the execution time of n tasks. (Another possible relation would be $\dfrac{T}{n} + g(n)C$). Function $g(n)$, $n > 1$ is the following for different interconnection structures (see Appendix for derivations):

ring

$$g_{ring}(n) = \frac{n(n-1)}{2}$$

tree

$$g_{tree}(n) = [(n+1)\log_2(n+1) - 2n]$$

binary k-cube

k is such as $n < 2^k$ (2^k is the number of processors in the binary k-cube). It is assumed that each task is created on different processor (valid if $n \ll 2^k$).

$$g_{cube}(n) = \frac{[n(k-1)+1]\log_k[n(k-1)+1] - kn}{(k-1)}$$

complete connection

$$g_{c-c}(n) = (n-1)$$

The number of communications is $O(n^2)$ for the ring, $O[n\log(n)]$ for the tree and the binary k-cube and $O(n)$ for the complete connection.

Maximizing the speedup

Let us find the number of tasks so as to maximize the speedup. Derivating (1) for different functions $g(n)$ and setting to zero gives the following relations:

ring

$$n_{opt} = \sqrt{\frac{2T}{C}}$$

This form of expression is often found in various optimization problems, in particular, it is the formula for the optimal checkpointing interval for programs with checkpoint duration T and failure rate C [11].

tree

n_{opt} verifies

$$n_{opt} - \frac{T}{C}\ln(2) = \ln(n_{opt} + 1)$$

binary k-cube

n_{opt} verifies

$$n_{opt}(k-1) - \frac{T}{C}(k-1)\ln(2) = \ln[n_{opt}(k-1) + 1]$$

complete connection

in this case the speedup is an increasing function of n: the speedup is maximal if $n \to \infty$.

The equations for the tree and the binary k-cube must be solved numerically.

Figure 1 presents the execution time versus the number of tasks for different interconnection structures. It can be seen from this figure that only for the ring the execution time has a sharp minimum. The tree and the binary k-cube have minima, however the execution time in the neighborhood of the minimum is flat. The execution time for the complete connection decreases rapidly for small n and then the decrease is slight. Figure 2 presents the speedup and we can observe a similar behavior. The figures suggest that in the case of the tree, the binary k-cube and

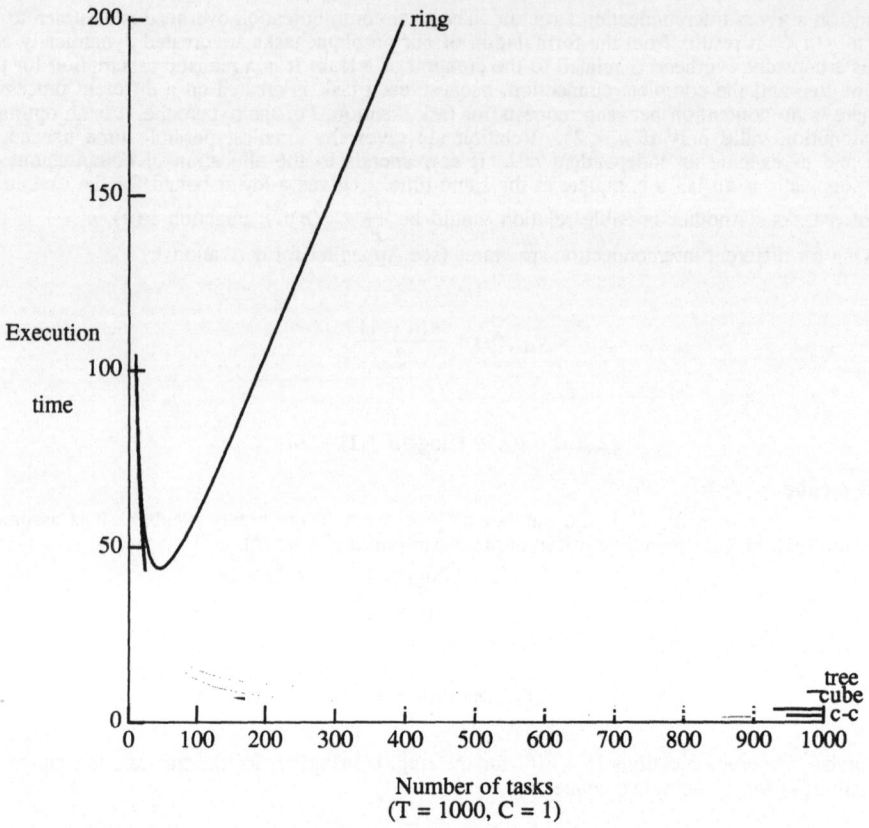

Figure 1. Execution time vs. number of tasks (deterministic model)

the complete connection it is preferable to have a reasonable small number of tasks because the further decrease of the execution time is obtained for a large number of tasks. To study qualitatively this phenomenon, we will consider another performance index - the quality.

Maximizing the quality

From the definition we obtain

$$Q_n = \frac{T^3}{n^2 t_n^3} \tag{2}$$

Figure 3 presents the quality versus the number of tasks for $T/C = 1000$. It can be seen from this figure that the quality attains a maximum for all interconnection structures. The maximum is attained for the smaller number of tasks then in the case of the speedup. The derivation of (2) for different functions $g(n)$ and setting to zero gives the following relations:

ring

$$n_{opt} = \frac{1}{5}(1 + \sqrt{\frac{C + 10T}{C}})$$

tree

n_{opt} verifies

$$T\ln(2) + n_{opt}C[4\ln(2) - 3] = C(2n_{opt} - 1)\ln(n_{opt}+1)$$

binary k-cube

n_{opt} verifies

$$T\ln(k)(k - 1) + n_{opt}C[k(2\ln(k) - 3) + 3] = C[2n_{opt}(k - 1) - 1]\ln[n_{opt}(k - 1) + 1]$$

326

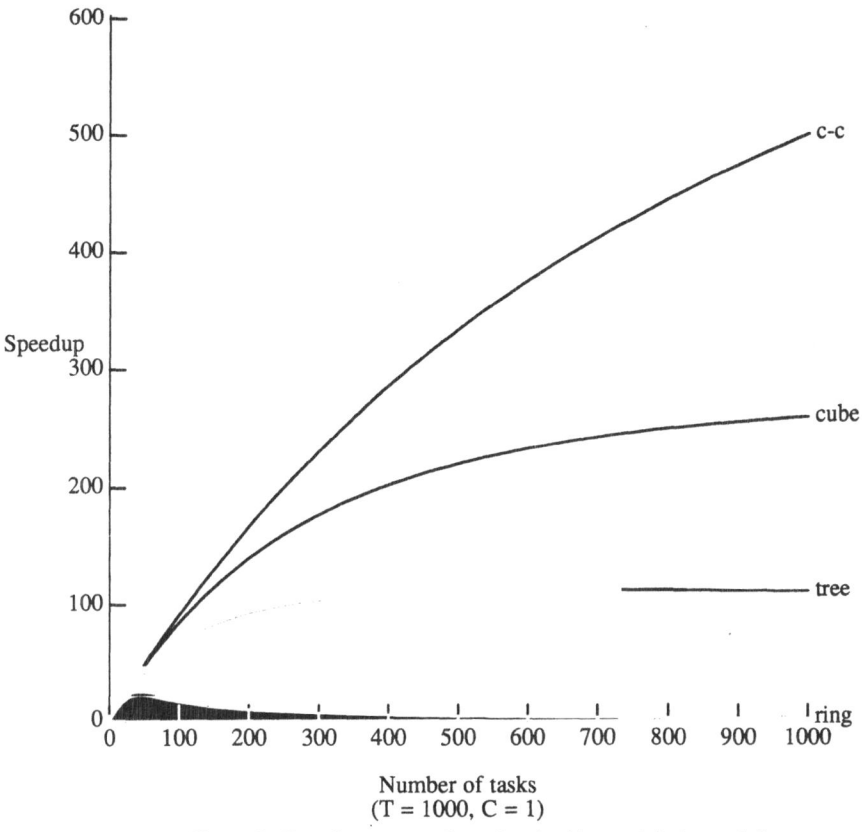

Figure 2. Speedup vs. number of tasks (deterministic model)

complete connection

$$n_{opt} = \frac{T - C}{2C}$$

STOCHASTIC MODEL - B

In this section we will assume random execution times of tasks and random communication delays. Let time τ has an infinitely divisible distribution with mean T (we will assume the gamma distribution). If we also assume that the communication overhead has the gamma distribution with mean C, the distribution of the sum of computation and communication (i.e. P_n) will be gamma with mean $T + g(n)C$. This results from the property of the gamma distribution: the sum of two gamma random variables has also the gamma distribution. Thus, the execution time of one task will have the gamma distribution with mean $\dfrac{T + g(n)C}{n}$. The total execution time of n tasks can be calculated as the maximum of n random variables distributed according to the gamma distribution. There is no simple expression for the mean of the maximum of gamma random variables [2]. Therefore, we will develop an approximation. Let us assume that the sum of computation and communication has the Erlang-n distribution with mean $T + g(n)C$. Recall that the Erlang-n distribution is a special case of gamma distribution. Therefore, the execution time of one task (denoted by τ_n) is exponentially distributed with mean $\dfrac{T + g(n)C}{n}$ and it is easy to find the mean execution time of n tasks i.e. the mean of the maximum of n exponentially distributed random variables [2]

$$t_n = E[\max_n \tau_n] = H_n \frac{T + g(n)C}{n} \tag{3}$$

where H_n denotes the harmonic series. Note that the assumption about random task execution times permits to take into account synchronization delays. The delays arise when one task finishes before other tasks and must wait until all tasks are terminated.

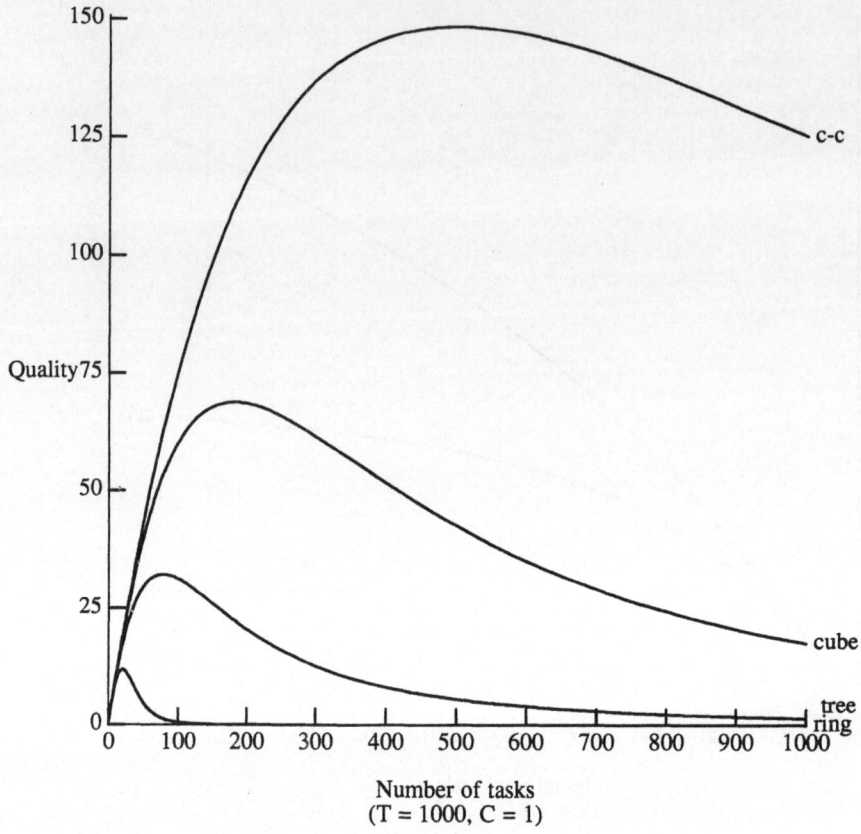

Figure 3. Quality vs. number of tasks (deterministic model)

The approximation yields an upper bound for the execution times: for small values of n, task execution times τ_n have a distribution with less variability than the exponential distribution. This smaller variability results in the mean of the maximum of n random variables smaller than for the exponential case. Relation (3) can be approximated by

$$t_n = [\ln(n) + \gamma] \frac{T + g(n)C}{n} \qquad (4)$$

where γ is the Euler constant. Now we are able to consider the optimization problem - find the optimal number of tasks that maximizes the speedup or the quality.

Maximizing the speedup

The speedup is the following

$$S_n = \frac{nT}{[\ln(n) + \gamma] [T + g(n)C]} \qquad (5)$$

Derivating (5) for different functions $g(n)$ and setting to zero gives the following relations:
ring

n_{opt} verifies

$$2T(1 - \gamma) - n_{opt}C + n_{opt}^2 C(1 + \gamma) = (2T - n_{opt}^2 C)\ln(n_{opt})$$

tree

n_{opt} verifies

$$T\ln(2)(\gamma - 1) - n_{opt}C(\gamma - 2\ln(2)) = [Cn_{opt} - T\ln(2)]\ln(n_{opt})$$
$$+ C[1 - \gamma - \ln(n_{opt}) + n_{opt}]\ln(n_{opt} + 1)$$

binary k-cube

328

n_{opt} verifies

$$T\ln(k)(k-1)(\gamma-1) - n_{opt}C[\gamma(k-1) - k\ln(k)] =$$
$$(k-1)[Cn_{opt} - T\ln(k)]\ln(n_{opt}) + C[1-\gamma-\ln(n_{opt}) + n_{opt}(k-1)]\ln[n_{opt}(k-1)+1]$$

complete connection

n_{opt} verifies

$$n_{opt}C + (T-C)(1-\gamma) = (T-C)\ln(n_{opt})$$

The equations must be solve numerically.

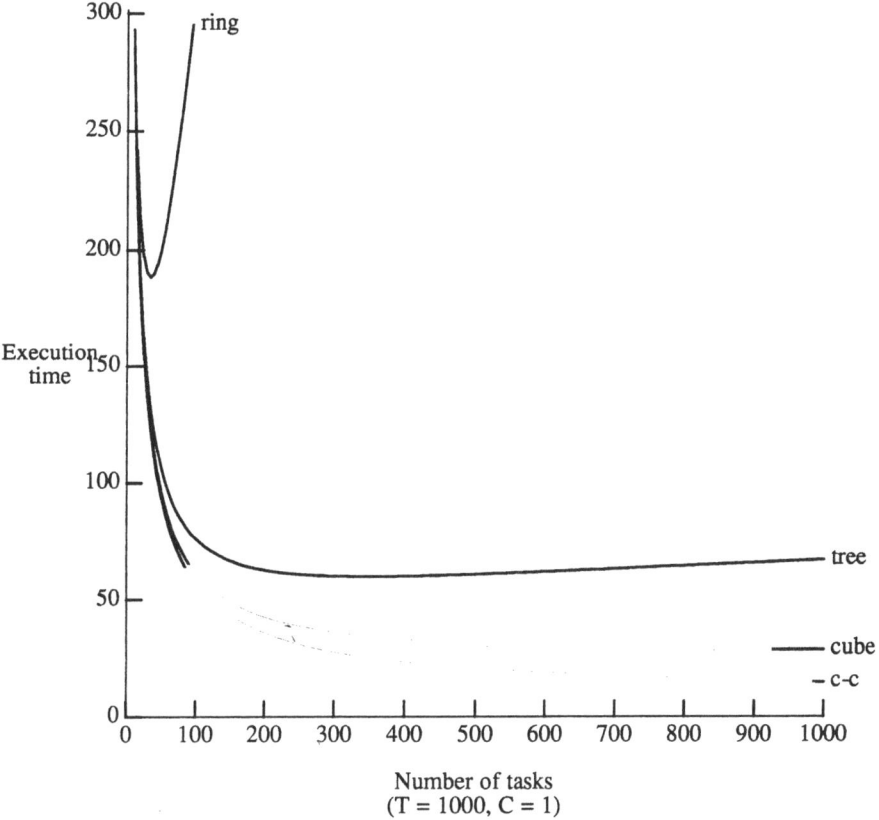

Number of tasks
(T = 1000, C = 1)

Figure 4. Execution time vs. number of tasks (stochastic model)

Figure 4 presents the execution time versus number of tasks for different interconnection structures ($T/C = 1000$). The figure is similar to Figure 1: for the tree, cube and the complete connection the execution time decreases rapidly for small n and then decreases slowly. For the four interconnection structures the minimum does exist and the optimal number of tasks is smaller than in the deterministic case. Figure 5 presents the speedup and we can observe a similar behavior. We consider now another performance index - the quality.

Maximizing the quality

From the definitions above we have

$$Q_n = \frac{T^3}{n^2 t_n^2 E[\tau_n]} \tag{6}$$

because $R_n = \dfrac{nE[\tau_n]}{T}$. Figure 6 presents the quality versus the number of tasks for $T/C = 1000$. The derivation of Eq.(6) for different functions $g(n)$ and setting to zero gives the following relations:

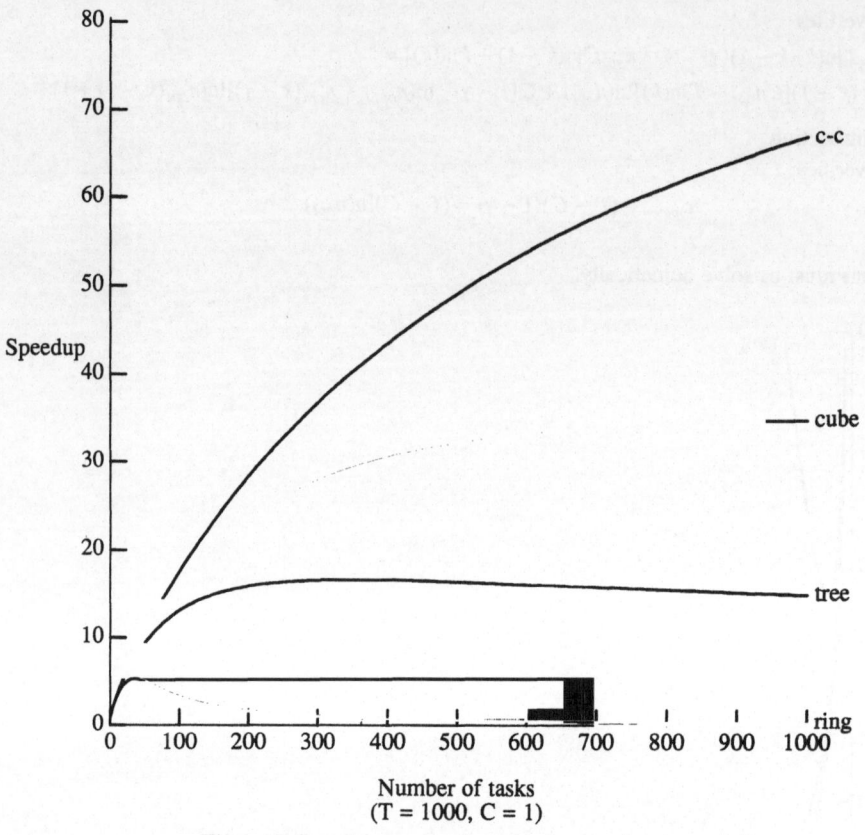

Figure 5. Speedup vs. number of tasks (stochastic model)

ring

n_{opt} verifies

$$n^2C(2 + 5\gamma) - 2nC(1 + \gamma) - 2T(\gamma - 2) = (2T - 5n^2C + 2nC)\ln(n)$$

tree

n_{opt} verifies

$$nC[4\ln(2)(\gamma + 1) - 3\gamma] + T\ln(2)(\gamma - 2) =$$
$$[3Cn - T\ln(2) - 4\ln(2)Cn]\ln(n) + C[(2n - 1)\ln(n) + 2n(\gamma + 1) + 2 - \gamma]\ln(n + 1)$$

binary k-cube

n_{opt} verifies

$$nC[2k\ln(k)(\gamma + 1) - 3\gamma(k - 1)] + T\ln(k)(k - 1)(\gamma - 2) =$$
$$[(k - 1)(3Cn - T\ln(k)) - 2k\ln(k)Cn]\ln(n) +$$
$$C[(2n(k - 1) - 1)\ln(n) + 2n(k - 1)(\gamma + 1) + 2 - \gamma]\ln[n(k - 1) + 1]$$

complete connection

n_{opt} verifies

$$2nC(1 + \gamma) - (T - C)(\gamma - 2) = (T - C - 2nC)\ln(n)$$

The equations must be solved numerically.

COMPARISONS

Figure 7 presents the optimal number of tasks versus the computation/communication ratio T/C for two models. The optimization criterion is the speedup. It can be seen from this figure that n_{opt} is almost linear in this scale. Note that only for the ring and the tree the optimal number

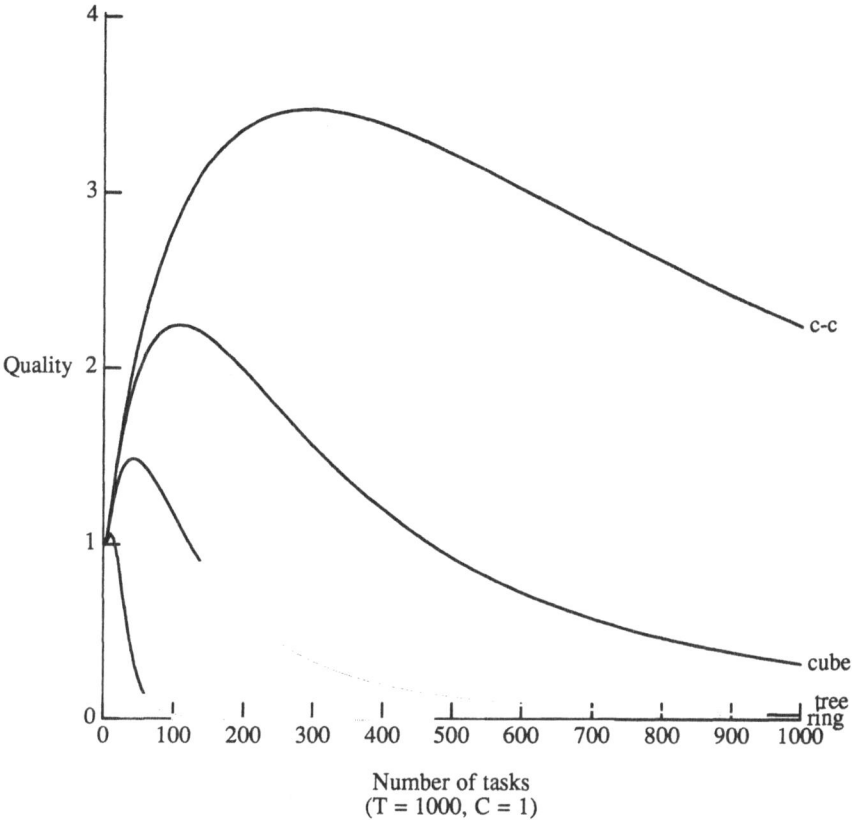

Number of tasks
(T = 1000, C = 1)

Figure 6. Quality vs. number of tasks (stochastic model)

of processors satisfies $n_{opt} < \dfrac{T}{C}$. Figure 8 presents the same function but now the optimization criterion is the quality. The optimal values are smaller than in the case of the speedup. An interesting property can be seen for all interconnection structures: $n_{opt} < \dfrac{T}{C}$. Remark also the influence of random execution times (model B) on the optimal number of tasks.

CONCLUSIONS

In the paper we have studied the problem of the optimal partitioning of a computation into parallel tasks. It is assumed that tasks are created dynamically and there is a cost associated with the creation and with the transfer of parameters and results. Several processor interconnection structures are considered: the ring, the tree, the binary k-cube, the complete connection. We have analyzed the optimal number of tasks that maximizes the speedup. For the interconnection structures other than the ring, the total execution time decreases rapidly for small number of tasks and then it decreases slowly. Therefore, it is preferable to have a reasonable number of tasks because the further decrease of the execution time is obtained for a large number of tasks. This behavior may be important in multiprogramming systems when several programs are executed simultaneously. It may be interesting to allocate a smaller number of processors to several programs than to give all processors to one program. To study qualitatively this phenomenon, we have considered another performance index - the quality. The quality attains a maximum for the smaller number of tasks then the speedup. The maximum exists even in the case of the complete connection. We have derived explicit formulae for the optimal number of processors whenever it was possible. Otherwise, equations are given that must be solved numerically. The application of the results to the decomposition of parallel programs will probably show that performance indices are situated between the values predicted by the two considered models.

Acknowledgments
This research has been supported by the French project C^3 of CNRS.

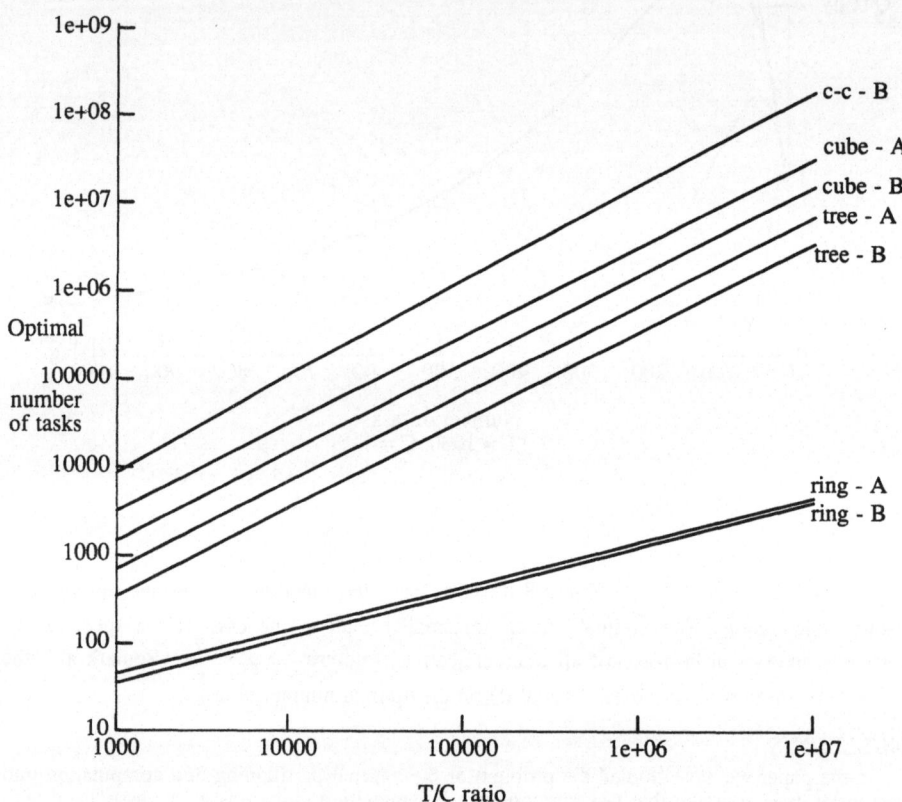

Figure 7. Optimal number of tasks vs. computation/communication ratio T/C
(optimization of the speedup)

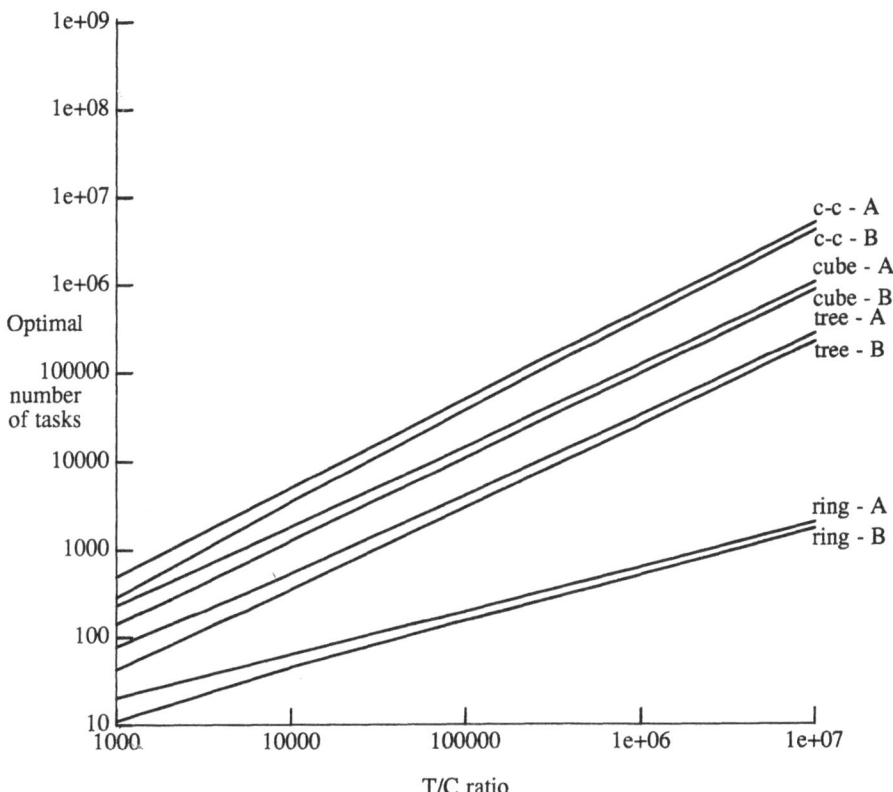

Figure 8. Optimal number of tasks vs. computation/communication ratio T/C
(optimization of the quality)

References

1. Axelrod, T.S., "Effects of Synchronization Barriers on Multiprocessor Performance," *Parallel Computing*, vol. 3, pp. 129-140, 1986.

2. David, H. A., *Order Statistics,* John Wiley, New York, 1970.

3. Dubois, M. and Briggs, F. A., "Performance of Synchronized Iterative Processes in Multiprocessor Systems," *IEEE Trans. on Soft. Eng.*, vol. SE-8, pp. 419-431, July 1982.

4. Kruatrachue, B. and Lewis, T., "Grain Size Determination for Parallel Processing," *IEEE Software*, no. 1, pp. 23-32, 1988.

5. Lee, R. B-L., "Empirical Results on the Speedup, Efficiency, Redundancy and the Quality of Parallel Computations," in *Int. Conf. Parallel Processing*, pp. 91-96, Aug. 1980.

6. Lint, B. and Agerwala, T., "Communication Issues in the Design and Analysis of Parallel Algorithms," *IEEE Trans. on Soft. Eng.*, vol. SE-7, pp. 174-188, March 1981.

7. Reed, D. A., "Performance Based Design and Analysis of Multimicrocomputer Networks," *Ph.D. Thesis, Purdue University*, May 1983.

8. Reed, D. A., "The Performance of Multimicrocomputer Networks Supporting Dynamic Workloads," *IEEE Trans. on Comp.*, vol. C-33, pp. 1045-1048, November 1984.

9. Reed, D. A. and Grunwald, D. C., "The Performance of Multicomputer Interconnection Networks," *IEEE Computer*, no. 6, pp. 63-73, June 1987.

10. Robinson, J. T., "Some Analysis Techniques for Asynchronous Multiprocessor Algorithms," *IEEE Trans. on Soft. Eng.*, vol. SE-5, pp. 24-31, January 1979.

11. Young, J.W., "A First-order Approximation to the Optimum Checkpoint Interval," *Comm. ACM*, vol. 17, no. 6, 1974.

APPENDIX

We present here the derivation of the communication cost function $g(n)$ for different interconnection structures.

ring

Each processor communicates only with its neighbor, thus $g(n)$ is the sum of $n - 1$ communications.

$$g_{ring}(n) = \frac{n(n - 1)}{2}$$

tree

Each processor communicates with two neighbors and $g_{tree}(n)$ can be derived from $g_{cube}(n)$ for the binary k-cube when $k = 2$.

binary k-cube

Each processor communicates with k neighbors. If m is such as $n = \sum_{i=0}^{m} k^i$, then $g_{cube}(n) = \sum_{i=1}^{m-1} ik^i$ which yields

$$g_{cube}(n) = \frac{k[(m - 1)(k - 1)k^{m-1} - k^{m-1}+1]}{(k - 1)^2}$$

Replacing m with $\log_k[n(k - 1) + 1] - 1$ gives

$$g_{cube}(n) = \frac{[n(k - 1) + 1]\log_k[n(k - 1) + 1] - kn}{(k - 1)}$$

Note that we suppose that tasks are created on different processors and there is no situation when two requests for creating a task arrive at the same processor. It is a realistic assumption if $n \ll 2^k$.

complete connection

All processors communicate with all other processors, so $g_{c-c}(n)$ is simply $n - 1$.

PROPER, A PERFORMABILITY MODELLING AND ANALYSIS TOOL

Boudewijn R.H.M. Haverkort and Ignas G.M.M. Niemegeers

Department of Computer Science, University of Twente

P.O. Box 217, 7500 AE Enschede, The Netherlands

Abstract — Performability modelling is a modelling technique which incorporates aspects of both performance and reliability modelling. It therefore provides means to trade-off between the two. In this paper we briefly discuss the mathematical background of performability modelling as a start-up for the main discussion topic: the PROPER system.

The PROPER system is a modelling tool for performability analysis. It allows its users to specify at a high level, via the language PDL, performability models which are automatically translated into low level Markov-Reward processes. Invisible for the end user, this translation incorporates multiple performance analyses for obtaining the rewards. The PROPER system combines a high level specification technique with a number of state-of-the-art calculation methods and forms in that sense a new approach in quantitative systems modelling.

We end with an example showing the strength of PROPER and with some indications for further research.

1 Introduction

Performability modelling originates from two separately existing modelling techniques: performance and reliability modelling. Performability modelling is concerned with questions about the ability of a computer system to process certain amounts of work, given that parts of the system may fail. With the advent of gracefully degradable computer systems, which can operate at different levels of computation power due to the occurence of failures and repairs, this integration of both modelling techniques will become more and more important.

The first papers which discuss the integrated approach to reliability and performance modelling are [Beau78] and [Gay79]. Later, Meyer [Meye80] set up a general framework for performability modelling which he used in a case study of a homogeneous multiprocessor system [Meye82]. Later papers (references are given in section 4) developed new calculation methods for solving performability models but the same basis is still used.

In this paper we introduce the performability modelling tool PROPER. As far as we know PROPER is the first modelling tool that combines performability analysis with a high level model description technique. In that way, PROPER allows its users, typically system designers, to obtain performability measures of their design alternatives without having to cope with mathematical or simulation details. In other words: system designers can specify PROPER models without having to alter their way of thinking about their designs.

Earlier work with respect to performability modelling tools is scarce. Performability lookalike measures, e.g. transient measures and cumulative sums (see section 4.3), can be obtained with the tool METFAC [Carr86A,B]. However, the reward values (see section 3) to be used in each structure state have to be specified by the tool user. Since this implies that the tool user has to have knowledge about rewards, structure states etc., the specification is not totally at a high level.

With the tool NUMAS [Muel84] performability lookalike measures can be obtained. However, these measures only concern steady state behaviour whereas PROPER also deals with the transient behaviour.

Finally, with the tool METAPHOR [Furc84A,B] "real" performability measures, i.e. probability distributions, can be obtained. However, also in METAPHOR the rewards have to be input "by hand". Furthermore, the used failure/repair models are restricted: only non-repairable systems, yielding a-cyclic (semi) Markov models, can be analyzed.

This paper is organized as follows. In section 2 we discuss some tools and backgrounds of performance as well as reliability modelling. In section 3 we address the mathematical background of performability modelling. The issues of these two sections come together in section 4 where we discuss the PROPER system, a tool for performability modelling. In section 5 we will give an example of the use of PROPER. Section 6 discusses the state of PROPER. In section 7 we draw some conclusions.

2 Tools for Quantitative Systems Modelling

Over the last 20 years, quantitative system modelling has become increasingly important in the design of computer systems. The methods and techniques became more accurate and more complex, therefore asking for computer aid. A number of program packages, generally known as "tools" have been made by universities and industries. In the quantitative system modelling area we can distinguish two main streams, each with their own purposes and methods. They will briefly be introduced in the following two subsections (for a thorough discussion, see [Triv82]).

2.1 Performance Modelling

Performance modelling is concerned with questions about how well a given system performs under the assumption that everything is functioning correctly. The above mentioned "well" is expressed in terms of steady state throughputs, response times etc. Two of the most prominent analytic approaches in performance modelling are queueing networks (QNs) and Markov models. A third approach is the simulation of queueing networks (we do not address simulation in this paper, see e.g. [Mitr82]). Since, in general, we are interested in steady state performance measures, sets of linear equations have to be solved. For certain classes of QN models special algorithms have been developed such as the Mean Value Analysis [Reis81] and the product-form algorithms [Bcmp75].

Over the last ten years, a number of tools for performance modelling has been developed. Examples are QNAP, RESQ, HIT, COPE (all briefly discussed in [Beil85]), NUMAS [Muel84], MAOS [Jobm85] and GSPN [Chio86]. The tools mentioned use as solution methods either simulation, specialized algorithms, Markov models or combinations thereof. They provide their users with a high level input medium, most commonly a high level model description language, which is translated into a lower level mathematical or simulation model before the solution takes place. This makes these tools relatively easy to use for system designers since they do not have to deal with mathematical or simulation modelling details.

2.2 Reliability Modelling

Reliability modelling is concerned with questions about how long a system will operate correctly (i.e. without failures) or about how often failures take place and how long failure states last. Today, the most widespread modelling approach is Markov modelling. Since in reliability modelling, transient (i.e. time-dependent) aspects of the sytem are of interest, often sets of differential equations have to be solved.

In the late seventies, the avionics industries initiated the development of reliability modelling tools. Example are ARIES, SURF, CARE III, HARP, SHARPE, SAVE and METFAC. These tools were recently discussed and compared in [Mula86]. A short introduction to these tools is given in [Have87]. In reliability modelling the level of model specification is generally lower than in performance modelling. An exception is the SAVE package [Goya86] where high level descriptions of systems are translated into continuous time, homogeneous Markov models.

3 Mathematical Performability Modelling

In the following two subsections we will briefly discuss the main ideas of performability modelling. Section 3.1 introduces some terminology, definitions and notation known from reliability modelling theory. Section 3.2 discusses the basic approach as introduced in [Meye80] and gives an example which resembles the example given in [Meye82] and many other, later papers on this topic.

3.1 Mathematical Reliabilty Modelling

Let us recall some reliability modelling terminology, notation and definitions which we will use in the remainder of the paper. Let X be a stochastic variable denoting the lifetime of a component C. X has a distribution $F(t)$. The reliability $R(t)$ of component C is defined as follows:

$$R(t) = \Pr\{X > t\} = 1 - F(t) \tag{1}$$

The mean time to failure ($MTTF$) is defined as:

$$MTTF = EX = \int_0^\infty t f(t) dt = \int_0^\infty R(t) dt \tag{2}$$

Commonly we assume $F(t)$ to be exponential, i.e. $F(t) = 1 - e^{-\lambda t}$. The parameter λ of $F(t)$ is called the failure rate of the component C. After the occurence of a failure, the component C can be repaired which takes Z units of time. Z has a (repair time) distribution $G(t)$. Now, let $a(t)$ equal 1 if C is operational at time t and 0 if not, then the accumulated uptime up to time t is defined as:

$$U(t) = \int_0^t a(s)ds \qquad (3)$$

and the availability as:

$$A(t) = \frac{1}{t}\int_0^t a(s)ds \qquad (4)$$

Note that both $U(t)$ and $A(t)$ are stochastic variables, since $a(t)$ is a stochastic variable. The ability of a system to reconfigure (e.g. start a repair action) after a failure has occured is expressed by the coverage factor c which is defined as $\Pr\{system\ reconfigures | system\ has\ failed\}$.

3.2 The Basic Approach in Performability Modelling

In performability modelling we are concerned with obtaining the performance of a system which is subject to failures and repairs, i.e. the performance of a system which changes its structure during operation. In order to come to an actual performability model two basic observations are made:

1- There are two stochastic processes involved:

    a- the arrival/departure process modelling arrivals of customers at and departures of customers from the system;

    b- the failure/repair process which changes the system structure due to the occurences of failures and repairs. This process will be called the structure state process and is denoted by $(X_t, t \geq 0)$;

2- There are time scale differences between the two stochastic processes of 1a and 1b; the time between structure state changes (due to failures and repairs) is so long that the arrival/departure process between those successive structure state changes can be considered to be in steady state most of the time. This is called *behavioural decomposition* as opposed to the more familiar *structural decomposition*. It is an example of the nearly completely decomposability (NCD) property discussed in [Cour77].

The second observation is the basis for the assumption that we can summarize the performance of the system within a structure state i (being an instance of the stochastic variable X_t) with one value, the so-called *reward* $\mathbf{R}(i)$. Note that we assume that there is only one reward per structure state. In section 4 we will remove this restriction by allowing multiple rewards per structure state, thus allowing "multiple class modelling". The rewards $\mathbf{R}(i)$ can be seen as generalized performance measures. Together with the structure state process $(X_t, t \geq 0)$, the reward matrix $\mathbf{R}$ is used to obtain performability measures. Now, let us consider an example which will clarify the concept of behavioural decomposition.

Consider a two server system with buffer space for storing two customers (figure 1). Individual servers may fail with rate f and may be repaired with rate r by a single repair entity. Customers arrive at the system with rate λ and are served with rate μ in one of the servers. Figure 2 gives the corresponding Markov chain. State i,j denotes the state with i operational servers and j jobs in the system (note that a

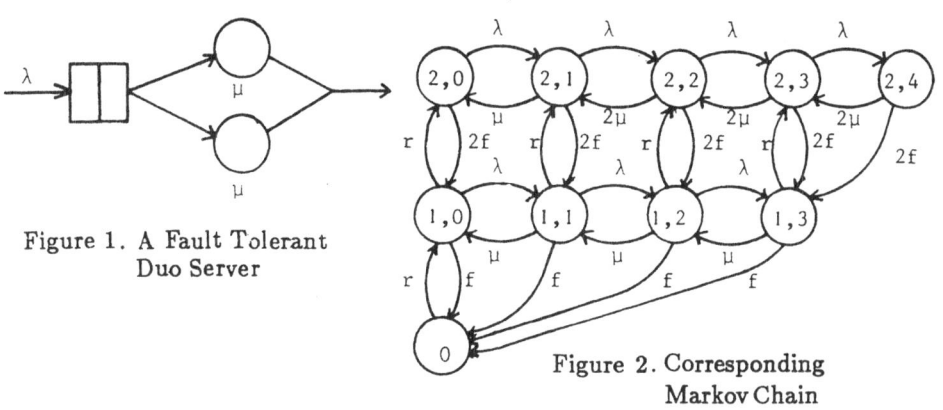

Figure 1. A Fault Tolerant
Duo Server

Figure 2. Corresponding
Markov Chain

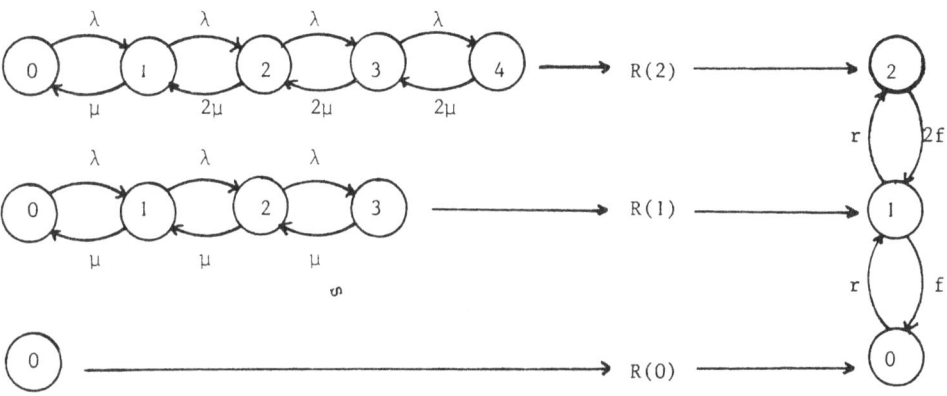

Figure 3. Isolated Performance
Models

Figure 4. Structure State
Process

lot of extra assumptions have been made). Since arrivals and departures occur much more frequently than failures and repairs we can approximate the whole behaviour of the system by the behaviour of the 3 arrival/departure processes in figure 3 and the structure state process in figure 4.

Now, we can define some performability measures. The cumulative reward $Y(t)$ is defined as:

$$Y(t) = \int_0^t \mathbf{R}(X_s)\,ds \qquad (5)$$

Since $(X_t, t \geq 0)$ is a stochastic process, $Y(t)$ has a distribution $F(t, x)$:

$$F(t, x) = \Pr\{Y(t) \leq x\} \qquad (6)$$

This distribution is called *the* performability. We can distinguish at least two special cases:

- $(X_t = Constant, t \geq 0)$. This means that there is only one accessible structure state, so there are no failures and repairs. This is exactly what was always the assumption in performance modelling, so we can still model solely for performance;

- $\mathbf{R}(i)$ is either 1 or 0. That is exactly what was assumed in section 3.1 via the function $a(t)$. So, we are also able to model solely for the availability and the reliability of a system.

339

4 The PROPER system

The PROPER system (a PRoject On PERformability) is a tool for the modelling of computer systems with respect to their performability. Consequently, it incorporates aspects of both performance and reliability modelling.

4.1 Overview of the PROPER system

Schematically, the PROPER system has the (simplified) structure shown in figure 5. A performability model is solved by the module LLMS (to be discussed in section 4.3). Input to this module is a Low Level Model Description (see section 4.2). This LLMD can either be input directly via the Low Level Input Module or can be the result of the compilation of a high level model description.

The high level model description is written in PDL (the PROPER Description Language; see section 4.4). The compilation consists of two steps:

1- the Q-matrix (to be discussed in section 4.2) is composed out of the failure/repair models of all the components in the model to be analyzed;

2- the reward matrix **R** is formed by repeated performance analyses: for each possible structure state of the model a performance analysis is required. Since we use an existing BCMP analyser (see [Bcmp75]) for obtaining the rewards, the PDL model class is also BCMP (with respect to the job arrival/departure process).

4.2 Low Level Model Description and Input

As is clear from section 3, the basic underlying mathematical model of a performability model is the Markov-Reward process $((X_t, t \geq 0), \mathbf{R})$. We call this a LLMD. The Markov process $(X_t, t \geq 0)$ is totally described by the infinitesimal Markov generator $\mathbf{Q}$, a square matrix with n rows and columns. The reward matrix **R** has size $n \times c$, where c is the number of customer classes in the model. Given the above mentioned matrices, a performability model is totally described and can be solved.

Since the matrices $\mathbf{Q}$ and R can be large ($n > 100$ is no exception) and since the matrix $\mathbf{Q}$ is generally sparse it is useful to have a convenient means to input these matrices. Furthermore, the matrix $\mathbf{Q}$ often contains entries which are the result of simple calculations of basic values such as $2f_1 + cf_2, f_1 + cf_2, \ldots$.

Keeping these considerations in mind we developed the Low Level Model Input module such that users could input a LLMD in the following way (not necessarily in this order):

- definition of basic values, such as failure rates, coverage factors etc., in a table. These definitions are stored in a file called "modelname.**T**";
- input of the non-zero, non-diagonal entries (diagonal entries are updated automatically) of the Q-matrix, either via symbolic expressions over the previously defined constants or directly. The matrix $\mathbf{Q}$ is stored sparsely (via the scheme RR(C)O, see [Curt71]) in a file called "modelname.**Q**";
- input of the non-zero entries of the matrix **R**, which is stored in the file "modelname.**R**".

Once a LLMD has been input, it can be edited and changed. When the model has to be analyzed, the .T-file is used for obtaining numerical-versions of the .R and the .Q files. It is also possible to combine different .T, .Q and .R. In this way different alternatives can easily be compared. Figure 6 displays the LLMD of the example of

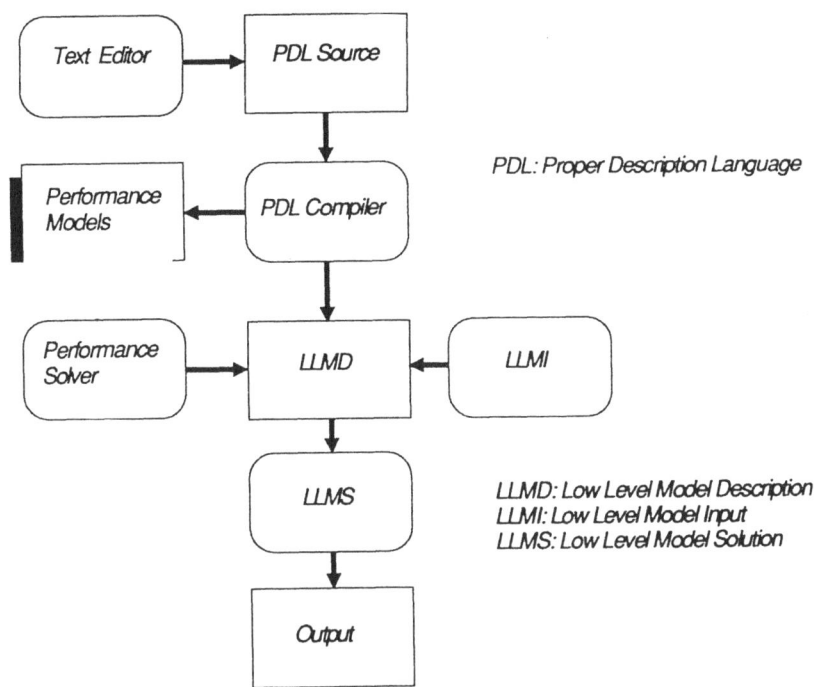

Figure 5. PROPER System Overview

model.T	model.Q			model.R
$\lambda = 5$	$-2f$	$2f$	0	$1 - p_2^{loss}$
$\mu = 3$	r	$-(r+f)f$		$1 - p_1^{loss}$
$r = 0.02$	0	r	$-r$	0
$f = 0.001$				

Figure 6. Low Level Model Description

figures 1–4. As rewards we choose the complement of the loss probabilities p_1^{loss} and p_2^{loss}. These probabilities can be obtained easily via a steady state analysis of the corresponding performance models and signify the probability of customer loss due to the limited queue size. For ease in reading, the matrices are shown as if they are stored directly instead of sparsely.

4.3 Low Level Model Solution

Once a Low Level Model Description has been made, the model can be analyzed. In the sequel we will use the subscript i for structure states and c for classes. Lets define the vectors $p(t) = [\ldots p_i(t) \ldots]$ and $p = [\ldots p_i \ldots]$. In PROPER we distinguish three main categories of measures which can be obtained: steady state measures, transient measures and performability measures.

Let us first discuss the **steady state measures**. They are labeled S1 through S5:

S1: Steady structure state probabilities:

$$p_i = \lim_{t \to \infty} p_i(t) \tag{7}$$

The p_i follow from the set of linear equations: $pQ = 0$ and $\sum p_i = 1$.

S2: Steady class availability:

$$A_c = \lim_{t \to \infty} A_c(t) = \sum_i p_i \mathbf{R}_A(i, c) \tag{8}$$

where the matrix $\mathbf{R}_A$ is defined as follows:

$$\mathbf{R}_A(i, c) = \begin{cases} 1 & \text{if } \mathbf{R}(i, c) > 0 \\ 0 & \text{if } \mathbf{R}(i, c) = 0 \end{cases}, \quad \forall i, c \tag{9}$$

Dual measure is the class unavailability: $U_c = 1 - A_c$. Note that we "extended" the rewards with a class index: in each structure state i there can be multiple rewards, one for each admissible class c. Note that, in section 3.2 we only addressed the single class case, thereby omitting, for ease in reading, the class index.

S3: Steady generalized class availability:

$$G_c = \lim_{t \to \infty} G_c(t) = \sum_i p_i \mathbf{R}_G(i, c) \tag{10}$$

The matrix $\mathbf{R}_G$ is defined as follows:

$$\mathbf{R}_G(i, c) = \frac{\mathbf{R}(i, c)}{\max_j \{\mathbf{R}(j, c)\}}, \quad \forall i, c \tag{11}$$

S4: Steady class performance:

$$Y_c = \lim_{t \to \infty} Y_c(t) = \sum_i p_i \mathbf{R}(i, c) \tag{12}$$

S5: Mean time to failure of class c:

$$MTTF_c = \int_0^\infty R_c(t)dt = \sum_{i \in Up(c)} \pi_i \tag{13}$$

The π_i are obtained by solving $\pi \mathbf{Q}_{Up(c)} = -[1, 0, ...]$ where $\mathbf{Q}_{Up(c)}$ is derived from $\mathbf{Q}$ by excluding all the failure states of class c (see [Carr86A,B]). The up states of class c are defined as those states in which class c jobs do get service: $Up(c) = \{i | \mathbf{R}(i, c) > 0\}$.

The steady state measures can be obtained by solving sets of linear equations of size less than or equal to the size of the $\mathbf{Q}$ matrix. These linear equations are the limiting case of sets of differential equations when t, the time parameter approaches infinity. Solving these sets of linear equations can be done in two ways:

- Directly, e.g. via the so-called Gaussian Elimination;
- Iteratively, e.g. via Gauss-Seidel iterations.

Direct methods are easily applicable for small models (say less than 250 equations) whereas iterative methods are especially suitable for large sparsely stored models.

The secound group of measures are the **transient measures**. They are labeled T1 through T5:

T1: Transient structure state probabilities: $p_i(t)$. The $p_i(t)$ follow from the set of differential equations: $p'(t) = p(t)\mathbf{Q}$.

T2: Transient class point availability:

$$A_c^\bullet(t) = \sum_i p_i(t)\mathbf{R}_A(i,c) \tag{14}$$

The dual measure is $U_c^\bullet(t) = 1 - A_c^\bullet(t)$.

T3: Transient generalized class point availability:

$$G_c^\bullet(t) = \sum_i p_i(t)\mathbf{R}_G(i,c) \tag{15}$$

T4: Transient class point performance:

$$Y_c^\bullet(t) = \sum_i p_i(t)\mathbf{R}(i,c) \tag{16}$$

T5: Transient class reliability $R_c(t)$:

$$R_c(t) = \sum_{i \in Up(c)} \pi_i(t) \tag{17}$$

Transient measures are obtained by solving sets of linear differential equations. This is done either by a fourth order Runge-Kutta procedure [Lamb73] or by the randomization approach. The latter is according to the literature one of the most promising generally applicable approaches for solving the transient behaviour of Markov processes [Gros84]. Apart from this approach, some specialized, easier but more restrictive approaches are known. A method restricted to acyclic Markov models yielding symbolic solutions (e.g. Simula or C procedures) is available [Mari87].

The last category of measures are the **performability measures**. They are listed below, labeled P1 through P3.

P1: Class performability:

$$F_{Y_c}(t,x) = \Pr\{Y_c(t) \le x\} \tag{18}$$

where $Y_c(t)$ is defined under P2.

P2: Cumulative class performance:

$$Y_c(t) = \int_0^t \mathbf{R}(X_s,c)\,ds \tag{19}$$

Note that P2 is a generalization of the following well known measures:

P2.1: Class availability: $A_c(t) = Y_c(t)/t$ with $\mathbf{R}(i,c)$ substituted by $\mathbf{R}_A(i,c)$.
P2.2: Generalized class availability: $G_c(t) = Y_c(t)/t$ with $\mathbf{R}(i,c)$ substituted by $\mathbf{R}_G(i,c)$.

343

P2.3: Class reliability: $R_c(t) = Y_c(t)$ with $\mathbf{Q}$ substituted by $\mathbf{Q}_{Up(c)}$.

P3: Moments of $F_{Y_c}(t, x)$:

$$m_c^n(t) = E[Y_c^n(t)] \qquad (20)$$

Note that P3 can be used to approximate P1.

These performability measures are an extension of the transient measures in that cumulative sums (say integrals) over the transient solutions are required. This observation can already serve as a basis for implementations. Furthermore, some specialized algorithms are available from the literature (see [Dona87], [Furc84A,B], [Goya86,87,88], [Iyer86], [Meye80,82], [Nico86,87] and [Smit88]).

4.4 High Level Model Description

Without going into all the details of PDL, we will by means of examples introduce the 4 basic building blocks of PROPER models: component types, load types, model types and evaluations. For a more detailed description of PDL and its implementation the reader is kindly referred to [Have88].

The first basic block in a PDL program is the **componenttype** (for ease in reading we print PDL keywords in boldface):

> **componenttype** $Ct =$
> **interface** $ReqA, ReqB$;
> **begin**
>   **servers** 3;
>   **schedule** $Fcfs$;
>   **frm** $BirthDeath([0.0012, 0.0008, 0.0004], [2, 2, 2])$;
> **end;**

This PDL fragment defines a component type, named Ct, which is able to provide service to two classes of customers (named $ReqA$ and $ReqB$). The component consists of three identical servers with one shared waiting queue. Jobs are served in $Fcfs$ order. Failures and repair take place in the component type according to the failure/repair model (frm), i.e. according to a pure $BirthDeath$ process with failure rates and repair rates as specified.

After having specified (a) component type(s), **loadtypes** can be defined. There are open and closed load types, just like there are open and closed chains in queueing networks. As an example, we define an openload type:

> **openloadtype** $Olt(ArrivalRate) =$
> **interface** $Serv$;
> **begin**
> $Serv(0.2)$;
> **end;**

This PDL fragment defines an open load type, named Olt which asks from its environment one type of service, named $Serv$. The mean service request is 0.2 seconds. The parameter $ArrivalRate$ will be set later.

After having defined component and load types, a **modeltype** can be defined:

> **modeltype** $Mt =$
> **begin**
>   **component** $C : Ct$;
>   **load** $La : Olt(2)$;

```
    Lb : Olt(3);
  alias La.Serv and C.ReqA;
  alias Lb.Serv and C.ReqB;
end;
```

This model type, named *Mt*, consists of 1 component, named *C* and of type *Ct* (according to the previous definition) and 2 loads, named *La* and *Lb*, both of type *Olt* (according to the previous definition) and with *ArrivalRates* equal to 2 and 3 respectively. Furthermore, any internal request in *La* (*Lb*) to *Serv* is handled by component *C* over the name *ReqA* (*ReqB*). What is clear from this approach is that there is a clear distinction between loads and components. The binding of the two takes place at a late stage in the modelling process. This approach is highly desirable in quantitative systems modelling (see [Beil85]) and is followed in the performance modelling tool HIT [Muel87].

The last step in a PDL model description is the **evaluation**:

```
evaluation e =
begin
  model M : Mt;
  measureperformability Moments(1)
  reward 1/ResponseTime
  classes La, Lb
  output Graph;
end.
```

The evaluation named *e*, indicates that the model named *M* (of previously defined type *Mt*) has to be analyzed. The output, in *Graph* form, consists of the first moment of the performability distribution of the overall failure/repair model of *M*. As reward 1/*ResponseTime* is chosen: the faster the service, the higher the reward.

5 An Example

In this section we present a model of a fault tolerant dual processor equipped with a fault tolerant dual I/O-processor. Computer systems of this class can typically be found in real-time control systems of e.g. chemical processes. The system can be depicted as in figure 7.

We have a *DualController* named *DC* connected to an external chemical process. There is a bidirectional flow of information between *DC* and the chemical process: on the one hand we have the sensing or sampling actions (information flow from the chemical process to the *DC*); on the other hand we have the trigger actions (information flow from *DC* to the chemical process). *DC* consists of two parts: a *Processor* named *P* and an *IOprocessor* named *IO*.

P models a *Fcfs M|M|s* system for one customer class (called *Request*) where *s* is the number of processing entities which ranges from 0 to 2, so *P* has 3 structure states. Changes in *s* are governed by the *BirthDeath* process which is indicated by the frm attribute of the component type *Processor*.

IO greatly resembles *P* however, *IO* allows two different classes of customers: *Sample* and *Trigger*. Since *IO* also has 3 structure states, the total number of structure states of *DC* equals 3 × 3 or 9.

The load on *DC* is formed by an infinite Measure-Calculate-Trigger cycle (MCT cycle). This infinite cycle is described by the body of *Clt*.

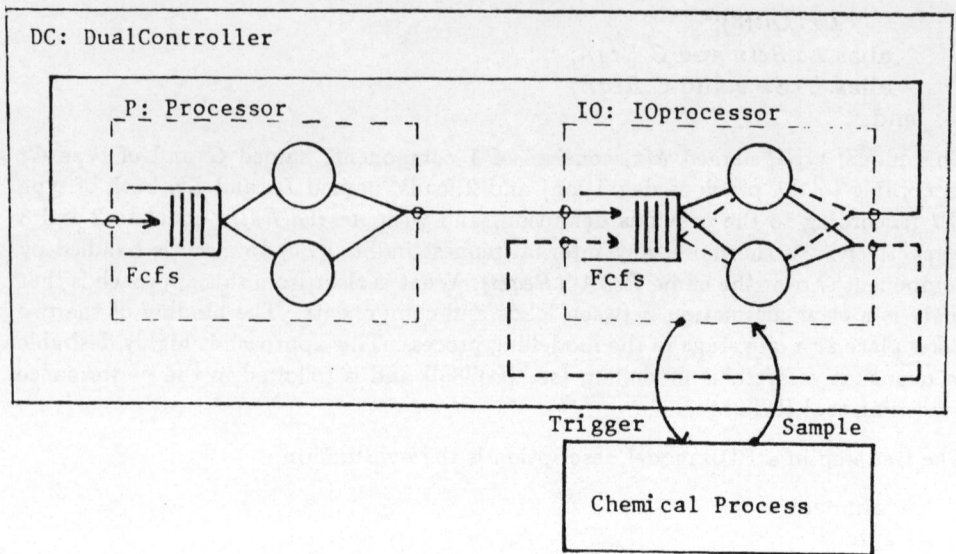

P: Processor

IO: IOprocessor

Fcfs

Fcfs

Trigger   Sample

Chemical Process

Figure 7. The Dual Controller System

The binding of the load to the components is expressed in the alias statements in the model type definition of *DualController*. Calculation actions in the load are mapped onto the *Processor P* and both *Sample* and *Trigger* actions are mapped onto the *IOprocessor IO*.

At system start the number of servers in both P and IO equals 2 so the system operates at maximum speed. However, after some time a failure of either P (with failure rate f_p) or IO (with failure rate $f_{i/o}$) will occur. The system will continue operation, albeit with degraded performance and less fault tolerance. This degradation process continues until the MCT cycle is broken. Then the system is said to be down.

properprogram *PdlDualController*;

$f_p = 0.0001$; (* server failure rate in fps for *Processor* *)
$f_{i/o} = 0.009$; (* server failure rate in fps for *IOprocessor* *)
$a = 1$; (* Population index *)

componenttype *Processor* =
interface *Request*;
begin
  servers 2;
  schedule *Fcfs*;
  frm *BirthDeath*$([2 \times f_p, f_p], [0, 0])$;
end;

componenttype *IOprocessor* =
interface *Sample, Trigger*;
begin
  servers 2;
  schedule *Fcfs*;

```
    frm BirthDeath([2 × f_{i/o}, f_{i/o}], [0, 0]);
end;

closedloadtype Clt(Population) =
interface Calculate, IOsample, IOtrigger;
begin
    IOsample(0.25);
    Calculate(0.2);
    IOtrigger(0.25);
end;

modeltype DualController =
begin
    component P : Processor;
                IO : IOprocessor;
    load L : Clt(a);
    alias L.Calculate and P.Request;
    alias L.IOsample and IO.Sample;
    alias L.IOtrigger and IO.Trigger;
end;

evaluation DualControlSystem =
begin
    model DC : DualController;
    measureperformability Moments(1)
    reward 1/CycleTime
    classes L
    output Graph;
end;
```

The above PDL program can be input to the PDL compiler which transforms it to a Markov-Reward process with 9 structure states. The reward vector (since there is only 1 class, **R** is a 9×1 matrix) is obtained via multiple performance analyses (actually, a CONVOL algorithm, being a direct implementation of the product form formulae of [Bcmp75] is used).

The $Moments(1)$, also often indicated with $EY(t)$, are solved via the ACE algorithm [Mari87]. The ACE algorithm calculates a symbolic solution of all the transient structure state probability functions as well as of the expected cumulative reward, i.e. $EY(t)$. Once this symbolic solution has been obtained, all types of graphs can be generated.

Now, we come to the interpretation of the results. Let us first address the rewards. The reward $1/CycleTime$ indicates the mean frequency with which a customer (a job) cycles through the system. One cycle conforms to one Measure-Calculate-Trigger or MCT sequence. If there is only 1 customer ($a = 1$), the reward equals the total number of MCT sequences per time unit. If $a = 2$, then the total number of MCT sequences per time unit equals 2 times $1/CycleTime$. In general, the total number of MCT-sequences per time unit equals the a parameter (i.e. the population index) times $1/CycleTime$.

The transient behaviour of the system is modelled via a Markov chain. Since there are no repairs (the repair rates in the frm attributes of the components are all zero) the system becomes worse in time. It is assumed that the whole system is functioning correctly at $t = 0$.

To be expected is the following behaviour: in the beginning of the operational period the expected cumulative reward will increase but the slope will decrease until it becomes zero after some time: the system is down. This is exactly what can be observed in figure 8. The a parameter in the figures conforms the a parameter of the PDL model description. We see, that when the population is smaller, the expected cumulative reward is higher: individual rewards are higher since there is less queueing. However, if we do not want the individual cycle frequency of 1 member of the population as reward but the total number of MCT sequences per time unit, we obtain the graph of figure 9. The total number of MCT sequences per time unit is an interesting measure since it determines how fast the total controller can react on (and influence) its environment, i.e. the chemical process. Now, we see that

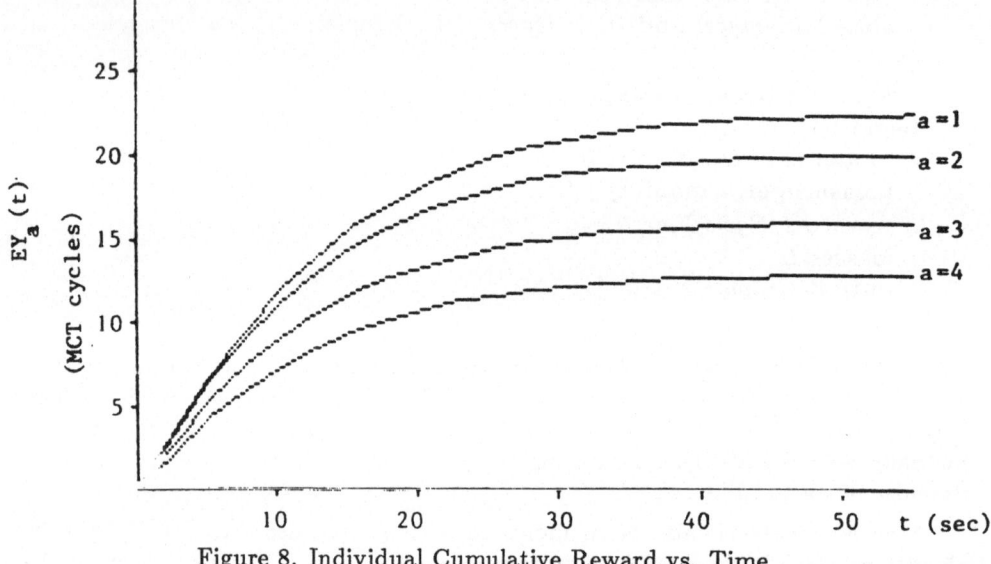

Figure 8. Individual Cumulative Reward vs. Time

for $a \leq 4$ the following holds: the greater the number of customers, the greater the expected cumulative reward. Of course, this is not true in general: when the number of customers increases there will be more queueing so individual rewards will possibly decrease more than can be compensated by the increase in their number. In this context it would also be interesting to include the influence of the number of customers on the failure rates and on the cumulative reward. However, this is not yet possible in the PROPER system. Finally, we come to figure 10. The graphs in figure 10 are obtained by dividing the cumulative reward of figure 9 by t. In this way, the mean number of MCT sequences per time unit over the interval $[0, t]$ is obtained. At $t = 0$ the function $aEY_a(t)/t$ equals the reward in its initial state times a. This is not only intuitively clear (in the interval $[0, t]$ for $t \to 0$, the system behaves as if failures can not occur) but can also be proved mathematically.

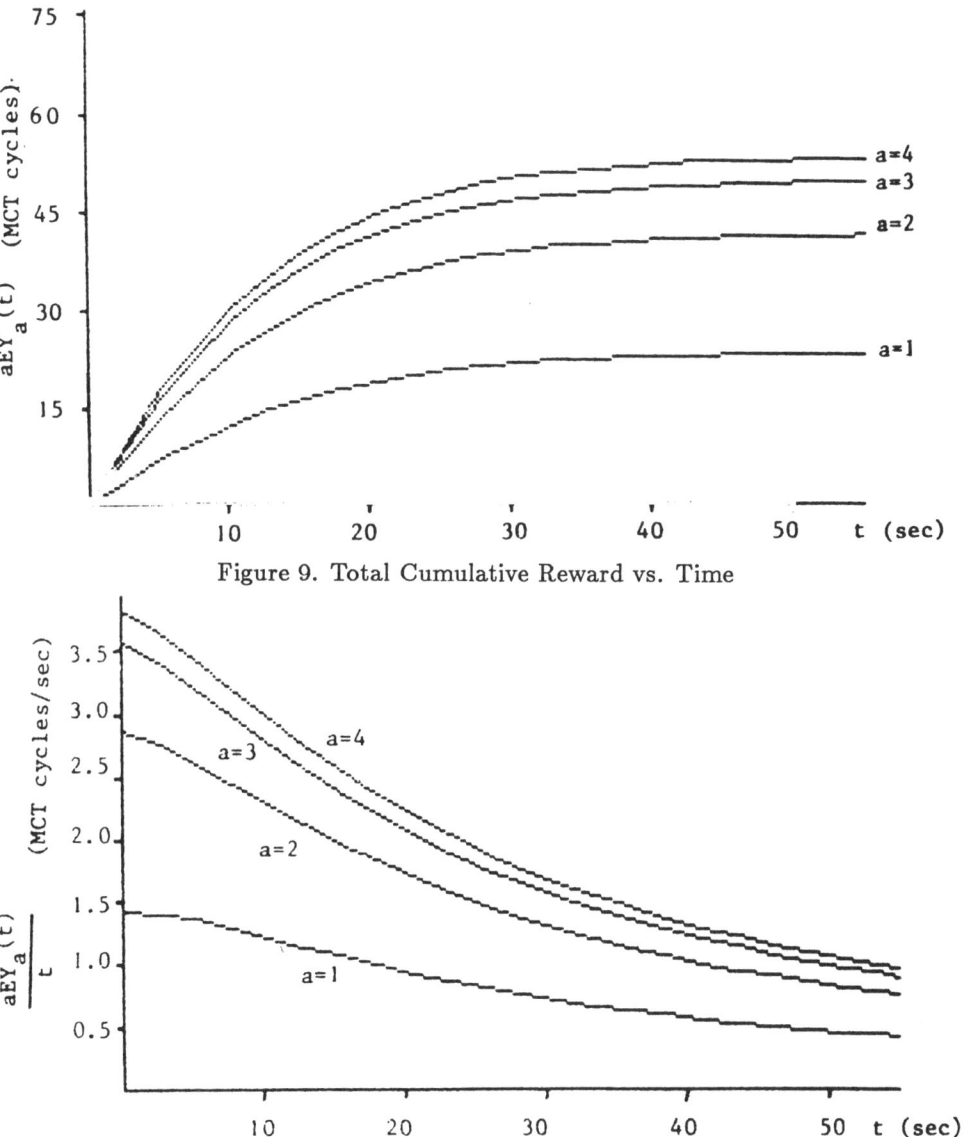

Figure 9. Total Cumulative Reward vs. Time

Figure 10. Mean number of MCT sequences per time unit vs. Time

6 The State of PROPER

The PROPER system is still under development. It is written in C and Simula and runs on a SUN 3 under UNIX BSD 4.2. We have not yet implemented all of the calculation methods mentioned in section 4.3. We are presently working on:

- the inclusion of more solution methods in the Low Level Model Solution module;
- the development of graphical input and an extension of the graphical output facilities;
- the development of menu-based input facilities for PDL;
- the inclusion of load dependent failure rates in the components;
- the inclusion of dependencies between repairs.

349

Furthermore we intend to extend PDL to allow for hierarchical modelling.

7 Concluding Remarks

In this paper we have given an overview of performability modelling in a broad sense. We have discussed the constituents of performability modelling, being performance and reliability modelling, as well as the basic mathematical theory about performability modelling. In section 4 we discussed the PROPER system, a performability modelling tool currently being developed at the University of Twente. The PROPER system allows its users to model for performability at a high level, i.e. via the language PDL. This combination (high level specification of the model and performability aspects) is, as far as we know, not yet seen in the literature. We demonstrated the tool by an example of a performability analysis for a class of computer systems which is becoming very important: the gracefully degradable multi-processor systems. PROPER is still under development. We indicated the directions which will be taken in the future.

Acknowledgements

The authors would like to thank Sietze Kloostra for implementing the Low Level Model Input and Solution modules of the PROPER system, as well as the referees for their useful comments on the draft version of the paper.

Literature

[Bcmp75]: F.Baskett, K.M.Chandy, R.R.Muntz, F.G.Palacios, *Open, Closed and Mixed Networks of Queues with Different Classes of Customers*, Journal of the ACM, Vol.22, No.2, April 1975, pp.248–260.

[Beau78]: M.D.Beaudry, *Performance Related Reliability Measures for Computing Systems*, IEEE Transactions on Computers, Vol.C-27, No.6, June 1978, pp.540–547.

[Beil85]: H.Beilner, *Workload characterisation and performance modelling tools*, Proceedings of the International Workshop on Workload Characterization of Computer Systems, Pavia, Italy, 23–25 Octobre, 1985.

[Carr86A]: J.A.Carrasco, J.Figueras, *METFAC: Design and Implementation of a Software Tool for Modeling and Evaluation of Complex Fault-Tolerant Computing Systems*, Proceedings FTCS, Vol.16, 1986, pp.424–429.

[Carr86B]: J.A.Carrasco, *Modelacion Y Evaluacion De La Tolerancia Fallos De Sistemas Distribuidos Con Capacidad De Reconfiguracion*, Ph.D.-Dissertation, University Catalunya, Spain, 1986.

[Chio86]: G.Chiola, *GSPN Users Manual*, Department of Computer Science, University of Turin, 1986.

[Cour77]: P.J.Courtois, *Decomposability: Queueing and Computer System Applications*, Academic Press, New York, 1977.

[Curt71]: A.R.Curtis, J.K.Reid, *The Solution of Large Sparse Unsymmetric Systems of Linear Equations*, J. Inst. Math. Appl., Vol. 10, 1971, pp.118–124.

[Dona86]: L.Donatiello, B.R.Iyer, *Analysis of a Composite Performance Reliability Measure for Fault Tolerant Systems*, Journal of the ACM, Vol.34, No.1, January 1986, pp.179–199.

[Furc84A]: D.G.Furchtgott, *Performability Models and Solutions*, Ph.D.-Dissertation, The University of Michigan, January 1984.

[**Furc84B**]: D.G.Furchtgott, J.F.Meyer, *A Performability Solution Method for Degradable Non-Repairable Systems*, IEEE Transactions on Computers, Vol. C-33, No.6, June 1984, pp.550–554.

[**Gay79**]: F.A.Gay, M.L.Ketelson, *Performance Evaluation for Gracefully Degradable Ssytems*, Proceedings FTCS 9, 1979, pp.51–58.

[**Goya86**]: A.Goyal, W.C.Carter, E. de Souza e Silva, S.S.Lavenberg, K.S.Trivedi, *The System Availability Estimator*, Proceedings FTCS 16, Vol.16, August 1986, pp.84–89.

[**Goya87**]: A.Goyal, A.N.Tantawi, *Evaluation of Performability for Degradable Computer Systems*, IEEE Transactions on Computers, Vol.C-36, No.6, June 1987, pp.738–744.

[**Goya88**]: A.Goyal, A.N.Tantawi, *A Measure of Guaranteed Availability and its Numerical Evaluation*, IEEE Transactions on Computers, Vol.C-37, No.1, January 1988, pp.25–32.

[**Gros84**]: D.Gross, D.R.Miller, *The Randomization Technique as a Modelling Tool and Solution Procedure for Transient Markov Processes*, Operations Research, Vol.32, No.2, March-April 1984, pp.343–361.

[**Have87**]: B.R.H.M.Haverkort, I.G.M.M.Niemegeers, *Probabilistic Modelling Of Reliability, Availability And Performability*, Internal Report INF-87-21, Department of Computer Science, University of Twente, May 1987.

[**Have88**]: B.R.H.M.Haverkort, *PDL, the PROPER Description Language; Concepts and Basic Language Elements*, Internal Report INF-88-4, Department of Computer Science, University of Twente, 1988.

[**Iyer86**]: B.R.Iyer, L.Donatiello, P.Heidelberger, *Analysis of Performability for Stochastic Models of Fault-Tolerant Systems*, IEEE Transactions on Computers, Vol.C-35, No. 10, October 1986, pp.902–907.

[**Jobm85**]: M.R.Jobmann, *Modellbildung und -analyse von Rechensystemen mit Hilfe des Programmsystems MAOS*, Proceedings of the 3rd GI/NTG Conference "Messung, Modellierung und Bewertung von Rechensystemen" (Ed.: H.Beilner), Dortmund 1985, pp.51–64, Springer Verlag.

[**Lamb73**]: J.D.Lambert, *Computational Methods in Ordinairy Differential Equations*, John Wiley & Sons, 1973.

[**Mari87**]: R.A.Marie, A.L.Reibman, K.S.Trivedi, *Transient Analysis of Acyclic Markov Chains*, Performance Evaluation 7, 1987, pp.175–194.

[**Mula86**]: M. Mulazzani, K.S. Trivedi, *Dependability Prediction, Comparison of Tools and Techniques*, Report CS-1986-20, Department of Computer Science, Duke University, 1986.

[**Meye80**]: J.F.Meyer, *On Evaluating the Performability of Degradable Computer Systems*, IEEE Transactions on Computers, Vol.C-29, No.8, August 1980, pp.720–731.

[**Meye82**]: J.F.Meyer, *Closed-Form Solutions of Performability*, IEEE Transactions on Computers, Vol.C-31, No.7, July 1980, pp.648–657.

[**Mitr82**]: I.Mitrani, *Simulation techniques for discrete event systems*, Cambridge University Press, 1982.

[**Muel84**]: B.Müller, *NUMAS – A Tool for the Numerical Analysis of Computer Systems*, in "Modelling Techniques and Tools for Performance Analysis" (Ed.: D.Potier), North Holland, 1985.

[**Muel86**]: B.Müller, *A Decomposition Approach for the Stationary Analysis of Fault Tolerant Queueing Systems*, The Journal of Systems and Software, Vol.6, No. 1&2, May 1986, pp.199– 204.

[**Muel87**]: B.Müller, *HIT – An Introduction*, Internal Report, University of Dortmund, 1988.

[**Nico86**]: V.F.Nicola, *Performance, Reliability and Queueing Analysis of Fault-Tolerant Computer Systems*, Ph.D.-Dissertation, Duke University, April 1986.

[**Nico87**]: V.F.Nicola, V.G.Kulkarni, K.S.Trivedi, *Queueing Analysis of Fault-Tolerant Computer Systems*, IEEE Transactions on Software Engineering, Vol.SE-13, No.3, March 1987, pp.363–375.

[**Reis81**]: M.Reiser, *Mean-Value Analysis and Convolution Methods for Queue-Dependent Servers in Closed Queueing Networks*, Performance Evaluation 1, 1981, pp.7–18.

[**Smit88**]: R.M.Smith, K.S.Trivedi, A.V.Ramesh, *Performability Analysis: Measures, An Algorithm, and a Case Study*, IEEE Transactions on Computers, Vol.C-37, No.4, April 1988, pp.406– 417.

[**Triv82**]: K.S.Trivedi, *Probability & Statistics with Reliability, Queueing and Computer Science Applications*, Prentice-Hall, Englewood Cliffs, NJ, 1982.

PETRI NETS GENERATING MARKOV REWARD MODELS FOR PERFORMANCE/RELIABILITY ANALYSIS OF DEGRADABLE SYSTEMS [1]

Andrea Bobbio

Istituto Elettrotecnico Nazionale Galileo Ferraris
Strada delle Cacce 91, 10135 Torino, Italy

ABSTRACT

This paper discusses how the formalism of Stochastic Petri Nets (SPN), with generally distributed transition times, can be used to generate Stochastic Reward Models (SRM) for the unified analysis of the performance and reliability of complex systems. In a SRM the working capacity (or performance level) of the system is modeled by attaching to each state of the process a real variable called the reward rate. The integral of the reward rate over a finite horizon provides the total amount of work accumulated by the system in a given time. An interesting and related figure of merit is the probability that an assigned task will be completed in a given time. We will refer to this problem as the completion time problem. The pictorial representation of the completion time problem at the Petri Net level is investigated. Two examples illustrate the application of the introduced modeling technique in simple cases.

1. INTRODUCTION

Stochastic Petri Nets (SPN)[2,1] have been extensively studied and applied to model systems whose behavior in time can be represented by a stochastic process. However, for degradable systems the classical tools of performance evaluation and reliability analysis are no more adequate and new modelling techniques and characterizing measures are needed.

In degradable systems the failure of one component reduces the working capacity of the system so that the overall performance degrades. The classical methods of the steady-state fault-free performance evaluation [15] overestimate the system capacity as a function of the time. On the other hand, the classical reliability theory is based on the assumption that each component, and the system as a whole, can be modelled by a binary variable [5] representing two possible states: functional or non-functional. This assumption implies that the state space of the system can be univocally partitioned

---

[1]Work partially supported by the Italian National research Council CNR under the Project "Materials and Devices for Solid State Electronics, Grant 87.02838.61

into two mutually exclusive subsets of states, one containing the up states, the other containing the down states. The classical reliability measures are defined on this binary partitioning of states.

A new methodology [26], proposed to face up the unified analysis of performance and reliability for degradable systems, consists in modeling the changing in the system configuration versus time by a discrete state stochastic process, and associating to each state a non-negative real variable representing the effective working capacity (or performance level) of the system in that state. The effective working capacity can be defined as the amount of useful computation per unit time in a computing system [6], or the amount of pieces produced per unit time in a manufacturing system. The stochastic process is called the structure-state process and the associated variable is usually referred to as the reward rate. The structure-state process, together with the reward assigned to each state form the Stochastic Reward Model (SRM). SRM's are formally introduced in section 2. They have been the subject of an extensive literature [20,8,16], but only recently have received attention as algorithmically feasible tools for system analysis [26,19,17].

Two main different points of view have been assumed in the literature when dealing with SRM for degradable systems: a system oriented point of view, and a task oriented point of view. In the system oriented point of view the most significant measure is the total amount of work done (or lost) by the system in a finite interval. This measure is often referred to as performability [21] and it is computed as the total accumulated reward [19,17].

In the task oriented point of view [12], the system is considered as a server whose service rate changes as the configuration changes; a task, that requires an assigned amount of work, is processed by the server and we want to evaluate the probability that the task will be completed in a given time interval, taking into account the possible system degradation. Moreover, the degradation may cause an error to occur in the execution of the task, and in the present formulation we consider two possible recovery policies [19,12].

When a change of state occurs in the structure-state process, the system keeps memory of the work already done and the task in progress is resumed in the new state. This policy will be called *preemptive resume (prs)*.

When a change of state occurs in the structure-state process, the system cannot keep track of the past; the task in progress is interrupted, and must be restarted from scratch in the new state. This policy will be called *preemptive repeat different (prd)*.

The distribution of the completion time depends on the preemptive policy, that needs to be defined as an input specification.

SPN are particularly suited for modeling conflict or concurrent interactions among resources, and a large number of examples and applications are available [2,1]. However, the use of SPN for generating SRM has never been discussed. In section 3 it is shown that the SPN formalism introduced in [4,3], and the semantics of the different execution policies, can be naturally extended to cover the case of the evaluation of the completion time when the underlying model is a SRM. Moreover, the general solution algorithm proposed in [4,9], when the distribution functions associated to the timed SPN transitions are of Phase (PH) type [22], can be invoked to computationally solve a class of completion time problems [7]. Sections 4 and 5 contain two examples intended to emphasize the compactness of the SPN formulation of completion time problems. In particular, the final example is introductory to the use of the above technique for planning the system capacity in order to achieve a prescribed accumulated amount of work over a finite horizon with a given probability.

2. STOCHASTIC REWARD MODELS

Let $Z(t)$ $(t \geq 0)$ denote a stochastic process defined over a discrete and finite state space Ω of cardinality n. Let f be a real valued function defined in Ω; then, $f[Z(t)]$ is a random variable [20]. In the present setting, $Z(t)$ represents the stochastic behavior of the system configuration in time (the structure-state-process), and f represents the rate (in some convenient unit) at which the work is performed by the system in each state; we further assume that the function f is non-negative and time-independent, so that we can write:

$$f[Z(t)] = r_j \geq 0 \qquad \text{if} \qquad Z(t) = j \qquad (1)$$

With the above definition $r_j \, dt$ provides the amount of work performed by the system in the interval t-$t + dt$ given that the system was in state j during that interval. The quantity r_j is called the reward rate. The structure state process $Z(t)$, together with the reward rates attached to each state, form the SRM.

The accumulated reward (or performability) is the random variable:

$$Y(t) = \int_0^t f[Z(x)] \, dx \qquad (2)$$

If $Z(t)$ is a Markov process, the expected value of $Y(t)$ is simply related to the state probabilities, thus can be computed by solving the transient Markov equation [26]. The distribution function $F_Y(t, x)$ of $Y(t)$ is defined as:

$$F_Y(t, x) = Prob\{Y(t) \leq x\} \qquad (3)$$

Computing $F_Y(t, x)$ is a more difficult task [19]. However the knowledge of the distribution function illuminates effects that are not detected by steady state values and by expected values [26]. Let us further suppose that the system must process a task whose execution requires B units of work. B is a random variable with distribution $\Psi(x)$ and density $\psi(x)$. The degenerate case in which B is deterministic and the distribution $\Psi(x)$ becomes the unit step function $U(B)$ located at $B = x$, can be considered as well. Given $B = x$, the task completion time $T(x)$ is the random variable representing the time to complete a task whose work requirement is x. The cumulative distribution function $F_T(t, x)$ is given by:

$$F_T(x, t) = Prob\{T(x) \leq t\} \qquad (4)$$

The unconditional completion time T is characterized by the following distribution:

$$F_T(t) = Prob\{T \leq t\} = \int_0^\infty F_T(t, x) \, d\,\Psi(x) \qquad (5)$$

In order to completely characterize the completion time problem, the interaction of the task in progress with the system must be specified. If in $Z(t)$ a transition from state i to state j occurs at time t and the transition is of prs type, the task execution resumes in state j at the new rate r_j. If the transition is of *prd* type, the task starts over again with rate r_j, and with a work requirement B resampled from the same distribution $\Psi(x)$.

When the structure-state process $Z(t)$ is a discrete-state homogeneous Markov process, the distribution of the completion time $F_T(t)$ (equation 5) has been expressed in [19] as two-dimensional Laplace transform equation. An algorithm for numerically inverting this equation has been presented in [25] when all the states are of *prs* type. In the case in which $\Psi(x)$ is of PH type, $F_T(t)$ is also of PH type [7], and can be computed as the distribution of the time to absorption of a suitable Markov chain. When the structure-state process $Z(t)$ is semi-Markov the distribution of the completion time has been investigated in [18].

3. PETRI NETS GENERATING STOCHASTIC REWARD MODELS

A marked Petri Net (PN) is the fourtuple $PN = (P, T, A, M)$, where:

- $P = \{p_1, p_2, \ldots, p_{np}\}$ is the set of places (drawn as circle in the graphical representation);

- $T = \{t_1, t_2, \ldots, t_{nt}\}$ is the set of transitions (drawn as bars);

- A is the set of directed arcs from places to transitions and from transitions to places;

- $M = \{m_1, m_2, \ldots, m_{np}\}$ is the marking. The generic entry m_i is the number of tokens (drawn as blak dots) in place p_i, in marking M.

A transition is enabled in a marking if all its input places carry at least one token; an enabled transition fires by removing one token from each input place and adding one token in each output place. The reachability set $\mathcal{R}(M_0)$ is the set of all the markings that can be generated from an initial marking M_0 by repeated application of the above rules.

A Stochastic Petri Net (SPN) [4,3] is a Marked PN in which:

- The set of transitions is partitioned into a subset of immediate transitions (thin bars) and a subset of timed transitions (thick bars). Immediate transitions fire in zero time and have higher priority over timed transitions.

- To each timed transition t_k is assigned a random variable modeling the time occurring to complete the activity associated to t_k.

- An execution policy is defined, which specifies the way in which a transition is selected to fire (among those enabled in a given marking), and the way in which the SPN keeps trace of its past history.

In the present paper the next transition to fire is selcted according to a *race policy*: if more than one transition (of the same priority level) is enabled in a given marking, the transition fires whose associated random delay is statistically the minimum.

For what concerns the conditioning on the past history we consider two alternatives:

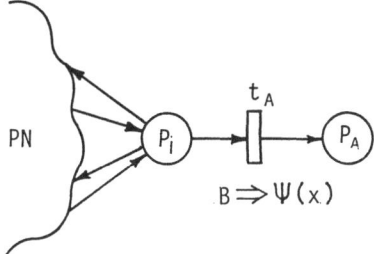

Figure 1 - A completion time problem represented as a first marking
time in place p_A

age memory: an age variable, associated to transition t_k, accumulates time since the
last firing of t_k;

enabling memory: the age variable accumulates time since the last epoch in which
t_k has been enabled.

When all the random variables associated to the SPN transitions are of PH type
[22], the SPN can be mapped into an equivalent homogeneous Markov chain [4,3]. The
implementation of the related algorithm is described in [9]; the expansion algorithm
is driven by the definition of the execution policy, and can accommodate marking
dependent transition rates. For further discussion on the semantics of the SPN model
considered in the present paper, we refer to [4,3].

3.1 Modeling the Completion Time Problem in a SPN

The completion time problem, formulated in the previous section, can be pictorially represented, at the SPN level, as a *first marking* problem. To this end, let us
suppose that the reward rate is equal to one ($r = 1$) in all the states producing useful
work. By this we physically mean that the task completes when the total accumulated
time spent in the markings producing useful work is greater than the requirement B.
We introduce in the basic net two supplementary places: an indicator place p_I and
an absorbing place p_A (figure 1).

The indicator place p_I is connected to the original SPN (indicated symbolically
as PN in figure 1) in such a way that it remains marked as long as the system is
producing useful work; on the other hand, the absorbing place p_A is inserted to stop
the execution of the net as soon as it becomes marked for the first time. The two places
p_I and p_A are connected with each other by a single timed transition t_A. Transition
t_A is assigned the random variable B (work requirement) with distribution $\Psi(x)$ (this
assignment is indicated as $B \Rightarrow \Psi(x)$ in figure 1).

From the semantics of the race policy, the epoch at which p_A becomes marked for
the first time is the epoch at which the time accumulated in p_I exceeds B, thus, by
construction, is the completion time. Sometimes, a place having the function of the
indicator place p_I is present in the SPN and need not to be added to the net. The role

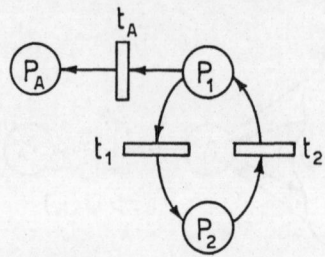

Figure 2 - PN modeling the task completion time problem with server breakdown.

of place p_A is to disable all the timed transitions in zero time when marked for the first time, so that the execution of the net stops. However, to realize the stopping property additional elements like immediate transitions or inhibitor arcs could be necessary. Using higher level nets like nets with enabling functions [10] or predicate/transition nets [13] the indicator and absorption property can be obtained by means of simpler and natural specifications.

The semantics of the execution policies of a SPN [4,3] is suited to model preemptive disciplines [19,12] in the task completion time problem. If transition t_A (figure 1) follows a race policy with age memory [4], it fires as the total marking time accumulated in p_I exceeds B (independently of the number of times place p_I has become enabled); from the point of view of the completion time problem, we realize a preemptive resume policy. If t_A follows a race policy with enabling memory [4], it fires the first time a continuous marked interval (without interruptions) exceeds B. The SPN models a completion time problem with preemptive repeat policy.

3.2 Modeling a Reward Function in a SPN.

In the present paper we discuss the case in which the reward rate can be expressed as a function of the marking. More formally we introduce a function $W(M)$ such that for any $M_i \in \mathcal{R}(M_0)$, $W(M_i) = r_i$ represents the reward rate in marking M_i. The markings M_i for which $r_i > 0$ correspond to states in which the system is producing useful work, while the markings M_j for which $r_j = 0$ correspond to states in which the system does not accumulate useful work. Let $\mathcal{S}(M_0) \subset \mathcal{R}(M_0)$ be the subset of the reachability set in which the SPN is producing useful work. By construction p_I is marked for any $M_i \in \mathcal{S}(M_0)$.

The case in which $r_i = 1$ for any $M_i \in \mathcal{S}(M_0)$, has been discussed in the previous paragraph. If $r_i = r$ for any $M_i \in \mathcal{S}(M_0)$, the work in place p_I is accumulated at a rate $r > 0$, but independent of M_i. In this case the completion time problem represented in figure 1 needs to be modified by associating to transition t_A the scaled random variable $B' = B/r$, with density [23]:

$$\psi'(x) = r\,\psi(r\,x) \qquad (6)$$

If $\psi(x)$ is PH, $\psi'(x)$ is obtained from equation (6) multiplying the transition rates

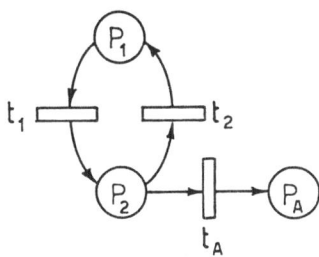

Figure 3 - PN modeling the attainment of a catastrophic failure subject
to the exceeding of a critical threshold in the down state.

of the representation [22] of $\psi(x)$ by the reward rate r. It turns out that, if $Z(t)$
is markovian and the distribution of the work requirement $\Psi(x)$ is of PH type, the
algorithm in [9] generates the equivalent Markov chain by scaling, in each marking
M_i, the transition rates of the PH representation by the corresponding reward rate
$W(M_i)$. The examples in the following sections illustrate the expansion technique.
The equivalence of the expansion technique with the closed form expression for the
distribution of the completion time $F_T(t)$ has been proved in [7] under various combination of preemption policies.

4. EXAMPLE 1: TASK COMPLETION TIME WITH SERVER BREAKDOWN

A server alternates between an up state (place p_1) and a down state (place p_2).
Transition t_1 represents the server failure (with distribution $F_U(x)$) and transition
t_2 the server repair (with distribution $F_D(x)$). The system produces useful work
only when place p_1 is marked (system up); in this case, $W(M) = r\, m_1$; thus either the
system works at rate r if p_1 is marked, or does not work if p_1 is not marked. Moreover,
p_1 can be used as the indicator place p_I (figure 2). If a task requires a work B with
distribution $\Psi(x)$ to be completed, we introduce, in figure 2, the absorbing place p_A
and transition t_A, with the associated scaled random variable $B' = B/r$ and density
given by equation (6). If, in the model specification, t_A follows an age memory policy,
the firing of t_A occurs only when the total accumulated up time is greater than B. In
the queueing language the failure of the server is preemptive resume: the work done
is not lost upon failure and is resumed as soon as the server becomes up again. If, on
the other hand, t_A follows an enabling memory policy, the server failure destroys the
work done, corresponding to a preemptive repeat different discipline.

A completely equivalent problem arises when we want to model a system that
reaches a catastrophic (unsafe) condition if and only if the time elapsed in the failed
state exceeds a tolerance threshold B. This problem is represented in figure 3, where
again place p_1 is the up state, place p_2 the down state and place p_A the absorbing
place representing the catastrophic condition.

If we specify a reward rate function $W(M) = m_2$, and assume p_2 as the indicator

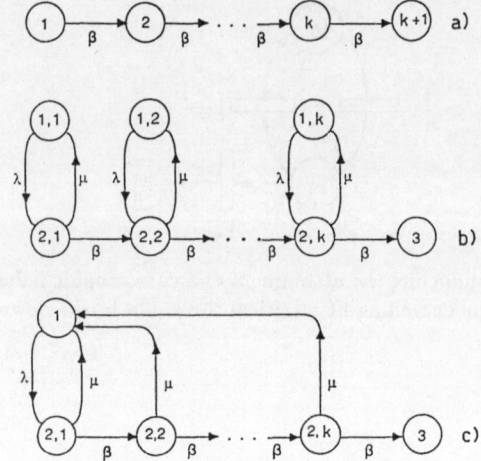

Figure 4 - a) The Erlang distribution with k states;
b) Equivalent Markov chain with t_A of *prs* type;
c) Equivalent Markov chain with t_A of *prd* type.

place p_I, the system accumulates *useful* work only when place p_2 is marked. Transition t_A is assigned the tolerance threshold B so that the catastrophic condition (token in p_A) is reached when the total down time exceeds B. Again, in this case, a preemptive resume or repeat policy can be assigned to transition t_A.

It should be emphasized that the stochastic formulation of both these problems (figures 2 and 3) is rather complex and has been examined in a number of papers [11,24,14]. The SPN formulation is, on the other hand, simple and straightforward. If $F_U(x)$ and $F_D(x)$ in figure 3 are exponential with parameters λ and μ respectively, and $\Psi(x)$ is an Erlang distribution $E(k,\beta)$ (figure 4a) of order k and rate $\beta = k/E[B]$ (being $E[B]$ the expected value), the corresponding completion time problem is evaluated as the absorption probability of the Markov chain of figure 4b when t_A is age memory (or *prs*) and of figure 4c when t_A is enabling memory (or *prd*).

5. EXAMPLE 2: PLANNING SYSTEM CAPACITY OVER A FINITE HORIZON

We have to produce an assigned amount of work B, over a finite horizon t. Knowing that a single resource can produce work at a rate r, we want to determine the number of resources to be installed, such that the probability that the work will be completed within t is $P(t, B) \geq 1 - \varepsilon$, being ε an acceptable risk level.

Resources fail independently with distribution $F_U(x)$, are repaired with distribution $F_D(x)$, and a single repair crew is available. The corresponding SPN is reported in figure 5. The number of tokens in place p_1 represents the number of available

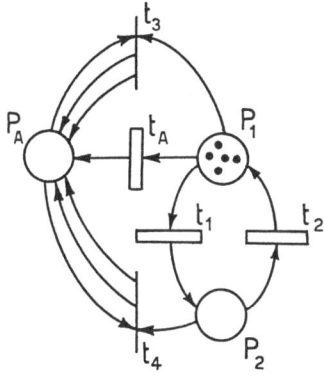

Figure 5 - Multiple resources working in parallel with failure and repair.

resources, while the number of tokens in place p_2 represents the number of resources under repair. Transition t_1 represents the failure and t_2 the repair. The system produces useful work only when place p_1 is marked and with a reward rate given by $W(M) = r\,m_1$. Since p_1 is marked as long as the system works, it acts as indicator place. Following the general pattern illustrated in section 3, we add to the basic SPN an absorbing place p_A connected to the indicator place p_1 by means of a single timed transition t_A with associated random variable B. In order to ensure the stopping property to place p_A, two extra immediate transitions t_3 and t_4 have been added. As soon as p_A becomes marked for the first time, t_3 and t_4 become enabled and fire with higher priority depleting instantaneously places p_1 and p_2, until all the tokens circulating in the net are confined in place p_A, and the net execution stops.

5.1 Numerical Results

Let $F_U(x)$ and $F_D(x)$ be exponential distributions with rates λ and μ respectively. Let the distribution $\Psi(x)$ of the task requirement B be an Erlang $E(k,\beta)$, where k is the number of stages and β the rate defined from the relation $\beta = k/E[B]$, where $E[B]$ is the expected value. The SPN of figure 5 is expanded into the Markov chain of figure 6 [9].

   The first component of the label inside each Markov state is the number m_1 of tokens in place p_1 (coincident with the number of working resources), while the second component denotes the stage of the Erlang distribution $E(k,\beta)$. Note that the rates of the Erlang distribution are multiplied by the reward rates of the corresponding state, so that the rates at which work accumulates become a function of the number of available resources. Since the algorithm in [9] can accommodate marking dependent transition rates, the above feature can be automatically incorporated by assigning t_A the marking dependent Erlang distribution $E(k, W(M)\beta)$.

   Results are reported for the following set of numerical values: $\lambda = 10^{-3}\ h^{-1}$,

$\mu = 0.1\ h^{-1}$ and $E[B] = 1000$. Figure 7 shows the distribution of the completion time $F_T(t)$ for different values of k ($k = 1, 2, 5, 10, 100, 1000$) given a fixed number of resources ($n = 2$). Figure 8 shows, for a fixed value of k ($k = 10$), the dependence of $F_T(t)$ on the number of resources n ($n = 3, 4, 5$ and 10 respectively). The curves of figure 8 allows us to answer the capacity planning problem since we can determine the minimum number of resources for which the production specifications are met at the assigned risk level ε. In particular the specifications are met in a time interval $t = 400\ h$ with probability $P = 0.95$ if we use 4 resources and with probability $P = 0.99$ if we use 5 resources.

If B is deterministic and $\Psi(x) = U(B)$, an approximate solution can be obtained by approximating $U(B)$ with an Erlang distribution with increasing number of stages. In this case, however, other solution techniques could be more effective [25].

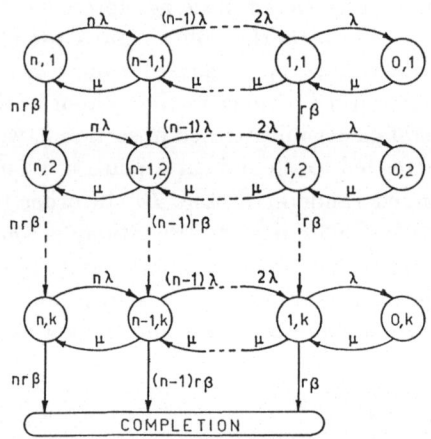

Figure 6 - Markov chain corresponding to the SPN of figure 5 when transition t_A is associated a work requirement B with distribution $E(k, W(M)\beta)$.

6 CONCLUSION

The paper has shown how the formalism and the semantics of the execution policies, already proposed for SPN with generally distributed transition times, can be adapted to generate SRM. In particular, the distribution of the completion time of a task processed by a degradable system can be pictorially represented at the SPN level, as a first marking problem into a suitably constructed absorbing place. The SPN representation of the completion time problem is rather compact and intuitive even if the

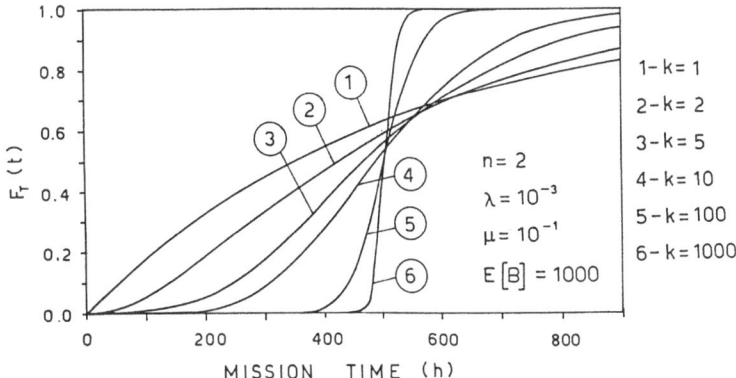

Figure 7 - Distribution of the completion time of a system with $n = 2$ parallel resources and different values of k.

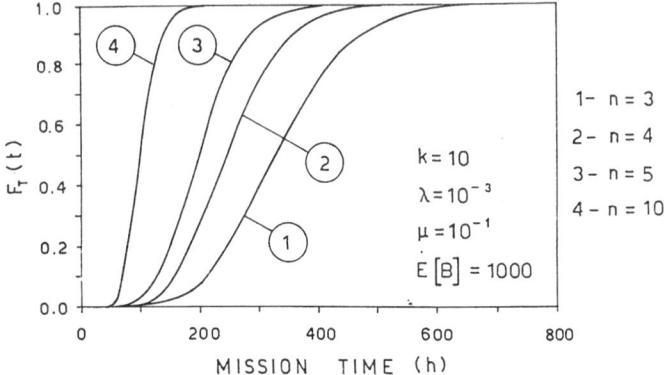

Figure 8 - Distribution of the completion time of a system with $k = 10$ for different values of the number of resources.

363

corresponding formulation as stochastic process is complex. The appealing feature of the SPN representation is that, the computation of the distribution of the completion time, can be automatically generated when the underlying process is Markov (or PH) and the work requirement is of PH type. In this way we have extended the SPN language to cover problems that, otherwise, require complex specification languages.

The reported examples show how typical problems, discussed in the literature, might find a natural description in the framework of SPN with reward.

References

[1] *International Workshop Petri Nets and Performance Models*, IEEE Computer Society Press No. 796, Madison, 1987.

[2] *International Workshop Timed Petri Nets*, IEEE Computer Society Press No. 674, Torino (Italy), 1985.

[3] M. Ajmone Marsan, G. Balbo, A. Bobbio, G. Chiola, G. Conte, and A. Cumani. The effect of execution policies on the semantics and analysis of stochastic Petri nets. *To be published on: IEEE Transactions on Software Engineering*, 1988.

[4] M. Ajmone Marsan, G. Balbo, A. Bobbio, G. Chiola, G. Conte, and A. Cumani. On Petri nets with stochastic timing. In *International Workshop on Timed Petri Nets*, pages 80–87, Torino (Italy), 1985.

[5] R.E. Barlow and F. Proschan. *Statistical Theory of Reliability and Life Testing*. Holt, Rinehart and Winston, New York, 1975.

[6] M.D. Beaudry. Performance-related reliability measures for computing systems. *IEEE Transactions on Computers*, C-27:540–547, 1978.

[7] A. Bobbio and K.S. Trivedi. *Computation of the distribution of the completion time when the work requirement is a PH random variable*. Technical Report, Accepted with revision on: Stochastic Models, 1988.

[8] E. Cinlar. Markov renewal theory. *Advances in Applied Probability*, 1:123–187, 1969.

[9] A. Cumani. Esp - A package for the evaluation of stochastic Petri nets with phase-type distributed transition times. In *Proceedings International Workshop Timed Petri Nets*, IEEE Comp Soc Press no. 674, Torino (Italy), 1985.

[10] J. Becta Dugan, A. Bobbio, G. Ciardo, and K. Trivedi. The design of a unified package for the solution of stochastic Petri net models. In *International Workshop on Timed Petri Nets*, pages 6–13, IEEE Comp Soc Press no. 674, Torino (Italy), 1985.

[11] A. Von Ellenrieder and A. Levine. The probability of an excessive non-functioning interval. *Operations Research*, 14:835–840, 1966.

[12] D.P. Gaver. A waiting line with interrupted service, including priorities. *Journal of the Royal Statistical Society*, B24:73–90, 1962.

[13] H.J. Genrich and K. Lautenbach. System modelling with high level Petri nets. *Theoretical Computer Science*, 13:109–136, 1981.

[14] A. Goyal, V.F. Nicola, A.N. Tantawi, and K.S. Trivedi. Reliability of systems with limited repair. *IEEE Transactions on Reliability*, R-36:202–207, 1987.

[15] P. Heidelberger and S.S. Lavenberg. Computer performance evaluation methodology. *IEEE Transactions on Computers*, C-33:1195–1220, 1984.

[16] R.A. Howard. *Dynamic Probabilistic Systems, Volume II: Semi-Markov and Decision Processes*. John Wiley and Sons, New York, 1971.

[17] B.R. Iyer, L. Donatiello, and P. Heidelberger. Analysis of performability for stochastic models of fault-tolerant systems. *IEEE Transactions on Computers*, C-35:902–907, 1986.

[18] V.G. Kulkarni, V.F. Nicola, and K. Trivedi. The completion time of a job on a multi-mode system. *Advances in Applied Probability*, 19:932–954, 1987.

[19] V.G. Kulkarni, V.F. Nicola, and K. Trivedi. On modeling the performance and reliability of multi-mode computer systems. *The Journal of Systems and Software*, 6:175–183, 1986.

[20] R.A. McLean and M.F. Neuts. The integral of a step function defined on a Semi-Markov process. *SIAM Journal of Applied Mathematics*, 15:726–737, 1967.

[21] J.F. Meyer. Closed form solution of performability. *IEEE Transactions on Computers*, C-31:648–657, 1982.

[22] M.F. Neuts. *Matrix Geometric Solutions in Stochastic Models*. John Hopkins University Press, Baltimore, 1981.

[23] A. Papoulis. *Probability, Random Variables and Stochastic Processes*. McGraw Hill, New York, 1965.

[24] S.M. Ross and J. Schechtman. On the first time a separately maintained parallel system has been down for a fixed time. *Naval Research Logistic Quarterly*, 26:285–290, 1979.

[25] R. Smith, K. Trivedi, and A.V. Ramesh. Performability analysis: measures, an algorithm and a case study. *IEEE Transactions on Computers*, C-37:406–417, 1988.

[26] K. Trivedi, A. Reibman, and R. Smith. Transient analysis of Markov and Markov reward models. In P. Courtois G. Iazeolla and O. Boxma, editors, *Computer Performance and Reliability*, pages 535–545, North Holland, 1988.

FAILURE DATA ANALYSIS OF A COMPUTER SYSTEM

B. Corby and H. Alaiwan

IBM France
CER La Gaude
06610 La Gaude - France

INTRODUCTION

Preliminary

The requirement for higher reliability in computer systems is having greater focus from the end user. This can be briefly explained by the fact that more and more vital applications, which require immediate service, are running on computerized machines. Therefore, the design of a new computer system is greatly influenced by its reliability objectives. One of the difficulties during the design phase, is the prediction of what would be the actual reliability of this new system once in full operation. We can find in the literature many papers for the prediction of some aspects of a system reliability [2,3,4], and we can note that most of them use a mathematical model obtained from the observation of similar systems in operation, and which present a set of parameters that should be adapted to the new one according to the new technologies used within. We say usually that the model is tuned to the future system.

The scope of our work falls in this context. Actually, we were first motivated by the prediction of the reliability of a new communication system, composed of both hardware and microcode components. Given the similarities between this new system and an already installed one, and assuming a common mathematical model, we observed the behavior of the latter in terms of number of failures, in order to tune the model to our new system. The model we assumed here was a Poisson distribution.

This type of procedure is well known today in the scientific community. The novelty of this paper lays in the fact that the field observation showed that the behaviour deviated from the model, and a revision of the model was necessary. Rather than trying to introduce in the model new parameters so the actual behaviour fits the one yielded by the model, we used a pragmatic approach, by revisiting the model assumptions and understanding where these assumptions were feeble with regard to the reality.

We began by 'relaxing' two assumptions in the model after a pragmatic analysis of the raw reliability data and the field reports. This yielded in the creation of an extension to the Poisson distribution, with two new parameters. When we ran the new model against the actual data, the results matched, but were valid only with a new assumption.

Not satisfied with the introduction of this new constraint, we pushed further our model using some concepts of the reliability theory related to the renewal process, and surprisingly succeeded in delivering a comprehensive model without the additional constraint.

The previous approach explains somehow the presence in this paper of two models, derived from the Poisson distribution.

Failure distribution

The failures we observe encompass both microcode and hardware component of the system, and correspond to ones that required an intervention by the customer engineer.

This paper deals with the distribution of the number of failures of a repairable machine when observed in the field [1], i.e. the proportion of machines with 0 failure, 1 failure, 2 failures, etc.. More specifically, the report studies the variance of this distribution.

The Poisson distribution is usually assumed. This means in particular that all machines have the same failure rate and the date of occurrence of one failure on one machine is independent of the date of occurrence of the previous failure on the same machine. "Poisson model" section recalls what does this mean in terms of variance.

However, the variance of field data is greater than the one of a Poisson distribution. After an "engineer" analysis of the previous data, we conclude that we may attribute this deviation to two different causes or a combination of them:

1. The population of machines may be heterogeneous, because it includes machines with different failure rates.

   A model exists that may describe this phenomenon. In this model, each machine follows a Poisson process, the failure rates are Gamma distributed, and the number of failures has a Negative Binomial distribution.

   A more general model is given in "Mixture of "good" and "bad" machines" section.

2. The failures may be clustered and appear in bursts.

In "Two parameter Burst model" section, a two parameter model is derived, which allows to account for the combination of the two above causes. This model assumes an heterogeneous population of machines, each with a Poisson burst occurrence rate, but is restricted to the case where the period of observation is large with respect to the burst duration.

In "Three parameter model" section, we generalize this model for any duration of observation, including durations which are small with respect to the burst duration (three parameter model).

The mathematical developments are in the appendices.

POISSON MODEL

We want to observe the behaviour of a machine[2] subject to failures.

---

[1] We assume that the repair duration is negligible with respect to the mean time between failures.

Let us call N(T) the random variable representing the number of failures observed during a time interval [0,T].

Let us call P(N(T) = k) the probability for N(T) to take the value k. If we assume that the failure distribution follows a Poisson process model, N(T) has the following distribution:

$$P(N(T) = k) = (\lambda T)^k \frac{e^{-(\lambda T)}}{k!} \qquad (1)$$

λ is the average rate of occurrence of failures within the time interval [0,T], or failure rate.

This Poisson distribution has the following mean and variance:

Mean $= (\lambda T)$ (2)

Variance = Mean   (3)

MIXTURE OF "GOOD" AND "BAD" MACHINES

Model description

Let us now observe the actual distribution of failures of a population of machines.

If equation 3 is representative of the field data, the machine behaviour can be modeled through a Poisson process.

If field data show more variance that the one determined by equation 3, we may try to explain this greater variance by the existence of "good" and "bad" machines:

1. Let's assume that for each machine, the number of failures in a time interval [0,T] is a Poisson distributed random variable with mean and variance given by equations 2 and 3, i.e. the machine failure rate is λ .

2. Let's also assume that the failure rate λ varies from machine to machine, i.e. there are "good" and "bad" machines in terms of failure rate.

To describe this variation of failure rate from machine to machine, we state that λ is a random variable, and we call E(λ) , for Expectation of λ, the mean of the distribution of λ, and V(λ) the variance of the distribution of λ .

Let's denote K the expression:

$$K = \frac{V(\lambda)}{E^2(\lambda)} \qquad (4)$$

Hence, K is the square of the coefficient of variation of the distribution of failure rates, i.e. the square of the ratio Standard Deviation/Mean of this distribution.

We shall call "Relative Variance" the square of a coefficient of variation. In particular, according to equations 2 and 3, the relative variance of a Poisson distribution is

---

[2] We shall use the term 'machine' instead of 'system' to adhere to the terminology of reliability theory.

equal to 1/Mean or $1/(\lambda T)$. In the present case, K is the relative variance of the distribution of failure rates. A small K corresponds to a small relative dispersion of the various λ around their mean $E(\lambda)$.

Let us take a machine at random amongst the total population of machines, and let X be the number of failures observed within a time interval [0,T].

Let's consider X as a random variable with mean $AVF(T)$ and variance $VAR(T)$. It can be shown (See appendix) that:

$$AVF(T) = T.E(\lambda) \tag{5}$$

and

$$VAR(T)/AVF^2(T) = 1/AVF(T) + K = 1/T.E(\lambda) + K \tag{6}$$

As a particular case of equations 5 and 6, if the failure rate distribution is expressed by a member of the Gamma family of distributions with mean value $E(\lambda)$ and relative variance K, then the distribution of the number of failures is negative binomial with mean and relative variance given by the equations 5 and 6.

Model interpretation and limiting cases

Model interpretation

1. The first term of the right side of equation 6, i.e. $1/T.E(\lambda)$ is the relative variance of a Poisson distribution with a fixed failure rate $E(\lambda)$, and an average number of failures $T.E(\lambda)$.
2. The second term K of the right side of equation 6 is the relative variance of the distribution of the failure rates (Equation 4).

Limiting cases

1. The first limiting case corresponds to K being negligible, in equation 6, with respect to $1/T.E(\lambda)$. In that case,

$$VAR(T)/AVF^2(T) = 1/T.E(\lambda)$$

which is the relative variance of a Poisson distribution. This may occur on two cases:

   a. On the one hand, K may be equal to 0; this represents the situation where all machines have an identical failure rate.

   b. On the other hand, the equation 6 also shows that for a given K different from 0, if we let T decrease so that $T.E(\lambda)$ tends towards zero, we reach the same effect, i.e. K becomes negligible with respect to $1/T.E(\lambda)$ in the limit.

   This is the case where the expected number of failures $T.E(\lambda)$ is small with respect to 1; one will observe a large proportion of machines with 0 failure, and a small proportion with one or more failures.

   In this case, the sample behaves as if all machines had an identical failure rate, whereas they have not.

2. In a second limiting case, if we let T increase so that $1/T.E(\lambda)$ becomes negligible with respect to K in equation 6, the relative variance of the number of failures tends towards K and mainly reflects the variation of failure rate from "bad" machines to "good" machines.

As a consequence, if this model is correct, the "deviation" behaviour, i.e. the fact that some machines encounter more failures that the average, is, for large T, mainly due to "bad" machine phenomenon, while the "deviation" behaviour for small T is purely random. As an example, let's see what happens if K = 0.5 and $E(\lambda)$ = 0.2 per Unit of time. For a large T = 50 Units of time, we get:

$$\frac{VAR(T)}{AVF^2(T)} = \frac{1}{T.E(\lambda)} + K = 1/(50).(0.2) + 0.5 = 1/10 + 0.5 = 0.6 \tag{6}$$

For this large T, the major contributor to the relative variance is K, which measures the "bad machine" phenomenon (we recall that should all machines be identical, K would be 0).

If the same machine population is observed within a small T = 1 Unit of time, we get:

$$\frac{VAR(T)}{AVF^2(T)} = \frac{1}{T.E(\lambda)} + K = 1/(1).(0.2) + 0.5 = 5 + 0.5 = 5.5 \tag{6}$$

For this small T, the major contributor to the relative variance is $1/T.E(\lambda)$, i.e. the Poisson distribution contributor. In other words, analysing machines which have failed for small T does not give any insights into the reasons why some machines will behave as "bad" machines when the period of observation T is large.

TWO PARAMETER BURST MODEL

Simple burst model

In the above model, we have seen in equation 6 that when $T.E(\lambda)$ tends towards 0, the relative variance of the distribution of failures should tend towards $1/T.E(\lambda)$.

If, however, actual data do not show this property, and if the relative variance noticeably exceeds $1/T.E(\lambda)$ for small values of $T.E(\lambda)$, then a phenomenon other than the heterogeneity between machines must be present.

This other phenomenon is the clustering of failures into bursts, i.e. the appearance of several failures in a short period. This behaviour is mathematically described in renewal theory (see Appendix).

In a first approach of the description of this burst phenomenon, we assume that a given machine has a given burst occurrence rate per Unit of time, and that there are "good" and "bad" machines in terms of burst occurrence rate. With these assumptions, we may apply to bursts the model previously developed for failures, i.e. assume that:

1. The number of bursts for a given machine is Poisson distributed.

2. The burst occurrence rate varies from machine to machine, and is itself a random variable.

We furthermore assume that, within a burst, Λ failures occur one after the other, the mean time between failures within a burst being small with respect to the period of observation.

Then the number of failures is always Λ times the number of bursts.

It can be shown (See appendix B) that equation 6 becomes:

371

$$\frac{VAR(T)}{AVF^2(T)} = \frac{A}{T.E(\lambda)} + K \tag{7}$$

Here, in the two limiting cases, K tending towards 0, and $T.E(\lambda)$ tending towards zero, the relative variance tends towards $A/T.E(\lambda)$.

This is A times the value $1/T.E(\lambda)$ that would take the relative variance if the distribution of failures was Poisson with the same failure rate $E(\lambda)$.

Generalized two parameter burst model

The above approach is not realistic: we do not expect all failures to be grouped by 2, or by 3. The appendix shows a generalisation of the use of equation 7, where Λ may take any value and is no longer limited to integer values, but still quantifies the tendency for failures to be clustered. The cases where $\Lambda < 1$ would correspond to a tendency for failures to be less clustered that in a Poisson process, i.e. to occur more regularly than in a Poisson Process.

Equation 7 can be rewritten as follows:

$$\frac{VAR(T)}{AVF(T)} = A + K.AVF(T) \tag{8}$$

which, in the case of a population of heterogeneous Poisson machines, becomes:

$$\frac{VAR(T)}{AVF(T)} = 1 + K.AVF(T) \tag{9}$$

Note: Equation 8 can be viewed in terms of variance, as:

$VAR(T) = VAR(\text{Poisson effect}) + VAR(\text{Burst effect}) + VAR(\text{Heterogeneous effect})$

where

$VAR(\text{Poisson effect}) = E(\lambda).T$

$VAR(\text{Burst effect}) = (\Lambda - 1).E(\lambda).T$

$VAR(\text{Heterogeneous effect}) = VAR(\lambda)$

First field data analysis

Equation 8 provides us a means to estimate the parameter Λ and K from the failure reports of the system in operation.

The process consists in selecting a wide sample of machines with their failure histories starting from a fixed date. Then we compute over increasing time periods T both VART(T) and AVF(T). Afterward, we plot $VAR(T)/AVF(T)$ versus $AVF(T)$ and we obtain A and K with a best fit with a straight line.

The estimates of $AVF(T)$ and $VAR(T)$ for various T are determined as follows:

Let Z be the total number of the observed machines. For a given T, we do the following:

One observes those machines over the time interval $[0,T]$.

Let $Z(n)$ be the number of machines having encountered n failures over the interval $[0,T]$, then we have:

$$AVF(T) = \frac{\sum_{n=0}^{\infty} n.Z(n)}{Z}$$

$$VAR(T) = E(n^2) - E^2(n) = \frac{\sum_{n=0}^{\infty} n^2 Z(n)}{Z} - AVF^2(T)$$

To see if the model applies, one plots the observation

$$(y(T); x(T)) = (\frac{VAR(T)}{AVF(T)}; AVF(T))$$

for different values of T.

This analysis yielded indeed a value of Λ which is superior to 1, and K different from zero, confirming the existence of both phenomena. Still, these results were obtained with some assumptions and we didn't know how much they influenced the obtained data. This leads us to the next section.

THREE PARAMETER MODEL

General

The two parameter model leading to equation 7 assumes that the observation period T is large with respect to the burst duration.

Let us consider what happens if, on the contrary, T is very small with respect to the burst duration. Let us assume that the failure occurrence within a burst is a Poisson process. Under these conditions, a machine observed while being in burst will appear as a "bad" Poisson machine, and a machine observed while being not in burst will appear as a "good" Poisson machine.

At this scale of observation, the clustering effect will be hidden, and the machines will behave as a population of heterogeneous Poisson machines (Equation 9). Therefore, one should introduce a third parameter K_2 in the model so that, for small T,

$$\frac{VAR(T)}{AVF(T)} = 1 + K_2.AVF(T) \tag{10}$$

while, for large T, we stay with

$$\frac{VAR(T)}{AVF(T)} = \Lambda + K.AVF(T) \tag{8}$$

We now describe such a model, disregarding its mathematical rationale which is explained in the appendices.

Homogeneous machines.

We first consider a population of homogeneous machines. All machines exhibit the same behaviour, which is as follows: After each failure, (and its repair, assumed to be immediate), the machine enters into one of two stages:

1. With probability P, the machine enters into a "burst" stage, where the failure rate is λ_1, i.e. the mean time to the next failure is $1/\lambda_1$.

2. With probability $(1 - P)$, the machine enters into a "no-burst" stage, where the failure rate is λ_2 with $\lambda_2 < \lambda_1$, i.e. the mean time to the next failure is $1/\lambda_2$ with $1/\lambda_2 > 1/\lambda_1$.

Therefore, the machine behaviour can be represented by a Markov state machine with 2 states, as shown in Figure 1.

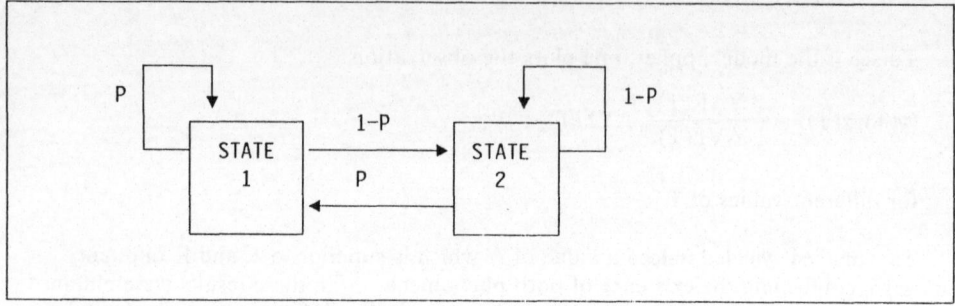

Figure 1. State transitions. State 1 characterizes the burst stage, and State 2 the 'no burst' stage.

The overall Mean Time Between Failure (μ) is

$$\mu = (P/\lambda_1) + ((1 - P)/\lambda_2) \qquad (11)$$

We furthermore assume that λ_1 is much greater than λ_2, so that μ is approximately $(1 - P)/\lambda_2$, the machine failure rate is

$$\lambda = \frac{1}{\mu} = \frac{\lambda_2}{1 - P} \qquad (12)$$

and λ_1 is much greater than λ

We believed a priori that the previous assumption was valid, because a rough analysis of the actual data showed indeed that there are long time periods during which most of the observed machines run without any failure. Applying this model to field data showed a posteriori that this assumption did actually agree with field data.

Population of heterogeneous machines

Three parameter model

We now consider a collection of heterogeneous machines all having the same burst structure, i.e. the same P and the same λ_1, but having different failure rates. The failure rate distribution has a Mean value $E(\lambda)$ and a relative variance K.

We introduce the two auxiliary parameters Λ and M_0 defined as

$$\Lambda = \frac{1 + P}{1 - P} \qquad (13)$$

$$M_0 = \frac{2.E(\lambda)}{(1 - P)\lambda_1} \qquad (14)$$

The reason why we choose these parameters will appear in the next two paragraphs.

We have, as shown in appendix A:

$$\frac{VAR(T)}{AVF(T)} = A - \frac{(A - 1).M_0(1 - e^{-2.AVF(T)/M_0})}{2.AVF(T)} + K.AVF(T) \qquad (15)$$

The asymptote when $AVF(T)$ tends to infinity is:

$$\frac{VAR(T)}{AVF(T)} = A + K.AVF(T) \qquad (8)$$

This is the two parameter model of section "Two parameter Burst model."

The asymptote when $AVF(T)$ tends to zero is:

$$\frac{VAR(T)}{AVF(T)} = 1 + (\frac{(A - 1)}{M_0} + K).AVF(T) \qquad (16)$$

The model therefore behaves as expected in equation 10.

The two above asymptotes intersect at the point with abscissa $AVF(T_0)$. Taking into account equations 8 and 16 we have:

$$AVF(T_0) = M_0 \qquad (17)$$

Graphical interpretation of the parameters

We see that K, A and M_0 have a graphical interpretation when plotting $VAR(T)/AVF(T)$ versus $AVF(T)$, since:

1. K in equation 8 is the slope of the asymptote when $AVF(T)$ tends to infinity,

2. A in equation 8 is the point where this asymptote crosses the Y axis, and

3. M_0 in equation 17 is the abscissa of the intersection between the above asymptote and the asymptote obtained when $AVF(T)$ tends to zero.

Physical interpretation of the parameters

In addition to having a graphical meaning, K, A and M_0 also have a physical meaning:

1. The parameter K quantifies the failure rate dispersion from machine to machine.

2. The parameters A and M_0 quantify the "clustering" or "burst" effect:

   a. The parameter A (related to P through equation 13) quantifies the probability P for a failure to be followed by a "clustered" failure.

   b. According to equation 14, the parameter M_0 is proportional to the mean time (i.e. $1/\lambda_1$) elapsing between two clustered failures. It is also the breakpoint for which the "deviation" phenomenon can be partly attributed to "bad machines"; before this point, no conclusion for this phenomenon can be made.

Second field data analysis

The process is very similar to that of section "First field data analysis" on page 7. Actually, equations 8, 15, 16 and 17 are used to compare the model with the data expressed as:

$$\frac{VAR(T)}{AVF(T)} \text{ versus } AVF(T)$$

The three coefficients Λ, K and M_0 are adjusted for best fit (See Figure 2):

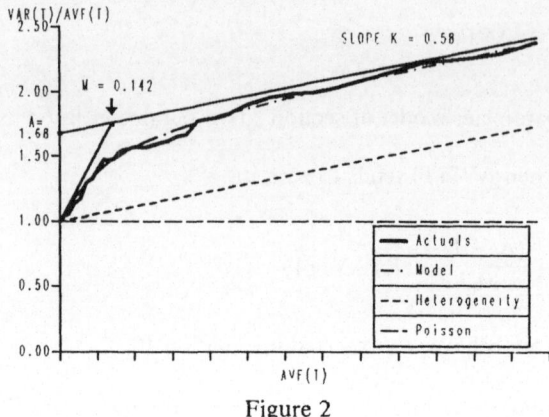

Figure 2

1. The asymptote for large T provides parameters Λ and K as per equation 8.

2. Its intersection with the asymptote for small T provides the parameter M_0 as per equation 17.

In that case, we obtain the best fit for: $\Lambda = 1.68$, $K = 0.58$, and $M_0 = 0.142$,

which correspond to the following model:

• Probability for next failure to be clustered (Derived from equation 13):

$$P = \frac{\Lambda - 1}{\Lambda + 1} = 0.25$$

• Ratio of λ_1 to $E(\lambda)$ (Derived from equation 14):

$$\frac{\lambda_1}{E(\lambda)} = \frac{2}{M_0(1 - P)} = 19$$

which shows a posteriori that the assumption leading to equation 12 was valid.

CONCLUSION

In this paper, we have shown that the behaviour of the machines cannot be assimilated to a simple Poisson distribution. The introduction of machines heterogeneity allowed the mathematical model to be closer to the reality; still this heterogeneity didn't explain the "deviation" phenomenon. Therefore, the introduction of the "burst" concept, with the ability to estimate it, resulted into a model that can be interpreted from an engineering point of view.

Thus, we have shown that the "deviation" behaviour of those machines encountering more failures than the average number of failures per machine, is due to three causes, whose contribution varies with the width of the observation period:

1. The random fluctuations due to the Poisson distribution is an important contributor

in any case, and is sufficient to explain "deviation" behaviour for very small observation periods (say, a week).

2. For larger observation period width (a month or so), a second cause intervenes, which is the tendency for failures to be clustered in bursts.

3. The third cause of High Flyer behaviour is the population heterogeneity: some machines have a higher failure rate than the other. As seen on the attached figure, this third cause is negligible for small observation periods, because it is hidden by the two above causes. It only becomes an important contributor when the observation periods is extended to around one year.

It should be mentioned that Confidence Intervals indicating the failure rate measurement precision are usually based upon the Poisson Distribution assumption, and are therefore optimistic, because they do not take take into account the additional dispersion brought by "burst" and "heterogeneity" phenomena.

REFERENCES

1. D.R.Cox, "Renewal theory", R.Cox, Ed. Methuen and Co. Ltd, Science Paperbacks, 1967.

2. B.S. Dhillon, "System reliability growth models", Proc. of International Conference on Policy Analysis and Information Systems, pp. 615-623 (1981).

3. A.L. Goel and K. Okumoto, "Time dependent error detection rate model for software reliability and other performance measures", IEEE Trans. on Reliability, VOL. R-28, No.3, AUGUST 1979.

4. S. Yamada and S. Osaki, "Reliability growth models for hardware and software systems based on nonhomogeneous Poisson processes: a survey", Microelectronic. Reliab., Vol. 23, No. 1, pp. 91-112 (1983).

APPENDIX. BURST MODEL WITH HOMOGENEOUS MACHINES

Renewal process

We shall recall some of the findings of Renewal theory [1], and we shall show how this can help to mathematically describe the failures clustering.

Consider a component with a time to failure distribution whose mean value is μ, and whose standard deviation is σ (in our case, the component is a machine).

Consider a renewal process by which the component, when it fails, is immediately renewed, i.e. replaced by a brand new one (in our case, the machine is repaired, but it behaves as if it were renewed).

Consider the random variable N(T), number of renewals in the time interval [0,T] for a given component. The distribution of N(T) has a mean value, called renewal function,

$$H(T) = E(N(T)) \tag{A1}$$

We may distinguish the "ordinary renewal process" when the component is new at time 0, and the "equilibrium renewal process", which can be regarded as an ordinary renewal process in which the system has been running a long time before it is first observed. To distinguish between these two processes, we shall use the subscripts o for ordinary and e for equilibrium.

As T tends to infinity, the variance and the mean of the distribution of N(T) for the equilibrium process tends to be normally distributed (Reference 1 page 40) with a Mean value:

$$E_e(N(T)) = H_e(T) = T/\mu \qquad (A2)$$

and a Variance $Var_e(T)$ such that:

$$\frac{Var_e(N(T))}{E_e(N(T))} = (\frac{\sigma}{\mu})^2 \qquad (A3)$$

This constant $(\sigma/\mu)^2$ corresponds to the clustering parameter Λ of section "Two parameter Burst model."

If the component failure rate decreases when the component age increases (wear-in phenomenon), Λ is superior to 1. The rationale is that the failure rate is high shortly after a renewal, hence a tendency for renewals to appear in bursts.

Conversely, if the failure rate increases with component age (wear-out phenomenon), Λ is inferior to 1. The rationale is that the failure time distribution is centered around its MTTF, hence a tendency for renewals to appear more regularly than with a Poisson distribution.

The intermediate case, $\Lambda = 1$ corresponds to a constant failure rate, which occurs for an exponential distribution of time to failure, and which leads to a Poisson renewal process with the familiar property of the Poisson distribution:

$$\frac{Variance}{Mean} = 1$$

Ideally, the superposition of renewal processes of the Field Replaceable Units (FRU) should lead to a Poisson Process at the machine level, if the number of FRU was large, and if the individual FRU renewal processes were independent.

However, that is not what is actually observed, and machine failures sometimes appear in bursts.

To determine the burst parameter of Section "Two parameter Burst model," we now wish to compute the ratio Variance/Mean of N(T) for any value of T, and not only when T tends to infinity.

It can be shown (Reference 1 page 57) that, for the equilibrium renewal process,

$$Var(N_e(T)) = \frac{2}{\mu} \int_0^T (H_o(t) - \frac{t}{\mu} + \frac{1}{2}) \, dt \qquad (A4)$$

We shall now proceed with determining $H_o(T)$, the renewal function for the ordinary renewal process; then we shall come back to equation A4.

Renewal function

To determine $H_o(T)$, we shall restrict ourselves to a family of time to failure distributions called "second type of General Erlang distribution (Reference 1 page 17). The p.d.f. is:

$$P\lambda_1 e^{-\lambda_1 t} + (1 - P)\lambda_2 e^{-\lambda_2 t} \qquad (A5)$$

with $\lambda_2 < \lambda_1$.

It can be shown that by suitable choice of P, λ_1, λ_2, we can produce distributions having any desired μ, and any relative variance between 1 and infinity. For this distribution:

$$\mu = \frac{P}{\lambda_1} + \frac{1 - P}{\lambda_2} \tag{A6}$$

$$A = \left(\frac{\sigma}{\mu}\right)^2 = \frac{2}{\mu^2}\left(\frac{P}{\lambda_1^2} + \frac{1 - P}{\lambda_2^2}\right) - 1 \tag{A7}$$

If we use the auxiliary parameter B:

$$B = (1 - P)\lambda_1 + P\lambda_2 \tag{A8}$$

it can be shown (Reference 1 page 50) that:

$$H_o(T) = \frac{T}{\mu} + \frac{(A - 1).(1 - e^{-B.T})}{2} \tag{A9}$$

Variance of the number of renewals

We may now compute $Var(N_e(T))$ as per equation A4, taking into account equation A9:

$$Var(N_e(T)) = \frac{2}{\mu}\int_0^T (H_o(t) - \frac{t}{\mu} + \frac{1}{2})\,dt \tag{A4}$$

$$= \frac{2}{\mu}\left(\frac{T^2}{2\mu} + \frac{(A - 1)}{2}.T - \frac{(A - 1)}{2.B}(1 - e^{-B.T}) - \frac{T^2}{2\mu} + \frac{T}{2}\right)$$

$$= \frac{A.T}{\mu} - \frac{(A - 1)(1 - e^{-B.T})}{B\mu} \tag{A10}$$

Taking into account the fact that:

$$E_e(N(t)) = H_e(T) = \frac{T}{\mu} \tag{A2}$$

we finally can compute the ratio Variance/Mean of the number of renewals:

$$\frac{Var_e(N(T))}{E_e(N(T))} = A - \frac{(A - 1).(1 - e^{-B.T})}{B.T} \tag{A11}$$

with the particular cases:

1. T tends to 0, Variance/Mean tends to

$$\frac{Var_e(N(T))}{E_e(N(T))} = 1 + \frac{(A - 1).B.T}{2} \tag{A12}$$

and

2. T tends to infinity, Variance/Mean tends to

$$\frac{Var_e(N(T))}{E_e(N(T))} = A \tag{A13}$$

From now on, we restrict our family of p.d.f. to the case where $\frac{\lambda_2}{\lambda_1}$ is small with respect to 1.

In that particular case, we have

$$\mu = \frac{1 - P}{\lambda_2} \tag{A14}$$

$$\Lambda = \frac{1 + P}{1 - P} \quad B = (1 - P)\lambda_1 \tag{A15}$$

We will consider in the next appendix a collection of heterogeneous machines with $\mu = (1 - P)/\lambda_2$ differing from machine to machine, but with the same burst structure for all machines, i.e. the same P and the same λ_1, hence the same Λ and the same B, and therefore a ratio Variance/Mean of the distribution of the number of renewals, given by equation A11, independent of μ.

INCLUSION OF MACHINE HETEROGENEITY

Definition of symbols

- We consider an interval of observation [0,T].

- We call λ the average failure rate of a specific machine during [0,T].

- If we take T as the Unit of time, we define the expression

  $$L = \lambda T \tag{B1}$$

  as the rate of failure per Unit of time T of a specific machine.

- We call P(L) the distribution of failure rates; this distribution has a mean E(L), and a variance V(L). We make no other assumption on this distribution.

- Let's denote K the relative variance of P(L):

  $$K = \frac{V(L)}{E^2(L)}$$

  If P is a member of the Gamma family of distributions, 1/K is its shape parameter. Decreasing K means decreasing machine to machine heterogeneity, with K = 0 being the particular case where all machines have the same failure rate.

- We denote

  N as the number of failures of a machine during T, and

  $\pi(N|L)$ as the distribution of N for a machine whose failure rate is L. This distribution has a mean

  $$E(N|L) = L \tag{B2}$$

- We call Var(N|L) the variance of $\pi(N|L)$. By definition,

  $$\mathrm{Var}(N|L) = (\sum_{n=0}^{\infty} N^2 \pi(N|L)) - E(L|N)^2$$

  which, combined with equation B2, gives:

  $$\mathrm{Var}(N|L) = (\sum_{n=0}^{\infty} N^2 \pi(N|L)) - L^2$$

  or

380

$$\sum_{n=0}^{\infty} N^2 \pi(N|L) = Var(N|L) + L^2 \qquad (B3)$$

Equation B3 will be used later-on.

We make no other assumption on $\pi(N|L)$ except that $Var(N|L)/L$ is independent of L as explained at the end of appendix A, with the particular case $Var(N|L) = 1$ if $\pi(N|L)$ is Poisson.

- Finally, we call $r(N)$ the distribution of N for a machine randomly chosen.

  $r(N)$ is the distribution whose relative variance $VAR(T)/AVF^2(T)$ is looked for.

  We call $AVF(T)$ and $VAR(T)$ the mean and variance of $r(N)$.

$$r(N) = \int_0^{\infty} \pi(N|L).P(L)\, dL \qquad (B4)$$

Computation of VAR(T)/AVF(T)

Computation of AVF(T)

$$AVF(T) = \sum_{n=0}^{\infty} N.r(N) = \sum_{n=0}^{\infty} N\int_0^{\infty} \pi(N|L).P(L)\, dL = \int_0^{\infty} \left(\sum_{n=0}^{\infty} N\pi(N|L) \right) P(L)\, dL \qquad (B5)$$

$$= \int_0^{\infty} L.P(L)\, dL = E(L)$$

Computation of VAR(T)

$$VAR(T) = \left(\sum_{n=0}^{\infty} N^2 r(N) \right) - \left(\sum_{n=0}^{\infty} N.r(N) \right)^2 \qquad (B6)$$

Taking into account equations B5 and B4, this can be rewritten

$$VAR(T) = \left(\sum_{n=0}^{\infty} N^2 r(N) \right) - E^2(L) \qquad (B7)$$

$$= \left(\sum_{n=0}^{\infty} N^2 \int_0^{\infty} \pi(N|L).P(L)\, dL \right) - E^2(L) = \int_0^{\infty} \left(\sum_{n=0}^{\infty} N^2 \pi(N|L).P(L) \right) dL - E^2(L)$$

Using equation B3, this becomes:

$$VAR(T) = \int_0^{\infty} (Var(N|L) + L^2).P(L)\, dL - E^2(L) \qquad (B8)$$

$$= \int_0^{\infty} Var(N|L).P(L)\, dL + \int_0^{\infty} L^2.P(L)\, dL - E^2(L)$$

$$= \int_0^{\infty} Var(N|L).P(L)\, dL + E(L^2) - E^2(L)$$

$$= \int_0^{\infty} Var(N|L).P(L)\, dL + (E(L^2) - E^2(L)) = \int_0^{\infty} Var(N|L).P(L)\, dL + V(L)$$

$$= \int_0^{\infty} \left(\frac{Var(N|L)}{L} \right).L.P(L)\, dL + V(L)$$

The first term being the average variance over L.

Now, since $Var(N|L)/L$ is assumed to be independent of L , equation B8 may be written:

$$VAR(T) = \frac{Var(N|L)}{L} \int_0^{\infty} L.P(L)\, dL + V(L) = \frac{Var(N|L)}{L}.E(L) + V(L) \qquad (B9)$$

Relative to the mean of r(N), equation B9 becomes:

$$\frac{VAR(T)}{AVF(T)} = \frac{Var(N|L)}{L} + \frac{V(L)}{E(L)} = \frac{Var(N|L)}{L} + \frac{V(L)}{E^2(L)} E(L) \tag{B10}$$

$$= \frac{Var(N|L)}{L} + K.E(L) = \frac{Var(N|L)}{E(N|L)} + K.E(L)$$

$$= \frac{Var(N|L)}{E(N|L)} + K.AVF(T)$$

We replace $Var(N|L)/E(N|L)$ by its value given by equation A11 and get:

$$\frac{VAR(T)}{AVF(T)} = A - (A - 1).\frac{(1 - e^{-B.T})}{B.T} + K.AVF(T) \tag{B11}$$

If we recall that

$$L = T\lambda \tag{B1}$$

we have

$$E(L) = E(T\lambda) = T.E(\lambda)$$

or

$$T = \frac{E(L)}{E(\lambda)} = \frac{AVF(T)}{E(\lambda)} \tag{B12}$$

we get

$$\frac{VAR(T)}{AVF(T)} = A - \frac{(A - 1).E(\lambda).(1 - e^{-B.AVF(T)/E(\lambda)})}{B.AVF(T)} + K.AVF(T) \tag{B13}$$

COMPARISON WITH FIELD DATA

Let us plot $VAR(T)/AVF(T)$ versus $AVF(T)$.

1. When $AVF(T)$ tends to zero, $VAR(T)/AVF(T)$ tends to

$$\frac{VAR(T)}{AVF(T)} = 1 + \left(\frac{(A - 1).B}{2.E(\lambda)} + K \right) AVF(T) \tag{C1}$$

which is a straight line as long as $E(\lambda)$ does not vary with T.

2. When $AVF(T)$ tends to infinity, $VAR(T)/AVF(T)$ tends to the straight line:

$$\frac{VAR(T)}{AVF(T)} = A + K.AVF(T) \tag{C2}$$

This is the 2 parameter model of Section "Two parameter Burst model."

The two above asymptotes intersect at the point with abscissa

$$M_0 = AVF(T_0) = \frac{2.E(\lambda)}{B} \tag{C3}$$

Taking into account equation C3, we may rewrite equation B13 as follows:

$$\frac{VAR(T)}{AVF(T)} = \Lambda - \frac{(\Lambda - 1).M_0(1 - e^{-2.AVF(T)/M_0})}{2.AVF(T)} + K.AVF(T) \qquad (C4)$$

The asymptote when $AVF(T)$ tends to zero is now the straight line:

$$1 + (\frac{(\Lambda - 1)}{M_0} + K).AVF(T) \qquad (C5)$$

The asymptote when $AVF(T)$ tends to infinity is still the straight line:

$$\frac{VAR(T)}{AVF(T)} = \Lambda + K.AVF(T) \qquad (C6)$$

FAST APPROXIMATE SOLUTION OF QUEUEING NETWORKS WITH MULTI-SERVER CHAIN-DEPENDENT FCFS QUEUES

Adrian E. Conway

GTE Laboratories Incorporated
40 Sylvan Road
Waltham, MA, USA

ABSTRACT

In this paper, we develop a Linearizer-type approximation technique for the analysis of large multiple-chain queueing networks that contain multi-server first-come, first-served queues with service times that are chain dependent. Use is made of a waiting time approximation based on Mean Value Analysis that has recently been developed by Souza e Silva and Muntz. The storage requirements of the iterative scheme are of the order of NR^2, and the computational requirements are of the order of NR^3, where N is the number of nodes and R is the number of closed routing chains. In comparing the results obtained with published empirical stress test results, the accuracy of the Linearizer-type approximation is found to be acceptable. An application in which the proposed iterative technique is found to be particularly useful is in the analysis of large queueing networks with nested passive resources and many closed routing chains, of the type arising in the modeling of computer systems with multi-programming constraints and of computer-communication networks with window flow controls.

1. INTRODUCTION

In this paper, we consider the fast approximate solution of large multiple-chain closed queueing networks of the BCMP type [BAS1] that contain multi-server first-come, first-served (FCFS) exponential queues with service times that are chain dependent. These queues are known to violate product-form conditions. There are several applications in which the solution to such queueing networks is required. One important application in which such queueing networks arise, and one which has received much attention in recent years, is in the solution of queueing networks that contain passive resources [LAV1], such as those which arise in the modeling of, for example, data base locking, computer systems with multi-programming constraints and computer-communication networks with window flow controls.

For the solution of queueing networks with passive resources, a variety of approximation techniques have been proposed that differ in the generality of their assumptions and in their computational requirements [BRA1, BRA2, JAC1, JAC2, KRZ2, LAZ1]. Recently, however, a relatively simple and accurate solution algorithm has been developed by Souza e Silva and Muntz [SOU1] which can accommodate more general forms of simultaneous resource possession than have previously been considered. This algorithm makes intensive use of queueing networks that contain multi-server FCFS queues with chain-dependent service times (to be abbreviated as MSFCFS). The solution methodology of Souza e Silva and Muntz can be used to analyze BCMP queueing networks with multiple passive resources that may be nested to an arbitrary degree and which may be shared among customers belonging to different routing chains.

In the solution approach of Souza e Silva and Muntz, the first step is to decompose the network into a set of smaller subnetworks according to the constrained (or flow controlled) domains that may be identified. The second step is to construct a reduced network around each subnetwork by including certain 'flow equivalent' queues [LAV1] of the infinite-server (IS) and MSFCFS type. The service times at these queues are defined by functions that are made to depend on the performance measures of the other reduced networks. The number of servers at each MSFCFS queue is made to correspond with the token population (or window size) of a particular passive resource (or flow control mechanism). In this manner, the flow equivalent queues are designed to represent approximately the complementary parts of the network. The final step is to solve the reduced networks in succession and iterate until certain convergence criteria have been satisfied. Since each reduced network may include MSFCFS flow equivalents, the algorithm of Souza e Silva and Muntz requires the repetitive application of a solution algorithm for BCMP queueing networks that contain MSFCFS queues. In order that the solution of each reduced network does not give rise to a computational bottleneck in the overall iterative solution algorithm, it is necessary that an efficient algorithm be employed for the analysis of the reduced networks. Our motivation for considering the fast approximate solution of BCMP queueing networks with MSFCFS queues arises from this application.

To analyze BCMP queueing networks with MSFCFS stations, Souza e Silva and Muntz [SOU1] have developed a Mean Value Analysis [REI1] (MVA)-based recursive approximation algorithm that makes use of the established exact MVA equations together with a newly developed MVA-type recursive approximation for the waiting times at MSFCFS queues. This recursive algorithm is similar in spirit to algorithms such as the one which has been proposed for the analysis of closed BCMP queueing networks that contain priority queues [BRY1]. Since the recursion in this approximation algorithm is over the chain populations, the computational requirements increase exponentially with the number of chains. By comparison with simulation results, Souza e Silva and Muntz show, in certain stress tests, that the accuracy of their MVA-based recursive approximation is acceptable. A limitation of the recursive approximation algorithm is, however, the computational cost. If, in a reduced network, there are many routing chains or chains with large populations, then a computational bottleneck will arise.

In this paper, we develop an iterative Linearizer [CHA1]-type approximation algorithm for the solution of BCMP queueing networks that contain MSFCFS queues. The storage requirements of the algorithm are of the order of NR^2, and the computational requirements are of the order of NR^3, where N is the number of queues and R is the number of closed routing chains. Our prime motivation for developing this fast approximation technique has been to enable the efficient solution of large BCMP queueing networks with multiple nested passive resources, shared passive resources, many routing chains, and large chain populations, using the general iterative solution methodology of Souza e Silva and Muntz, as has been outlined above.

There are several approaches that may be followed in the development of an iterative approximation technique for BCMP queueing networks that contain MSFCFS queues. We have chosen to develop an iterative approximation technique where we employ the exact MVA equations, together with the new recursive waiting time approximation of Souza e Silva and Muntz, and employ the Linearizer methodology to reduce the set of recursive equations into a set of simultaneous nonlinear equations. (This appears to be a reasonable approach in view of the extensive empirical evidence found in the literature [CHA1, KRZ1, NEU1] demonstrating the accuracy of the Linearizer algorithm for closed BCMP queueing networks, and in view of the reported accuracy of the recursive approximation method of Souza e Silva and Muntz for BCMP networks with MSFCFS queues.) An approximate solution to the set of nonlinear equations is found by successive substitution. This results in a computational procedure having, in general, substantially lower costs than the hitherto developed recursive approximation method. In comparing the results obtained with the stress test results published in [SOU1], we find that the accuracy of our iterative scheme is acceptable. Furthermore, the accuracy is found to be comparable to that of the recursive method.

The following section describes the recursive approximation method of Souza e Silva and Muntz for the solution of BCMP queueing networks with MSFCFS queues and Section 3 presents the proposed iterative Linearizer-type approximation method. Finally, Section 4 compares the accuracy of the two methods against the stress test simulation results that have been published in [SOU1].

2. THE SOUZA e SILVA – MUNTZ MVA APPROXIMATION

We consider a BCMP queueing network with multiple closed routing chains. There are N nodes and R routing chains. The visit ratio and the mean service requirement for chain r customers at node i are denoted by e_{ir} and t_{ir}, respectively. The population of chain r is K_r. The population vector of the network is $\mathbf{K}=(K_1,...,K_R)$. The mean performance measures, which include the mean waiting time (queueing time + service time), throughput, and mean queue length of chain r customers at node i, are denoted by $W_{ir}(\mathbf{K})$, $T_{ir}(\mathbf{K})$, and $Q_{ir}(\mathbf{K})$, respectively. The marginal probability that there are j customers at node i is denoted by $P_i(j,\mathbf{K})$. The number of servers at node i is M_i. Each server is assumed to work at unit rate. The probability that all M_i servers at node i are busy is denoted by $PB_i(\mathbf{K})$. We denote a unit vector pointing in the direction i by $\mathbf{1}_i$, and an all zero vector by $\mathbf{1}_0$.

The exact MVA algorithm, for the computation of the mean performance measures of a closed BCMP queueing network, consists of solving the following set of recursive equations [REI1] (in the following, LCFSPR and PS stand for last-come, first-served preempt resume and processor sharing, respectively):

$$W_{ir}(\mathbf{K}) = \begin{cases} t_{ir}, & \text{if node i is IS,} \\[2mm] t_{ir}[1+Q_i(\mathbf{K}-\mathbf{1}_r)], & \text{if node i is single-server FCFS, LCFSPR, or PS,} \\[2mm] t_{ir}[1+Q_i(\mathbf{K}-\mathbf{1}_r)+\sum_{j=0}^{M_i-2}(M_i-1-j)P_i(j,\mathbf{K}-\mathbf{1}_r)]/M_i, & \\ & \text{if node i is a multi-server queue,} \end{cases} \quad (2.1)$$

$$T_{ir}(\mathbf{K}) = e_{ir}K_r/\sum_{j=1}^{N}e_{jr}W_{jr}(\mathbf{K}), \quad (2.2)$$

$$Q_{ir}(\mathbf{K}) = T_{ir}(\mathbf{K})W_{ir}(\mathbf{K}), \quad (2.3)$$

$$P_i(j,\mathbf{K}) = \sum_{s=1}^{R}t_{is}T_{is}(\mathbf{K})P_i(j-1,\mathbf{K}-\mathbf{1}_s)/j, \; j=1,...,M_i-1, \quad (2.4)$$

$$PB_i(\mathbf{K}) = \sum_{s=1}^{R}t_{is}T_{is}(\mathbf{K})[PB_i(\mathbf{K}-\mathbf{1}_s)+P_i(M_i-1,\mathbf{K}-\mathbf{1}_s)]/M_i, \quad (2.5)$$

$$P_i(0,\mathbf{K}) = 1-\sum_{j=1}^{M_i-1}P_i(j,\mathbf{K}) - PB_i(\mathbf{K}), \quad (2.6)$$

where $i=1,...,N$, $r=1,...,R$, $Q_i(\mathbf{K})=\sum_{s=1}^{R} Q_{is}(\mathbf{K})$ and the initial conditions are $Q_{ir}(\mathbf{0})=0$, $PB_i(\mathbf{0})=0$, $P_i(j,\mathbf{0})=0$ for $j=1,...,M_i-1$ and $P_i(0,\mathbf{0})=1$. The computational costs to solve the above exact equations are of the order of $N\prod_{r=1}^{R}(K_r+1)$.

In a BCMP queueing network, it is required that t_{ir} be independent of r when service center i is a FCFS single-server or multi-server queue [BAS1]. In order to analyze queueing networks that contain multi-server FCFS queues with *chain-dependent* service times, of the type arising in the solution of queueing networks with passive resources, Souza e Silva and Muntz [SOU1] have recently proposed the following MVA-type recursive approximation for the mean waiting times at such queues:

$$W_{ir}(\mathbf{K}) = t_{ir} + \sum_{s=1}^{R} XE_{irs}(\mathbf{K})Q^*_{is}(\mathbf{K}-\mathbf{1}_r) + PB_i(\mathbf{K}-\mathbf{1}_r)XR_{ir}(\mathbf{K}). \tag{2.7}$$

In the above, $Q^*_{is}(\mathbf{K}-\mathbf{1}_r)$ is the mean number of chain s customers at node i, excluding those in service, in a network with population vector $(\mathbf{K}-\mathbf{1}_r)$, that is

$$Q^*_{is}(\mathbf{K}-\mathbf{1}_r) = Q_{is}(\mathbf{K}-\mathbf{1}_r) - T_{is}(\mathbf{K}-\mathbf{1}_r)t_{is},$$

$$XE_{irx}(\mathbf{K}) = \sum_{\mathbf{n} \in A_{xr}} PS_{ir}(\mathbf{n},x,\mathbf{K})(n_1\mu_{i1}+...+n_R\mu_{iR})^{-1},$$

$$XR_{ir}(\mathbf{K}) = \sum_{\mathbf{n} \in B_r} PS_{ir}(\mathbf{n},\mathbf{K})(n_1\mu_{i1}+...+n_R\mu_{iR})^{-1},$$

$$\mathbf{n} = (n_1,...,n_R), \qquad \mu_{ir} = t_{ir}^{-1},$$

$$PS_{ir}(\mathbf{n},\mathbf{K}) = A_i(\mathbf{n},\mathbf{K}-\mathbf{1}_r)/C_i(\mathbf{K}-\mathbf{1}_r),$$

$$PS_{ir}(\mathbf{n},x,\mathbf{K}) = A_i(\mathbf{n},\mathbf{K}-\mathbf{1}_r)/C_{ix}(\mathbf{K}-\mathbf{1}_r),$$

$$A_{xr} = \{\mathbf{n}|\ n_1+...+n_R = M_i,\ n_s \geq 0,\ s=1,...,R,\ \mathbf{n} \leq (\mathbf{K}-\mathbf{1}_r),\ n_x \geq 1\},$$

where $\mathbf{n} \leq (\mathbf{K}-\mathbf{1}_r)$ is true if each component of $\mathbf{n}$ is less than or equal to the corresponding component of $(\mathbf{K}-\mathbf{1}_r)$,

$$B_r = \{\mathbf{n}|\ n_1+...+n_R = M_i,\ n_s \geq 0,\ s=1,...,R,\ \mathbf{n} \leq (\mathbf{K}-\mathbf{1}_r)\},$$

$$C_i(\mathbf{K}-\mathbf{1}_r) = \sum_{\mathbf{n} \in B_r} A_i(\mathbf{n},\mathbf{K}-\mathbf{1}_r),$$

$$C_{ix}(\mathbf{K}-\mathbf{1}_r) = \sum_{\mathbf{n} \in A_{xr}} A_i(\mathbf{n},\mathbf{K}-\mathbf{1}_r),$$

$$A_i(\mathbf{n},\mathbf{K}-\mathbf{1}_r) = M_i![\prod_{s=1}^{R} F_{is}^{n_s}(\mathbf{K}-\mathbf{1}_r)]/[n_1!n_2!...n_R!],$$

$$F_{is}(\mathbf{K}-\mathbf{1}_r) = T_{is}(\mathbf{K}-\mathbf{1}_r)t_{is}/[\sum_{a=1}^{R} T_{ia}(\mathbf{K}-\mathbf{1}_r)t_{ia}]. \tag{2.8}$$

The waiting time approximation, as given by Eq. 2.7, is based on three assumptions [SOU1]. The first is that the *Arrival Theorem* for product-form queueing networks [LAV2] holds approximately when there are MSFCFS queues. The second is that at the arrival epoch of a chain r customer at a MSFCFS queue i, the probability density of the number of customers n_r, $1 \leq r \leq R$, of chain r being served, given that all M_i servers are occupied, is multi-nomial and given by $PS_{ir}(\mathbf{n},\mathbf{K})$. The final assumption is that when a particular customer of chain x (call it customer x) starts service, a customer of chain r which arrived at i while customer x was *in queue* sees the probability density $PS_{ir}(\mathbf{n},x,\mathbf{K})$ for the vector $\mathbf{n}$ of customers in service at node i.

The recursive approximation method, which has been developed by Souza e Silva and Muntz for the analysis of BCMP queueing networks with MSFCFS queues, makes use of Eq. 2.7 and consists of solving the original set of exact MVA equations, as given by Eqs. 2.1–2.6, but with Eq. 2.1 replaced by Eq. 2.7 for those queues that are of the MSFCFS type. The computational costs of the approximation method are at least as high as those of the exact MVA algorithm. For queueing networks with many chains or large chain populations, these costs may be excessive.

In order to enable the analysis of large BCMP queueing networks with MSFCFS queues so as to be able to efficiently analyze large queueing networks with many nested passive resources and many routing chains using the decomposition based approach of Souza e Silva and Muntz, we have developed a Linearizer-type approximation algorithm that makes direct use of Eq. 2.7. In the following section, we briefly review the original Linearizer algorithm and show how it may be used in conjunction with Eq. 2.7 to yield an efficient computational scheme for networks with MSFCFS queues.

3. FAST APPROXIMATE SOLUTION OF QUEUEING NETWORKS WITH MSFCFS QUEUES

Chandy and Neuse [CHA1] have developed a so-called Linearizer algorithm for the approximate solution of large BCMP queueing networks. The storage requirements of the algorithm are of the order of NR^2 and the computational costs are of the order of NR^3. The Linearizer algorithm makes use of the exact "forward" MVA equations, as given by Eqs. 2.1–2.6. In addition, use is made of certain approximate "backward" estimation equations which serve to reduce the set of exact recursive equations into a set of approximate simultaneous nonlinear equations. The following backward estimation equations are customarily used:

$$P_i(j,\mathbf{K}-\mathbf{1}_r) = P_i(j,\mathbf{K}), \text{ for } j=0,\dots,M_i-1,$$

$$PB_i(\mathbf{K}-\mathbf{1}_r) = PB_i(\mathbf{K}),$$

$$Q_{ir}(\mathbf{K}-\mathbf{1}_s) = (\mathbf{K}-\mathbf{1}_s)_r[(Q_{ir}(\mathbf{K})/K_r)+\Delta_{irs}(\mathbf{K})].$$

In the above, $\Delta_{irs}(\mathbf{K}) = (Q_{ir}(\mathbf{K}-\mathbf{1}_s)/(\mathbf{K}-\mathbf{1}_s)_r)-(Q_{ir}(\mathbf{K})/K_r)$, and $(\mathbf{K}-\mathbf{1}_s)_r$ denotes the r'th component of the vector $(\mathbf{K}-\mathbf{1}_s)$.

The Linearizer algorithm consists essentially of solving, by successive substitution, the set of forward *exact* MVA equations together with the set of *approximate* backward equations. Initially $\Delta_{irs}(\mathbf{K})$ is set to zero. After a certain number of iterations, $\Delta_{irs}(\mathbf{K})$ is updated in an attempt to improve upon the accuracy of the backward equations. The

Linearizer algorithm may be summarized as follows [KRZ1]. A detailed explanation may be found in [CHA1].

Linearizer:
Call **Initialize**
Do Pass = 1,2
Do k = 0,R
$N=K-1_k$
Call **Core(N)**
End
Call **Update_Δ**
End
Call **Core(K)**
Call **List_Performance_Measures**
Stop
End **Linearizer**

Initialize:
Do i = 1,N
$\Delta_{irs}(K) = 0$, r=1,...,R, s=1,...,R
$Q_{ir}(K) = N_r/N$, r=1,...,R
$pop = (N_1+...+N_R)$
$Q_i(K) = pop/N$
If queue i is multi-server FCFS Then Do
$P_i(j,K) = 2Q_i(K)/(pop(pop+1))$, j=1,...,$M_i-1$
$PB_i(K) = 2Q_i(K)(pop+1-M_i)/(pop(pop+1))$
$$P_i(0,K) = 1-PB_i(K)- \sum_{j=1}^{M_i-1} P_i(j,K)$$

End
End
End **Initialize**

Update_Delta:
$\Delta_{irs}(N) = (Q_{ir}(N-1_s)/(N-1_s)_r)-(Q_{ir}(N)/N_r)$, i=1,...,N, r=1,...,R, s=1,...,R
End **Update_Delta**

Estimate:
Do i = 1,N
If queue i is multi-server FCFS Then Do
$P_i(j,N-1_r) = P_i(j,N)$, for j=0,...,M_i-1, r=1,...,R
$PB_i(N-1_r) = PB_i(N)$, r=1,...R
End
$Q_{ir}(N-1_s) = (N-1_s)_r[(Q_{ir}(N)/N_r)+\Delta_{irs}(N)]$, r=1,...,R, s=1,...,R
End
End **Estimate**

Core:
While not converged Do
Call **Estimate**
Call **Forward_MVA**
End
End **Core**

Forward_MVA:
Update $\overline{W}_{ir}(N)$, $T_{ir}(N)$, $Q_{ir}(N)$, $P_i(j,N)$, $PB_i(N)$ and $P_i(0,N)$, $i=1,...,N$, $r=1,...,R$, $j=1,...,M_i-1$, using the forward MVA equations (Eqs. 2.1–2.6)
End **Forward_MVA**

The iterative technique that we have developed for the fast approximate solution of BCMP queueing networks with MSFCFS queues and many routing chains is essentially the same as the original Linearizer algorithm, as has been summarized above, except that in the **Forward_MVA** routine, Eq. 2.1 is replaced by Eq. 2.7 for those queues i that are of the MSFCFS type. In addition, as can be seen from Eq. 2.8, a supplementary backward equation is required in the **Estimate** routine for the estimation of $T_{is}(K-1_r)$. We have chosen to adopt the following simple backward estimation equation:

$$T_{is}(K-1_r) = (K-1_r)_s[(Q_{is}(K)/K_s)+\Delta_{isr}(K)]/W_{is}(K).$$

Furthermore, in the **Initialize** routine it is necessary to provide initial estimates for $T_{ir}(K)$. This is done using a method that has been used in [SOU2], as follows:

$$T_{ir}(K) = e_{ir}K_r/\{\ \sum_{i \in I_1} e_{ir}t_{ir}[1+(Q_i(K)-Q_{ir}(K)/K_r)]$$

$$+ \sum_{i \in I_2} e_{ir}t_{ir}[1+(Q_i(K)-Q_{ir}(K)/K_r)/M_i] + \sum_{i \in I_3} e_{ir}t_{ir}\ \}.$$

In the above, I_1 is the set of queues in the network that have a single server, I_2 is the set of multi-server queues, and I_3 is the set of IS queues. We have also chosen to initialize $Q_{ir}(K)$ according to the method given in [SOU2], as follows:

$$Q_{ir}(K) = e_{ir}t_{ir}K_r/\sum_{i=1}^{N} e_{ir}t_{ir}.$$

The convergence criterion we use in the **Core** routine is to terminate if

$$|Q_{ir}(K)^{(j)}-Q_{ir}(K)^{(j-1)}|/K_r < 10^{-4}$$

for $i=1,...,N$ and $r=1,...,R$, where the superscript indicates the iteration number. We also terminate the **Core** routine if the number of iterations in the routine has reached 50, as is done in [KRZ1].

Our iterative approximation algorithm has been programmed in VS FORTRAN and can be used for the solution of large networks. In the following section, we compare the results obtained by our iterative algorithm with the stress test results documented in [SOU1] for BCMP networks with MSFCFS queues.

4. EMPIRICAL STRESS TEST COMPARISONS

In [SOU1], Souza e Silva and Muntz have considered two queueing network examples which stress their MVA-based recursive approximation technique. In their examples, they compare the results of Monte Carlo simulations with the results obtained by their recursive solution algorithm. In both networks, there are two service centers ($N=2$) and two closed routing chains ($R=2$). In one of the networks, the first queue has the PS service discipline, while in the other network, the first queue is of the IS type. The second queue, in both networks, is a MSFCFS queue with two servers ($M_2=2$). In the following, we compare the results obtained by our iterative algorithm with the approximation results and simulation results of Souza e Silva and Muntz.

In the first example, the first queue is PS and the parameters are $t_{11}=1$, $t_{12}=2$, $t_{21}=1$, $t_{22}=\alpha$ (a variable), $K_1=5$, $K_2=2$, $e_{11}=1$, $e_{12}=1$, $e_{21}=1$, and $e_{22}=1$. In Figures 1 and 2, we compare the utilizations at the second queue for chains 1 and 2, respectively, as a function of α, the mean service time for chain 2 customers at node 2 (**SM approx** denotes the results for the Souza e Silva – Muntz recursive approximation, **lin. approx** denotes the results of our iterative algorithm and **sim. lower** and **sim. upper** denote the lower and upper confidence limits, with a 90% confidence level, of the simulation results of Souza e Silva and Muntz). In Figures 3 and 4, we compare the mean waiting times at the second queue for chains 1 and 2, respectively.

In the second example, the parameters are the same as in the first, except that $K_2=1$. The utilizations and mean waiting times at the second queue are compared in Figures 5–8.

In the third example, the first queue is changed to IS, and we have $K_2=2$, $t_{11}=6$, $t_{12}=3$, $t_{21}=1$, and $t_{22}=\alpha$. The utilizations and mean waiting times at the second queue are compared in Figures 9–12.

In the final example, the parameters are the same as in the third example, except that $K_2=1$. The utilizations and mean waiting times at the second queue are compared in Figures 13–16.

From Figures 1–16, we see that the approximate results obtained by our iterative algorithm usually compare quite favourably with the approximate results of Souza e Silva and Muntz and the simulation results. In Figures 3, 11, and 15, we see that for high values of α, the mean waiting time of chain 1 customers is overestimated significantly. This may be explained by observing that in these situations, the chain 2 utilizations at the MSFCFS queue are relatively high, and a small error in the probability distribution of chain 2 customers at the servers can give rise to relatively large errors in the waiting times of chain 1 customers. However, the magnitudes of these errors can be considered acceptable for a stress test.

5. CONCLUSION

In this paper, we have developed an iterative approximation algorithm for the efficient analysis of large multiple-chain BCMP queueing networks that contain multi-server first-come, first-served (MSFCFS) queues with chain-dependent service times. The algorithm may be applied to the analysis of queueing networks of the BCMP type that contain MSFCFS queues, such as those that arise in the solution method of Souza e Silva and Muntz for multiple-chain queueing networks that contain nested passive resources. This enables the efficient solution of queueing networks with passive resources when there are a large number of routing chains or large chain populations.

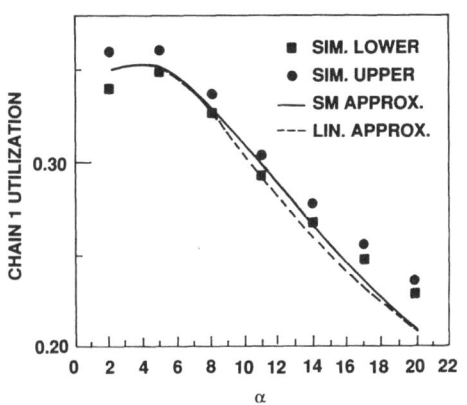

Figure 1. Utilization of chain 1 at the second queue in example 1 as a function of α.

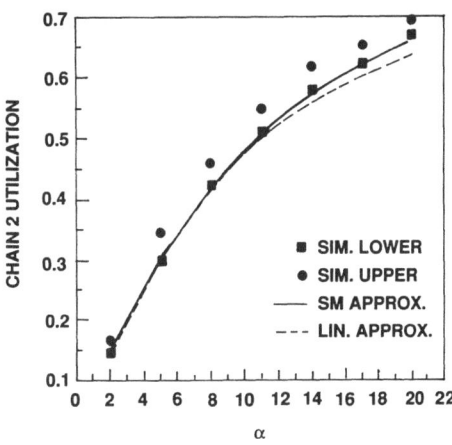

Figure 2. Utilization of chain 2 at the second queue in example 1 as a function of α.

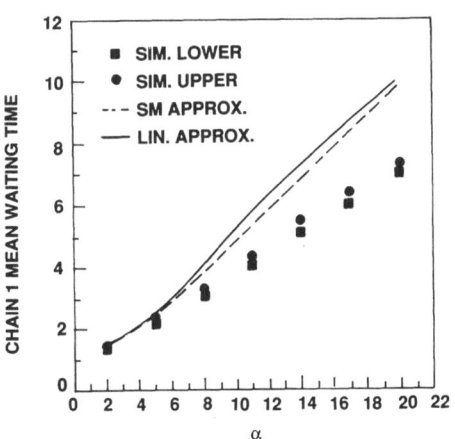

Figure 3. Mean waiting time of chain 1 at the second queue in example 1 as a function of α.

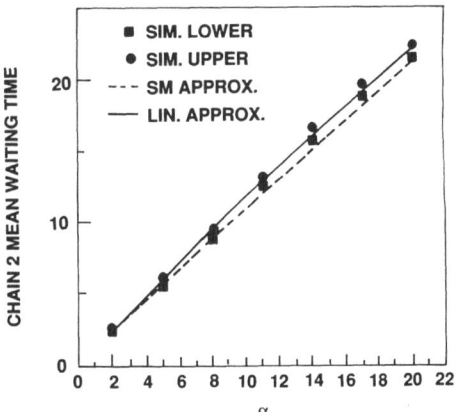

Figure 4. Mean waiting time of chain 2 at the second queue in example 1 as a function of α.

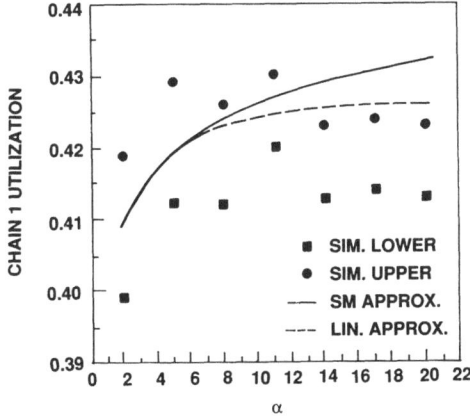

Figure 5. Utilization of chain 1 at the second queue in example 2 as a function of α.

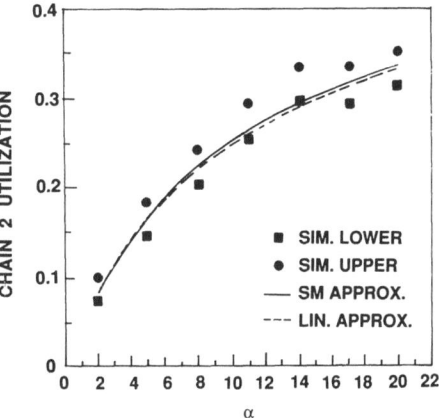

Figure 6. Utilization of chain 2 at the second queue in example 2 as a function of α.

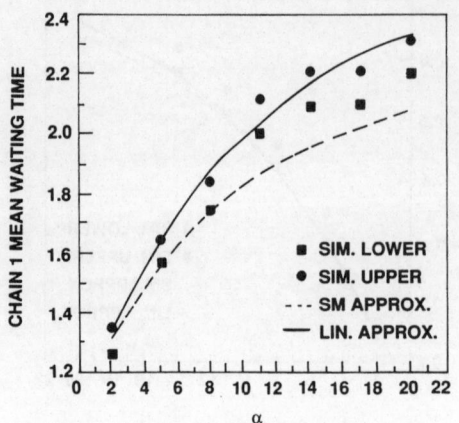

Figure 7. Mean waiting time of chain 1 at the second queue in example 2 as a function of α.

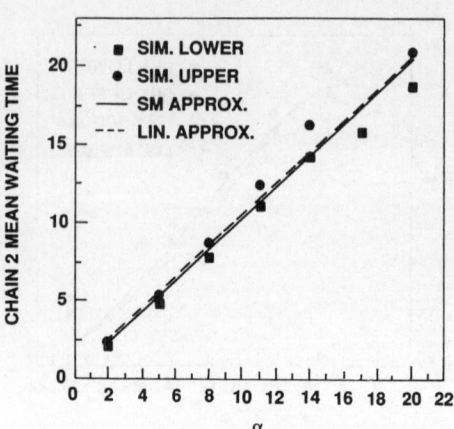

Figure 8. Mean waiting time of chain 2 at the second queue in example 2 as a function of α.

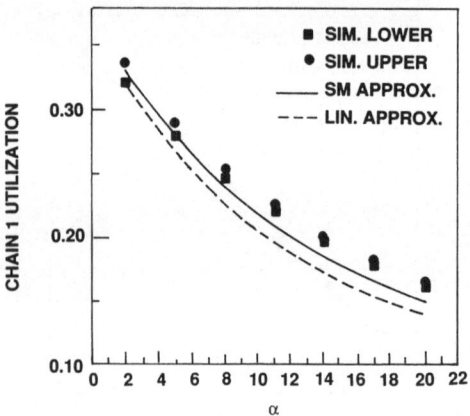

Figure 9. Utilization of chain 1 at the second queue in example 3 as a function of α.

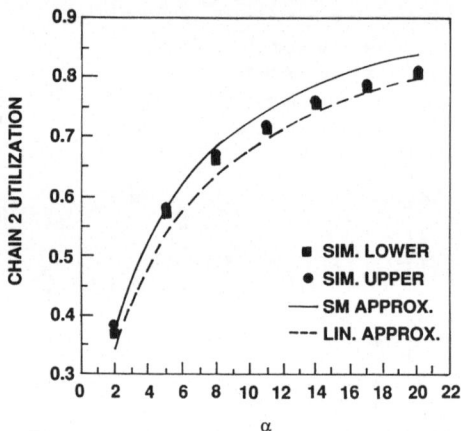

Figure 10. Utilization of chain 2 at the second queue in example 3 as a function of α.

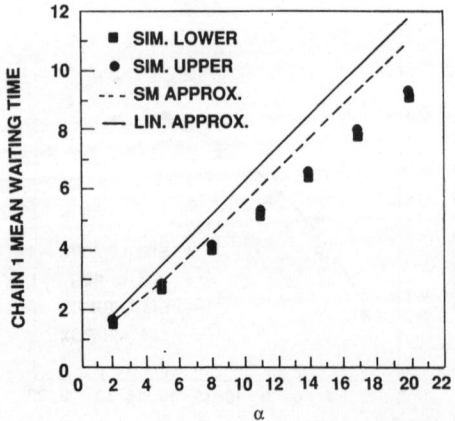

Figure 11. Mean waiting time of chain 1 at the second queue in example 3 as a function of α.

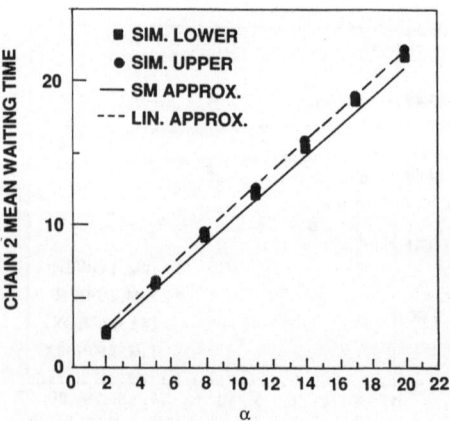

Figure 12. Mean waiting time of chain 2 at the second queue in example 3 as a function of α.

394

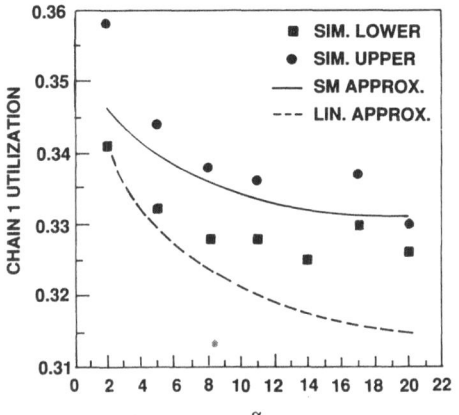

Figure 13. Utilization of chain 1 at the second queue in example 4 as a function of α.

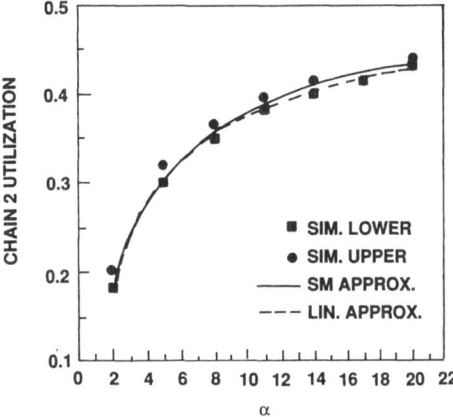

Figure 14. Utilization of chain 2 at the second queue in example 4 as a function of α.

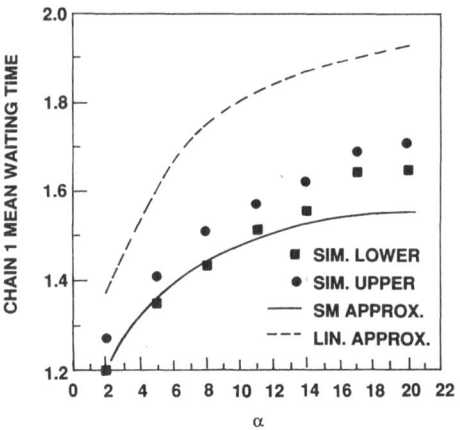

Figure 15. Mean waiting time of chain 1 at the second queue in example 4 as a function of α.

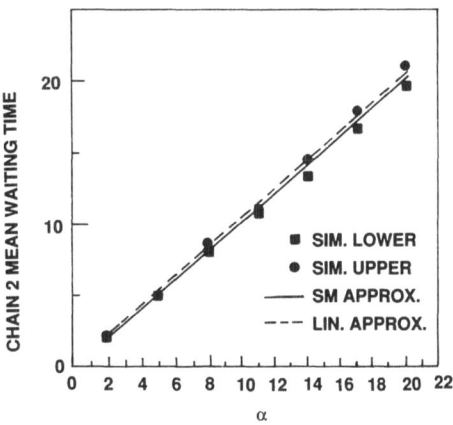

Figure 16. Mean waiting time of chain 2 at the second queue in example 4 as a function of α.

REFERENCES

[BAS1] F. Baskett, K.M. Chandy, R.R. Muntz, and F. Palacios, "Open, Closed and Mixed Networks of Queues with Different Classes of Customers," *J. ACM* 22, pp. 248-260, 1975.

[BRA1] A. Brandwajn, "A Model of a Time-Sharing System Solved Using Equivalence and Decomposition Methods," *Acta Informatica* 4, 1, pp. 11-47, 1974.

[BRA2] A. Brandwajn, "Fast Approximate Solution of Multiprogramming Models," *Proc. 1982 ACM SIGMETRICS Conf. Meas. Mod. Comp. Sys.*, pp. 141-149, 1982.

[BRY1] R.M. Bryant, A.E. Krzesinski, M.S. Lakshmi, and K.M. Chandy, "The MVA Priority Approximation," *ACM Trans. Computer Systems* 2, 4, pp. 335-359, 1984.

[CHA1] K.M. Chandy, and D. Neuse, "Linearizer: A Heuristic Algorithm for Queueing Network Models of Computing Systems," *Commun. ACM* 25, 2, pp. 126-134, 1982.

[JAC1] P.A. Jacobson, and E.D. Lazowska, "Analyzing Queueing Networks with Simultaneous Resource Possession," *Comm. ACM* 25, pp. 142-151, 1982.

[JAC2] P.A. Jacobson, and E.D. Lazowska, "A Reduction Technique for Evaluating Queueing Networks with Serialization Delays," in *Performance '83*, North-Holland, Amsterdam, 1983.

[KRZ1] A. Krzesinski, and J. Greyling, "Improved Linearizer Methods for Queueing Networks with Queue Dependent Centers," *Proc. 1984 ACM SIGMETRICS Conf. Meas. Mod. Comp. Sys.*, pp. 41-50, 1984.

[KRZ2] A. Krzesinski, and P. Teunissen, "Multiclass Queueing Networks with Population Constrained Subnetworks," *Proc. 1985 ACM SIGMETRICS Conf. Meas. Mod. Comp. Sys.*, pp. 128-139, 1985.

[LAV1] S.S. Lavenberg (Ed.), *Computer Performance Modeling Handbook*, Academic Press, New York, 1983.

[LAV2] S.S. Lavenberg, and M. Reiser, "Stationary State Probabilities at Arrival Instants for Closed Queueing Networks with Multiple Types of Customers," *J. Appl. Prob.* 17, pp. 1048-1061, 1980.

[LAZ1] E.D. Lazowska, and J. Zahorjan, "Multiple Class Memory Constrained Queueing Networks," *Proc. 1982 ACM SIGMETRICS Conf. Meas. Mod. Comp. Sys*, pp. 130-140, 1982.

[NEU1] D. Neuse, "Approximate Analysis of Large and General Queueing Networks," *Ph.D. Dissertation*, The University of Texas at Austin, 1982.

[REI1] M. Reiser, and S.S. Lavenberg, "Mean Value Analysis of Closed Multichain Queueing Networks," *J. ACM* 27, pp. 313-322, 1980.

[SOU1] E. de Souza e Silva, and R.R. Muntz, "Approximate Solutions for a Class of Non-Product Form Queueing Network Models," *Performance Evaluation* 7, pp. 221-242, 1987.

[SOU2] E. de Souza e Silva, S.S. Lavenberg, and R.R. Muntz, "A Clustering Approximation Technique for Queueing Network Models with a Large Number of Chains," *IEEE Trans. Computers* 35, 5, pp. 419-430, 1986.

A UNIVERSAL MAXIMUM ENTROPY ALGORITHM FOR GENERAL

MULTIPLE CLASS OPEN NETWORKS WITH MIXED SERVICE DISCIPLINES*

Demetres D. Kouvatsos
Panagiotis H.E. Georgatsos and Nasreddine M. Tabet-Aouel

Postgraduate School of Studies in Computing
University of Bradford
Bradford, BD7 1DP, UK

The principle of maximum entropy (ME) is used to characterise a new product-form approximation for the analysis of arbitrary open networks of queues at equilibrium with infinite capacities, single servers, multiple job classes, distinct general exogeneous interarrival-time and service-time distributions per class, non-priority (first-come-first-served, processor-sharing, last-come-first-served with or without pre   or priority (preemptive-resume, non-preemptive head-of-line) service disciplines and random routing under class switching. The ME approximation suggests a decomposition of the open network into individual multiple class G/G/1 queues at equilibrium with a revised arrival process for each class of jobs. A universal implementation of the ME solution is achieved by making use of the Generalised Exponential (GE) distribution to model the service and flow processes of each G/G/1 queue per class. As a consequence, the ME analysis of open queueing networks can be interpreted in terms of bulk-arrival and bulk-service queues with geometrically distributed bulk sizes. The credibility of 'the ME approximation is demonstrated by some illustrative examples and favourable comparisons with simulation and other approximate methods are made. Comments on the extension of the work to multiple server queues and general closed networks are included.

1.   INTRODUCTION

Open queueing network models with multiple classes of jobs are widely recognised as powerful tools for analysing large-scale computer and communication systems and optimising their performance. Exact queueing theory, operational analysis and approximate methods provide conventional frameworks for formulating and solving open queueing network models. However, despite persistent attempts for extension and generalisation some problems have remained without a satisfactory solution.

Exact product-form solutions for a wide class of open networks of queues without priorities have been proposed under restrictions on the behaviour of the jobs and the type of resources (e.g. [1]). For example, exogeneous

* This research work was sponsored in part by the Science and Engineering Research Council (SERC) UK, under grant GR/D/12422, and in part by the Ministry of Higher Education of the Algerian Government.

arrivals follow a Poisson pattern while all jobs must have the same exponential service-time distribution under a first-come-first-served (FCFS) discipline. Similar comments apply to operational results, based on necessary assumptions such as homogeneity (e.g. [2]), which are analogous to those obtained in classical queueing theory (c.f. exponentiality).

Approximate methods apply to more general and, therefore, more realistic models. However, their relative accuracy may be affected when intuitive heuristics are used. In the case of FCFS open networks without priorities, diffusion and other approximations (e.g. [3-8]) require certain restrictive assumptions, such as non-preemptive queueing disciplines, and are based on class composition and disaggregation. In this context, the first two moments of the effective interarrival-time and service-time distributions of an aggregated class of jobs are estimated prior to the network being decomposed into individual infinite capacity queues. Moreover, a number of heuristic approximations (e.g. [9-12]) have been proposed to analyse open Markovian networks with priorities, based on the method of reduced occupancy approximation (ROA) [9]. Roughly, it is assumed that class r jobs are served by a "dedicated" virtual exponential server whose "occupancy" (i.e. perceived service) time is the class r service-time inflated to account for degradation due to the use of the actual server by higher priority jobs. Unfortunately, these techniques do not quite capture the variability of the effective service-time for low priority classes of jobs (which often has coefficient of variation greater than 1 [10]). Consequently, significant errors may be experienced, particularly when a priority queue has very high utilisation mostly attributed to high priority classes. To the knowledge of the authors, work on open queueing networks with priorities and general service times has not yet been reported in the literature.

The principle of maximum entropy (ME) [13,14] is a uniquely correct, self-consistent method of inference for estimating a discrete probability distribution based on information in the form of expected values. The principle has been employed [8] to analyse approximately general FCFS open queueing networks with multiple job classes and class switching, subject to aggregated class constraints on the utilisation and the mean queue length per station. The ME solution is applied by making use of the robust generalised exponential (GE) probability density function of the form

$$f(t) = \left[\frac{C^2 - 1}{C^2 + 1}\right]u_0(t) + \frac{4v}{(C^2 + 1)^2} \exp\left\{-\frac{2vt}{C^2 + 1}\right\}, \quad t \geqslant 0, \qquad (1)$$

in approximating general distributions with known mean value, $1/v$, and coefficient of variation, C ($u_0(t)$ being the unit impulse function) [15]. As a consequence, ME analysis of general networks can be interpreted in terms of either

i)   extremal two-phase interarrival-time and service-time distributions, where one of the two phases has zero interevent time, or

ii) Poissonian bulk-arrival and exponential bulk-service queues with geometrically distributed bulk sizes.

Note that although the GE distribution is improper for $C^2 < 1$, it still represents a robust and versatile model in approximating general distributions with known v and $C^2 < 1$ (c.f. [16]). The ME algorithm has been experimentally tested against simulation [8,17] and favourable comparisons against other approximations (e.g. [3-6]) were made. However, this algorithm needs to be extended or redesigned in order to include mixed service disciplines with priorities and general service times.

The foregoing discussion indicates that although much progress has been made in the analysis of general open queueing networks with multiple classes, there is still a need to search for new analytic tools in order to enhance the applicability and improve the accuracy of ME and other approximate methods. Note that further details on the justification and use of the principle of ME as applied to general queueing systems can be found in [8,15,17,18].

In this paper, the principle of ME is used to characterise a new product-form approximation for arbitrary open networks of queues with

i)   infinite capacities
ii)   single servers
iii) multiple job classes
iv)   distinct general exogeneous interarrival-time and service-time distributions per class
v)   non-priority (FCFS), processor-sharing (PS), last-come-first-served (LCFS) with or without preemption) and/or priority (preemptive resume (PR), non-preemptive head-of-line (HOL)) service disciplines, and
vi)   random routing under class switching.

The ME solution implies a class-by-class decomposition of the open network into individual G/G/1 queues at equilibrium within tandem, split and merged configurations. This solution is implemented in a universal fashion by using the GE model to approximate the interarrival-time and service-time distributions per class.

A universal ME queue length distribution (qld) of an abstract but stable multiple class G/G/1 queue and the GE-type ME implementations are presented, as building blocks, in Section 2. The ME product-form solution for general open queueing networks and GE-type flow approximations per class are given in Section 3. Numerical validation results, involving ME, simulation and other known approximate methods are included in Section 4. Final remarks and comments on the extension of the work follow in Section 5.

2.   AN ABSTRACT ME G/G/1 QUEUE

Consider a stable G/G/1 queue (or station) i with R ($\geqslant$ 2) classes of jobs under an abstract service discipline. In the case of a priority based discipline, job classes are indexed in decreasing order of priority. For each class r job, r = 1, 2,..., R, let

$\lambda_{i,r}$ be the mean arrival rate,

$C_{ai,r}$ be the interarrival-time coefficient of variation,

$\mu_{i,r}$ be the mean service rate,

$C_{si,r}$ be the service-time coefficient of variation.

The state of the queue is described by a vector $\underline{n}_i = (n_{i,1}, n_{i,2}, \ldots, n_{i,R})$ where $n_{i,r}$, r = 1, 2,..., R is the number of class r jobs in the queue (waiting for or receiving service) such that $0 \leqslant n_i < +\infty$. Moreover, let

$P_i(\underline{n}_i)$ be the state probability,

$P_{i,r}(n_{i,r})$ be the marginal queue length distribution (qld) for jobs of class r, r = 1, 2,..., R.

$<\theta_{i,r}>$ be the non-zero marginal state probability for class r jobs i.e., $<\theta_{i,r}> = 1 - P_{i,r}(0)$,

$<n_{i,r}>$ be the mean queue length (mql) of class r.

The analytic (exact or approximate) treatment of a stable multiple class G/G/1 queue depends, in principle, on the type of service discipline employed and the characterisation of the G-type distributions for each class of jobs, usually known in terms of their first two moments. What is the best way to utilise this kind of a priori knowledge in approximating the form of the state probability $p_i(n_i)$?

ME formalism can be used to provide an answer to this question. For a specified G/G/1 queue with multiple job classes, it may be generally possible to approximate analytically expected values of the qld per class, $P_{i,r}(n_{i,r})$, in terms of the first two moments of the G-type distributions of all classes. Given these expected values as marginal class constraints, the principle of ME can be applied to provide an estimate for the state probability $p_i(n_i)$. Thus, in this way, a fruitful correspondence can be established between the performance analysis of a multiclass G/G/1 queue and the principle of ME.

2.1 Prior Information

Suppose that the following mean value constraints about the state probability $p_i(n_i)$ are known to exist:

i)   The normalisation (norm),

$$\sum_{n_i} p_i(n_i) = 1. \tag{2}$$

ii)   The "existence" of class r (exist), $<\theta_{i,r}> = 1 - p_{i,r}(0)$, with $<\theta_{i,r}> \in (0, 1)$, written as

$$\sum_{n_i} h(n_{i,r}) \, p(n_i) = <\theta_{i,r}>, \quad r = 1, 2, .., R, \tag{3}$$

where $h(n_{i,r}) = 0$, if $n_{i,r} = 0$ or 1, if $n_{i,r} > 0$.

iii) The mql per class r, $<n_{i,r}>$, $<n_{i,r}> \geqslant <\theta_{i,r}>$,

$$\sum_{n_i} n_{i,r} \, p(n_i) = <n_{i,r}>, \quad r = 1, 2, .., R. \tag{4}$$

Note that although at this stage the expected values $<\theta_{i,r}>$ and $<n_{i,r}>$ are not explicitly known in terms of system parameters $\lambda_{i,r}$, $C_{ai,r}$, $\mu_{i,r}$ and $C_{si,r}$, they can be incorporated into the ME formalism in order to determine the form of the ME solution $p_i(n_i)$.

2.2 The ME State Probability

The principle of ME states [13] that of all distributions satisfying the constraints supplied by the given information (2)-(4), the form of the minimally biased distribution which should be chosen is the one that maximises the system's entropy function

$$H(p_i) = - \sum_{n_i} p_i(n_i) \log p_i(n_i). \tag{5}$$

The maximisation of (5), subject to constraints (2)-(4), can be carried out analytically by using the Lagrange method of undetermined multipliers [13] leading to the general solution

$$p_i(\underline{n}_i) = \frac{1}{Z_{p_i}} \prod_{r=1}^{R} g_{i,r}^{h(n_{i,r})} x_{i,r}^{n_{i,r}}, \tag{6}$$

where Z_{p_i} is the partition function (or, normalising constant), $g_{i,r} = ex[\{-\beta_{1i,r}\}$, $x_{i,r} = exp\{-\beta_{2i,r}\}$ and $\{\beta_{ji,r}\}$, $j = 1, 2$, are the Lagrangian multipliers corresponding to constraints (3) and (4), respectively. It can be clearly seen that (6) is rewritten as

$$p_i(\underline{n}_i) = \prod_{r=1}^{R} p_{i,r}(0) \, g_{i,r}^{h(n_{i,r})} x_{i,r}^{n_{i,r}}. \tag{7}$$

But the expression in the product is equivalent to the well-known ME solution of a stable single class G/G/1 queue viewed here as a virtual G/G/1 queue at equilibrium dedicated exclusively to class r jobs, subject to a "new" utilisation, $<\theta_{i,r}>$, and mql, $<n_{i,r}>$, constraints (c.f., Kouvatsos [15,19]). It is therefore implied that the following theorem clearly holds.

Theorem 1. The ME joint state probability, $p_i(\underline{n}_i)$, of an abstract but stable G/G/1 with R classes of jobs given by (6), subject to norm, exist, $<\theta_{i,r}>$, and mql, $<n_{i,r}>$, $r = 1, 2,..., R$ constraints, is decomposed into a product-form class-by-class solution

$$p_i(\underline{n}_i) = \prod_{r=1}^{R} p_{i,r}(n_{i,r}), \tag{8}$$

where the marginal qld per class r, $p_{i,r}(n_{i,r})$, is equivalent to the ME solution of a virtual stable G/G/1 queue of class r jobs only, subject to a "new" utilisation, $<\theta_{i,r}>$, and mql, $<n_{i,r}>$, constraints, given by

$$p_{i,r}(n_{i,r}) = \begin{cases} 1 - <\theta_{i,r}>, & \text{if } n_{i,r} = 0, \\ <\theta_{i,r}>(1 - x_{i,r}) x_{i,r}^{n_{i,r}-1}, & \text{if } n_{i,r} > 0, \end{cases} \tag{9}$$

with Lagrangian coefficients $g_{i,r}$ and $x_{i,r}$, $r = 1, 2,..., R$ given by

$$g_{i,r} = \frac{(1 - x_{i,r})<\theta_{i,r}>}{(1 - <\theta_{i,r}>)x_{i,r}}, \tag{10}$$

and

$$x_{i,r} = \frac{<n_{i,r}> - <\theta_{i,r}>}{<n_{i,r}>}, \tag{11}$$

respectively.

Note that the proofs of formulae (9)–(11) follow similar steps to those in [15, 19].

In order to implement the ME solution of Theorem 1, it is first necessary to provide new closed-form (exact or approximate) expressions for the statistics $<\theta_{i,r}>$ and $<n_{i,r}>$, $r = 1, 2,..., R$, respectively. For this purpose the GE-type approximation is presented next.

2.3 The GE-type Approximation

Consider an abstract but stable GE/GE/1 with GE-type interarrival-time and service-time distributions and R (≥ 2) classes of jobs. The bulk interpretation and the pseudo-memoryless properties of the GE distributional model can be applied to determine analytically new (exact or approximate) expressions for $<\theta_{i,r}> = 1 - p_{i,r}(0)$ and $<n_{i,r}>$, $r = 1, 2,$ ..., R, respectively. These statistics depend on the particular service discipline (SD) and are functions of the parameters $\lambda_{i,r}$, $C^2_{ai,r}$, $\mu_{i,r}$ and $C^2_{si,r}$, $r = 1, 2,.., R$, namely

$$<n_{i,r}> = F^{(SD)}_{i,r}(\lambda_{i,r}, C^2_{ai,r}, \mu_{i,r}, C^2_{si,r}, r = 1, 2,..., R), \quad (12)$$

and

$$<\theta_{i,r}> = G^{(SD)}_{i,r}(\lambda_{i,r}, C^2_{ai,r}, \mu_{i,r}, C^2_{si,r}, r = 1, 2,..., R), \quad (13)$$

where $F^{(SD)}_{i,r}$ and $G^{(SD)}_{i,r}$, $r = 1, 2,...,$ R are suitable functions for each SD, where SD = FCFS, PS, LCFS with preemption, LCFS without preemption, PR, non-preemptive HOL. Analytic expressions for these functions can be found in Appendix I, while details of proofs can be seen in [20].

The ME solution of Theorem 1, in conjunction with the new GE-type expressions of the form (12), (13) can be used as building blocks for the ME approximation of arbitrary open networks in the next section.

3. GENERAL OPEN QUEUEING NETWORKS

Consider an arbitrary open queueing network at equilibrium with M infinite capacity queues (or nodes) containing one server. Jobs of the network belong to R classes under abstract service disciplines and they may switch class membership as they move from one queue to another. For each class r, $r = 1, 2,...,$ R and queue i, $i = 1, 2,...,$ M, the notation of Section 3 applies and, in addition, let

$\lambda_{0,r}$ be the mean external arrival rate,

$C_{0,r}$ be the coefficient of variation of the external interarrival-times,

$\lambda_{0;i,r}$ be the mean external arrival rate to queue i,

$C_{ao;i,r}$ be the coefficient of variation of the external interarrival-times to queue i,

$\{P_{i,r;j,u}\}$ $i, j = 0, 1,...,$ M (0 indicates outside world), $r, u = 1, 2,$ ..., R be a transition (1st order Markov chain) matrix describing the routing in the network such that $P_{i,r;j,u}$ is the probability of a class r job having just completed service at queue i joins queue j in class u.

The joint state of the network is described by a vector $\underline{n} = (\underline{n}_1, \underline{n}_2,..., \underline{n}_M)$ where $\underline{n}_i$ is the state of an individual queue i (i.e., $\underline{n}_i = (n_{i,1}, n_{i,2},..., n_{i,R})$, $n_{i,u} \geqslant 0$, $u = 1, 2,...,$ R). The joint state probability, $p(\underline{n})$, is characterised below by using the principle of ME.

3.1 The ME Product-Form Solution

Suppose all that is known about the probability, $p(\underline{n})$, is the existence of the norm,

$$\sum_{\underline{n}} p(\underline{n}) = 1, \quad (14)$$

and the marginal constraints of exist, $<\theta_{i,r}>$, and mql, $<n_{i,r}>$ (c.f., (3), (4)), $r = 1, 2, \ldots, R$, $i = 1, 2, \ldots, M$.

The form of the ME solution, $p(\underline{n})$, can be completely specified by maximising the entropy functional of $p(\underline{n})$, i.e.,

$$H(p) = -\sum_{\underline{n}} p(\underline{n}) \log p(\underline{n}),\qquad(15)$$

subject to norm, exist and mql constraints, leading to the solution

$$p(\underline{n}) = \frac{1}{Z_p} \prod_{i=1}^{M} \prod_{r=1}^{R} h(n_{i,r}) \, g_{i,r}^{n_{i,r}} \, x_{i,r}^{n_{i,r}},\qquad(16)$$

where Z_p is the partition function and $g_{i,r}$, $x_{i,r}$ are the Lagrangian coefficients corresponding to $<\theta_{i,r}>$ and $<n_{i,r}>$ constraints, respectively. Proceeding as in Section 2, it can be clearly seen that the following theorem holds.

Theorem 2. The ME joint state probability, $p(\underline{n})$, of an arbitrary open queueing network at equilibrium with R classes of jobs, subject to norm, exist, $<\theta_{i,r}>$, and mql, $<n_{i,r}>$, constraints, is decomposed into a product-form station-by-station and class-by-class solution

$$p(\underline{n}) = \prod_{i=1}^{M} p_i(\underline{n}_i) = \prod_{i=1}^{M} \prod_{r=1}^{R} p_{i,r}(n_{i,r}),\qquad(17)$$

where the marginal qld $p_{i,r}(n_{i,r})$ has an equivalent form to the ME solution given by (9).

3.2 The Universal GE-type Flow Approximation

The ME approximation (17) suggests a decomposition of the network into individual multiple class G/G/1 queues with a revised arrival process for each class of jobs. In order to implement the ME solution under an abstract service discipline, the flow processes in the general network should be determined. For each queue i, $i = 1, 2, \ldots, M$, it is assumed that the arriving and departing streams per class r jobs, $r = 1, 2, \ldots, R$ form renewal processes conforming with GE-type underlying interarrival-time and service-time distributions (with known first two moments). The task is now to compute the mean rates and coefficients of variation of the (overall) interarrival and interdeparture processes of class r jobs in queue i.

3.2.1 The Interdeparture Process

For each queue i, $i = 1, 2, \ldots, M$, the mean rate, $\lambda_{di,r}$, and coefficient of variation, $C_{di,r}$, of the interdeparture-time per class r can be approximated under an abstract service discipline by considering a virtual FCFS GE/G/1 queue i_r exclusively dedicated to jobs of class r with a qld identical to the marginal ME qld $p_{i,r}(n_{i,r})$, $r = 1, 2, \ldots, R$, of the original multiple class G/G/1 queue given by (9) (c.f., Theorem 1). Defining the z-transform of $p_{i,r}(n_{i,r})$ and using the generalised Pollaczek-Khinchin transform equation it can be verified, in a similar fashion to that employed in Kouvatsos [19], that the perceived service-time

403

at the virtual queue i_r is also of GE type of the form (1) with mean, $1/\hat{\mu}_{i,r}$, where $\hat{\mu}_{i,r} = \lambda_{i,r}/<\theta_{i,r}>$ and squared coefficient of variation, $\hat{C}^2_{si,r}$, $C^2_{si,r} = (2 - \hat{\tau}_{i,r})/\hat{\tau}_{i,r}$, where

$$\hat{\tau}_{i,r} = \frac{2g_{i,r}x_{i,r}/(1 + C^2_{ai,r})}{x_{i,r} - [1 - 2/(1 + C^2_{ai,r})](1 + g_{i,r}x_{i,r})} . \tag{18}$$

To this end, following from Kouvatsos [8,19], the first two moments of the interdeparture-time distribution of the resulting GE/GE/1 queue can be determined, namely, $\lambda_{di,r} = \lambda_{i,r}$ and

$$C^2_{di,r} = (1 - <\theta_{i,r}>)<\theta_{i,r}> + <\theta_{i,r}>^2 \hat{C}^2_{si,r} + (1 - <\theta_{i,r}>)C^2_{ai,r}. \tag{19}$$

By using the mql, $<n_{i,r}>$, formula for the virtual (single-class) GE/GE/1 queue i_r [8,19], a universal approximation for $C^2_{di,r}$ is obtained via the following proposition.

Proposition 1. Given an arbitrary open network with M infinite capacity queues at equilibrium and R classes of jobs under an abstract service discipline, a universal approximation for the squared coefficient of variation of the interdeparture-time distribution, $C^2_{di,r}$, is given by

$$C^2_{di,r} = 2<n_{i,r}>(1 - <\theta_{i,r}>) + C^2_{ai,r}(1 - 2<\theta_{i,r}>), \tag{20}$$

where $<n_{i,r}>$ and $<\theta_{i,r}>$ are dependent on the particular service discipline used and are expressed by (12) and (13), respectively.

Note that formula (20) does not depend explicitly on the perceived service-time coefficient of variation, $\hat{C}^2_{si,r}$. Moreover, the effect of each service discipline is reflected via the particular form of the statistics $<n_{i,r}>$ and $<\theta_{i,r}>$.

3.2.2 The Split Process

For each queue j, any departing class u stream denoted by (j, u)-stream, can produce MR potential streams (denoted by (j, u; i,r)-streams) directed to queue i as class r. Let $\lambda_{dj,u,i;r}$, $C^2_{dj,u;i,r}$ be the mean rate and coefficient of variation for such departing streams. Assuming that the interdeparture process per class is a renewal process, these parameters can be determined directly by using the splitting formulae per class, namely

$$\lambda_{dj,u;i,r} = \lambda_{j,u}p_{j,u;i,r}, \tag{21}$$

$$C^2_{dj,u;i,r} = 1 + p_{j,u;i,r}(C^2_{dj,u} - 1), \quad u, r = 1, 2,.., R. \tag{22}$$

3.2.3 The Merging Process

The (overall) arrival process of class r jobs to queue i, i = 1, 2,..., M, is clearly the merging process of MR + 1 potential streams of class r. Assuming that the interevent-time distribution of such streams is approximated by the GE distributional model with parameters $\lambda_{dj,u;i,r}$ and $C_{dj,u;i,r}$, it follows from Kouvatsos [8] that the merging stream has also a GE-type interarrival-time distribution with parameters

$$\lambda_{i,r} = \lambda_{0,i,r} + \sum_{j=1}^{M} \sum_{u=1}^{R} \lambda_{dj,u;i,r}, \quad u, r = 1, 2, \ldots, R, \qquad (23)$$

$$c_{ai,r}^2 = -1 + \left\{ \sum_{j=1}^{M} \sum_{u=1}^{R} \frac{\lambda_{dj,u;i,r}}{\lambda_{i,r}} \left[c_{dj,u;i,r}^2 + 1 \right]^{-1} \right.$$

$$\left. + \frac{\lambda_{0;i,r}}{\lambda_{i,r}} \left[c_{a0;i,r}^2 + 1 \right]^{-1} \right\}^{-1}. \qquad (24)$$

Note that is now possible, due to the common underlying structure of the GE-type flow approximations (20)-(24), to treat all classes of jobs under various service disciplines in a direct and universal manner, thus avoiding techniques based on class composition and disaggregation (e.g. [3-5]) or ROA (e.g. [9,10]). A universal ME algorithm for the approximate analysis of general multiple class open networks is proposed next.

3.3 A Universal ME Algorithm

A universal ME algorithm general multiple class open network of queues with mixed service disciplines is based on the previous analytic approximations and involves the following steps:

BEGIN

STEP 1   Obtain $\lambda_{i,r}$, $i = 1, 2, \ldots, M$, $r = 1, 2, \ldots, R$ from the linear system of MR equations (23).

STEP 2   Compute $\rho_{i,r} = \lambda_{i,r}/\mu_{i,r}$ and $\lambda_{dj,u;i,r}$ from (21), $i, j = 1, 2, \ldots,$ M and $r, u = 1, 2, \ldots, R$.

STEP 3   Obtain $c_{ai,r}^2$, $i = 1, 2, \ldots, M$, $r = 1, 2, \ldots, R$ from flow equations (22)-(24).

   STEP 3.1   Compute $<n_{i,r}>$, $<\theta_{i,r}>$, $i = 1, 2, \ldots, M$, $r = 1, 2, \ldots, R$ using formulae (I1)-(I14) (Appendix I) for SD = FCFS, LCFS with or without preemption, PS, PR and HOL, as appropriate.

   STEP 3.2   Obtain $c_{di,r}^2$, $i = 1, 2, \ldots, M$, $r = 1, 2, \ldots, R$ from (20).

   STEP 3.3   Compute a new value of $c_{ai,r}^2$, $i = 1, 2, \ldots, M$, $r = 1, 2, \ldots, R$ from (24) and repeat from Step 3.1 until convergence in $c_{ai,r}^2$.

STEP 4   Obtain performance measures for $<n_{i,r}>$, $<\theta_{i,r}>$, $P_{i,r}(n_{i,r})$ etc.

END

It is interesting to note that the universal ME algorithm for general open networks with mixed service disciplines provides, to the knowledge of the authors, the only tool available to date for calculating analytically an approximate solution for the marginal qld per class, $P_{i,r}(n_{i,r})$, $i = 1, 2, \ldots, M$. Furthermore, it is the first algorithm of its kind, being implemented via the GE distributional model, that is applicable to bulk arrivals and bulk service queues in an open network.

4. NUMERICAL RESULTS

In this section numerical results are presented to demonstrate the credibility of the universal multiple-class ME algorithm (UME1) for GE-type open networks in relation to simulation (SIM) and other approximate methods.

For FCFS service disciplines the methods of Kuehn (KUEHN) [5], Reiser and Kobayashi (RK) [3], Gelenbe and Pujolle (GP) [4], Sevcik et al. (SEA) [6], Whitt (WHITT) [7] and Kouvatsos (UME2) [8], based on class composition and disaggregation, are included in the study. The extension of these methods to apply to LCFS with or without preemption and PS service disciplines clearly depends on analytic formulae for the mql, $\langle n_{i,r} \rangle$, and flow equations which, unfortunately, are not readily available, with the exception of UME2 which has been adjusted [21] to utilise the new GE-type results of Sections 2 and 3. Moreover, based on the reduced occupancy approximation technique [9], the UME2 has also been extended [21] to analyse PR or HOL general open networks and is included in the numerical tests together with the approximate techniques proposed by Sevcik (ROA) [9], Kaufman (m-ROA) [10] and Bryant et al. (MVA) [12] (which only apply to Markovian type networks). The simulation results quoted are produced by using the queueing network analysis package QNAP-2 [22].

The comparative study focuses on the marginal mql's, $\langle n_{i,r} \rangle$ for various open networks of the type displayed in Fig. 1a with coefficients of variation $\geqslant 1$ and mixed service disciplines (see Tables 1-6). Figs. 1b-6 either display % differences of UME1, UME2 and other approximations from SIM or exhibit the absolute mql's, as appropriate. Note that the simulation is based on the GE distribution representing general distributions with known first two moments.

It can be generally observed in Fig. 1b-6 that the UME1 and UME2 results are comparable to those obtained by SIM both under light or heavy traffic conditions. For moderate class utilisations and with even high flow coefficients of variation, the UME1 and UME2 are considerably closer to SIM in comparison to other methods (e.g. Fig. 2). In heavier traffic involving job classes of similar behaviour all methods perform relatively well (e.g. Fig. 3). However, the UME1 and UME2 become superior when there exists high variability discrepancy amongst different classes of jobs (e.g. Fig. 1b). In the latter case, the UME1 is relatively more accurate than the UME2 (e.g. Figs. 1b, 4, 6). For Markovian networks of queues with PR or HOL service disciplines and high server utilisation(s), mostly attributed to high priority jobs, the UME1 and UME2 methods provide an improvement in accuracy over the other approximate techniques (e.g. Fig. 5). Note that the ME algorithms produce exact results when appropriate conditions for separability apply [1].

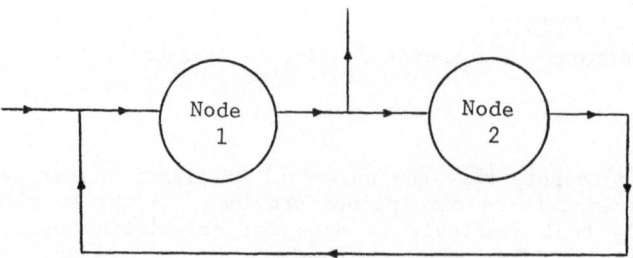

Figure 1a. Two-stage cyclic open queueing network

TABLE 1. Raw data for network 1 (Fig. 1)

Class r	$\lambda_{0;1,r}$	$C^2_{a0;1,r}$	Node 1 [FCFS]			Node 2 [FCFS]			$\rho_{1,r;2,r}$
			$\mu_{1,r}$	$\rho_{1,r}$	$C^2_{s1,r}$	$\mu_{2,r}$	$\rho_{2,r}$	$C^2_{s2,r}$	
1	0.4	3	4	0.5	9	5	0.32	11	0.8
2	0.15	5	1.875	0.2	3	0.9	0.25	25	0.6
3	0.1	1	2	0.1	5	1	0.1	3	0.5
4	0.2	11	2.5	0.1	1	1	0.05	7	0.2

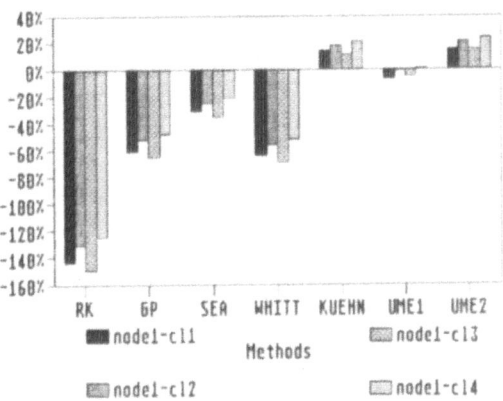

Figure 1b.   Percentage Difference from Mean Dueue Length (Simul).

TABLE 2. Raw data for network 2 (Fig. 2)

Class r	$\lambda_{0;1,r}$	$C^2_{a0;1,r}$	Node 1 [LCFS–NON–PR]			Node 2 [FCFS]			$\rho_{1,r;2,r}$
			$\mu_{1,r}$	$\rho_{1,r}$	$C^2_{s1,r}$	$\mu_{2,r}$	$\rho_{2,r}$	$C^2_{s2,r}$	
1	1	3	6.25	0.4	2	3.75	0.4	3	0.6
2	1	5	25	0.08	3	5	0.2	5	0.5

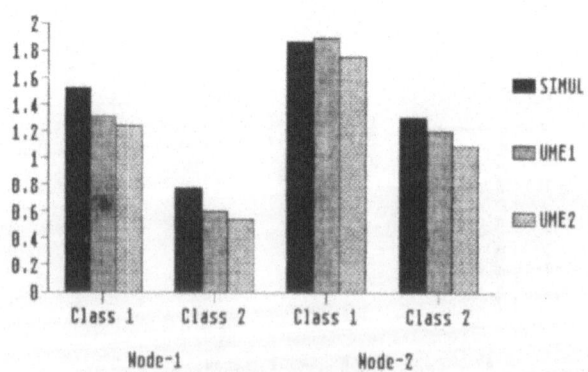

Figure 2. Mean Dueue Length Per Node and Per Class.

TABLE 3. Raw data for network 3 (Fig. 3)

Class r	$\lambda_{0;1,r}$	$C^2_{a0;1,r}$	Node 1 [LCFS-PR]			Node 2 [FCFS]			$\rho_{1,r;2,r}$
			$\mu_{1,r}$	$\rho_{1,r}$	$C^2_{s1,r}$	$\mu_{2,r}$	$\rho_{2,r}$	$C^2_{s2,r}$	
1	3	2	25	0.4	3	23.333	0.3	4	0.7
2	2	6	12.5	0.4	3	6	0.5	5	0.6

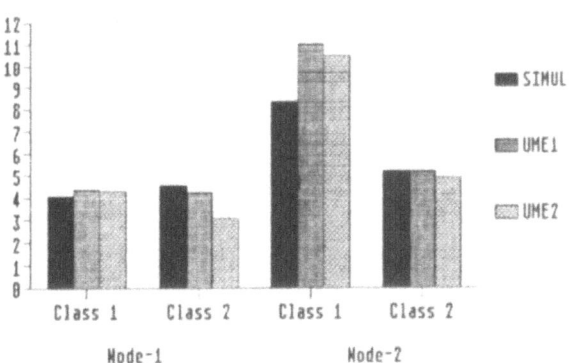

Figure 3. Mean Dueue Length Per Node and Per Class.

TABLE 4. Raw data for network 4 (Fig. 4)

Class r	$\lambda_{0;1,r}$	$C^2_{a0;1,r}$	Node 1 [PS]			Node 2 [FCFS]			$\rho_{1,r;2,r}$
			$\mu_{1,r}$	$\rho_{1,r}$	$C^2_{s1,r}$	$\mu_{2,r}$	$\rho_{2,r}$	$C^2_{s2,r}$	
1	1	3	6.25	0.4	2	3.75	0.4	3	0.6
2	1	5	25	0.08	3	5	0.2	5	0.5

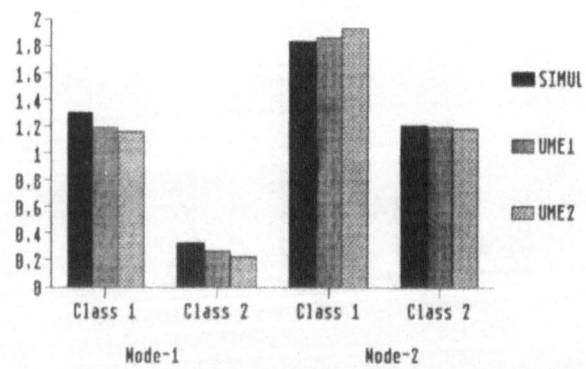

Figure 4.   Mean Dueue Length Per Node and Per Class.

TABLE 5. Raw data for network 5 (Fig. 5)

Class r	$\lambda_{0;1,r}$	$C^2_{a0;1,r}$	Node 1 [PR]			Node 2 [FCFS]			$\rho_{1,r;2,r}$
			$\mu_{1,r}$	$\rho_{1,r}$	$C^2_{s1,r}$	$\mu_{2,r}$	$\rho_{2,r}$	$C^2_{s2,r}$	
1	1	1	6.25	0.8	1	5	0.8	1	0.8
2	1	1	25	0.1	1	15	0.1	1	0.6

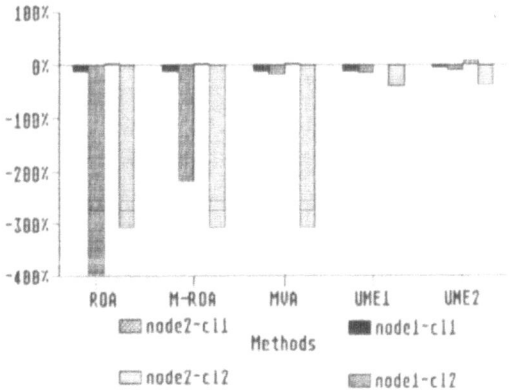

Figure 5. Percentage Difference from Mean Dueue Length (SIMUL).

411

TABLE 6. Raw data for network 6 (Fig. 6)

Class r	$\lambda_{0;1,r}$	$C^2_{a0;1,r}$	Node 1 [PR]			Node 2 [HOL]			
			$\mu_{1,r}$	$\rho_{1,r}$	$C^2_{s1,r}$	$\mu_{2,r}$	$\rho_{2,r}$	$C^2_{s2,r}$	$\rho_{1,r;2,r}$
1	3	2	25	0.4	4	23.333	0.3	3	0.7
2	2	6	12.5	0.4	5	6	0.5	5	0.6

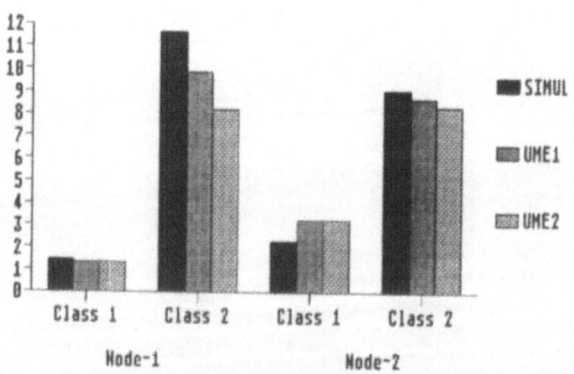

Figure 6. Mean Dueue Length Per Node and Per Class.

The relatively good accuracy of the UME1 and UME2 methods is attributed to the robust and versatile flow formulae of the GE distributional model. In particular, the UME1 method provides the best overall approximation for GE-type open networks by capturing the influences amongst the various classes of jobs in a more direct fashion to that provided by the other methods such as class composition and disaggregation or ROA. Moreover, the computational costs of UME1 and UME2 are comparable in terms of flow iterations when non-priority disciplines apply, otherwise the UME2 is clearly less efficient using empirically $(ck/R) + k$ iterations, where c is the number of priority queues $(c < M)$, and k is the corresponding number of iterations for UME1.

Finally, marginal mql's, $\langle n_{i,r} \rangle$, of an open network (Table 7) are depicted in Fig. 7, where curves are grouped according to $C^2_{si,r}$ ranging from 0.5 to 9. Note that the distributional models of Erlang-2 (E_2) and Hyper-exponential-2 (H_2) with different tuning parameters k, $k \in (1, +\infty)$ [15], are taken into account in representing G-type distributions (with known first two moments) for carrying out simulations. It can be seen that the UME1 algorithm for GE-type queues generally provides for $\langle n_{i,r} \rangle$ upper bounds (pessimistic) when $C^2_{ao;i,r}$, $C^2_{ai,r} > 1$ and lower bounds (optimistic) when $C^2_{ao;i,r} = C^2_{si,r} = 0.5$ (and, generally, less than 1). This is a typical situation in many experiments, leading to the following conjecture.

Conjecture 1. Consider an arbitrary open network of queues with multiple classes and mixed service disciplines including FCFS, LCFS with or without preemption, PS, PR and HOL. The marginal mql's $\langle n_{i,r} \rangle$ obtained by the UME1 algorithm, given the first two moments of the external interarrival and service times per class at each queue i, generally define pessimistic (optimistic) bounds on the corresponding quantities, obtained from simulation models, when representing external interarrival and service times by H_2 (E_2, Hypoexponential) distributions with the same first two moments.

Note that the bounding behaviour of the GE-type mql's may be attributed to the extremal nature of the GE distributional model [19]. Performance bounds of GE-type for FCFS single-class non-exponential closed networks with service time coefficients of variation greater than one have been first observed in [17].

5. CONCLUSIONS AND FURTHER COMMENTS

The principle of ME, viewed as an inference procedure, is used to characterise a new product-form solution for the approximate analysis of arbitrary multiple class open networks of queues at equilibrium with infinite capacities, single servers and mixed service disciplines. The ME approximation implies a decomposition of the open network into individual multiple class G/G/1 queues at equilibrium with a revised arrival process for each class of jobs.

The GE distributional model provides (under renewal assumptions) new analytic expressions for the $p_{i,r}(0)$ and $\langle n_{i,r} \rangle$, $i = 1, 2, .., M$, $r = 1, 2,$ ..., R, constraints under various service disciplines (see Appendix I), and it is used to establish a universal approximation of the flow processes in the network in terms of their first two moments. The new UME1 algorithm via the GE-type implementation offers the only analytic tool available in the literature for calculating approximately marginal qld's per class and

Table 7   Raw data for network 7 (fig. 7)

Station i	Class r	$\lambda_{0;i,r}$	$C^2_{ao;i,r}$ GE, E_2	M	$C^2_{ao;i,r}$ $H_2(k=2,10)$, GE	$\mu_{i,r}$	$C^2_{si,r}$ GE, E_2	M	$C^2_{si,r}$ $H_2(k=2,10)$, GE	$P_{i,r;j,r}$
1 [PR]	1	0.40	0.5	1	3	4	0.5	1	9	0.6
	2	0.15	0.5	1	5	1.875	0.5	1	3	0.5
	3	0.10	0.5	1	1	2	0.5	1	5	0.8
2 [HOL]	1	0	–	–	–	2	0.5	1	5	1
	2	0	–	–	–	0.75	0.5	1	2	1
	3	0	–	–	–	1.6	0.5	1	3	1

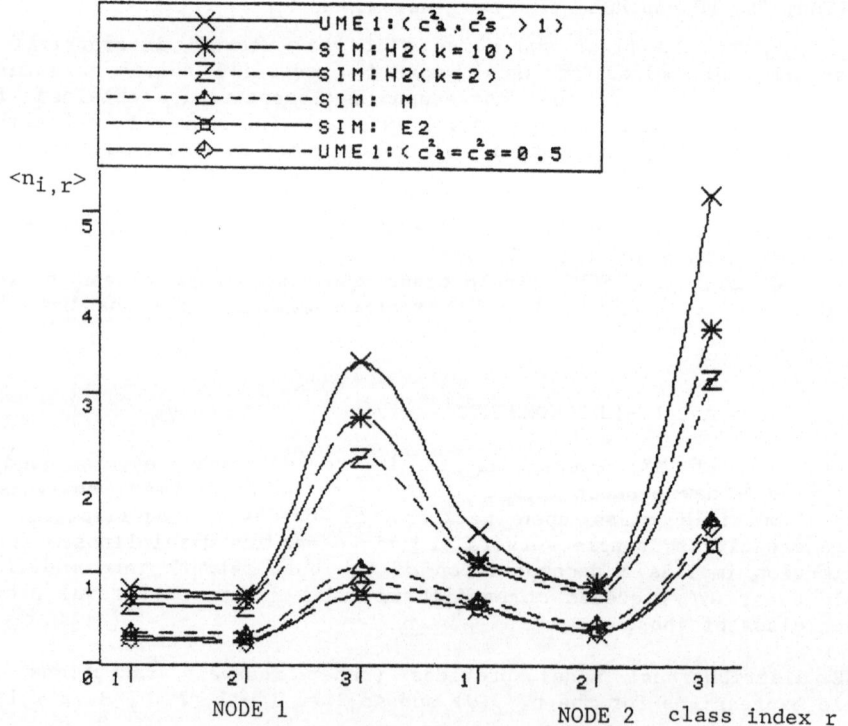

Fig. 7   Performance bounds for the two-stage
cyclic open queueing network of Fig. 0

also analysing bulk-type open queueing networks with mixed service disciplines.

The credibility of the UME1 method is demonstrated by making use of some illustrative GE-type networks and favourable comparisons with other approximate techniques (including a modified version of an earlier ME algorithm, UME2, described in [21]) are made relative to simulation. The new ME algorithm seems to capture in a better fashion the influences amongst the various classes in comparison to other approximate methods which are based on class composition and disaggregation (only for GE-type networks with FCFS disciplines) or ROA (only for Markovian Networks). Furthermore, GE-type performance bounds for the mql for each queue per class are defined.

The ME method can be extended to analyse general networks of queues with multiple and/or infinite servers, based on the robust GE model and the universal flow approximations. For example, an infinite server queue i can be immediately incorporated into the ME algorithms by using the formulae $C_{ai,r}^2 = C_{di,r}^2$ and $\langle n_{i,r} \rangle = \rho_{i,r}$. In addition, multiple server queues can be included, by applying ME analysis of a GE/GE/c queue with multiple classes and mixed disciplines, where the departure process is determined under the stipulation that "when the queue i is busy, then all c servers are busy". Moreover, the GE-type results of open networks can be used to analyse the corresponding closed networks with multiple chains, in a similar fashion to that of [8]. Problems of this nature are currently the subject of further study.

6. REFERENCES

[1] Baskett, F., Chandy, K.M., Muntz, R.R. and Palacios, F.G., Open Closed and Mixed Networks with Different Classes of Customers, JACM 22, No. 2 (1975) 248-260.

[2] Denning, P.J. and Buzen J.P., The Operational Analysis of Queueing Network Models, Computing Serveys 10, No. 3 (1978) 225-261.

[3] Reiser, M. and Kobayashi, H., Accuracy of the Diffusion Approximation for Some Queueing Systems, IBM J. Res. & Dev., 18 (1974) 110-124.

[4] Gelenbe, E. and Pujolle, G., The Behaviour of a Single Queue in a General Queueing Network, Acta Informatica, 7 (1976) 123-160.

[5] Kuehn, P.J., Approximate Analysis of General Queueing Networks by Decomposition, IEEE Trans. Comp., COM-27 (1979) 113-126.

[6] Sevcik, K.C., Levy, A.I., Tripathi, S.K. and Zahorjan, J.L., Improving Approximation of Aggregated Queueing Network Subsystems, Chandy, K.M. and Reiser, M. (Eds.), Comp. Performance, North-Holland, New York (1977) 1-22.

[7] Whitt, W., The Queueing Network Analyser, Bell System Tech. J., 62 (1983) 2779-2815.

[8] Kouvatsos, D.D., Maximum Entropy Methods for General Queueing Networks, Proc. of Modelling Techniques and Tools for Performance Analysis, May 1984, Potier, D. (Ed.), North-Holland (1985) 589-608.

[9] Sevcik, K.C., Priority Scheduling Disciplines in Queueing Network Models of Computer Systems, Info. Proc. 77 (Gilchrist, B., Ed.), IFIP, North-Holland (1977) 565-570.

[10] Kaufman, J.S., Approximation Methods for Networks of Queues with Priorities, Perf. Eval., 4 (1984) 183-198.

[11] Schmitt, W., Approximation Methods for Networks of Queues with Priorities, Proc. of 10th Int. Tel. Congress, Montreal (1983).

[12] Bryant, R.M., Krzesinski, E., Seetha Lakshmi M., Chandy, K.U., The MVA Priority Approximation, ACM Trans. on Comp. Systems, 2 (1984) 335-359.

[13] Jaynes, E.T., Prior Probabilities, IEEE Trans. Syst. Sci. and Cyber., SSC-4, 4 (1968) 227-241.

[14] Shore, J.E. and Johnson, R.W., Axiomatic Derivation of the Principle of Maximum Entropy and the Principle of Minimum Cross-Entropy, IEEE Trans. Info. Theory, IT-26 (1980) 26-37.

[15] El-Affendi, M.A. and Kouvatsos, D.D., A Maximum Entropy Analysis of the M/G/1 and G/M/1 Queueing Systems at Equilibrium, Acta Informatica, 19 (1983) 339-355.

[16] Sauer, C., Configuration of Computing Systems: An Approach Using Queueing Network Models, Ph.D. Thesis, University of Texas, Austin (1975).

[17] Walstra, R.J., Iterative Analysis of Networks of Queues, Ph.D. Thesis, University of Toronto, Dec. 1984.

[18] Shore, J.E., Information Theoretic Approximations for M/G/1 and G/G/1 Queueing Systems, Acta Informatica, 17 (1982) 43-61.

[19] Kouvatsos, D.D., A Maximum Entropy Analysis of the G/G/1 Queue at Equilibrium, J. Opl. Res. Soc., Vol. 39, No. 2 (1988) 183-200.

[20] Kouvatsos, D.D., Georgatsos, H.E.P. and Tabet-Aouel, N.A., General Multiple Class Open Networks with Mixed Service Disciplines, Tech. Rep. DK/PG/NT-A/1, University of Bradford (1988).

[21] Kouvatsos, D.D. and Tabet-Aouel, N., Maximum Entropy Analysis of General Queueing Networks with Priorities, Papers of Int. Conf. on the Analysis and Control of Large Scale Stochastic Systems, University of North Carolina, Chapel Hill, USA, May 23-25, 1988.

[22] Veran, M. and Potier, D., QNAP-2: A Portable Environment for Queueing Network Modelling, Proc. Int. Conf. on Modelling Techniques and Tools for Performance Analysis, INRIA (1984).

Appendix I

Consider a stable GE/G/1 queue with R (≥ 2) classes of jobs and distinct GE interarrival-time and general service-time distributions per class. The mql, $\langle n_{i,r} \rangle$, and $\langle \theta_{i,r} \rangle = 1 - p_{i,r}(0)$, r = 1, 2,..., R can be determined for each service discipline of interest as follows:

i)   The FCFS GE/G/1 queue

$$\langle n_{i,r} \rangle = \frac{\rho_{i,r}}{2}\left[C_{ai,r}^2 + 1\right] + \frac{\sum_{u=1}^{R} \frac{\lambda_{i,r}}{\lambda_{i,u}} \rho_{i,u}^2 \left[C_{si,u}^2 + C_{ai,u}^2\right]}{2(1 - \rho_i)}, \qquad (I1)$$

where $\rho_{i,r} = \lambda_{i,r}/\mu_{i,r}$, $\rho_i = \sum_{r=1}^{R} \rho_{i,r}$,

$$p_{i,r}(0) = S_{i,r}^*(\lambda_{i,r}\sigma_{i,r}) = \frac{\lambda_{i,r}\sigma_{i,r}(1 - \rho_i)B_{i,r}^{b*}(\lambda_{i,r}\sigma_{i,r})}{\lambda_{i,r}\sigma_{i,r} + \Lambda_R^b B^{b*}(\lambda_{i,r}\sigma_{i,r}) - \Lambda_R^b}, \qquad (I2)$$

where

$$\sigma_{i,r} = 2/\left[1 + C_{ai,r}^2\right], \qquad \Lambda_R^b = \sum_{r=1}^{R} \lambda_{i,r}\sigma_{i,r},$$

$$B^{b*}(\theta) = \sum_{r=1}^{R} \frac{\lambda_{i,r}\sigma_{i,r}}{\Lambda_R^b} B_{i,r}^{b*}(\theta),$$

$$B_{i,r}^{b*}(\theta) = \frac{\sigma_{i,r}B_{i,r}^{*}(\theta)}{1 - (1 - \sigma_{i,r})B_{i,r}^{*}(\theta)} \quad ,$$

$S_{i,r}^{*}(\theta)$ is the Laplace-Stieljes (L-S) transform of the response time distribution and $B_{i,r}^{*}(\theta)$ is the L-S transform of a distinct G-type service-time distribution per class r, r = 1, 2,..., R.

ii)   The LCFS GE/G/1 queue with preemption

$$<n_{i,r}> = \rho_{i,r}\frac{c_{ai,r}^2 + 1}{2(1 - \rho_i)} \quad , \tag{I3}$$

$$p_{i,r}(0) = \frac{1 - \rho_i}{1 - (\rho_i - \rho_{i,r})} \quad . \tag{I4}$$

iii) The LCFS GE/G/1 queue without preemption

$$<n_{i,r}> = \rho_{i,r}\frac{c_{ai,r}^2 + 1 - 2\rho_i}{2(1 - \rho_i)} + \sum_{u=1}^{R}\left[\frac{\rho_{i,u}^2\lambda_{i,r}}{\lambda_{i,u}}\right]\left[\frac{c_{si,u}^2 + 1}{2(1 - \rho_i)}\right] \quad , \tag{I5}$$

and $p_{i,r}(0)$ is approximated by (I2).

iv)   The PS GE/G/1 queue

$$<n_{i,r}> = \rho_{i,r}\left[\frac{1 + c_{ai,r}^2}{2} + \frac{\sum\limits_{u=1}^{R}\rho_{i,u}w_{i,u}\left[1 + c_{ai,u}^2\right]/2}{w_{i,r}(1 - \rho_i)}\right], \tag{I6}$$

where $w_{i,r}$ is a known weight allocated to class r jobs so that they receive a fraction of the server's capacity at a rate $w_{i,r}/\sum\limits_{u=1}^{R}w_{i,u}n_{i,u}$ (n.b. when the non-discriminatory PS policy is applied, the value of $w_{i,r}$ is equal to 1 for all r = 1, 2,.., R).

$$p_{i,r}(0) = \frac{1 - \rho_i}{1 - (\rho_i - \rho_{i,r})} \quad , \quad r = 1, 2,.., R. \tag{I7}$$

v)   The PR GE/G/1 queue

$$<n_{i,r}> = \frac{\rho_{i,r}}{1 - \gamma_{i,r-1}} +$$

$$\frac{\rho_{i,r}^2\left[c_{si,r}^2 + 1\right] + \sum\limits_{u=1}^{r-1}\frac{\lambda_{i,r}}{\lambda_{i,u}}\rho_{i,u}^2\left[c_{si,u}^2 + c_{ai,u}^2\right] + \rho_{i,r}\left[c_{ai,r}^2 - 1\right]\left[1-\gamma_{i,r-1}\right]}{2\left[1 - \gamma_{i,r-1}\right]\left[1 - \gamma_{i,r}\right]}, \tag{I8}$$

where $\gamma_{i,r} = \sum\limits_{u=1}^{r}\rho_{i,u}$, $\gamma_{i,0} \equiv 0$ and

$$P_{i,r}(0) = S^*_{i,r}\left[\lambda_{i,r}\sigma_{i,r}\right]$$

$$= \left[1 - \gamma_{i,r}\right]\left[1 + \frac{\Lambda^b_{i,r-1}}{\lambda_{i,r}\sigma_{i,r}}\left[1 - G^*_{i,r-1}\left[\lambda_{i,r}\sigma_{i,r}\right]\right]\right] \quad (I9)$$

where $S^*_{i,r}(\theta)$ is the L-S transform of the response time distribution, $\Lambda^b_{i,r-1} = \sum_{u=1}^{r-1}\lambda_{i,u}\sigma_{i,u}$, and $G^*_{i,r-1}(\theta)$ is the L-S transform of the busy period attributed to job classes $1, 2,.., r - 1$.

vi)   The HOL GE/G/1 queue

$$<n_{i,r}> = \rho_{i,r} + \frac{\rho_{i,r}(C^2_{ai,r} - 1)}{2(1 - \gamma_{i,r})}$$

$$+ \frac{\sum_{u=1}^{r-1}\frac{\lambda_{i,r}}{\lambda_{i,u}}\rho^2_{i,u}\left[C^2_{si,u} + C^2_{ai,u}\right] + \sum_{u=r}^{R}\frac{\lambda_{i,r}}{\lambda_{i,u}}\rho^2_{i,u}\left[C^2_{si,u} + 1\right]}{2\left[1 - \gamma_{i,r}\right]\left[1 - \gamma_{i,r-1}\right]}, \quad (I10)$$

$$P_{i,r}(0) = \frac{B^*_{i,r}(\lambda_{i,r}\sigma_{i,r})}{\lambda_{i,r}\sigma_{i,r}C^*_{i,r}(\lambda_{i,r}\sigma_{i,r})}$$

$$\times \left[(1 - \rho_i)\left[\Lambda^b_{i,r} - \Lambda^b_{i,r-1}G^*_{i,r-1}(\lambda_{i,r}\sigma_{i,r})\right]\right.$$

$$\left. + \sum_{u=r+1}^{R}\lambda_{i,u}\left[1 - B^*_{i,u}\left[\Lambda^b_{i,r} - \Lambda^b_{i,r-1}G^*_{i,r-1}(\sigma_{i,r}\lambda_{i,r})\right]\right]\right] \quad (I11)$$

where $\quad C^*_{i,r}(\theta) = B^*_{i,r}\left[\theta_{i,r} + \Lambda^b_{i,r-1} - \Lambda^b_{i,r-1}G^*_{i,r-1}(\theta)\right]$

is the L-T transform of the completion time for jobs of class r, $G^*_{i,r-1}(\theta)$ is the L-S transform of the busy period attributed to job classes $1, 2, ..., r - 1$ and $B^*_{i,r}(\theta)$ is the L-T of the class r job's service-time.

Formulae (I1)-(I11) are applied when the service-time distribution is of GE-type.   In this case the L-S transform of the service-time, $B^*_{i,r}(\theta)$, is given by (e.g., [15])

$$B^*_{i,r}(\theta) = 1 - \tau_{i,r} + \frac{\tau^2_{i,r}\mu_{i,r}}{\tau_{i,r}\mu_{i,r} + \theta}, \quad (I12)$$

where $\tau_{i,r} = 2/(1 + C^2_{si,r})$.   Moreover, the L-S transform of the busy period attributed to job classes $1, 2, ..., r - 1$ of a stable GE/GE/1 queue with R classes under PR or HOL service disciplines, $G^*_{i,r-1}(\theta)$, can be established by using the bulk interpretation of the GE distribution and are given by

i) For r = 1,

$$G^*_{i,1}(\theta) = \frac{\varphi_{i,1} - \psi_{i,1}}{\omega_{i,1}}, \tag{I13}$$

where

$$\varphi_{i,1} = \tau_{i,1}\mu_{i,1}\sigma_{i,1} + (\tau_{i,1} + \sigma_{i,1} - \tau_{i,1}\sigma_{i,1})\theta$$
$$+ 2\lambda_{i,1}\sigma^2_{i,1} + \tau_{i,1}\lambda_{i,1}\sigma_{i,1}(1 - 2\sigma_{i,1}),$$

$$\psi_{i,1} = \left\{\left[\tau_{i,1}\sigma_{i,1}(\mu_{i,1} + \lambda_{i,1}) + (\tau_{i,1} + \sigma_{i,1} - \tau_{i,1}\sigma_{i,1})\theta\right]^2\right.$$
$$\left. - 4\lambda_{i,1}\mu_{i,1}\tau^2_{i,1}\sigma^2_{i,1}\right\}^{\frac{1}{2}},$$

$$\omega_{i,1} = 2\lambda_{i,1}\sigma_{i,1}(\tau_{i,1} + \sigma_{i,1} - \tau_{i,1}\sigma_{i,1}),$$

and

ii) For r > 1,

$$G^*_{i,r}(\theta) = \frac{\lambda^b_{i,r}}{\Lambda^b_{i,r}} G^*_{i,r_1}(\theta) + \frac{\Lambda^b_{i,r-1}}{\Lambda^b_{i,r}} G^*_{i,r_2}(\theta), \tag{I14}$$

where

$$G^*_{i,r_1}(\theta) = B^{b*}_{i,r}\left[\theta + \Lambda^b_{i,r} - \Lambda^b_{i,r-1}G^*_{i,r-1}\left[\theta + \lambda^b_{i,r} - \lambda^b_{i,r}G^*_{i,r_1}(\theta)\right]\right.$$
$$\left. - \lambda^b_{i,r}G^*_{i,r_1}(\theta)\right],$$

$$G^*_{i,r_2}(\theta) = G^*_{i,r-1}\left[\theta + \lambda^b_{i,r} - \lambda^b_{i,r}G^*_{i,r_1}(\theta)\right]$$

where $\lambda^b_{i,r} = \lambda_{i,r}\sigma_{i,r}$ and $\Lambda^b_{i,r} = \sum\limits_{u=1}^{r}\lambda_{i,u}\sigma_{i,u}$.

The various values of $G^*_{i,r}(\theta)$, $r = 1, 2,\ldots, R$ can be calculated recursively using formulae (I13) (initially) and (I14), respectively.

Note that formulae (I1) — (I14) are exact for $C^2_{ai,r}$, $C^2_{si,r} \geqslant 1$ and details of the proofs can be seen in [22]. When $C^2_{ai,r}$ or $C^2_{si,r} < 1$, these results can be effectively used as heuristic approximations.

PIECEWISE APPROXIMATION OF DENSITIES

APPLYING THE PRINCIPLE OF MAXIMUM ENTROPY:

WAITING TIMES IN G/G/1-SYSTEMS

Christoph Strelen

Institut für Informatik
Universität Bonn
Römerstr. 164
D-5300 Bonn
Germany

Abstract

Two methods are proposed for the calculation of the densities of the waiting times in G/G/1 queues. The densities are approximated by distributions with maximum entropy or minimum cross-entropy. Begining with a given distribution for the first job, the distributions for the succeeding jobs are computed until equilibrium is reached, thus not only obtaining a solution in case of equilibrium. Both methods determine the necessary moments by themselves, no other approximations are needed. Comparing sample results to exact values and other approximations, the accuracy of the methods is demonstrated. The first method is suited for systems with medium or high utilization. In the second method the real axis is partitioned suitably, and densities over the subsets are considered. This allows to control the accuracy.

1. INTRODUCTION

The principle of maximum entropy for probability distributions can be applied in order to analyse stochastic models. In a series of papers this is done for systems in equilibrium: based on some expectations of random variables which represent interesting features of the model, distributions of maximum entropy (DME) can be calculated. The expectations must be provided from other sources, e.g. from other approximate formulae. In most cases, discrete distributions are considered. Queueing systems are discussed in [AK] (M/G/1, G/M/1),[K2], [TZ], [T], [S] (G/G/1, M/G/1), e.g., and queueing networks in [K1], [W], [TZ], [T]. Recently, Kouvatsos proposed an approximate maximum entropy analysis for G/G/1 queues in equilibrium which is based on the first and the second moments of the interarrival time and the service time.

In this paper we deal with the approximate determination of densities for the waiting times of G/G/1 queues by distributions with maximum entropy or minimum cross-entropy (DMC). Beginning with the first job's waiting time, densities for the waiting times of the succeeding jobs are calculated by evaluating the Chapman-Kolmogorov equations. To this end we need three or five moments, resp., of the interarrival time and the service time for method 1, or some conditional expectations of these r.v. for method 2. After some jobs, the equilibrium waiting time distribution is also found. The following are important properties of our methods: DMEs and DMCs for densities are computed; the methods calculate the necessary expectations by themselves, they need not be provided; the transient behavior is also considered.

A numerical analysis as we propose requires more programming effort and computing time than the application of simple approximate formulae, but the results are more accurate, and the system is analysed more in detail.

In Section 2 the principles of maximum entropy and minimum cross-entropy are applied to the calculation of densities, in Section 3 such densities are used to approximate waiting time densities (method 1), in Section 4 examples are given, and in Section 5 method 2 is proposed.

2. THE PRINCIPLES OF MAXIMUM ENTROPY AND MINIMUM CROSS-ENTROPY, APPLIED TO DENSITIES

The priciples of maximum entropy and minimum cross-entropy are used to define probability distributions [SJ]: Firstly, a set of distributions is defined by fixing the sample space and some expectations. Secondly, one of them, say P, is selected by requiring its entropy to be maximum or a cross-entropy to be minimum. We call the resulting distribution *distribution with maximum entropy* (DME) or *distribution with minimum cross-entropy* (DMC), resp. For the latter, additional prior information about the distribution is taken into account.

This procedure can be interpreted as an approximation of a distribution: Let a sample space be given, a distribution P_X over it, and some expectations. The just defined distribution P is used as approximation of P_X.

First we consider the principle of maximum entropy. Let X be a r.v. with the unknown distribution P_X, and known expectations,

$$E(g_k(X)) = G_k, \quad k \in [0:K], \quad K \in I\!N_0. \tag{1}$$

Here, g_k are known funcions, $g_0(x) = 1$, and $G_k \in I\!R$, $G_0 = 1$.

From the set of distributions defined by (1), the one posessing the maximum entropy is chosen. If the sample space Ω is discrete, $\Omega \subseteq Z\!\!\!Z$, the entropy of a distribution $(p_n, n \in \Omega)$ is defined by

$$H \stackrel{\text{def}}{=} -\sum_{n \in \Omega} p_n \ln p_n, \tag{2}$$

and in the density case where $\Omega \subseteq \bar{I\!R}$ $(I\!R \cup \{-\infty\} \cup \{\infty\})$, it is defined by

$$H \overset{\text{def}}{=} - \int_\Omega f(x) \ln f(x) dx \tag{2'}$$

$(y \ln y \to 0 \text{ for } y \to 0)$.

Clearly, for discrete distributions

$$p_n \geq 0 \text{ for all } n \in \Omega, \text{ and } \sum_{n \in \Omega} p_n = 1,$$

and for densities

$$f(x) \geq 0 \text{ for all } x \in \Omega, \text{ and } \int_\Omega f(x) dx = 1$$

must hold. We assume in the sequel, that every DME lies in the inner of these domains, because DMEs on the boundary need a specific treatment. In [HA] it is considered how the former can be verified for distributions over discrete sample spaces, and how a DME on the boundary can be approximated uniformly.

Here we are interested in densities. Let $\Omega \subseteq \bar{I\!R}$ be the sample space, and the moments

$$M_j = \int_\Omega x^j f_X(x) dx, \quad j \in [0 : K], \tag{3}$$

of an unknown density $f_X(x)$ are given, where $M_0 = 1$. An approximation $f(x)$ of the density with the same moments is searched by maximizing the entropy

$$H = - \int_\Omega f(x) \ln f(x) dx. \tag{4}$$

We say, it is of the *order* K.

This is an isoperimetric variation problem, see [SM]. A solution $y = f(x)$ satisfies Euler's partial differential equation,

$$h_y - y'' h_{y'y'} - y' h_{y'y} - h_{y'x} = 0 \tag{5}$$

($'$ denotes a total derivation, e.g. $y' = \frac{d}{dx} f(x)$, and an index denotes a partial derivation, e.g. $h_y = \frac{\partial}{\partial y} h$). $h(x, y, y')$ is the sum of the integrands from the integral to be maximized and the integrals defining the constraints, the latters being multiplied with Lagrangian multipliers, here

$$h(x, y, y') = -y \ln y + \sum_{j=0}^{K} \lambda_j^* x^j y, \tag{6}$$

where λ_j^* are the multipliers. Euler's DE degenerates to

$$-\ln y - 1 + \sum_{j=0}^{K} \lambda_j^* x^j = 0,$$

and we have as solution

$$f(x) = e^{-\lambda(x)}, \tag{7}$$

where

$$\lambda_0 \stackrel{\text{def}}{=} 1 - \lambda_0^*, \quad \lambda_j \stackrel{\text{def}}{=} -\lambda_j^*, \quad j \in [1 : K],$$

$$\lambda(x) \stackrel{\text{def}}{=} \sum_{j=0}^{K} \lambda_j x^j. \tag{8}$$

These matters can be found in the book of Kagan et al. [KA].

The real problem is the calculation of the parameters λ_j from the non-linear equations

$$M_k = \mu_k \stackrel{\text{def}}{=} \int_\Omega x^k e^{-\lambda(x)} dx, \quad k \in [0 : K], \tag{9}$$

which follows from (3). We consider only such parameter values, for whom the integrals exist.

We now present three examples.

Example 1. Let $\Omega = \bar{I\!R}_+ = [0, \infty) \cup \{\infty\}$, $K = 1$, and M_1 be given. Then $f(x) = \lambda_1 e^{-\lambda_1 x}$, where $\lambda_1 = 1/M_1$, i.e. the exponential distribution.

Example 2. Let $\Omega = \bar{I\!R}$, $K = 2$, and $M_2 \neq 0$ be given. After some manipulations one gets

$$e^{-\lambda_0} = e^{-M_1^2/(2\sigma^2)}/\sqrt{2\pi\sigma^2},$$

$$\lambda_1 = -M_1/\sigma^2, \tag{10}$$

$$\lambda_2 = \frac{1}{2\sigma^2},$$

where

$$\sigma^2 = M_2 - M_1^2.$$

Thus

$$f(x) = \frac{1}{\sqrt{2\pi\sigma^2}} e^{-(x-M_1)^2/(2\sigma^2)},$$

i.e. the Gaussian distribution $N(M_1, \sigma)$.

Example 3. Let $\Omega = [0, 1], K = 0$ or $1, M_1 = 1/2$. Then

$$f(x) = 1,$$

the uniform distribution. The first moment is not necessary.

The prior information of a DMC is a distribution, here denoted by $(v_n, n \in \Omega)$ in the discrete case, and by $v(x), x \in \Omega$, in the density case. The cross-entropy is defined by

$$H^+ \overset{\text{def}}{=} \sum_{n \in \Omega} p_n(\ln p_n - \ln v_n) \tag{11}$$

or

$$H^+ \overset{\text{def}}{=} \int_\Omega f(x)[\ln f(x) - \ln v(x)]dx, \tag{11'}$$

respectively.

A DMC is selected by requiring H^+ to be minimum.

In the density case, this leads again to an isoperimetric variation problem where

$$h = y \ln y - y \ln v + \sum_{j=0}^{K} \lambda_j^* x^j y. \tag{12}$$

The solution of Euler's DE is

$$f(x) = v(x)e^{-1-\lambda_0^* - \lambda_1^* x - \ldots - \lambda_K^* x^K}. \tag{13}$$

For practical reasons, we choose

$$v(x) = x^{p-1}e^{c_0 + c_1 x + \ldots + c_K x^K}, p > 0,$$

without fixing p. Thus we get

$$f(x) = x^{p-1}e^{a_0 + a_1 x + \ldots + a_K x^K} \tag{14}$$

as DMC with the parameters p and $a_0, a_1, \ldots, a_K$.

Example 4. Let $\Omega = \bar{\mathbb{R}}_+$, $K = 1$, and the Moments M_1 and M_2 be given. One gets

$$\lambda_1 = \frac{M_1}{M_2 - M_1^2}$$

and

$$p = \frac{M_1^2}{M_2 - M_1^2};$$

$f(x)$ is the Gamma distribution.

There are no error bounds for the approximation of distributions by DMEs, but we wish to exhibit two obstacles to accuracy. Firstly, a DME of the form (7) has at most $K - 1$ extrema, and it is continuous and smooth. A density not having these properties is not accurately approximated.

The second point concerns conditional distributions. Let P be a DME over Ω. In general, the relative errors of $P\{A\}$ are not of the same order of magnitude for any $A \subset \Omega$: If $|A|$ is not small compared to $|\Omega|$, but $P\{A\}$ is small, the conditional probabilities $P\{B|A\}$, $B \subset \Omega$, tend to be inaccurate. Later on one observes, that this situation occurs in our method 1 for small utilization factors ρ, where $A = \bar{I\!R}_+$ and $P\{A\} = \rho$. Therefore method 1 is not suited for small ρ.

In method 1 we apply DMEs of the order 1 and 2, i.e. exponential and Gaussian distributions, and DMCs of the form (14), order 1, i.e. Γ-distributions.

3. WAITING TIMES IN G/G/1 QUEUES

We consider G/G/1 queues fitting the usual assumptions, see [KL], e.g. Let the interarrival times be distributed as a r.v. T, and the service times as a r.v. S, both over $\bar{I\!R}_+$. Let $C \overset{\text{def}}{=} S - T$, and $W^{(n)}, n \in I\!N$, be the waiting times of the nth job. Defining the following *pseudo waiting times*,

$$\widetilde{W}^{(n)} \overset{\text{def}}{=} W^{(n-1)} + C, \tag{1}$$

one has

$$W^{(n)} = \max(0, \widetilde{W}^{(n)}), \ n = 2, 3, \ldots. \tag{2}$$

We assume that S and T have densities, and that the necessary moments exist.

In this section we describe our method 1 for calculating approximatly the densities of the waiting times $W^{(n)}$, beginning with the known density of the first job's waiting time density.

Let $T_j, S_j, C_j, \widetilde{W}_j^{(n)}$ and $W_j^{(n)}, j \in I\!N_0$, denote the jth moments of the just introduced r.v., and $\tilde{w}^{(n)}(t), t \in \bar{I\!R}$, the densities of the pseudo waiting times. The distributions of the waiting times $W^{(n)}$ are described by the probabilities $p_0^{(n)} \overset{\text{def}}{=} P\{W^{(n)} = 0\}$ and the densities $w^{(n)}(t), t > 0$, where

$$w^{(n)}(t) = \tilde{w}^{(n)}(t), \ t > 0,$$

$$p_0^{(n)} = \int\limits_{-\infty}^{0} \tilde{w}^{(n)}(t)dt. \tag{3}$$

Now we state an algorithm for approximating these quantities. To this end we define r.v. U over $\bar{I\!R}_- = (-\infty, 0] \cup \{-\infty\}$ and V over $\bar{I\!R}_+$,

$$U \overset{\text{def}}{=} \min(0, \widetilde{W}^{(n)}), \ V \overset{\text{def}}{=} \max(0, \widetilde{W}^{(n)}),$$

and

$$\alpha^{(n)} \overset{\text{def}}{=} P\{\widetilde{W}^{(n)} \le 0\}, \ \beta^{(n)} \overset{\text{def}}{=} 1 - \alpha^{(n)}.$$

Let $u(t)$ and $v(t)$, resp., denote the densities of these r.v. conditioned that they are different from 0, and U_j and $V_j, j \in I\!N_0$, their moments. Then

$$\widetilde{W}_j = \alpha U_j + \beta V_j,$$

$$\tilde{w}(t) = \alpha u(t) + \beta v(t) \text{ for } t \ne 0, \ \tilde{w}(0) = \lim_{\tau \uparrow 0} u(\tau) \tag{4}$$

holds (we often omit the upper indices $^{(n)}$). In the sequel we use this partition of $\widetilde{W}$ for two reasons: the densities $\widetilde{w}(t)$ are not smooth at $t = 0$, and by this we have more free parameters for better fitting $\widetilde{w}(t)$; this aspect is discussed later on. $u(t)$ and $v(t)$ are approximated by DMEs of the order 1 - in this case we call the results M-approximations - or by DMCs of the order 1 - and we call the results Γ-approximations.

As DMEs of order 1 we take exponential distributions,

$$u(t) = ae^{at}, \ v(t) = be^{-bt}, \tag{4'}$$

where $a > 0$ and $b > 0$ must hold, and as DMCs Γ-distributions,

$$u(t) = \frac{a^p}{\Gamma(p)}(-t)^{p-1}e^{at},$$

$$v(t) = \frac{b^q}{\Gamma(q)}t^{q-1}e^{-bt}, \tag{4''}$$

where $p, a, q, b > 0$. Thus the moments are

$$U_j = (-1)^j \frac{j!}{a^j}, \ V_j = \frac{j!}{b^j}$$

or

$$U_j = (-1)^j \frac{p(p+1)\ldots(p+j-1)}{a^j},$$

$$V_j = \frac{q(q+1)\ldots(q+j-1)}{b^j}, \ j \in \mathbb{N},$$

resp., and

$$U_0 = 1, V_0 = 1.$$

If the parameters a, b, α or p, a, q, b, α, resp., are known, one has the desired approximations by means of (4) and (3).

For the calculation of these parameters, we define functions φ_j of them,

$$\varphi_j \overset{\text{def}}{=} \alpha U_j + \beta V_j - \widetilde{W}_j,$$

which are

$$\varphi_j \overset{\text{def}}{=} \alpha(-1)^j \frac{j!}{a^j} + (1-\alpha)\frac{j!}{b^j} - \widetilde{W}_j$$

in the case of DMEs.

$$\varphi_j = 0, \quad j = 1, 2, 3, \tag{5'}$$

are non-linear equations for the parameters a, b, α. These equations are solved for every job, in turn, observing the constraints

$$a > 0, \ b > 0, \ 0 < \alpha < 1. \tag{6'}$$

The necessary moments $\widetilde{W}_j^{(n)}$ can be obtained as follows, because the waiting time of the $(n-1)$th job, its service time, and the succeeding interarrival times are independent:

$$\widetilde{W}_j^{(n)} = \sum_{i=0}^{j} \binom{j}{i} W_{j-i}^{(n-1)} C_i \tag{7}$$

where

$$C_j = \sum_{i=0}^{j} \binom{j}{i} (-1)^i S_{j-i} T_i$$

and

$$W_j^{(n-1)} = (1 - \alpha^{(n-1)}) V_j^{(n-1)}, \ j = 1, 2, \ldots.$$

When U and V are approximated with DMCs, we take

$$\varphi_j \stackrel{\text{def}}{=} \alpha(-1)^j \frac{p(p+1)\ldots(p+j-1)}{a^j} + (1-\alpha) \frac{q(q+1)\ldots(q+j-1)}{b^j} - \widetilde{W}_j,$$

and

$$\varphi_j = 0, \quad j = 1, \ldots, 5, \tag{5''}$$

is a system of non-linear equations for the parameters p, a, q, b, α. The constraints are

$$p, a, q, b > 0, \ 0 < \alpha < 1. \tag{6''}$$

If one approximates the pseudo waiting time density of every job by one single DME of the order 2,

$$\widetilde{w}^{(n)}(t) = e^{-\lambda_0 - \lambda_1 t - \lambda_2 t^2},$$

one gets a very simple algorithm, because the non-linear equations for the parameters can be solved explicitly according to (10), Sec.2, using the moments $\widetilde{W}_j^{(n)}$, $j = 1, 2$, which are known from (7). The moments of the waiting time are

$$W_j^{(n)} = \int_0^\infty t^j \widetilde{w}^{(n)}(t) dt.$$

We call these approximations *N-approximations*.

For the other approximations we calculate the parameters a, b, α or p, a, q, b, α, resp., by solving the non-linear equations (5') or (5") with a Newton method. For its description, we combine the unknown parameters in the tuple

$$x = (x_1, \ldots, x_K) = \begin{cases} (a, b, \alpha) & \text{for M-approximations,} \\ (p, a, q, b, \alpha) & \text{for } \Gamma\text{-approximations,} \end{cases}$$

and write the non-linear equations in the form

$$\varphi_j(x) = 0, \ j \in \mathcal{K}, \tag{5}$$

where $\mathcal{K} = [1 : K]$, and $K = 3$ or $K = 5$, resp. The constraints are

$$x_i > 0, \ i \in \mathcal{K}, \ x_K < 1. \tag{6}$$

428

To solve (5), we start with an approximate parameter vector x_{old} which fulfills the constraints. In one iteration step of the Newton method, a new vector x_{new} is determined from an old one, x_{old}, by

$$x_{new} := x_{old} - c\delta. \tag{8}$$

The number c is useful to the constraints and to speeding up the convergence of the iterations; it is explained later on. $\delta = (\delta_1, \ldots, \delta_K)$ is the solution of a system of linear equations,

$$J\delta = \varphi(x_{old}), \tag{9}$$

where J is the Jacobian of the system (5) for $x = x_{old}$, and φ denotes $(\varphi_1, \ldots, \varphi_K)$. The elements of the $K \times K$-matrix J are approximated by difference-quotients, observing the constraints (6):

$$J_{j,i} = \frac{\varphi_j(y) - \varphi_j(x)}{y_i - x_i}$$

where

$$x = x_{old},$$
$$y_k = x_k, \; k \in \mathcal{K} \setminus \{i\},$$
$$y_i = (1 - \epsilon)x_i, \quad j, i \in \mathcal{K},$$
$$\epsilon > 0, \; \epsilon << 1.$$

The number $c \in (0, 1]$ is chosen such that x_{new} fulfills the constraints (6), and that the Euclidian norm of the defect deminishes,

$$\|\varphi(x_{new})\|_E < \|\varphi(x_{old})\|_E. \tag{10}$$

To accomplish the first, we determine a number c' as follows: For all $j \in \mathcal{K}$ with $x_j - \delta_j \leq 0$, we choose numbers $c_j = (x_j - \epsilon)/\delta_j$, and if $x_K - \delta_K \geq 1$, we take $c_{K+1} = (x_K - 1 + \epsilon)/\delta_K)$, where $\epsilon > 0$, $\epsilon << 1$. c' is the minimum of these numbers. To cause the defect to decrease, we apply bisection (see [ST], e.g.):

$$c = 2^{-k}c'$$

where $k \in \mathbb{N}_0$ is the smallest integer for which (10) holds.

In our examples we choose $\epsilon = 10^{-4}$, and restrict k by 13. The Newton iterations were performed until $\|\varphi\|_E < 10^{-4}$, at most 20 times.

It is important to start the Newton iteration with rather accurate starting parameter vectors x_{old}. For the 3rd job and its successors, we take the predecessor's parameters as starting values. If a Γ-approximation for the 2nd job is to be calculated, we start the iterations with $x_{old} = (1, a, 1, b, \alpha)$, where a, b, α are the parameters of the corresponding M-approximation, or with an N-approximation. The starting vectors for the M-approximation of the 2nd job are given later on, see (11) and (12).

The waiting time distribution of the first job must be given in advance. We consider two distributions: $W^{(1)} = 0$ or $W^{(1)} = Y^{(s)}$. $Y^{(s)}$ denotes the equilibrium waiting time of the *corresponding* M/M/1 queue; by this we mean the M/M/1 queue with the same mean interarrival and service times.

In an M/M/1 queue with a zero waiting time for the first job, the pseudo waiting times of the 2nd job and in equilibrium have exactly the form (4), (4'):

$$a = 1/T_1, \ b = 1/S_1, \ \alpha = \frac{T_1}{T_1 + S_1}, \tag{11}$$

and

$$a = 1/T_1, \ b = 1/S_1 - 1/T_1, \ \alpha = \frac{T_1 - S_1}{T_1}, \tag{12}$$

resp. We take these parameters of the corresponding M/M/1 queue as starting values for the M-approximation of the 2nd job.

Our choice of DMEs and DMCs as approximating densities also has practical aspects. Clearly, a greater number of parameters result in more accurate solutions: M-approximations are better than N-approximations, and Γ-approximations are still better. This is the reason why we consider DMCs.

One can increase the number of parameters by taking DMEs or DMCs of higher order K, but this leads to problems. Firstly, the integrations for the calculation of the moments cannot be done by formulae. Secondly, serious numerical problems occur: The coefficient of x_K in (8) and (12), Sec.2, is small, in general, but it must be evaluated very accuratly (if its sign is wrong, and $I\!R_+$ is the sample space, the moments don't exist, e.g.). We tried higher orders K, but we did not succeed.

For the M- and Γ-approximations, we split the sample space up into parts, $\bar{I\!R}_+$ and $\bar{I\!R}_-$, for two reasons:
-   to take account for the kink of $\tilde{w}(t)$ at $t = 0$,
-   to have more parameters.

The second seems to be more important, as the following demonstrates. $\tilde{w}(t)$ is continuous at $t = 0$; therefore we tried the continuous approximation

$$\tilde{w}(t) = \frac{ab}{a+b} \begin{cases} e^{at}, \ t \le 0, \\ e^{-bt}, \ t > 0, \end{cases} \tag{13}$$

instead of the density (4),(4') being not continuous, in general. This density (13) is also of the order 1, but has one parameter less. The results were far less accurate. It is even possible to use an approximation for $\tilde{w}(t)$ with just one parameter because the angle at $t = 0$ is known from the desities of the interarrival time and the service time. But, the results are still worse. Thus, it seems to be good for the accuracy to ignore known but less important properties of $\tilde{w}(t)$ in order to have more parameters.

Since we realized that more parameters are favorable to accuracy, and that higher orders of the DMEs are unpractical, we tried to divide the sample space $I\!R$ into even more pieces and to consider DMEs of low order over them, which resulted in a large number of parameters. This consideration turned out to be successful; the result is our method 2, described in Section 5.

4. EXAMPLES

We tested our method 1 applying it to various examples. The obtained results were compared with other approximate solutions and - if possible - with the exact values. We found medium sized and small errors for the first K moments; the results for the probability of a zero waiting time, $p_0 = P\{W = 0\}$, were not so accurate but better than those obtained by the formula of Krämer and Langenbach-Belz [KLB].

The table on the next page contains an overview of some examples. Here we considered 13 G/G/1 queues, each with four values of the utilization factor ρ. The table shows the greatest errors we observed among the 13 queues, and the according maximum errors of three other approximate methods which we explain later on.

The densities of the interarrival time and service time are of the following types: exponential distribution (M), Gamma (Erlang) distribution (Γ_p or E_p, resp.) with the parameters b and p,

$$\frac{b^p}{\Gamma(p)} t^{p-1} e^{-bt},$$

hyperexponential distribution (H) with the parameters λ_1, λ_2, q,

$$q\lambda_1 e^{-\lambda_1 t} + (1-q)\lambda_2 e^{-\lambda_2 t},$$

and uniform distribution (U) over $[0, c]$, $c \in \mathbb{R}_+$. These are the 13 queues:
M/G/1 for $G \in \{M, H, U, \Gamma_{0.5}, E_4\}$ and
G/G'/1 for $G \in \{H, U, \Gamma_{0.5}, E_4\}$ and $G' \in \{M, E_2\}$.

Greatest observed relative errors [%]:

	$\rho = 0.5$	$\rho = 0.6$	$\rho = 0.8$	$\rho = 0.9$
M-Approximations:				
W_1	24.6	13.3	5.6	2.7
W_2	102	27.7	2.1	1.6
W_3	451	88.4	6.0	0.7
p_0 (abs. error [%])	21.8	16.4	5.6	2.0
Γ-Approximations:				
W_1	3.9	3.6	1.8	0.8
W_2	11.1	2.6	1.2	0.7
W_3	4.0	1.0	1.1	0.7
W_4	20.3	4.5	1.3	0.7
W_5	42.4	11.6	1.7	0.7
p_0 (abs. error [%])	22.4	12.7	3.0	3.9
W_{AC}	67.6	42.6	14.9	6.5
W_{KLB}	26.9	21.0	10.2	5.1
W_{MG}	17.3	13.2	5.9	2.8
p_{KLB} (abs. error [%])	28.8	33.4	46.8	54.9

We calculated the waiting time distributions for a series of succeeding jobs, until "equilibrium was reached". We defined this to happen when the according moments of two succeeding jobs differ from one another by a small amount, i.e. when $\Delta < 10^{-5}$, where

$$\Delta \stackrel{\text{def}}{=} \sum_{j \in \mathcal{K}} \left| \frac{W_j^{(n)} - W_j^{(n-1)}}{W_j^{(n)}} \right|. \tag{1}$$

In order to speed up this procedure, we consider transformed series of the parameters x_j, applying Aitken's Δ^2-method (see [ST], e.g.). These transformed series always converged more rapidly.

For the comparison we used approximations for the expectation of the waiting time by Allen and Cunneen [AC], by Krämer and Langenbach-Belz [KLB], and by Marchall and Gross (MG):

$$W_{AC} = \frac{\rho S_1}{2(1-\rho)}(C_T^2 + C_S^2),$$

$$W_{KLB} = \frac{S_1}{2(1-\rho)}(C_r^2 + C_S^2) \begin{cases} e^{\frac{-2(1-\rho)(1-C_T^2)}{3\rho(C_T^2+S_S^2)}}, & C_T^2 \leq 1, \\ e^{\frac{-(1-\rho)(C_T^2-1)}{C_T^2+4C_S^2}}, & C_T^2 \geq 1, \end{cases}$$

and

$$W_{MG} = \frac{1+C_S^2}{1/\rho^2 + C_S^2} \frac{\sigma_T^2 + \sigma_S^2}{2T_1(1-\rho)}$$

where

$$\sigma_T^2 = T_2 - T_1^2, \ \sigma_S^2 = S_2 - S_1^2,$$
$$C_T^2 = \sigma_T^2/T_1^2, \ C_S^2 = \sigma_S^2/S_1^2,$$

and we used the formula of Krämer and Langenbach-Belz approximating $p_0 = P\{W = 0\}$ [KLB],

$$p_{KLB} = 1 - \rho + \rho(1-\rho)(C_T^2 - 1) \begin{cases} \frac{1+C_T^2+\rho C_S^2}{1+\rho(C_S^2-1)+\rho^2(4C_T^2+C_S^2)}, & C_T^2 \leq 1, \\ \frac{4\rho}{C_T^2+\rho^2(4C_T^2+C_S^2)}, & C_T^2 \geq 1. \end{cases}$$

We tested our method 1 with further examples, including the case $\rho > 1$. For a $\Gamma_{0.5}/E_2/1$ queue we present the results more detailed:
If $T_1 = 1$, $S_1 = 0.6$, $\rho = 0.6$, the exact moments and p_0 are

$$W_1 = 1.29 \quad W_2 = 4.39 \quad W_3 = 22.32 \quad W_4 = 151.2 \quad W_5 = 1281$$

$$P\{W = 0\} = 0.274$$

Results: M-Approximations

$x_1^{(2)} = 0.597$	$x_2^{(2)} = 2.546$	$x_3^{(2)} = 0.384$
$W_1^{(2)} = 0.242$	$W_2^{(2)} = 0.190$	$W_3^{(2)} = 0.224$
$x_1^{(3)} = 0.584$	$x_2^{(3)} = 1.729$	$x_3^{(3)} = 0.322$
$W_1^{(3)} = 0.392$	$W_2^{(3)} = 0.454$	$W_3^{(3)} = 0.787$
$x_1^{(77)} = 0.597$	$x_2^{(77)} = 0.610$	$x_3^{(77)} = 0.239$

$$W_1^{(AIT)} = 1.25 \qquad W_2^{(AIT)} = 4.11 \qquad W_3^{(AIT)} = 20.3$$

$W_j^{(AIT)}$ denotes the moments calculated using the quoted Aitken series. The relative errors compared to the exact values are:

$$2.9\% \qquad\qquad 6.3\% \qquad\qquad 9.2\%$$

$$|P\{W = 0\} - x_3^{(77)}| = 0.035$$

Γ-Approximations:

$$x_1^{(2)} = 0.609 \qquad x_2^{(2)} = 0.509 \qquad x_3^{(2)} = 2.450 \qquad x_4^{(2)} = 4.040 \qquad x_5^{(2)} = 0.558$$
$$W_1^{(2)} = 0.268 \qquad W_2^{(2)} = 0.229 \qquad W_3^{(2)} = 0.252 \qquad W_4^{(2)} = 0.340 \qquad W_5^{(2)} = 0.542$$
$$x_1^{(3)} = 0.630 \qquad x_2^{(3)} = 0.510 \qquad x_3^{(3)} = 2.488 \qquad x_4^{(3)} = 3.000 \qquad x_5^{(3)} = 0.465$$
$$W_1^{(3)} = 0.443 \qquad W_2^{(3)} = 0.515 \qquad W_3^{(3)} = 0.771 \qquad W_4^{(3)} = 1.410 \qquad W_5^{(3)} = 3.048$$
$$x_1^{(109)} = 0.716 \qquad x_2^{(109)} = 0.521 \qquad x_3^{(109)} = 1.101 \qquad x_4^{(109)} = 0.611 \qquad x_5^{(109)} = 0.291$$
$$W_1^{(AIT)} = 1.28 \qquad W_2^{(AIT)} = 4.39 \qquad W_3^{(AIT)} = 22.3 \qquad W_4^{(AIT)} = 149.8 \qquad W_5^{(AIT)} = 1252$$

Relative errors of the $W_j^{(AIT)}$:

$$0.9\% \qquad\qquad 0.1\% \qquad\qquad\qquad 0.1\% \qquad\qquad\qquad 1\% \qquad\qquad\qquad 2.4\%$$

$$|P\{W = 0\} - x_5^{(109)}| = 0.017$$

Relative errors of the comparative formulae: W_{AC}: 12.7%, W_{KLB}: 21.0%, W_{MG}: 3.3%.

We applied the maximum entropy solution for a GE/GE/1 queue of Kouvatsos to this example, namely

$$W_{KOU} = \frac{h\rho + g(1 - h)}{hg\mu(1 - \rho)},$$

$$p_{KOU} = \frac{h(1 - \rho)}{h + g(1 - h)},$$

where $g = 2/(1 + C_S^2)$ and $h = 2/(1 + C_T^2)$. We got the following good results: The relative error of W_{KOU} is 9.5%, and $|P\{W = 0\} - p_{KOU}| = 0.034$.

If $\rho \leq 0.6$, Newton's iteration of the equations (5), Sec.3, did not converge in some rare examples for one or two jobs; in this case we applied the N-Approximation for these jobs. Other numerical problems were sometimes observed if the moments differ by orders of magnitude. This could be handled by scaling. A third type of problem occured when the calculated parameters become smaller than ϵ. This can happen if the utilization factor is greater than 1: $P\{W^{(n)} = 0\} \approx a = x_K$ becomes arbitrarily small, and the equations (5), Sec.3, do not depend on a and p any longer. In this case the moments can be calculated easily by $W^{(n)} \approx W^{(n-1)} + C$, using (7), Sec.3, or by N-approximations.

5. APPROXIMATING THE DENSITIES PIECEWISE

At the end of Section 3 we remarked that a large number of parameters of the approximating densities are beneficial. This cannot be achieved by increasing the order of the DMEs. Therefore we consider in this section approximations for densities, consisting of some DMEs over pairwise disjunct intervals of the sample space, i.e.

$$X_{-\infty} \stackrel{\text{def}}{=} (-\infty, -Nd),$$

$$X_i \stackrel{\text{def}}{=} [id, (i+1)d), \ i \in \mathcal{L},$$

$$X_\infty \stackrel{\text{def}}{=} [Ld, \infty),$$

where $d \in I\!R^+ = (0, \infty)$, $N, L \in I\!N_0$, $\mathcal{L} \stackrel{\text{def}}{=} [-N : L-1]$. The DME over $X_{-\infty}$ has the order K_1, the DME over X_∞ the order K_3, and the other ones the order K_2. We call such densities "$K_1 K_2 K_3$-densities".

Here we get a method, which has some advantages compared with our first method:
-   There is no non-linear equation to be solved
-   The accuracy of the results can be controlled by choosing appropriate parameters N, L, d, but we are not able to estimate the approximation errors. Naturally, larger values of N and L lead to more computing time.
-   There is no restriction with respect to the utilization factor ρ.

In the sequel we consider the simplest case, i.e. 101-densities, denoted by γ:

$$\gamma(t) = \begin{cases} c'e^{\lambda't}, & \text{if } t \in X_{-\infty}, \\ f_i, & \text{if } t \in X_i, \ i \in \mathcal{L}, \\ ce^{-\lambda t}, & \text{if } t \in X_\infty. \end{cases}$$

These densities are represented by the parameters $c', \lambda', c, \lambda, N, L, d$ and $f_i, i \in \mathcal{L}$, where $f_i, c', \lambda', c, \lambda \in I\!R_+ = [0, \infty)$.

If the order K_2 is 1 or greater, non-linear equations must be solved to get the parameters for the densities over the $X_i, i \in \mathcal{L}$. But in [STR] a method is proposed, how to do this approximatly by linear equations. Orders K_1 and K_3 greater than 1 lead also to non-linear equations, and impose serious numerical problems.

Now we define some operations concerning 101-densities, which we shall need in order to describe the algorithm.

Γ_{101} is the operator which transforms a density into a 101-density where the parameters N, L and d are given. It is defined as follows. Let $f(t)$ be a given density, and

$$F(t) \stackrel{\text{def}}{=} \int_{-\infty}^{t} f(x)dx, \quad M(t) \stackrel{\text{def}}{=} \int_{-\infty}^{t} xf(x)dx, \quad t \in I\!R.$$

Then we choose the remaining parameters:

$$\lambda' := \frac{1}{-Nd - \frac{M(-Nd)}{F(-Nd)}}, \quad c' := \lambda' F(-Nd) e^{\lambda' Nd} \quad \text{if } F(0) > 0,$$

$$\lambda' := 1 \ (\text{any constant} > 0), \quad c' := 0 \quad \text{otherwise};$$

$$\lambda := \frac{1}{\frac{M(\infty) - M(Ld)}{1 - F(Ld)} - Ld}, \quad c := \lambda\big(1 - F(Ld)\big) e^{\lambda Ld} \quad \text{if } F(0) < 1,$$

$$\lambda := 1, \quad c := 0, \quad \text{otherwise};$$

$$f_i := \Big(F((i+1)d) - F(id)\Big)/d, \quad i \in \mathcal{L}.$$

This means, that the 101-densities over $X_{-\infty}$ and X_{∞} are DMEs of the order 1, for which the probabilities $P\{X_{-\infty}\}$ and $P\{X_{\infty}\}$ and the first moments agree with those of the initial density $f(t)$. For the densities f_i, only the probabilities $P\{X_i\}$ agree.

$\otimes_{101}$ is the operator, which delivers a 101-density, say $\gamma(t)$, as an approximation for the convolution of two 101-densities, say $\gamma_1(t)$ and $\gamma_2(t)$. If the parameters N, L and d of γ are given, $\otimes_{101}$ is defined as follows:

$$\gamma_1 \otimes_{101} \gamma_2 = \gamma \stackrel{\text{def}}{=} \Gamma_{101}(\gamma_1 \otimes \gamma_2).$$

Here $\otimes$ denotes the usual convolution. This formula looks very simple, but it is rather cumbersome to write it down explicity, which fills lots of pages with formulae, and to program them, which gives some hundred lines of code.

MAX_{101} is the operator, which delivers the distribution of the r.v. $max(X, 0)$, where X is a r.v. with a 101-density, say $\gamma(t)$:

$$MAX_{101}\gamma = (\tilde{\gamma}, \, p_0),$$

where $\tilde{\gamma}$ is the 101-density with the paramaters $c, \lambda, L, (f_i, i \in [0 : L-1])$ being the same as for γ, and

$$c' = 0, \ \lambda' = 1, \ N = 0.$$

$\tilde{\gamma}$ is not really a density, but it is $\gamma_{X|X>0}(t) P\{X > 0\}$. Nevertheless, we shall denominate it an 101-density. The other part is the probability $P\{X \le 0\}$:

$$p_0 = \int\limits_{-\infty}^{0} \gamma(t)dt.$$

Now we are prepared to write down the algorithm for the calculation of the distributions of the waiting times, successively for the 2nd, 3rd, 4th, ... job. They are of the type just introduced when explaining the MAX_{101} operator.

Algorithm for the calculation of 101-densities of the waiting times of the 2nd, 3rd, 4th, ... job. (f_X denotes the density of a r.v. X)
choose the parameters N, L, d for all 101-densities;
$\gamma_{-T} := \Gamma_{101} f_{-T}$;

$\gamma_S := \Gamma_{101} f_S;$

$\gamma_C := \gamma_S \otimes_{101} \gamma_{-T};$

$n := 2; \quad \{\text{ number of the job}\}$

$\gamma_{\widetilde{W}} := \gamma_C; \quad \{\text{pseudo waiting time of the 2nd job}\}$

repeat

$\quad (\gamma_W, p_0) := MAX_{101} \, \gamma_{\widetilde{W}}; \quad \{\text{waiting time of the } n\text{th job}\}$

$\quad n := n + 1;$

$\quad \gamma_{\widetilde{W}} := \Gamma_{101}(p_0 \gamma_C + \gamma_W \otimes_{101} \gamma_C); \quad \{\text{pseudo waiting time of the } n\text{th job}\}$

until equilibrium.

The equilibrium is stipulated according to (1), Sec.4.

We conclude this section by presenting some numerical results. We executed an experiment with 10 queues, every one with four values of the utilization factor ρ:
M/G/1 for G $\in$ {M, H, U, E$_4$ } and
G/G'/1 for G $\in$ {H, U, E$_4$ } and G' $\in$ {M, E$_2$}.

An overview of the results is contained in the subsequent table. Let N_q, L_q, $q \in \{T, S, C\}$, and d, denote the parameters N, L, d of the 101-densities of the interarrival times, the service times, and their difference C, respectively. We fixed $L_T + L_S = 50$, $N_S = 0$, $N_T = 0$, $N_C = L_T$, and $L_C = L_S$, and determined L_T, L_S, d heuristically: $L_S/L_T \approx S_1/T_1$, and the value of d by some trials - not very systematically.

Greatest observed relative errors [%]:

	$\rho = 0.1$	$\rho = 0.3$	$\rho = 0.5$	$\rho = 0.9$
101-Approximations:				
W_1	11.1	3.5	2.2	2.9
W_2	14.2	4.6	3.0	5.4
W_3	17.7	6.6	4.0	7.9
p_0 (abs. error [%])	0.4	0.5	0.3	0.3
W_{AC}	1904	197	67.6	6.5
W_{KLB}	95.4	49.7	20.1	1.2
W_{MG}	917	67.6	17.4	2.8
p_{KLB} (abs. error [%])	11.0	23.8	16.2	38.7

As can be seen, the results are accurate, particularly the computed values of $P\{W = 0\}$. The accuracy does not strongly depend on the utilization factor ρ. No numerical problems occurred.

We were able to improve significantly the accuracy of the results by searching better values of L_S/L_T and d. From this we conclude that a careful treatment of these matters should be done. Another useful development concerning $K_1 K_2 K_3$-densities would be considering higher orders K_2.

CONCLUSION

We showed how to analyze a special Markov process, the waiting times of a G/G/1 queue, approximating the densities piecewise by DMEs or DMCs, and iterating the Chapman-Kolmogorov equations. These densities are defined by some parameters: either moments, or the proper parameters of the DMEs (DMCs).

It was demonstrated that the considered processes can be analysed accurately and in detail.

A serious problem is the calculation of the parameters of a DME from given moments. To this end, non-linear equations must be solved in general. Method 1 proceeds in this manner, but some open questions remain: How great are the errors? Can conditioned DMEs be accurate? What about existence and uniqueness of the solutions of the non-linear equations? Are the Newton iterations convergent?

Some of these problems are solved by method 2, where the solution of non-linear equations is not necessary, and where the remark concerning the inaccuracy of conditioned DMEs does not apply. The question of accuracy remains open, of course.

LITERATURE

[AC] A.O. Allen: Probability, Statistics, and Queueing Theory. Academic Press, New York, 1978

[AK] M.A. El-Affendi and D.D. Kouvatsos: A Maximum Entropy Analysis of the M/G/1 and G/M/1 Queueing Systems at Equilibrium. Acta Informatica 19 (1983), p. 339

[GK] Gnedenko, König: Handbuch der Bedienungstheorie, Band 2. Akademie-Verlag, Berlin, 1984

[HA] G. Haßlinger: Das Näherungsverfahren nach dem Prinzip der maximalen Entropie für Warteschlangen-Verteilungen in geschlossenen Netzwerken. Thesis, Technische Hochschule Darmstadt, 1986

[KA] A.M. Kagan, Yu.V. Linnik, and C.R. Rao: Characterization Problems in Mathematical Statistics. J. Wiley, New York, 1973

[KL] L. Kleinrock: Queueing Systems, Vol. 1. J. Wiley, New York, 1975

[KLB] W. Kämer and M. Langenbach-Belz: Approximate Formulare for the Delay in the Queueing System G/G/1. In: Proc. 8th Intern. Teletraffic Congr. (ITC8), Melbourne, 1976, p. 235-1

[K1] D.D. Kouvatsos: A Universal Maximum Entropy Algorithm for the Analysis of General Closed Networks. In: T.Hasegawa, H.Takagi, Y.Takahashi (Hrsg.), Computer Networking and Performance Evaluation, Elsvier Science Publishers, Amsterdam, 1986, p. 113

[K2] D.D. Kouvatsos: A Maximum Entropy Queue Length Distribution for a G/G/1 Finite Capacity Queue. ACM Performance Evaluation Review, Vol.14, No.1 (1986), p. 224

[S] J. E. Shore: Information Theoretic Approximations for M/G/1 and G/G/1 Queueing Systems. Acta Informatica 17, 1982, p. 43

[SJ] J. E. Shore and R. W. Johnson: Axiomatic Derivation of the Principle of Maximum Entropy and the Principle of Minimum Cross-Entropy. IEEE Trans. Inf. Theory, Vol. IT-26, No. 1, Jan 1980, p. 26-37

[SM] W. J. Smirnow: Lehrgang der höheren Mathematik, Teil IV, Berlin 1961.

[ST] J. Stoer: Einführung in die Numerische Mathematik. Springer, Berlin, Heidelberg, New York, 1976

[STR] J. Ch. Strelen: Lineare Berechnungsverfahren für Wahrscheinlichkeitsverteilungen mit maximaler Entropie. Interner Bericht II/86/1, Institut für Informatik, Universität Bonn, 1986

[TZ] H. Tzschach: The Principle of Maximum Entropy applied to Queueing Systems. Bericht TI-2, Fachbereich Informatik, Technische Hochschule Darmstadt, 1983.

[T] H. Tzschach: Information Theoretic Approximations of Queueing Systems and Queueing Networks. Bericht des Fachbereichs Informatik, Technische Hochschule Darmstadt, 1986

[W] R.J. Walstra: Nonexponential Networks of Queues: A Maximum Entropy Analysis. ACM Sigmetrics, 1985, p. 27

TWO-STAGE CYCLIC NETWORK WITH BLOCKING :

CYCLE TIME DISTRIBUTION AND EQUIVALENCE PROPERTIES

S.Balsamo and L.Donatiello

Dipartimento di Informatica
University of Pisa
Pisa, Italy

ABSTRACT

An efficient algorithm is provided to compute the cycle time distribution for a cyclic two-stage queueing network with exponential servers and blocking. Blocking phenomenon occurs when a job attempting to enter a full stage is forced to remain in its source stage, thus blocking the source server until the destination stage releases a job. By using some equivalence properties between models with different finite capacity sizes, we derive the conditions under which the cycle time distribution is independent of the relative values of the finite capacity sizes.

1. INTRODUCTION

The finite capacity queue can be used to represent significant characteristics such as memory constraints or software resource constraints in computer systems, as well as window flow control in communication networks [1,8,13,17]. In systems with finite capacity, when a job attempts to enter a full queue, it is rejected and the blocking phenomenon arises. An extensive bibliography on queueing networks with blocking can be found in [16]. Queueing networks with blocking are in general difficult to treat. All the known results concern the steady-state queue length distribution and average performance indices like throughput, utilization, etc. [1,2,8,13,14,15,17,18], while no solution is known on cycle time distribution.

In the literature several types of blocking have been considered, corresponding to different application fields. We shall consider the blocking type which is defined as follows. A job upon completion of its service in a node (i) attempts to enter a new node (j) which is full. The job is forced to wait in the server of source node i until it is allowed to enter destination node j. The server of source node i stops processing jobs, i.e., it is blocked, until destination node j releases a job. In other words, the service will be resumed as soon as a departure occurs from queue j. This blocking mechanism has been used to model production systems and disk I/O subsystems [1,14,17,18,19].

In this paper we provide an efficient algorithm to compute the cycle time distribution (CTD) for a closed cyclic exponential two-stage network where both the nodes have finite capacity. The solution technique is based on a recursive scheme with the number of users (N) in the network, and its computational complexity is of the order of N^3. Moreover, we provide an equivalence relation for the CTD between models with different finite capacity sizes.

This work has been partially supported by M.P.I. Research Project Found.

Consequently, we prove that the CTD depends only on the sum of the two finite capacity sizes while it is independent of their relative values.

The paper is organized as follows. In section 2 the model is introduced. An expression for the cycle time distribution is given in section 3, while the computational details are reported in Appendix. Equivalence relations between models with different finite capacity sizes are presented in section 4, while section 5 provides a numerical example.

2. THE MODEL

Consider a two-stage cyclic closed queueing network where N users are cycling, as shown in Fig.1. Service times at servers 1 and 2 are exponentially distributed with parameters

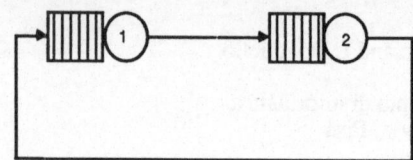

Fig. 1 - Two-stage closed cyclic network

μ_1 and μ_2, respectively. Both nodes are single server queue with FCFS discipline. Let $M_i < N$ denote the finite capacity of node i, where i=1,2. In order to avoid empty state space we assume that $M_1 + M_2 \geq N$.

When a job (x) completes its service at node 2 (1) attempts to enter node 1 (2) ; if node 1 (2) is full (with a job (y) in service), then job (x) is forced to wait in node 2 (1), thus blocking its service. When node 1 (2) releases job (y) the following transition takes place: job (y) is placed in node 2 (1) and, at the same time, job (x) is placed in node 1 (2), while node 2 (1) service is resumed.

In order to simplify state notation, we assume an extra position in both the queues. In this case when job (x) completes its service at node 2 (1) while node 1 (2) is full, then it is placed in the extra queue position of node 1 (2). As a consequence, $B_1 = M_1 + 1$ and $B_2 = M_2 + 1$ become the new finite capacity sizes of the two nodes.

We are interested in the cycle time distribution, i.e., the time between two consecutive departures of a particular customer (tagged job) from node 2 (i.e., arrivals to node 1) *. In the case of infinite capacity queues, i.e., $B_i = N$, for i = 1, 2, the cycle time distribution has been derived by Chow as a closed form solution [10]. Successively, Shassenberger and Daduna [20] and Boxma et alt. [6] obtained a closed form for the Laplace-Stieltjes transform (LST) for a cyclic model with more than two queues in tandem. Related works are [4,5,7,9,11,12]. Under the assumption of a node with finite capacity, the cycle time distribution is not known. We provide a closed form solution which works in the time domain, and an efficient algorithm for the computation of formula coefficients.

3. CYCLE TIME DISTRIBUTION

In order to compute the cycle time distribution we first derive the steady-state probabilities at arrival times at node 1 in the network with N customers and finite capacities B_1 and B_2.

Consider the queueing network at arrival times of a job at node 1. Let (n,q) denote the state (just after the arrival of a job at node 1) of the network when there are n and q jobs in the first and second queue, respectively. Then (n,q) is an irreducible homogeneous aperiodic discrete time Markov process, with state space A_0 defined as follows :

---

* Note that, if we consider the time between two consecutive arrivals to node 1 without considering the extra queue position, we define a different cycle time, which can be still analyzed by using a similar technique.

$$A_0 = \{ (n,q) \mid n+q=N, \ q=N-B_1,...,B_2-1 \}$$

and matrix $S = \| S[(n,q),(n',q')] \|$ of transition probabilities is defined as follows:

$$S[(j,N-j),(k,N-k)] = \frac{\mu_2}{\mu_1 + \mu_2} \qquad \text{if } k=j+1$$

$$S[(j,N-j),(k,N-k)] = \frac{\mu_1^{j+1-k} \mu_2}{(\mu_1 + \mu_2)^{j+2-k}} \qquad \text{if } k=j,...,N-B+2$$

$$S[(j,N-j),(k,N-k)] = \frac{\mu_1^{j-(N-B)}}{(\mu_1 + \mu_2)^{j-(N-B)}} \qquad \text{if } k=N-B+1$$

for $j=N-B_2+1,...,\ B_1-1$ and $B=B_1+B_2-N$, and

$$S[(B_1,N-B_1),(k,N-k)] = S[(B_1-1,N-B_1+1),(k,N-k)] \qquad \text{for } k=N-B_2+1,...,B_1 .$$

One can prove [3] that the steady-state probabilities $P_A=\{P_A(n,q), (n,q) \in A_0\}$ can be computed as steady-state probabilities at random time in a system with N-1 customers and finite capacities B_1 and B_2-1, at nodes 1 and 2, respectively. Therefore probabilities P_A yield the following product form solution [1] :

$$P_A(n,q)= C_1^{-1} \mu_1^{q'} \mu_2^{B-1-q'} \qquad \forall (n,q)\in A_0 \qquad (1)$$

where : $q' = q-N+B_1$, $B = B_1+ B_2-N$, and

$$C_1 = \sum_{q' = 0}^{B-1} \mu_1^{q'} \mu_2^{B-1-q'}$$

In order to compute the cycle time distribution, let us introduce a new transient Markov process T with state space E defined as follows:

$$E = \{ (n,q,p) \mid n+q=N , \ p=0,...,N , \ q=N-B_1,...,\min\{N-B_1+p, B_2\} \} \qquad (2)$$

where (n,q,p) denote the state of the network when there are n and q jobs in the first and second queue, respectively, and p jobs which must be served by node 2 before the end of the cycle of the tagged job. In other words, component p represents the position of the tagged job during its cycle. Transition rate matrix $R = \| R[(n,q,p),(n',q',p')] \|$, with $(n,q,p),(n',q',p')\in E$, is defined as follows:

$$\begin{aligned} R[(n,q,p), (n',q',p')] &= \mu_1 & &\text{if } p'=p, \ n'=n-1, \ q'=q+1 \\ R[(n,q,p), (n',q',p')] &= \mu_2 & &\text{if } p'=p-1, \ n'=n+1, q'=q-1 \\ R[(n,q,p), (n',q',p')] &= 0 & &\text{otherwise} \end{aligned}$$
$$(3)$$

We shall use this stochastic process T, represented in Fig.2, to evaluate the cycle time distribution. Set E_0 (subset of E), defined as

$$E_0 = \{ (n,q,p) \mid n+q=N, \ p=N, \ q=N-B_1,...,B_2-1 \}$$

contains all the possible initial states, i.e., all those system states (n,q,p) that arise at arrival times of the tagged job at node 1, and set $E-E_0$ contains all the intermediate states of the evaluation process. Finally, when the tagged job completes its service at node 2, then process T is in the absorbing state $(B_1,N-B_1,0)$.

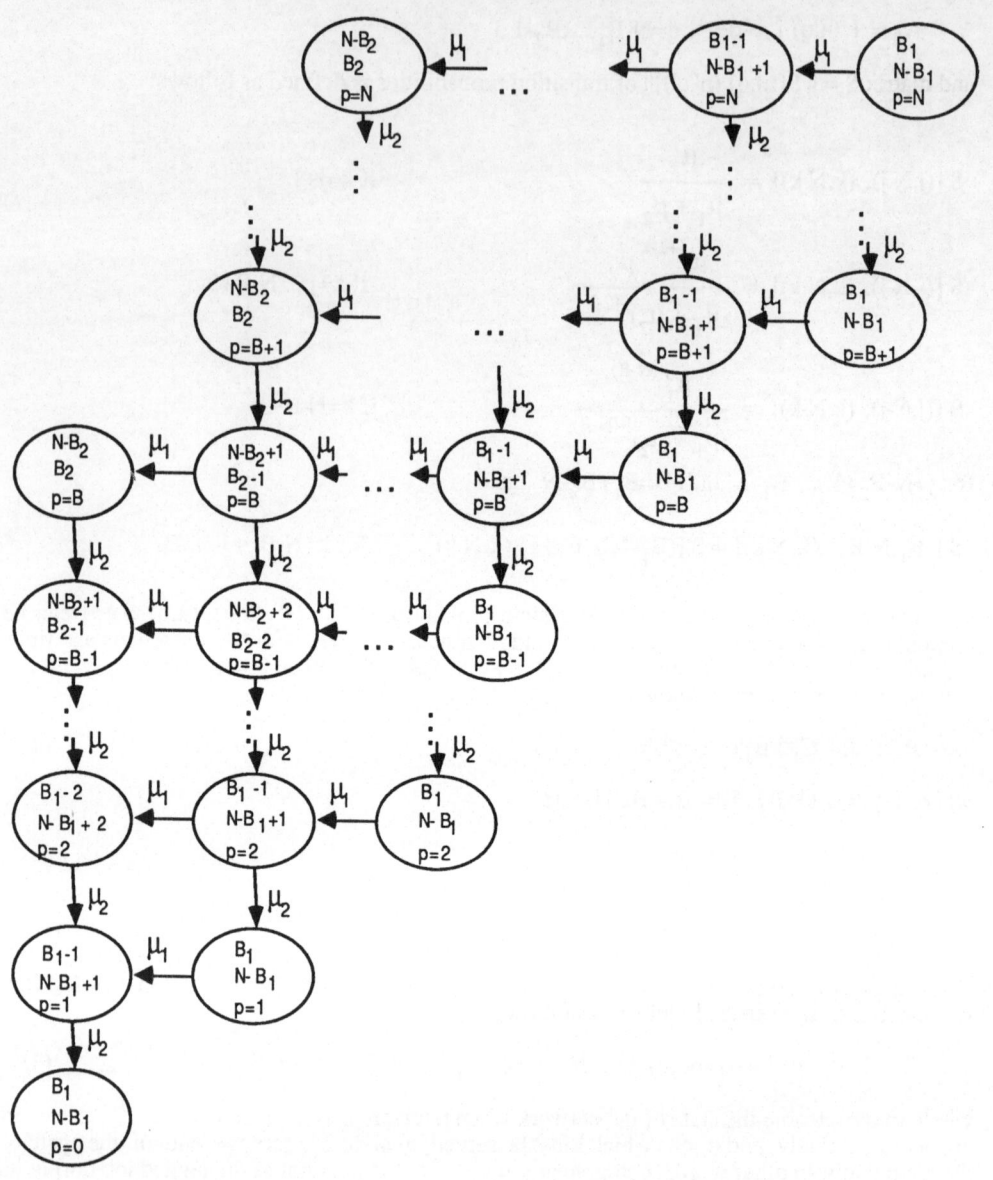

Fig. 2 - Stochastic process T: state transition graph representation

In conclusion, the evaluating problem of the cycle time distribution is reduced to the evaluation of the first hitting time distribution of process T to state $(B_1, N-B_1, 0)$, starting from any state in E_0. Steady-state probabilities $P=\{P(n,q,N), (n,q,N) \in E_0\}$ of the tagged job at arrival time at node 1 can be computed by formula (1), i.e., $P(n,q,N)=P_A(n,q), \forall (n,q)\in A_0$.

Let $T(n,q,p,s)$ denote the LST of the passage time distribution from state (n,q,p) to state $(B_1, N-B_1, 0)$. By using definition (3) we can write the following recursive relations:

$$T(n, q, p, s) = \frac{\mu_2}{\mu_2 + s} T(n+1, q-1, p-1, s) \quad \text{for } n = N - B_2, ..., B_1 - 1; \quad q = N - n \text{ and } p = B_1 - n$$

$$\text{(4)}$$

$$T(N - B_2, B_2, p, s) = \frac{\mu_2}{\mu_2 + s} T(N - B_2 + 1, B_2 - 1, p - 1, s) \quad \text{for } p = B + 1, ..., N$$

$$T(n, q, p, s) = \frac{\mu_1}{\mu_3 + s} T(n - 1, q + 1, p, s) + \frac{\mu_2}{\mu_3 + s} T(n + 1, q - 1, p - 1, s) \quad \text{(5)}$$

for $p = 2, ..., B$, and $n = B_1 + 1 - p..., B_1 - 1$, and

for $p = B + 1, ..., N$, and $n = N - B_2 + 1, ..., B_1 - 1$

$$T(B_1, N - B_1, p, s) = \frac{\mu_1}{\mu_1 + s} T(B_1 - 1, N - B_1 + 1, p, s) \quad \text{for } p = 1, ..., N \quad \text{(6)}$$

with $T(B_1, N-B_1, 0, s) = 1$ and $\mu_3 = \mu_1 + \mu_2$.

Let $F_{N,B1,B2}(s)$ denote the LST of the cycle time distribution of the two-stage closed cyclic network with N customers and finite capacities B_1 and B_2, which is defined as follows:

$$F_{N,B1,B2}(s) = \sum_{(n,q,p) \in E_0} P(n,q,p) \, T(n,q,p,s) \quad \text{(7)}$$

where probabilities $P(n,q,p)$ are given by (1), and $T(n,q,p,s)$ are recursively defined by (4)-(6). Let $F_{N,B1,B2}(t)$ denote the cycle time distribution for the two-stage closed cyclic network with N customers and nodes with finite capacites B_1 and B_2, respectively. Hereafter we shall assume that $B>2$. Cases $B=1,2$ have a trivial solution. By inverting formula (7) and by using recursive relations (4)-(6), an explicit expression in the time domain is obtained as follows:

Theorem 1

$$F_{N,B1,B2}(t) = \sum_{j=1}^{3} \left\{ \sum_{i=1}^{k_j} \frac{c_{ji}}{\mu_j^i} - e^{-\mu_j t} \sum_{z=0}^{k_j-1} \frac{t^z}{z!} \sum_{i=1}^{k_j-z} \frac{c_{j\,i+z}}{\mu_j^i} \right\}$$

$$\text{(8)}$$

with $k_1 = k_2 = N$ and $k_3 = 2N-3$; coefficients c_{ji} are recursively computed, for each i and j, as reported in Appendix.
Proof. see Appendix.

Formula (8) requires the evaluation of coefficients c_{ji} , for a total computational complexity of $O(N^3)$, as shown in Appendix.

Note that the proposed solution provides the result directly in the time domain.

4. EQUIVALENCE PROPERTIES

In this section we show an equivalence relation for the CTD between the model with only

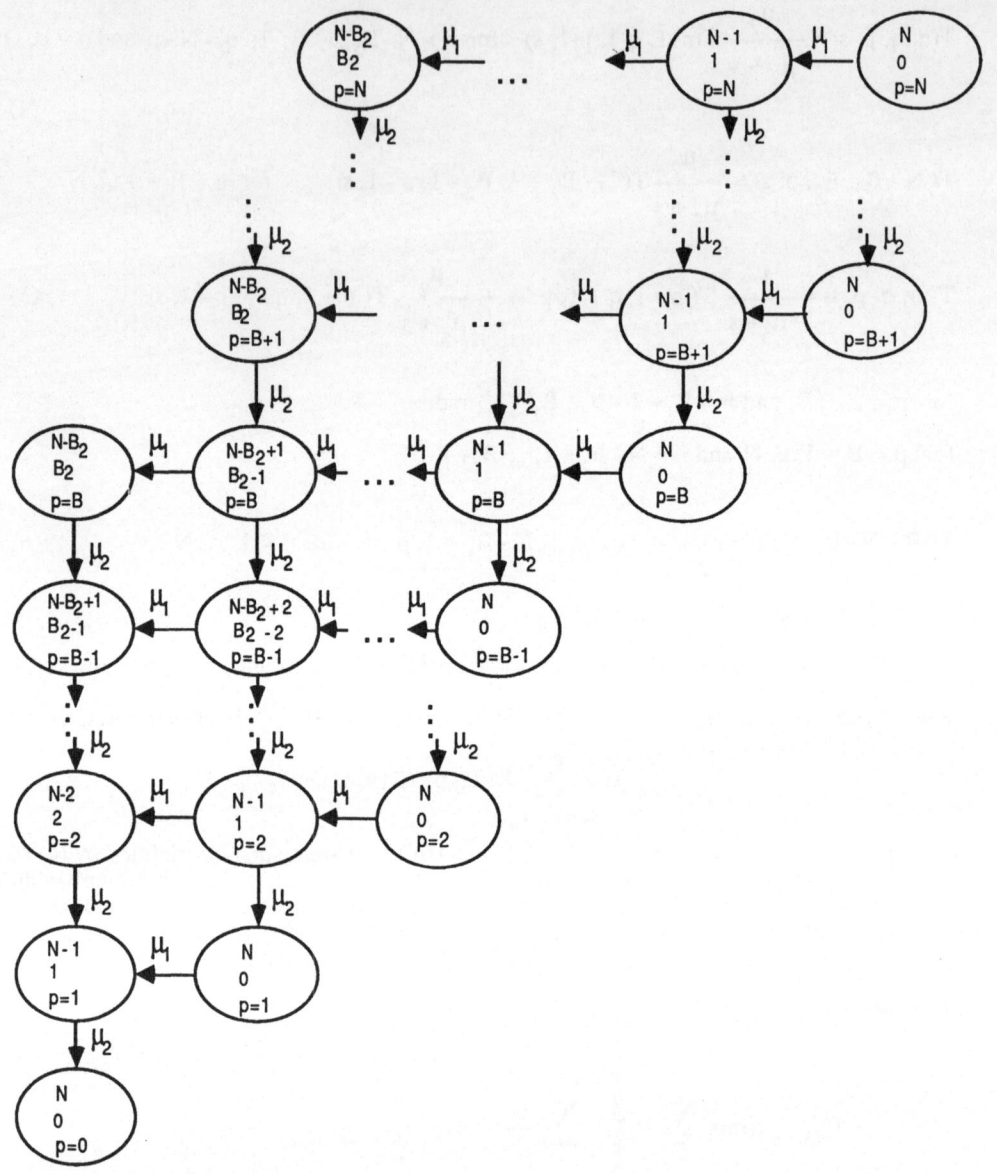

Fig. 3 - Stochastic process T of model 2 : state transition graph representation

one node of finite capacity and the model with both the nodes of finite capacity.

Consider a two-stage cyclic closed queueing network with N users and where only node 2 has finite capacity, i.e., $B_1 = N$ and $B_2 < N$. In order to compute the CTD (i.e., the time between two consecutive arrivals at node 1) we apply the same solution technique of the previous model. Hence, set E_0 of all possible initial states is given by:

$$E_0 = \{ (n,q,p) \mid n+q=N, p=N, q=0,...,B_2-1 \}$$

The steady-steate probabilities $P=\{P(n,q,p), (n,q,p) \in E_0\}$ at arrivals time can be computed by formula (1) where $B=B_2$. State space E becomes:

$$E = \{ (n,q,p) \mid n+q=N , p=0,...,N , q=0,...,\min\{p, B_2\} \}$$

and transition rate matrix is defined by (3). Therefore, the evaluation of the CTD is reduced to the evaluation of the first hitting time distribution of process T to state $(N,0,0)$ starting from any state in E_0. Hence, one can apply formula (8) to compute the CTD in a model with $B_1=N$ and $B_2 < N$.

We shall now define an equivalence relation between the following models:

Model 1) N customers, service rates μ_1 and μ_2, and both nodes with finite capacities B_1 and B_2 respectively.

Model 2) N customers, service rates μ_1 and μ_2, and only node 2 with finite capacity $B=B_1+B_2-N$.

By comparing the two models, one can observe that the two processes T, defined to compute the CTD, are isomorphic (see Fig. 2 and Fig. 3). Therefore the following relation between model 1 and model 2 holds:

Theorem 2

$$F_{N,B1,B2}(s) = F_{N,N,B}(s)$$

An immediate consequence of Theorem 2 is that the cycle time distribution $F_{N,B1,B2}(t)$

depends only on values N and B, given service rates μ_1 and μ_2, while it is independent of the single values of the finite capacities B_i, with $i=1,2$. In other words, the CTD for the same network with different finite capacity values B_1' and B_2' is equal to $F_{N,B1,B2}(t)$, provided that $B_1'+B_2' = B_1+B_2$. This property is expressed by the following corollary.

Corollary

$$F_{N,B1,B2}(s) = F_{N, B1 + i, B2 - i}(s)$$

for $i=B_2-N,..., N-B_1$.

5. NUMERICAL EXAMPLE

Consider the two-stage cyclic network with $N=10$ customers, service rates $\mu_1=1$ and $\mu_2=2$, and finite capacities B_1 and B_2 such that $B = B_1 + B_2- N = 1,...,10$. The comparison between the CTD among the different values of B is shown in Fig.4.

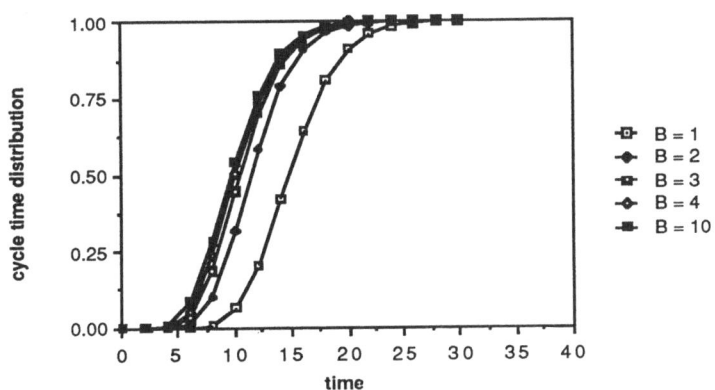

Fig. 4 - Influence on the cycle time distribution of factor B.

Note that as factor B increases, the relative CTD approaches CTD with B=N, which corresponds to the model with only one node with finite capacity, equal to B. Moreover, starting from the value $B^{\wedge}=5$ the difference between the distributions is negligible. In other words, increasing values B_1 and B_2 more than value such that $B>B^{\wedge}$ does not provide a substantial improvement in the CTD. Such a parametric analysis on the blocking factor can be helpful in determining the minimum B which guarantees a required cycle time level (value). For example, from Fig.4, one can derive that the cycle time is guaranteed to be less than or equal to 13.5 with 0.75 probability for the minimum B=2, and for B=2,...,10 with probability greater than or equal to 0.75.

6. CONCLUSIONS

An efficient algorithm is provided to compute the cycle time distribution for a cyclic two-stage queueing network with exponential servers and blocking. The algorithm is based on a recursive scheme with the number of customers, and is characterized by a computational complexity of $O(N^3)$. An equivalence relation is proved between the CTD of the model with one finite capacity queue and the model with both queues of finite capacity. Moreover, the CTD has been shown to depend only on values N and B, while it is independent of the relative values of finite capacities B_i, i=1,2.

APPENDIX

The cycle time distribution for the two-stage network with N customers and finite capacities B_1 and B_2 given by expression (8) requires the recursive computation of coefficients c_{ji} for each i and j, as follows :

$$c_{1i} = \sum_{z=N-B+1}^{N} P(n, N-n, N)\, \delta_i^z(N) \qquad\qquad i = 1,..., N-B+1$$

$$c_{1i} = \sum_{z=i}^{N} P(n, N-n, N)\, \delta_i^z(N) \qquad\qquad i = N-B+2,..., N$$

$$c_{2i} = \sum_{z=N-B+1}^{N} P(n, N-n, N)\, \beta_i^z(N) \qquad\qquad i = 1,..., N$$

$$c_{3i} = \sum_{z=N-B+1}^{N} P(n, N-n, N)\, \gamma_i^z(N) \qquad\qquad i = 1,..., 2N-B-1$$

$$c_{3i} = \sum_{z=i+2-N}^{N} P(n, N-n, N)\, \gamma_i^z(N) \qquad\qquad i = 2N-B,...,2N-3$$

$$(A.1)$$

where $B=B_1+B_2-N$, $n=z-N+B_1$, probabilities $P(n,N-n,p)$ at arrival time in node 1 are given by formula (1), and coefficients $\beta_i^z(N)$, $\gamma_i^z(N)$, and $\delta_i^z(N)$, for each i and z are recursively computed as follows:

1) for k+1=2,...,B and z=1,...,k , and for k+1=B+1, ...,N and z=k+2-B,...,k :

$$\beta_i^z(k+1) = \beta_i^{z-1}(k+1) + \frac{1}{\mu_1}\left\{ \mu_2\,\beta_i^z(k) - \beta_{i+1}^z(k+1) \right\} \qquad i = 1,...,k$$

$$\beta_i^z(k+1) = \beta_{k+1}^{z-1}(k+1) \qquad\qquad\qquad i = k+1$$

$$\delta_i^z(k+1) = \delta_i^z(k) + \frac{1}{\mu_2}\left\{ \mu_1\,\delta_i^{z-1}(k+1) - \delta_{i+1}^z(k+1) \right\} \qquad i = 1,...,z-1$$

$$\delta_i^z(k+1) = \delta_i^z(k) \qquad\qquad\qquad i = z$$

$$\gamma_i^z(k+1) = \sum_{j=1}^{k+1} (-1)^j \frac{\beta_j^{z-1}(k+1)}{\mu_1^{j-1}} + \sum_{j=1}^{k} (-1)^j \frac{\mu_2\,\beta_j^z(k)}{\mu_1^j} + \sum_{j=1}^{z}(-1)^j \frac{\delta_j^z(k)}{\mu_2^{j-1}} + \sum_{j=1}^{z-1} (-1)^j \frac{\mu_1\,\delta_j^{z-1}(k+1)}{\mu_2^j}$$

$$i=1$$

and if k>1

$$\gamma_i^z(k+1) = \mu_2\,\gamma_{i-1}^z(k) + \mu_1\,\gamma_{i-1}^{z-1}(k+1) \qquad\qquad \text{for } i=2,...,k-1+z \text{ and } z=2,...,k-1,$$
$$\text{and for } i=2,...,k-2+z \text{ and } z=k$$

$$\gamma_i^z(k+1) = \mu_2\,\gamma_{i-1}^z(k) \qquad\qquad\qquad \text{for } i=k-1+z \text{ and } z=k$$

$$\gamma_i^z (k+1) = \mu_1 \, \gamma_{i-1}^{z-1} (k+1) \qquad\qquad \text{for } i=2,\ldots,k-1+z \text{ and } z=1$$

2) for k+1=1,...,N and z= k+1 :

$$\beta_i^{k+1} (k+1) = \frac{1}{\mu_1 - \mu_2} \left\{ \mu_1 \beta_i^k (k+1) - \beta_{i+1}^{k+1} (k+1) \right\} \qquad i = 1,\ldots,k$$

$$\beta_i^{k+1} (k+1) = \frac{\mu_1}{\mu_1 - \mu_2} \beta_i^k (k+1) \qquad\qquad i = k+1$$

$$\delta_i^{k+1} (k+1) = \mu_1 \left\{ \sum_{j=1}^{k+1} \frac{\beta_j^k (k+1)}{(\mu_2 - \mu_1)^j} + \sum_{j=1}^{\lim(k+1,k)} \frac{\gamma_j^k (k+1)}{\mu_2^{\,j}} \right\} \qquad i=1$$

$$\delta_i^{k+1} (k+1) = \mu_1 \, \delta_{i-1}^k (k+1) \qquad\qquad i=2,\ldots,k+1$$

where function lim(k,j) is defined as follows :

$$\lim (k, 0) = 0 \qquad\qquad \text{for } k=1,\ldots,B$$

$$\lim (k, k-B) = 2k-B-3 \qquad\qquad \text{for } k=B+1,\ldots,N$$

$$\lim (k, j) = k-2+j \qquad\qquad \begin{array}{l} \text{for } k=1,\ldots,B \text{ and } j=1,\ldots,k-1 \text{ and} \\ \text{for } k=B+1,\ldots,N \text{ and } j=k-B+1,\ldots,k-1 \end{array}$$

$$\lim (k, k) = 2k-3 \qquad\qquad \text{for } k=1,\ldots,N$$

3) for k+1=2,...,N and z= k+1 :

$$\gamma_i^{k+1}(k+1) = \frac{1}{\mu_2} \left\{ \gamma_{i+1}^{k+1} (k+1) - \mu_1 \gamma_i^k (k+1) \right\} \qquad i = 1,\ldots,\lim(k+1,k+1)-1$$

$$\gamma_i^{k+1} (k+1) = - \frac{\mu_1}{\mu_2} \gamma_i^k (k+1) \qquad\qquad i = \lim(k+1,k+1)$$

4) for z=k-B and k=B+1,...,N :

$$\beta_i^{k-B}(k) = \mu_2 \left\{ \sum_{j=1}^{\lim(k-1,k-B)} \frac{\gamma_j^{k-B} (k-1)}{\mu_1^{\,j}} + \sum_{j=1}^{k-B} \frac{\delta_j^{k-B} (k-1)}{(\mu_1 - \mu_2)^j} \right\} \qquad i=1$$

$$\beta_i^{k-B}(k) = \mu_2 \, \beta_{i-1}^{k-B} (k-1) \qquad\qquad i = 2,\ldots,k$$

$$\gamma_i^{k-B} (k) = - \frac{1}{\mu_1} \left\{ \mu_2 \gamma_i^{k-B} (k-1) - \gamma_{i+1}^{k-B} (k) \right\} \qquad i = 1,\ldots,\lim(k,k-B)-1$$

$$\gamma_i^{k-B} (k) = - \frac{\mu_2}{\mu_1} \gamma_i^{k-B} (k-1) \qquad\qquad i = \lim(k,k-B)$$

448

$$\delta_i^{k\text{-}B}(k) = \frac{1}{\mu_2 - \mu_1} \left\{ \mu_2 \, \delta_i^{k\text{-}B}(k\text{-}1) - \delta_{i+1}^{k\text{-}B}(k) \right\} \qquad\qquad i = 1,\dots,k\text{-}B\text{-}1$$

$$\delta_i^{k\text{-}B}(k) = \frac{\mu_2}{\mu_2 - \mu_1} \, \delta_{k\text{-}B}^{k\text{-}B}(k\text{-}1) \qquad\qquad\qquad\qquad i = k\text{-}B$$

$$(A.2)$$

and with initial conditions for states $(B_1\text{-}k, N\text{-}B_1\text{+}k, k)$, for $k=1,\dots,B$:

$$\gamma_i^0(k) = \delta_i^0(k) = 0 \quad \forall i$$

$$\beta_i^0(k) = 0 \quad i = 1,\dots,k\text{-}1$$

$$\beta_k^0(k) = \mu_2^k$$

Proof of Theorem 1

The Laplace transform $T(n,q,p,s)$ of the first hitting time to state $(B_1, N\text{-}B_1, 0)$ of process T starting from state (n,q,p) is computed by the recursive scheme (4)-(6), from which one can derive

$$T(B_1\text{-}k, N\text{-}B_1\text{+}k, k, s) = \frac{\mu_2^k}{(\mu_2 + s)^k} \qquad\qquad \text{for } k=1,\dots,B \text{ ;}$$

$$T(n, N\text{-}n, k, s) = \sum_{i=1}^{k} \frac{\beta_i^j(k)}{(\mu_2 + s)^i} + \sum_{i=1}^{k\text{-}2\text{+}j} \frac{\gamma_i^j(k)}{(\mu_3 + s)^i} + \sum_{i=1}^{i} \frac{\delta_i^j(k)}{(\mu_1 + s)^i}$$

with $j=n+k\text{-}B_1$ and for $j=1,\dots,k\text{-}1$ if $k=2,\dots,B$ and for $j=k\text{-}B\text{+}1,\dots,k\text{-}1$ if $k=B\text{+}1,\dots,N$;

$$T(B_1, N\text{-}B_1, k, s) = \sum_{i=1}^{k} \frac{\beta_i^k(k)}{(\mu_2 + s)^i} + \sum_{i=1}^{2k\text{-}3} \frac{\gamma_i^k(k)}{(\mu_3 + s)^i} + \sum_{i=1}^{k} \frac{\delta_i^k(k)}{(\mu_1 + s)^i}$$

for $k=1,\dots,N$;

$$T(N\text{-}B_2, B_2, k, s) = \sum_{i=1}^{k} \frac{\beta_i^{k\text{-}B}(k)}{(\mu_2 + s)^i} + \sum_{i=1}^{2k\text{-}B\text{-}3} \frac{\gamma_i^{k\text{-}B}(k)}{(\mu_3 + s)^i} + \sum_{i=1}^{k\text{-}B} \frac{\delta_i^{k\text{-}B}(k)}{(\mu_1 + s)^i}$$

for $k=B\text{+}1,\dots,N$.

$$(A.3)$$

and where coefficients $\beta_i^z(N)$, $\gamma_i^z(N)$, and $\delta_i^z(N)$ are given by (A.2), as one can prove by induction. A more detailed proof can be found in [3].

The LST of cycle time distribution $F_{N,B1,B2}(s)$, defined by (7), can by (A.2) be rewritten as

$$F_{N,B1,B2}(s) = \sum_{j=1}^{3} \sum_{i=1}^{k_j} \frac{c_{ji}}{(\mu_j + s)^i} \qquad\qquad (A.4)$$

where $k_1 = k_2 = N$, $k_3 = 2N\text{-}3$, and coefficients c_{ji} are given by formula (A.1).

By inverting expression (A.4) one obtains immediately the cycle time density, from which, by integration and with some algebra, formula (8) can be derived for the CTD $F_{N,B1,B2}(t)$.

The overall computational complexity of coefficients c_{ji} is determined by the computational effort required by coefficients $\beta_i{}^z(.)$, $\gamma_i{}^z(.)$, and $\delta_i{}^z(.)$, evaluated for each state in state space E. The computational complexity of these coefficients for each state (n,q,p) is given by $O(p)$, as one can derive by formula (A.3). Therefore, since the state space E cardinality is of $O(N^2)$, the total computational complexity becomes of $O(N^3)$.

REFERENCES

[1]   Akyildiz I.F. 'Exact product form solution for queueing networks with blocking', IEEE Trans. on Comp., vol. C-36, 1, 1987, pp.122-125;

[2]   Balsamo S., De Nitto Personé V., Iazeolla G. 'Identity and reducibility properties of some blocking and non-blocking mechanisms in congested networks' in "Flow Control of Congested Networks", Nato ASI Series, Comp. Sys. and Sciences, vol.38, (A.R.Odoni, L.Bianco, G.Szegö eds.), Springer-Verlag 1987, pp.243-254;

[3]   Balsamo S., Donatiello L. 'On the cycle time distribution in a two-stage cyclic network with blocking', University of Pisa, Computer Science Dept., Research Report S-87-17, November 1987;

[4]   Boxma O.J. 'The cyclic queue with one general and one exponential server', Adv. in Applied Probability, vol.15, 1983, pp.857-873;

[5]   Boxma O.J., Donk P. 'On response time and cycle time distribution in a two-stage cyclic queue', Performance Evaluation, 2, 1982, pp.181-194;

[6]   Boxma O.J., Kelly F., Kohneim A.G. 'The product form sujourn time distribution in cyclic exponential queues', J. of ACM, vol.31, 1984, pp.128-133;

[7]   Boxma O.J. 'Models of two queues: a few new views', Teletraffic Analysis and Computer Performance Evaluation, (O.J. Boxma, L.Cohen, H.C. Tijms eds.), North-Holland 1986, pp.75-98;

[8]   Boxma O.J., Konheim A.G. 'Approximate Analysis of Exponential Queueing Systems with Blocking', Acta Informatica, Vol 15, 1981, pp.19-66;

[9]   Carbini S., Donatiello L., Iazeolla G. 'An efficient algorithm for the cycle time distribution in two-stage cyclic network with a non-exponential server', Teletraffic Analysis and Computer Performance Evaluation, (O.J. Boxma, L.Cohen, H.C. Tijms eds.), North-Holland 1986, pp. 99-115;

[10]   Chow W.M. 'The cycle time distribution of exponential cyclic queues', J. of ACM, 27, 1980, pp.281-286;

[11]   Daduna H. 'The cycle time distribution of cyclic two-stage queues with a non-exponential servers', in Modelling and Performance Evaluation Methodology, (F.Baccelli, G. Fayolle, eds), Springer, Berlin, 1984, pp.641-653;

[12]   Daduna H. 'Two-stage queues with non-exponential servers: steady-state and cycle time', Oper. Research, vol.34, 3, 1986, pp.445-459;

[13]   Gershwin S., Berman U. 'Analysis of Transfer Lines Consisting of two Unreliable Machines With Random Processing Times and Finite Storage Buffers', AIIE Trans., vol.13,1, 1981, pp. 2-11;

[14]   Latouche G., Neuts M. 'Efficient Algorithmic Solution to Exponential Tandem Queues with Blocking', SIAM, Alg. Dis. Meth., vol.1, March 1980;

[15]   Onvural R.O., Perros H.G. 'On equivalences of blocking mechanisms in queueing networks with blocking', Operation Research Letters, vol.5, n.2, 1986, pp.293-297;

[16]   Perros H.G. 'Queueing Networks with Blocking: a bibliography', ACM Sigmetrics, Performance Evaluation Review, August 1984;

[17]   Perros H. G. 'A symmetrical exponential open queue network with blocking and feedback', IEEE Trans. on Soft. Eng., vol SE-7, 1981, pp. 395-402;

[18]   Perros H.G., Altiok T. 'Approximate Analysis of Open Networks of queues with blocking : tandem configuration', IEEE Trans. on Soft. Eng., vol. SE-12, 1986, pp.450-462;

[19]   Suri R., Diehl G.W. 'A variable buffer-size model and its use in analyzing closed queueing networks with blocking', Manag. Science, vol 32, n.2, 1986, pp. 206-225;

[20]   Shassenberger R., Daduna H. 'The time for a round trip in a cycle of exponential queues', J. of ACM, vol.30, 1983, pp.181-194.

INDEX